VOLUME EIGHTY

ADVANCES IN PHARMACOLOGY

VOLUME EIGHTY

ADVANCES IN PHARMACOLOGY

Cannabinoid Pharmacology

Edited by

DAVID KENDALL

PharmNovo UK Ltd. and School of Pharmacy, Liverpool John Moores University, Liverpool, United Kingdom

STEPHEN P.H. ALEXANDER

Life Sciences, University of Nottingham Medical School, Nottingham, United Kingdom

Serial Editor

S.J. ENNA

University of Kansas Medical Center, Kansas City, Kansas, United States

Managing Editor

LYNN LECOUNT

University of Kansas Medical Center, School of Medicine, Kansas City, Kansas, United States

ELSEVIER

ACADEMIC PRESS

An imprint of Elsevier

Academic Press is an imprint of Elsevier
50 Hampshire Street, 5th Floor, Cambridge, MA 02139, United States
525 B Street, Suite 1800, San Diego, CA 92101-4495, United States
The Boulevard, Langford Lane, Kidlington, Oxford OX5 1GB, United Kingdom
125 London Wall, London, EC2Y 5AS, United Kingdom

First edition 2017

ISBN: 978-0-12-811232-8
ISSN: 1054-3589

For information on all Academic Press publications
visit our website at https://www.elsevier.com/books-and-journals

Publisher: Zoe Kruze
Acquisition Editor: Zoe Kruze
Editorial Project Manager: Shellie Bryant
Production Project Manager: Vignesh Tamil
Cover Designer: Greg Harris

Typeset by SPi Global, India

CONTENTS

CONTRIBUTORS

Ghayth Abdulrazzaq
Life Sciences, University of Nottingham Medical School, Nottingham, United Kingdom

Mary E. Abood
Center for Substance Abuse Research, Lewis Katz School of Medicine at Temple University, Philadelphia, PA, United States

Stephen P.H. Alexander
Life Sciences, University of Nottingham Medical School, Nottingham, United Kingdom

Angel Arevalo-Martin
Laboratory of Neuroinflammation, Hospital Nacional de Paraplejicos (SESCAM), Toledo, Spain

Heather B. Bradshaw
Indiana University, Bloomington, IN, United States

Sue L.F. Chan
Life Sciences, University of Nottingham Medical School, Nottingham, United Kingdom

Colin Davidson
School of Pharmacy and Biomedical Sciences, University of Central Lancashire, Preston, United Kingdom

Luciano De Petrocellis
National Research Council of Italy, Institute of Biomolecular Chemistry, Endocannabinoid Research Group, Naples, Italy

Patrick Doherty
Wolfson Centre for Age-Related Disease, King's College London, London, United Kingdom

David P. Finn
Pharmacology and Therapeutics, School of Medicine, Galway Neuroscience Centre and Centre for Pain Research, NCBES, National University of Ireland, Galway, Ireland

Christopher J. Fowler
Umeå University, Umeå, Sweden

Daniel Garcia-Ovejero
Laboratory of Neuroinflammation, Hospital Nacional de Paraplejicos (SESCAM), Toledo, Spain

Michelle Glass
Faculty of Medical and Health Sciences, University of Auckland, Auckland, New Zealand

Euan S. Graham
School of Medical Sciences, Faculty of Medical and Health Sciences, University of Auckland, Auckland, New Zealand

Jenni Harvey
Division of Neuroscience, Ninewells Hospital and Medical School, University of Dundee, Dundee, Scotland, United Kingdom

Burkhard Hinz
Institute of Pharmacology and Toxicology, Rostock University Medical Center, Rostock, Germany

Wing S.V. Ho
Vascular Biology Research Centre, St George's University of London, London, United Kingdom

Allyn C. Howlett
Center for Research on Substance Use and Addiction, Wake Forest University Health Sciences, Winston-Salem, NC, United States

Andrew Irving
The Conway Institute, School of Biomolecular and Biomedical Science, University College Dublin, Dublin, Ireland

Melanie E.M. Kelly
Dalhousie University, Halifax, NS, Canada

David Kendall
PharmNovo UK Ltd. and School of Pharmacy and Biomolecular Sciences, Liverpool John Moores University, Liverpool, United Kingdom

Dan T. Kho
School of Medical Sciences, Faculty of Medical and Health Sciences, University of Auckland, Auckland, New Zealand

Alessia Ligresti
National Research Council of Italy, Institute of Biomolecular Chemistry, Endocannabinoid Research Group, Naples, Italy

Jahan Marcu
Americans for Safe Access, Patient Focused Certification, Washington, DC, United States

Eduardo Molina-Holgado
Laboratory of Neuroinflammation, Hospital Nacional de Paraplejicos (SESCAM), Toledo, Spain

Francisco Molina-Holgado
Health Science Research Centre, University of Roehampton, London, United Kingdom

Massimo Nabissi
School of Pharmacy, University of Camerino, Camerino, Italy

Jolanta Opacka-Juffry
Health Science Research Centre, University of Roehampton, London, United Kingdom

Saoirse E. O'Sullivan
School of Medicine, Faculty of Medicine & Health Sciences, University of Nottingham, Royal Derby Hospital Centre, Derby, United Kingdom

June Penman
Division of Neuroscience, Ninewells Hospital and Medical School, University of Dundee, Dundee, Scotland, United Kingdom

Fabiana Piscitelli
Endocannabinoid Research Group, Istituto di Chimica Biomolecolare-Consiglio Nazionale delle Ricerche (ICB-CNR), Pozzuoli, Italy

Marco Pistis
University of Cagliari, Cittadella Universitaria di Monserrato, Cagliari, Italy

Richard Priestley
Alzheimer's Research UK Drug Discovery Institute, University of Oxford, Oxford, United Kingdom

Robert Ramer
Institute of Pharmacology and Toxicology, Rostock University Medical Center, Rostock, Germany

Ethan B. Russo
PHYTECS, Los Angeles, CA, United States

Giorgio Santoni
School of Pharmacy, University of Camerino, Camerino, Italy

Katarzyna Starowicz
Institute of Pharmacology, Polish Academy of Sciences, Laboratory of Pain Pathophysiology, Krakow, Poland

PREFACE

Preparations of the *Cannabis* plant have been used by man for multiple purposes for millennia; however, a pharmacological understanding of the plant's unique metabolites has only come about in the last 60–70 years. A key landmark in cannabinoid science was the work of Raphael Mechoulam identifying the nature of many of these unique metabolites, notably Δ^9-tetrahydrocannabinol (THC) in the early 1960s. In the late 1980s, William Devane and Allyn Howlett provided evidence for the existence of a cannabinoid receptor in the brain, where THC predominantly acts. Molecular identification of this CB_1 cannabinoid receptor and a "peripheral" CB_2 cannabinoid receptor was reported in the early 1990s by Tom Bonner and Sean Munro, respectively. At about that time, Raphael Mechoulam and Roger Pertwee expanded the field further with identification of the two major endogenous agonists at the cannabinoid receptors, paving the way for characterization of the multiple constituents of the endocannabinoid system.

Today, a simple interrogation of PubMed reveals tens of thousands of published articles relating to *Cannabis* and the cannabinoids.

The breadth of involvement of cannabinoids and their receptors in basic physiology and pathophysiology is immense ranging from roles in the most basic aspects of gene expression to suspected mediation of complex disease processes including chronic pain, cancer, schizophrenia, and neurodegeneration.

Getting to grips with such a massive and diverse subject requires some signposting and the *Pharmacology of Cannabinoids* aims to do just that. The chapters are authored by combinations of experienced and well-published experts in the field who have not, in the main, worked together previously, a strategy which we think facilitates fresh approaches to the topics covered.

The scene is set with reviews of the pharmacology of the plant-derived cannabinoids and the diverse range of endogenous lipids that underpin cannabinoid signaling in the body. How these endocannabinoids are practically analyzed and quantified is also explained, as well as descriptions of the mechanisms of their turnover. The multiple targets for the endogenous and exogenous cannabinoids are discussed in chapters covering the G protein-coupled CB_1 and CB_2 receptors, cannabinoid-receptor-like orphan GPCR, ion channels (particularly the transient receptor potential channels), and nuclear receptors; postreceptor signaling mechanisms are described within these chapters. It is now clear that agonist signaling in general is more dynamic than previously thought and a chapter on cannabinoid agonist bias is included.

Understanding the roles of cannabinoids in the pathophysiology of important disease states and the potential for developing new therapies based on an expanded knowledge base is crucial and chapters are devoted to in-depth accounts of cannabinoid involvement in pain, cancer, and cardiovascular and neuroinflammatory diseases.

We are sincerely grateful to our friends and colleagues who have contributed to this volume which we trust will be a useful reference source and, hopefully, an inspiration to scientists, be they novices in the field or cannabinoid aficionados.

David Kendall
PharmNovo UK Ltd. and School of Pharmacy,
Liverpool John Moores University,
Liverpool, United Kingdom

Stephen P.H. Alexander
Life Sciences, University of Nottingham Medical School,
Nottingham, United Kingdom

CHAPTER ONE

Endocannabinoid Analytical Methodologies: Techniques That Drive Discoveries That Drive Techniques

Fabiana Piscitelli*,[1], Heather B. Bradshaw†
*Endocannabinoid Research Group, Istituto di Chimica Biomolecolare-Consiglio Nazionale delle Ricerche (ICB-CNR), Pozzuoli, Italy
†Indiana University, Bloomington, IN, United States
[1]Corresponding author: e-mail address: fpiscitelli@icb.cnr.it

Contents

Advances in Pharmacology, Volume 80
ISSN 1054-3589
http://dx.doi.org/10.1016/bs.apha.2017.04.003

Abstract

Identification of the two major endogenous cannabinoid ligands, known as endocannabinoids, *N*-arachidonoyl-ethanolamine (anandamide, AEA) and 2-arachidonoyl-glycerol (2-AG), opened the way for the identification and isolation of other lipid congeners, all derivatives of fatty acids and related to the Endocannabinoid System. The nomenclature of this anandamide-type class of lipids is evolving as new species are discovered all the time. However, they each fall under the larger umbrella of lipids that are a conjugation of a fatty acid with an amine through and amide bond, which we will refer to as lipoamines. Specific subspecies of lipoamines that have been discovered are the *N*-acyl-ethanolamides (including AEA), *N*-acyl-dopamines, *N*-acyl-serotonins, *N*-acyl-GABA, *N*-acyl-taurines, and a growing number of *N*-acyl amino acids. Emerging data from multiple labs also show that monoacylglycerols (including 2-AG), COX-2 metabolites, and fatty acid esters of hydroxyl fatty acids are interconnected with these lipoamines at both the biosynthetic and metabolic levels. Understanding the molecular relatedness of these lipids is important for studying how they act as signaling molecules; however, a first step in this process hinges on advances in being able to accurately measure them.

ABBREVIATIONS

APCI atmospheric pressure chemical ionization
DAGs diacylglycerols
eCBs endocannabinoids
ESI electrospray ionization
GC gas chromatography
GPCRs G protein-coupled receptors
LC liquid chromatography
MAGs monoacylglycerols
MS mass spectrometry
NAEs *N*-acyl-ethanolamides
TRPV1 transient receptor potential vanilloid type-1

1. INTRODUCTION

Discovery of Δ^9-tetrahydrocannabinol (Δ^9-THC; Fig. 1) and the chemical synthesis of its analogues (Gaoni & Mechoulam, 1971) provided a foundation for modern *Cannabis* research. That research and a growing body of evidence have emerged on the role of the Endocannabinoid System (ECS) in numerous diseases and disorders. In general, the ECS is defined as the endogenous signaling system comprised of: (1) cannabinoid receptors, (2) endogenous cannabinoid receptor ligands, also known as endocannabinoids (eCBs), and (3) enzymes responsible for the production and degradation of eCBs (*for review, see* De Petrocellis & Di Marzo, 2009). In

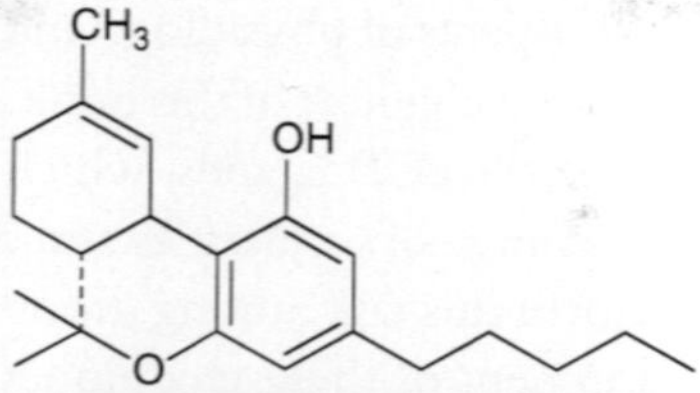

Δ⁹-Tetrahydrocannabinol (Δ⁹-THC)

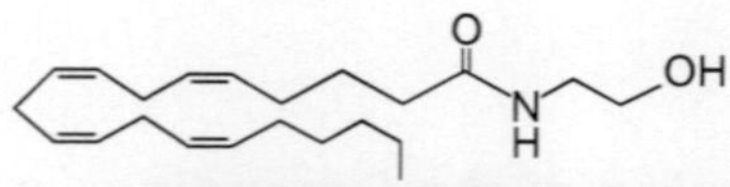

***N*-Arachidonoyl-ethanolamine (Anandamide, AEA)**

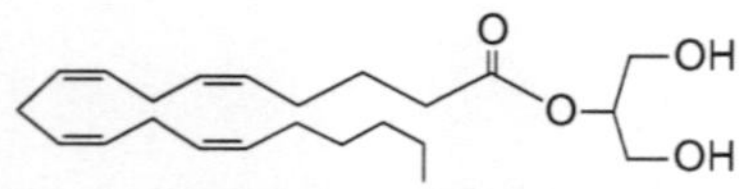

2-Arachidonoyl-glycerol (2-AG)

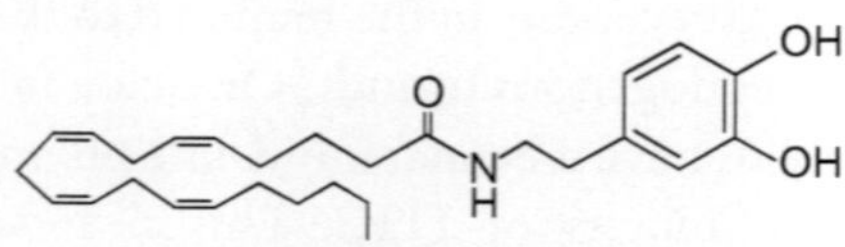

***N*-Arachidonoyl-dopamine (NADA)**

Fig. 1 Structures of Δ^9-tetrahydrocannabinol and major endocannabinoids, anandamide, 2-arachidonoyl-glycerol, and *N*-arachidonoyl-dopamine.

1990, the screening of a series of "orphan" (i.e., without a known ligand) G protein-coupled receptors (GPCRs) led to the molecular characterization of a specific receptor for THC, or "cannabinoid receptor" (Devane, Dysarz, Johnson, Melvin, & Howlett, 1988; Matsuda, Lolait, Brownstein, Young, & Bonner, 1990). In 1993, this was renamed "cannabinoid receptor type-1" (CB_1) because of the discovery, by homology cloning, of a second GPCR for THC, the "cannabinoid receptor type-2" (CB_2) (Munro, Thomas, & Abu-Shaar, 1993). Over the last decade additional GPCRs such as GPR55 (Lauckner et al., 2008; Moreno et al., 2014; Pertwee, 2007) and GPR18 (Console-Bram, Brailoiu, Brailoiu, Sharir, & Abood, 2014; McHugh, Page, Dunn, & Bradshaw, 2012; McHugh, Roskowski, Xie, & Bradshaw, 2014; Miller et al., 2016) as well as multiple members of the TRPV channels (Darmani et al., 2014; De Petrocellis et al., 2012; Espejo-Porras, Fernandez-Ruiz, Pertwee, Mechoulam, & Garcia, 2013; Silvestri et al., 2015) have been associated with CB (cannabinoid) signaling by THC and a growing list of other phytocannabinoids. These discoveries have fundamental importance for the growing field of CB pharmacology and for a broad range of aspects of physiology and pathology and will be discussed more deeply in other chapters of this book. Here, we will focus on the techniques for measuring the eCB ligands, which are structurally small molecule lipids. There are a range of similarities and differences in methodological approaches to perform this task among groups of scientists. It is through the continuous development of these techniques to measure the eCBs that other endogenous structural analogs have been discovered, which is opening up more avenues of research within and beyond the fields of cannabinoid signaling.

1.1 Endocannabinoids: The Beginning of the Expanding Universe

Activity of THC at CB receptors in the brain led to the search and discovery of the receptor's endogenous ligands. One clue in this search was that while it was unlikely to have a cannabinoid-like chemical structure, it did likely shared the lipophilicity of THC. This clear logic resulted in the screening of lipid fractions from mammalian brain that led to the isolation, in 1992, by Devane and coworkers in the laboratory of Raphael Mechoulam of the first endogenous CB_1/CB_2 ligand, *N*-arachidonoyl-ethanolamine also known as anandamide (AEA; Fig. 1; Devane et al., 1992; Lin et al., 1998). Three years after the discovery of AEA, a second endogenous ligand for cannabinoid receptors named 2-arachidonoyl-glycerol (2-AG; Fig. 1) was identified (Mechoulam et al., 1995; Sugiura et al., 1995). Both AEA and 2-AG contain in their chemical structure an arachidonate acyl chain and a polar alcohol functional group and share some common features with THC: lipophilicity and the same sterical organization of the *n*-pentyl chain and of the hydroxyl group. They belong to the family of *N*-acyl-ethanolamides (NAEs) and monoacylglycerols (MAGs), respectively. *N*-Arachidonoyl-dopamine (NADA; Fig. 1), which is one of the first identified endogenous AEA lipoamine congeners, has affinities for both CB_1 and CB_2, though it appears to be produced only in the striatum and hippocampus (Bradshaw, Rimmerman, Krey, & Walker, 2006; Huang et al., 2002), and like AEA (Zygmunt, Julius, Di Marzo, & Hogestatt, 2000) and 2-AG (Zygmunt et al., 2013), has activity at the TRPV1 (transient receptor potential vanilloid type-1) channel, a ligand-gated Ca^{2+}-permeable nonselective cation channel that is activated by multiple noxious stimuli, including heat, protons, and capsaicin

(Caterina et al., 1997). Moreover, NADA is 40 times more selective for CB_1 than for CB_2 (Bisogno et al., 2000). Modulatory roles of additional 2-acylglycerol species at CB_1 are also coming to light, suggesting a more molecular basis for what was previously referred to as "entourage effects" (Murataeva et al., 2016). As more lipids species are discovered and more CB-responsive receptors and channels are identified, the full understanding of the roles each of them plays in cellular signaling will be revealed. Here, we will highlight some of the techniques for measuring these that are providing us with novel lipid species to examine in the context of eCB signaling.

2. MASS SPECTROMETRY-BASED TECHNIQUES FOR LIPIDOMICS APPROACHES APPLIED TO THE ENDOCANNABINOIDOME

Mass spectrometric (MS) equipment and techniques enjoyed an explosion of innovation in the 1990s including the development of electrospray ionization (ESI), which was awarded a Nobel Prize in 2001. While this evolution in MS is largely thought of in terms of the proteomics revolution, lipid analysis using these tools was also underway. Through the initial discovery of the two major eCBs at the end of the 1990s, the complexity of lipids related to the ECS increased and the scenario is in constant evolution. The wide nature of eCB-like lipids have been discovered mainly thanks to considerable advances in MS techniques coupled to gas chromatography (GC) or liquid chromatography (LC). In Table 1, we summarized some of the most prominent lipidomics approaches reported for eCBs and related lipids.

3. OVERVIEW OF ANALYTICAL METHODOLOGIES FOR eCBs EXTRACTION AND QUANTIFICATION

For nearly two decades, eCBs content has been quantified by lipid extraction and purification from bulk tissue and subsequent analysis by LC-MS or GC-MS. To date, several analytical approaches have been reported for eCBs measurement in biological matrices, and the steps more relevant analytically are lipid extraction technique that take into

Table 1 Overview of the Lipidomics Approaches Reported so far for Endocannabinoids and Related Molecules

Technique	Types	Analytes	Key Features	References
GC-based	Electron impact (EI) GC-MS	AEA		Devane et al. (1992)
	EI GC-MS	NAEs (arachidonyl-; eicosenoyl-; linoleoyl-; γ-inolenoyl-; lignoceroyl-; behenoyl-; arachidoyl-; stearoyl-; palmitoyl-; miristoyl-; lauroyl-ethanolamide)	Selected-ion monitoring (SIM) from rat brain homogenates, primary cultures of striatal and cortical rat neurons	Fontana, Di Marzo, Cadas, and Piomelli (1995)
	EI GC-MS	AEA	Isotope dilution, rat brain tissue	Kempe, Hsu, Bohrer, and Turk (1996)
	EI GC-MS	NAEs (16:0, 18:0, 18:1n-9, 18:1n-7, 18:2n-6, 20:4n-6)	Isotope dilution, mouse peritoneal macrophages	Schmid, Kuwae, Krebsbach, and Schmid (1997)
	EI GC-MS	MAGs [1(3)-14:0 + 1(3)-16:1 (n-7); 2-14:0 + 2-16:1(n-7) + 1 (3)-18:2(n-6); 1(3)-16:0 + 1(3)-18:1 (n-7, n-9); 2-16:0 + 2-18:1(n-7, n-9); 1(3)-18:0; 2-18:2(n-6); 1(3)-20:4(n-6); 2-20:4(n-6); 1(3)-22:6(n-3); 2-22:6(n-3)], 2-AGE	Isotope dilution, various rat tissues	Kondo et al. (1998) and Oka et al. (2003)
	EI GC-MS	AEA, PEA, and OEA	Isotope dilution, rat blood plasma	Giuffrida and Piomelli (1998)
	EI GC-MS	AEA	Isotope dilution, various rat tissues	Yang et al. (1999)

	EI or PICI (positive-ion detection) GC-MS	AEA, 2-AG	Isotope dilution, various rat or mice, and human tissues	Hardison, Weintraub, and Giuffrida (2006), Kirkham, Williams, Fezza, and Di Marzo (2002), Maccarrone, Attina, Cartoni, Bari, and Finazzi-Agro (2001), Muccioli and Stella (2008), Obata, Sakurai, Kase, Tanifuji, and Horiguchi (2003), and Schmid et al. (2000)
	ECNICI (negative-ion chemical ionization) GC-MS/MS	AEA	Isotope dilution, human plasma	Zoerner et al. (2009)
LC-based	APCI, ESI +, ESI-LC-MS, and LC-MS/MS	NAEs, 2-AG, 2-AGE, and NADA	Isotope dilution, various biological matrices	Astarita et al. (2006), Balvers, Verhoeckx, and Witkamp (2009), Bystrowska, Smaga, Tyszka-Czochara, and Filip (2014), Chen, Paudel, Derbenev, Smith, and Stinchcomb (2009), De Filippis et al. (2010), Felder et al. (1996), Huang, Strangman, and Walker (1999), Kantae et al. (2017), Kirkwood, Broeckling, Donahue, and Prenni (2016), Ligresti et al. (2003), Richardson, Ortori, Chapman, Kendall, and Barrett (2007), and Sergi et al. (2013)

Continued

Table 1 Overview of the Lipidomics Approaches Reported so far for Endocannabinoids and Related Molecules—cont'd

Technique	Types	Analytes	Key Features	References
	ESI-FTMS, ESI-MS/MS, ESI +MS/MS	NATs	Discovery metabolite profiling, untargeted metabolomics, several mice tissues	Saghatelian, McKinney, Bandell, Patapoutian, and Cravatt (2006) and Sasso et al. (2016)
	ESI- and + MS/MS	Lipoamines including NAEs and over 60 *N*-acyl amino acids; 2-acylglycerols; free fatty acids; and prostaglandins	Broad-scale lipidomics of brain, spinal cord, plasma, lung, bone, uterus, and additional organs; Drosophila; and cooking oils	Balakrishna et al. (2014), Bradshaw and Leishman (2016), Bradshaw, Rimmerman, Hu, Burstein, and Walker (2009), Smoum et al. (2010), Tan et al. (2010), Tortoriello et al. (2013), and Wolfson et al. (2015)
	ESI + MS/MS	*N*-Acyl-serotonins	Isotope dilution, gastrointestinal tract of pigs and mice	Verhoeckx et al. (2011)
	ESI-MS and MS/MS	FAHFAs	Untargeted and targeted approach, mice adipose tissue	Yore et al. (2014)
	ESI MS/MS; ESI-IT-TOF MS/MS	COX-2 derivatives	Cell cultures; rat spinal cord	Gatta et al. 2012, Hu, Bradshaw, Chen, Tan, and Walker (2008), and Kingsley and Marnett (2007)

accounts sample storage, tissue homogenization, internal standards, protein precipitation, purification of the extracts, and analysis by GC-MS, LC-MS, or LC-MS/MS.

3.1 Sample Storage, Tissue Homogenization, Internal Standards, Protein Precipitation, and Lipid Extraction Technique

Sample storage is the first and the most crucial aspect of the entire extraction process. Generally, eCBs are unstable since biological matrices contain degradative enzymes for eCBs. Indeed, in a study from Willoughby and coworkers, authors showed that the half-life of AEA in vivo is of the order of few minutes (Willoughby, Moore, Martin, & Ellis, 1997).

Once tissue to be analyzed is frozen in liquid nitrogen, it can be stored at −80°C before analysis. Before homogenization, tissues have to be weighed very quickly, to avoid postmortem change in metabolite amounts that may be generated during thawing. Different approaches have been reported for homogenization step. In particular, silanized glass homogenizer (Richardson et al., 2007), electric homogenizer (Hardison et al., 2006; Lehtonen et al., 2011; Nucci et al., 2007), or bead beater with glass beads (Kilaru et al., 2010). This step is performed rapidly and on ice, and internal standards are added at the beginning of this process. Particularly in LC-based methods, protein precipitation is commonly performed by acetone prior to solvent extraction (Giuffrida & Piomelli, 1998; Lam et al., 2008; Schreiber et al., 2007; Williams et al., 2007; Wood et al., 2008). Acetone (Giuffrida & Piomelli, 1998; Lam et al., 2008; Schreiber et al., 2007; Williams et al., 2007; Wood et al., 2008), acetonitrile (Balvers et al., 2009; Palandra, Prusakiewicz, Ozer, Zhang, & Heath, 2009; Patel, Rademacher, & Hillard, 2003; Vogeser et al., 2006), methanol (Huang et al., 1999; Opitz et al., 2007), or methanol–acetonitrile mixtures (Bradshaw et al., 2006) are the most used solvents. Precipitated proteins are then eliminated by centrifugation, and supernatants containing eCBs are collected. However, recent studies have demonstrated that evaporation protocols for supernatants facilitate 2-AG/1-AG isomerization, and it is not recommended for LC-MS/MS analysis (Zoerner et al., 2012).

The internal standards most used for eCBs quantification for MS-based analysis are deuterated analogs. AEA and 2-AG are commercially available as two forms: d^4 and d^8. The d^4 molecules are labeled with four deuterium atoms in the ethanolamide and in the glycerol moieties, for AEA and 2-AG, respectively. Whereas for d^8 standards, deuterium atoms are on the acyl chain.

Regarding lipid extraction techniques, the most widely used are chloroform-based (Bligh & Dyer, 1959; Folch, Lees, & Sloane Stanley, 1957) combined with methanol in different ratios. However, also chloroform alone or methanol (Tan et al., 2009) alone and ethyl acetate/hexane mixture (Richardson et al., 2007) have been reported. Repeated extraction usually significantly increases lipid yield.

3.2 Purification of the Extracts

Extraction from biological matrices requires, usually, a purification process to achieve a fraction enriched in eCBs. The most used techniques are solid phase extraction (SPE)-based (Zoerner et al., 2011) or thin layer chromatography (TLC)-based (Zoerner et al., 2011). However, SPE are most frequently used because it can be fully automated which is more suitable for high-throughput analysis. SPE can be divided into two categories, based on the nature of the phase that can be reverse (C8 or C18) or direct.

3.3 Mass Spectrometric Analysis Coupled to GC or LC

eCBs analysis by GC/MS techniques requires previous steps of derivatization, and it is not so largely used, especially with the introduction of HPLC coupled to electrospray (LC-ESI-MS) or atmospheric pressure chemical ionization MS (LC-APCI-MS). LC/MS and LC/MS/MS methodologies, instead, do not require derivatization and provide best analytical performance in terms of accuracy, sensitivity, and precision. LC/MS methodologies, usually, utilize the selection ion monitoring (SIM) mode to select the molecular ions ($[M + H]^+$), sodium adducts ($[M+ Na]^+$), or potassium adducts ($[M + K]^+$) in positive ion mode (Schreiber et al., 2007; Zoerner et al., 2011). On the other hand, in LC-MS/MS analysis the selected reaction monitoring or the multiple reaction monitoring (MRM) are the most used approaches. For AEA, when $[M + H]^+$ is subjected to collision-induced decomposition, the mass transition of m/z 348 $\rightarrow$ 62 is formed due to loss of ethanolamine moiety (Balvers et al., 2009). For 2-AG, the transition observed is m/z 379 $\rightarrow$ 287 that correspond to the fragment $[M - C_3H_8O_3]^+$ due to the loss of glycerol (Bradshaw et al., 2006).

4. ADVANCES IN EXPANDING THE COVERAGE OF THE ENDOCANNABINOIDOME USING "ENDOCANNABINOIDOMICS"

Vincenzo Di Marzo's lab has made history in the field eCBs quantification, starting from GC-MS analysis, switching to a more modern single quadrupole LC-MS until the advanced technology of LC-MS-IT-TOF. As stated earlier the world of eCB-like molecules is enlarging, and the application of lipidomics approaches is necessary to identify these lipid mediators and to understand their biological significance. The targeted lipidomics approach applied is called "endocannabinoidomics" and includes all the methodologies needed to investigate the metabolomic, proteomic, and genomic components of the "endocannabinoidome" (Bisogno, Piscitelli, & Di Marzo, 2009). In these years several targeted lipidomics methodologies have been developed to detect novel bioactive lipids as well as monitor known simultaneously eCB-like molecules and their biosynthetic precursors. In this section a typical workflow for endocannabinoidomic analysis of biological samples is provided, including sample preparation, MS-based analysis, and data processing (Fig. 2).

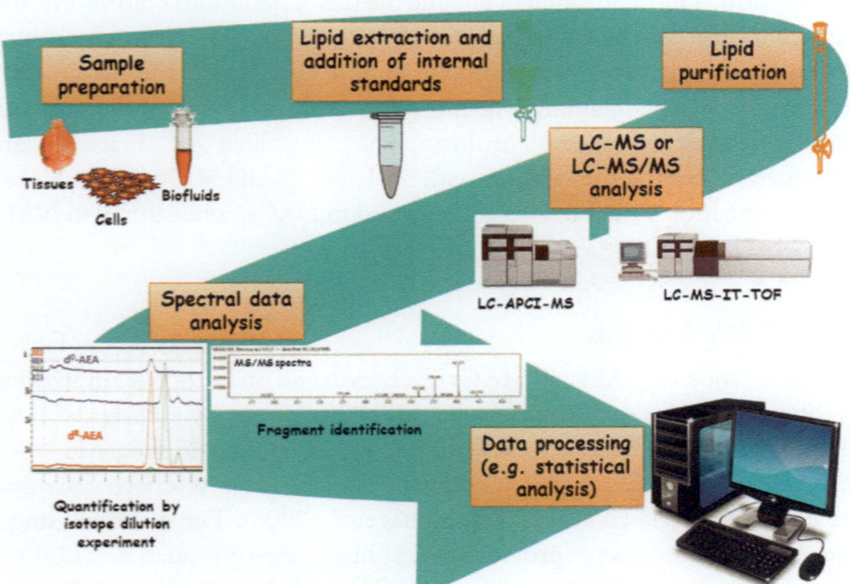

Fig. 2 Typical workflow for an "endocannabinoidomics" experiment.

4.1 Lipid Extraction Technique

Sample preparation protocols for endocannabinoidomics approach exploit the hydrophobic nature of lipids to extract them while eliminating other components of the biological matrix (i.e., proteins, sugars, inorganic salts) that could potentially interfere with the chromatographic separation and MS analysis.

Traditionally, lipid extraction technique is chloroform-based, as originally described by Folch et al. (1957) and Bligh and Dyer (1959). A modified Folch extraction protocol, based on liquid–liquid partitioning using chloroform and methanol in a 2:1 (v/v) ratio, is the most widely used in Di Marzo's lab for extraction of NAEs, MAGs, and diacylglycerols (DAGs). First, frozen tissues are weighted and extracted with chloroform/methanol/TRIS–HCl (2:1:1, v/v, 10 mM, pH 7.2). Samples are cooled on ice for the homogenization and extraction processes. The homogenate is spiked with internal standards, deuterium-labeled standards (e.g., for eCBs $[^2H]_8$ AEA 10 pmol, $[^2H]_5$2-AG, $[^2H]_4$ PEA (*N*-palmitoyl ethanolamide), $[^2H]_4$ OEA (*N*-oleoyl ethanolamide) 50 pmol each), or external standards (e.g., for DAGs quantification 1,2-heptadecanoin (17:0–17:0)) (Bisogno et al., 1997; Di Marzo et al., 2001; Matias et al., 2006; Piscitelli et al., 2011), depending on the nature of lipids to extract, and extracted with chloroform. The disadvantages include the use of hazardous chloroform and the collection of chloroform extract from the bottom layer (which may cause the carry-over of water soluble impurities and difficulty in automation). The lipid-containing organic phase is dried down, weighted, and prepurified by open bed chromatography on silica gel. Fractions are obtained by eluting the column with 99:1, 90:10, and 50:50 (v/v) chloroform/methanol. 99:1 fractions are enriched in DAGs, while 90:10 in NAEs and MAGs.

4.2 LC-MS Analysis

Quantification of NAEs and MAGs levels are based on isotope dilution using a Shimadzu high-performance liquid chromatography apparatus (LC-10ADVP) coupled to a Shimadzu (LCMS-2020) quadrupole MS via a Shimadzu atmospheric pressure chemical ionization interface (Bisogno et al., 1997; Di Marzo et al., 2001; Matias et al., 2006). The use of this single quadrupole instrument provided very high sensitive analysis (LOD = 10 fmol) for the simultaneous detection of AEA, 2-AG, PEA, and OEA from several biological matrices. Same sensitivity is observed for NADA detection, even if in neural precursor cells it has not been detectable in any samples (Stock et al., 2012). Very recently, other n-3 and n-6 NAEs and MAGs (NAEs: DHA-EA *N*-docosahexaenoylethanolamine, EPA-EA *N*-eicosapentaenoylethanolamine, 18:2 EA *N*-linoleylethanolamine; MAG: 2-22:6-G 2-docosahexaenoilglycerol) are identified and quantified, as well as simultaneous monitoring of the above mentioned eCBs, using the same technology (Zamberletti et al., 2017). In particular, MS detection is performed by using *m/z* values of 356 and 348 (molecular ions +1 for d^8-AEA and AEA), 304 and 300 (molecular ions +1 for d^4-PEA and PEA), 328 and 326 (molecular ions +1 for d^2-OEA and OEA), 376 and 372 (molecular ions +1 for d^4-DHA-EA and DHA-EA), 384 and 379 (molecular ions +1 for d^5-2-AG and 2-AG), 346 (molecular ions +1 for EPA-EA), 324 (molecular ions +1 for 18:2-EA), 314 (molecular ions +1 for 17:0-EA), 403 (molecular ions +1 for 2-22:6-G), and 345 (molecular ions +1 for 2-17:0-G). AEA, PEA, OEA, DHA-EA, and 2-AG levels are therefore calculated on the basis of their area ratios with the internal deuterated standard signal areas. EPA-EA, 18:2-EA and 2-22:6-G are quantified against 17:0-EA and 2-22:6-G, respectively. The setup of this targeted and accurate method allowed to prove that an imbalanced dietary n-3 and n-6 PUFA content associated with a number of neurological deficits in rats is probably due in part to an alteration of eCBs and eCB-like levels in brain regions involved in mood and cognition.

4.3 LC-MS-IT-TOF Analysis

As stated earlier also the profiling of eCBs biosynthetic precursors could be included into endocannabinoidomics and a very sensitive and highly resolutive method to quantify DAGs (the biosynthetic precursors of 2-AG and other 2-acylglycerols) and NAPEs (*N*-acyl-phosphatidylethanolamines, the biosynthetic precursors of anandamide, and other NAEs, as PEA and OEA) is set up in peripheral tissues of mice fed with Krill oil (KO), a dietary ω-3-PUFA supplementation (Piscitelli et al., 2011). These data have shown that in mice n-3 PUFA dietary content influences eCB precursors and biosynthesis, and the use of this novel-targeted lipid profiling methodology could allow to understand the regulation of eCB levels under physiopathological conditions, also by assessing their precursor availability.

Quantification of cyclooxygenase-2 (COX-2) derivatives of eCBs, prostaglandin ethanolamides (prostamides or PM) and prostaglandin glyceryl esters (PG-GEs), has been carried out by setting up a novel analytical technique for the unequivocal identification and quantification of these lipid species (Gatta et al., 2012). This analysis is performed by LC-MS-IT-TOF technology and using MRM approach. The method has been set up for PME_2, $PMF_{2\alpha}$, PGE_2-GE, and $PGF_{2\alpha}$-GE, and analysis provided high-resolution $[M + Na]^+$ adducts, and PM and PG-GE quantification is performed by isotope dilution. The fragmentation of the ion $[M + Na]^+$ yielded the characteristic loss of water. The LC-ESI-IT-TOF method described in this study for the first time provided a novel tool of analysis to investigate the biological role of these lipids.

5. MEASURING eCBs DROVE DISCOVERY OF LIPOAMINES AND ADDITIONAL MONO ACYLGLYEROLS

5.1 NAEs and Other *N*-Acyl Amines

As eCB measurements have become more routine in labs around the world, many labs are simultaneously also measuring the NAE lipoamine AEA congeners revealing novel signaling roles. NAEs are related to the eCB ligands through biosynthetic and metabolic pathway; however, they do not have the same activity at the active sites of the CB receptors. The following is a short list of the publications involving these NAEs (Fig. 3) to provide a general overview of what we are learning from the analysis of more than AEA in a sample. In particular, endogenous levels of PEA and OEA have been found to change together with eCB levels in several diseases, such as metabolic disorders (Starowicz, Cristino, & Di Marzo, 2008), whereas all NAEs measured in most areas of the brain were upregulated in an acute model of inflammatory pain (Raboune et al., 2014). In contrast, all NAEs measured significantly decreased after mating in female rats, but only in the midbrain, brainstem, and hippocampus (Stuart, Paris, Frye, & Bradshaw, 2013). PEA has emerged as an important analgesic, anti-inflammatory and neuroprotective mediator, acting at several molecular targets in both central and sensory nervous systems as well as immune cells (Petrosino, Iuvone, & Di Marzo, 2010). Whereas, OEA is an anorectic mediator and regulates food intake through peroxisome proliferator-activated receptor (PPAR)-α (Izzo et al., 2010). Moreover, PEA and OEA are able to potentiate the effect of anandamide on cannabinoid receptors or TRPV1 presumably through some as yet unknown allosteric effects (Ben-Shabat et al., 1998; De Petrocellis, Davis, & Di Marzo, 2001; Lambert & Di Marzo, 1999). Other NAEs discovered in mammalian tissues

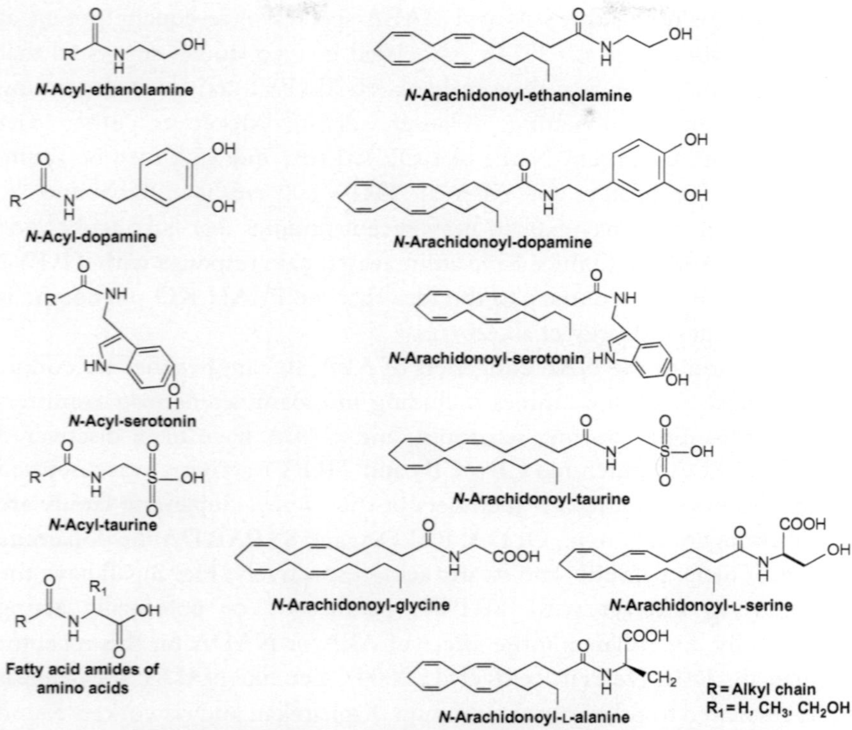

Fig. 3 Chemical structures of different classes of endocannabinoids and endocannabinoid-like molecules.

were *N*-stearoyl ethanolamine (SEA) and *N*-linoleoyl ethanolamine (LEA) found in brains and peripheral tissue of rats and guinea pigs and in infracted dog heart muscle (Bachur, Masek, Melmon, & Udenfriend, 1965; Epps, Schmid, Natarajan, & Schmid, 1979; Hansen & Diep, 2009; Stuart et al., 2013), as well as NAEs, *N*-eicosapentaenoyl ethanolamine (EPEA) and *N*-docosahexaenoyl ethanolamine (DHEA) (Artmann et al., 2008; Carey et al., 2016; Leishman, Cornett, et al., 2016; Lucanic et al., 2011; Raboune et al., 2014).

EPEA and DHEA have been proposed to be cannabinoid receptor agonists (Brown et al., 2010) and able to activate PPAR-γ receptor (Rovito et al., 2013), although their mechanism of action still remain controversial. One of the ways in which the NAEs may be involved in CB-related signaling is through TRPV1. OEA and PEA were shown to have some activity at TRPV1, though not at the same potency as AEA. It has been reported that LEA and DHEA have a similar potency to AEA and that six additional lipoamines including three *N*-acyl GABA species were equally potent at TRPV1 (Raboune et al., 2014). Associated in vivo studies suggested that OEA can induce pain as well as analgesia via TRPV1 activation depending on the experimental settings (Hansen, 2010). Moreover, other data suggested that less potent NAEs like OEA, PEA, and SEA may be acting as allosteric modulators for AEA at TRPV1 (Bradshaw, Raboune, & Hollis, 2013). This may explain most recent findings that fatty acid amide hydrolase (FAAH) KO mice have an increased pain response with TRPV1 activation, which is contrary to the idea that the FAAH KO phenotype is globally analgesic (Carey et al., 2016).

In addition to the NAE congeners of AEA, lipoamines that are conjugates of fatty acids and amines including monoamines neurotransmitters such as dopamine, taurine, serotonin, and GABA have been discovered (Fig. 3). NADA, which has CB_1/CB_2 and TRPV1 activity, was discussed earlier; however, additional members of the *N*-acyl-dopamine family are found endogenously (e.g., OLDA, PALDA, and STEARDA the dopamine amides of oleic, palmitic, and stearic acid, respectively; Fig. 3); all have the capability to interact with TRPV1, or directly or potentially acting allosterically, by enhancing the effect of AEA or NADA on this receptor (Chu et al., 2003; De Petrocellis et al., 2004). Yet, like NADA, they appear to be restricted to primarily the striatum. Saghatelian and coworkers found taurine-conjugated fatty acids in the CNS and peripheral tissues like testes, kidney, and liver of mice (Saghatelian & Cravatt, 2005; Saghatelian et al., 2006, 2004), called *N*-acyl-taurines (NATs; Fig. 3). *N*-Arachidonoyl-taurine is able to activate TRPV1 and TRPV4 calcium channels in mouse kidney (EC_{50} 28 and 21 μM, respectively), and Saghatelian showed that NAT levels in tissues are regulated by FAAH by applying a discovery metabolite profiling strategy (Saghatelian et al., 2006). In 2011, Long and collaborators found in liver and plasma of mice treated with FAAH inhibitor (PF-3845) very high levels of *N*-linoleoyl taurine, *N*-arachidonoyl-taurine, and *N*-docosahexaenoyl taurine (C18:2-Tau, C20:4-Tau, and C22:6-Tau, respectively) (Long, LaCava, Jin, & Cravatt, 2011). Contrary to this, we found that C20:4-Tau was significantly decreased in FAAH KO brains (C18:2-Tau and C22:6-Tau were not measured), suggesting there are likely differences in central and peripheral regulation of these lipids (Leishman, Cornett, et al., 2016). The biosynthetic pathways that produce these lipoamines remain poorly characterized; however, lipidomics techniques will likely play a role in elucidating their regulation. Likewise, many of these lipoamines have been well described in rodent species, but their presence in humans remains largely unknown, though this might be a function of lipid extraction techniques and sample availability. Indeed, it was assumed for years that the *N*-acyl-serotonins were not endogenous; however, modified techniques and equipment were able to show that multiple species are produced endogenously. Verhoeckx reported the isolation of six different *N*-acyl-serotonins (Fig. 3) in the gastrointestinal tract of pigs and mice: *N*-palmitoylserotonin (PA-5-HT), *N*-stearoylserotonin (SA-5-HT), *N*-oleoylserotonin (OA-5-HT), *N*-arachidonoylserotonin (AA-5-HT), *N*-eicosapentaenoylserotonin (EPA-5-HT), and *N*-docosahexaenoylserotonin (DHA-5-HT) (Verhoeckx et al., 2011).

5.2 *N*-Acyl Amino Acids

The largest family of AEA congener lipoamines discovered to date are the *N*-acyl amino acids (Fig. 3). One of the first to be isolated was NAGly in Michael Walker's laboratory (Huang et al., 2001). At low concentrations, NAGly is able to activate GPR18, an orphan receptor coupled to G proteins (Kohno et al., 2006) and GPR92 (Oh et al., 2008). Importantly, GPR18 is also activated by THC (Console-Bram et al., 2014; McHugh et al., 2012, 2014), suggesting the GPR18 and NAGly are additional eCBs. Other endogenous *N*-acyl glycines have been identified: *N*-palmitoyl glycine (PalGly), *N*-oleoyl glycine (OlGly), *N*-stearoyl glycine (StrGly), *N*-linoleoyl glycine (LinGly), and *N*-docosahexaenoyl glycine (DocGly) (Bradshaw, Rimmerman, Hu, Burstein, & Walker, 2009; Rimmerman et al., 2008). Each *N*-acyl glycine is ubiquitous throughout the body with similar distributions as NAEs (Bradshaw et al., 2009). However, the relative amounts changed were dependent on the tissue (Bradshaw et al., 2009). PalGly was shown to drive calcium mobilization in DRG neurons and suppress spinal nociceptive transmission through an as-yet unknown receptor (Rimmerman et al., 2008). However, the signaling properties of the additional *N*-acyl glycine species are still under active investigation.

It is only thanks to improvements in separation techniques and more sensitive MS equipment that have allowed to use targeted lipidomics approaches in which Bradshaw's lab can consistently measure ~60 additional novel endogenous *N*-acyl amino acids in a variety of tissues consistantly (Balakrishna et al., 2014; Leishman, Cornett, et al., 2016; Raboune et al., 2014; Tan et al., 2010, 2009; Tortoriello et al., 2013). Milman et al. isolated and characterized *N*-arachidonoyl-L-serine (AraS) from bovine brain, acting as a relaxing factor in isolated mesenteric arteries in rats (Milman et al., 2006). Some of this activity of Ara may be due to its ability to act as an endogenous antagonist at GPR18 (McHugh et al., 2010). An additional *N*-acyl alanine has been studied by Burstein et al., showing that *N*-linoleoyl-D-alanine increased the production of an antiinflammatory agent (Burstein, McQuain, Salmonsen, & Seicol, 2012). Using TRPV-HEK cell screens, Raboune and coworkers identified 20 novel lipoamines that are active at TPRV1–4 including endogenous antagonists at TRPV3 (Raboune et al., 2014), suggesting that this class of lipids is particularly suited to interact with TRP receptors.

5.3 Products of the Oxidative Metabolism of eCBs and Related Lipids

Multiple investigations into eCB metabolic pathway have been carried out and accumulating data suggest that these lipids act as good substrates of several fatty acid oxygenases. The presence of an arachidonate moiety in both AEA and 2-AG raised the possibility that these molecules might function also as substrate for the same enzymes implicated in arachidonic acid metabolism. The increasing evidence on the role of eCBs in both physiological and pathological conditions and in a plenty of cellular mechanisms prompted many researchers that multiple ways for eCB metabolic dispositions should exist. Such studies have identified a number of novel, eCB-derived lipids, which suggest the possibility that these molecules, additionally to the well-studied hydrolytic metabolism, undergo also oxidative metabolism by a number of fatty acid oxygenases. These include the COX-2 (Kozak & Marnett, 2002), the lipoxygenases-12 and -15 (LOX-12 and LOX-15) (Kozak & Marnett, 2002), and cytochrome P450 oxygenases (Kozak & Marnett, 2002), known to be involved in eicosanoid production from arachidonic acid.

Although kinetic studies indicate that AEA has less affinity than arachidonic acid as substrate, at high concentration (100 μM), it has been shown that the inducible isoform of COX is able to oxygenate AEA at similar rates than its "natural" substrate. Similarly, it has been demonstrated that 2-AG can be selectively oxygenated by this enzyme. The oxygenation of eCBs by COX-2 leads to the formation of prostaglandin-ethanolamides (prostamides, PMs) and prostaglandin-glyceryl esters with unique pharmacological properties (Fig. 4; Kozak & Marnett, 2002). COX-2 oxygenates AEA first to PGH_2-ethanolamide, which, probably through the action of prostaglandin E synthase, is then converted PGE_2-ethanolamide (PME_2), the first prostamide to be discovered (Yu, Ives, & Ramesha, 1997). Yu and coworkers showed that PME_2 was the major product when human

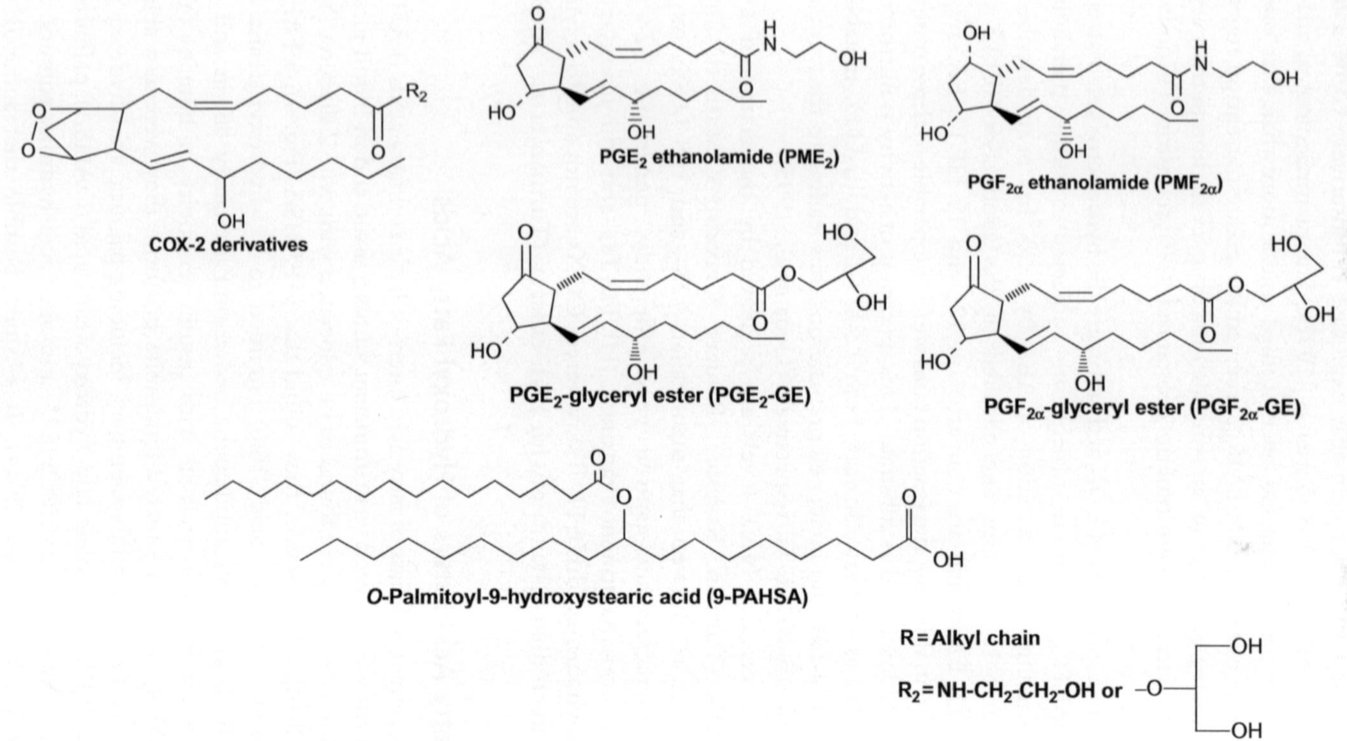

Fig. 4 Chemical structures of COX-2 derivatives and FAHFA.

recombinant COX-2 or cells that expressed constitutively COX-2 have been incubated with AEA (Yu et al., 1997). The pharmacological characterization of prostamides has been studied much more than that one of PG-glyceryl esters. In fact, $PMF_{2\alpha}$ received the greatest attention together with its analog bimatoprost, an antiglaucoma drug, even though their action is not mediated by homomeric prostanoid (FP) receptors (Woodward et al., 2008).

The main products of LOX activation are the hydroperoxyeicosatrenoic acids (HpETEs) which are subsequently subjected to further metabolism. Correspondingly, the oxidation of AEA by LOX has been described in the 12 and 15 positions and resulted in the production of 12- and 15-HpETE-EA which are converted in 12- and 15-HETE-EA, respectively. Also in this case, the reaction rates were comparable to those observed with arachidonic acid as substrate. This spectrum of activity is mirrored by using 2-AG as substrate; in fact, both 12-LOX and 15-LOX metabolize 2-AG in cell-free and intact cell preparations thus leading to the formation of 12- and 15-HETE-G, respectively (Ueda et al., 1995).

Moreover, also NAT levels are regulated by the action of LOX and COX (Turman, Kingsley, Rouzer, Cravatt, & Marnett, 2008). Turman et al. showed that mammalian 12S- and 15S-LOXs oxygenated *N*-arachidonoyl-taurine very efficiently, generating 12- and 15-hydroxyeicosatetraenoyltaurines (HETE-Ts) and dihydroxyeicosa tetraenoyltaurines (diHETE-Ts), whereas COXs are not able to oxygenate *N*-arachidonoyl-taurine with high efficacy (Turman et al., 2008).

5.4 Fatty Acid Esters of Hydroxyl Fatty Acids

An emerging lipid class of fatty acid esters of hydroxyl fatty acids (FAHFA) was recently discovered in mammalian adipose tissue and in blood plasma, and some FAHFAs were found to be associated with type 2 diabetes (Yore et al., 2014). In particular, they found that 9-PAHSA (Fig. 4), a FAHFA comprised of palmitic acid (16:0) esterified to a 9-hydroxyl stearic acid (9-O-18:0), promotes antidiabetic and antiinflammatory effects and that its levels are highly correlated with insulin sensitivity in humans (Yore et al., 2014). Using a targeted lipidomics platform, they were also able to identify 16 FAHFA family members, including palmitic acid-hydroxy palmitic acid (PAHPA), oleic acid-hydroxy stearic acid (OAHSA), palmitoleic acid-hydroxy stearic acid (POHSA), and oleic acid-hydroxy palmitic acid (OAHPA) (Yore et al., 2014). It is quite possible that some of the biosynthetic processes regulating these lipids will be shared with some of the small molecule lipids discussed here.

6. CONCLUSION

The advancing analytical technology and novel bioinformatic strategies has greatly driven the lipidomics field in all biological and biomedical areas. The application of lipidomics approaches to the expanding world of eCB and eCB-related compounds has led us to identify new signaling molecules, to better understand their physiopathological roles and their metabolic pathways, to discover potential biomarkers for early diagnosis and prognosis of diseases, to screen drug targets and/or test drug efficacy, and to achieve personalized medicine. We have summarized the state of current knowledge and traditional techniques applied for eCB quantification.

In conclusions, despite the need of dealing with an increasingly complex "endocannabinoidome" has led us to use novel and more modern and complex analytical approaches, has not discouraged all those who have been fascinated by this system, and has directed us to new exciting discoveries.

CONFLICT OF INTEREST

The authors declare there are no conflicts of interest.

REFERENCES

Artmann, A., Petersen, G., Hellgren, L. I., Boberg, J., Skonberg, C., Nellemann, C., et al. (2008). Influence of dietary fatty acids on endocannabinoid and N-acylethanolamine levels in rat brain, liver and small intestine. *Biochimica et Biophysica Acta*, *1781*(4), 200–212. http://dx.doi.org/10.1016/j.bbalip.2008.01.006.

Astarita, G., Rourke, B. C., Andersen, J. B., Fu, J., Kim, J. H., Bennett, A. F., et al. (2006). Postprandial increase of oleoylethanolamide mobilization in small intestine of the Burmese python (*Python molurus*). *American Journal of Physiology. Regulatory, Integrative and Comparative Physiology*, *290*(5), R1407–R1412. http://dx.doi.org/10.1152/ajpregu.00664.2005.

Bachur, N. R., Masek, K., Melmon, K. L., & Udenfriend, S. (1965). Fatty acid amides of ethanolamine in mammalian tissues. *The Journal of Biological Chemistry*, *240*, 1019–1024.

Balakrishna, S., Song, W., Achanta, S., Doran, S. F., Liu, B., Kaelberer, M. M., et al. (2014). TRPV4 inhibition counteracts edema and inflammation and improves pulmonary function and oxygen saturation in chemically induced acute lung injury. *American Journal of Physiology. Lung Cellular and Molecular Physiology*, *307*(2), L158–L172. http://dx.doi.org/10.1152/ajplung.00065.2014.

Balvers, M. G., Verhoeckx, K. C., & Witkamp, R. F. (2009). Development and validation of a quantitative method for the determination of 12 endocannabinoids and related compounds in human plasma using liquid chromatography-tandem mass spectrometry. *Journal of Chromatography B, Analytical Technologies in the Biomedical and Life Sciences*, *877*(14–15), 1583–1590. http://dx.doi.org/10.1016/j.jchromb.2009.04.010.

Ben-Shabat, S., Fride, E., Sheskin, T., Tamiri, T., Rhee, M. H., Vogel, Z., et al. (1998). An entourage effect: Inactive endogenous fatty acid glycerol esters enhance 2-arachidonoyl-glycerol cannabinoid activity. *European Journal of Pharmacology, 353*(1), 23–31. http://dx.doi.org/10.1016/S0014-2999(98)00392-6 [pii].

Bisogno, T., Melck, D., Bobrov, M. Y., Gretskaya, N. M., Bezuglov, V. V., De Petrocellis, L., et al. (2000). N-Acyl-dopamines: Novel synthetic CB(1) cannabinoid-receptor ligands and inhibitors of anandamide inactivation with cannabimimetic activity in vitro and in vivo. *The Biochemical Journal, 351*(Pt. 3), 817–824.

Bisogno, T., Piscitelli, F., & Di Marzo, V. (2009). Lipidomic methodologies applicable to the study of endocannabinoids and related compounds: Endocannabinoidomics. *European Journal of Lipid Science and Technology, 111*(1), 10.

Bisogno, T., Sepe, N., Melck, D., Maurelli, S., De Petrocellis, L., & Di Marzo, V. (1997). Biosynthesis, release and degradation of the novel endogenous cannabimimetic metabolite 2-arachidonoylglycerol in mouse neuroblastoma cells. *The Biochemical Journal, 322*(Pt. 2), 671–677.

Bligh, E. G., & Dyer, W. J. (1959). A rapid method of total lipid extraction and purification. *Canadian Journal of Biochemistry and Physiology, 37*(8), 911–917. http://dx.doi.org/10.1139/o59-099.

Bradshaw, H. B., & Leishman, E. (2016). Levels of bioactive lipids in cooking oils: Olive oil is the richest source of oleoyl serine. *Journal of Basic and Clinical Physiology and Pharmacology, 27*(3), 247–252. http://dx.doi.org/10.1515/jbcpp-2015-0104.

Bradshaw, H. B., Raboune, S., & Hollis, J. L. (2013). Opportunistic activation of TRP receptors by endogenous lipids: Exploiting lipidomics to understand TRP receptor cellular communication. *Life Sciences, 92*(8-9), 404–409. http://dx.doi.org/10.1016/j.lfs.2012.11.008.

Bradshaw, H. B., Rimmerman, N., Hu, S. S., Burstein, S., & Walker, J. M. (2009). Novel endogenous N-acyl glycines identification and characterization. *Vitamins and Hormones, 81*, 191–205. http://dx.doi.org/10.1016/S0083-6729(09)81008-X.

Bradshaw, H. B., Rimmerman, N., Krey, J. F., & Walker, J. M. (2006). Sex and hormonal cycle differences in rat brain levels of pain-related cannabimimetic lipid mediators. *American Journal of Physiology. Regulatory, Integrative and Comparative Physiology, 291*(2), R349–R358. http://dx.doi.org/10.1152/ajpregu.00933.2005.

Brown, I., Cascio, M. G., Wahle, K. W., Smoum, R., Mechoulam, R., Ross, R. A., et al. (2010). Cannabinoid receptor-dependent and -independent anti-proliferative effects of omega-3 ethanolamides in androgen receptor-positive and -negative prostate cancer cell lines. *Carcinogenesis, 31*(9), 1584–1591. http://dx.doi.org/10.1093/carcin/bgq151.

Burstein, S., McQuain, C., Salmonsen, R., & Seicol, B. (2012). N-Amino acid linoleoyl conjugates: Anti-inflammatory activities. *Bioorganic & Medicinal Chemistry Letters, 22*(2), 872–875. http://dx.doi.org/10.1016/j.bmcl.2011.12.040.

Bystrowska, B., Smaga, I., Tyszka-Czochara, M., & Filip, M. (2014). Troubleshooting in LC-MS/MS method for determining endocannabinoid and endocannabinoid-like molecules in rat brain structures applied to assessing the brain endocannabinoid/endovanilloid system significance. *Toxicology Mechanisms and Methods, 24*(4), 315–322. http://dx.doi.org/10.3109/15376516.2014.898356.

Carey, L. M., Slivicki, R. A., Leishman, E., Cornett, B., Mackie, K., Bradshaw, H., et al. (2016). A pro-nociceptive phenotype unmasked in mice lacking fatty-acid amide hydrolase. *Molecular Pain, 12*, 1–23. http://dx.doi.org/10.1177/1744806916649192.

Caterina, M. J., Schumacher, M. A., Tominaga, M., Rosen, T. A., Levine, J. D., & Julius, D. (1997). The capsaicin receptor: A heat-activated ion channel in the pain pathway. *Nature, 389*(6653), 816–824. http://dx.doi.org/10.1038/39807.

Chen, J., Paudel, K. S., Derbenev, A. V., Smith, B. N., & Stinchcomb, A. L. (2009). Simultaneous quantification of anandamide and other endocannabinoids in dorsal vagal complex of rat brainstem by LC-MS. *Chromatographia*, *69*(1-2), 1–7. http://dx.doi.org/10.1365/s10337-008-0841-x.

Chu, C. J., Huang, S. M., De Petrocellis, L., Bisogno, T., Ewing, S. A., Miller, J. D., et al. (2003). N-oleoyldopamine, a novel endogenous capsaicin-like lipid that produces hyperalgesia. *The Journal of Biological Chemistry*, *278*(16), 13633–13639. http://dx.doi.org/10.1074/jbc.M211231200.

Console-Bram, L., Brailoiu, E., Brailoiu, G. C., Sharir, H., & Abood, M. E. (2014). Activation of GPR18 by cannabinoid compounds: A tale of biased agonism. *British Journal of Pharmacology*, *171*(16), 3908–3917. http://dx.doi.org/10.1111/bph.12746.

Darmani, N. A., Chebolu, S., Zhong, W., Trinh, C., McClanahan, B., & Brar, R. S. (2014). Additive antiemetic efficacy of low-doses of the cannabinoid CB(1/2) receptor agonist Delta(9)-THC with ultralow-doses of the vanilloid TRPV1 receptor agonist resiniferatoxin in the least shrew (Cryptotis parva). *European Journal of Pharmacology*, *722*, 147–155. http://dx.doi.org/10.1016/j.ejphar.2013.08.051.

De Filippis, D., D'Amico, A., Cipriano, M., Petrosino, S., Orlando, P., Di Marzo, V., et al. (2010). Levels of endocannabinoids and palmitoylethanolamide and their pharmacological manipulation in chronic granulomatous inflammation in rats. *Pharmacological Research*, *61*(4), 321–328. http://dx.doi.org/10.1016/j.phrs.2009.11.005.

De Petrocellis, L., Chu, C. J., Moriello, A. S., Kellner, J. C., Walker, J. M., & Di Marzo, V. (2004). Actions of two naturally occurring saturated N-acyldopamines on transient receptor potential vanilloid 1 (TRPV1) channels. *British Journal of Pharmacology*, *143*(2), 251–256. http://dx.doi.org/10.1038/sj.bjp.0705924.

De Petrocellis, L., Davis, J. B., & Di Marzo, V. (2001). Palmitoylethanolamide enhances anandamide stimulation of human vanilloid VR1 receptors. *FEBS Letters*, *506*(3), 253–256. http://dx.doi.org/10.1016/S0014-5793(01)02934-9 [pii].

De Petrocellis, L., & Di Marzo, V. (2009). An introduction to the endocannabinoid system: From the early to the latest concepts. *Best Practice & Research. Clinical Endocrinology & Metabolism*, *23*(1), 1–15. http://dx.doi.org/10.1016/j.beem.2008.10.013.

De Petrocellis, L., Orlando, P., Moriello, A. S., Aviello, G., Stott, C., Izzo, A. A., et al. (2012). Cannabinoid actions at TRPV channels: Effects on TRPV3 and TRPV4 and their potential relevance to gastrointestinal inflammation. *Acta Physiologica (Oxford, England)*, *204*(2), 255–266. http://dx.doi.org/10.1111/j.1748-1716.2011.02338.x.

Devane, W. A., Dysarz, F. A., 3rd, Johnson, M. R., Melvin, L. S., & Howlett, A. C. (1988). Determination and characterization of a cannabinoid receptor in rat brain. *Molecular Pharmacology*, *34*(5), 605–613.

Devane, W. A., Hanus, L., Breuer, A., Pertwee, R. G., Stevenson, L. A., Griffin, G., et al. (1992). Isolation and structure of a brain constituent that binds to the cannabinoid receptor. *Science*, *258*(5090), 1946–1949.

Di Marzo, V., Goparaju, S. K., Wang, L., Liu, J., Batkai, S., Jarai, Z., et al. (2001). Leptin-regulated endocannabinoids are involved in maintaining food intake. *Nature*, *410*(6830), 822–825. http://dx.doi.org/10.1038/35071088.

Epps, D. E., Schmid, P. C., Natarajan, V., & Schmid, H. H. (1979). N-acylethanolamine accumulation in infarcted myocardium. *Biochemical and Biophysical Research Communications*, *90*(2), 628–633. http://dx.doi.org/10.1016/0006-291X(79)91281-6 [pii].

Espejo-Porras, F., Fernandez-Ruiz, J., Pertwee, R. G., Mechoulam, R., & Garcia, C. (2013). Motor effects of the non-psychotropic phytocannabinoid cannabidiol that are mediated by 5-HT1A receptors. *Neuropharmacology*, *75*, 155–163. http://dx.doi.org/10.1016/j.neuropharm.2013.07.024.

Felder, C. C., Nielsen, A., Briley, E. M., Palkovits, M., Priller, J., Axelrod, J., et al. (1996). Isolation and measurement of the endogenous cannabinoid receptor agonist, anandamide, in brain and peripheral tissues of human and rat. *FEBS Letters*, *393*(2–3), 231–235. http://dx.doi.org/10.1016/0014-5793(96)00891-5 [pii].

Folch, J., Lees, M., & Sloane Stanley, G. H. (1957). A simple method for the isolation and purification of total lipides from animal tissues. *The Journal of Biological Chemistry*, *226*(1), 497–509.

Fontana, A., Di Marzo, V., Cadas, H., & Piomelli, D. (1995). Analysis of anandamide, an endogenous cannabinoid substance, and of other natural N-acylethanolamines. *Prostaglandins, Leukotrienes, and Essential Fatty Acids*, *53*(4), 301–308.

Gaoni, Y., & Mechoulam, R. (1971). The isolation and structure of delta-1-tetrahydrocannabinol and other neutral cannabinoids from hashish. *Journal of the American Chemical Society*, *93*(1), 217–224.

Gatta, L., Piscitelli, F., Giordano, C., Boccella, S., Lichtman, A., Maione, S., et al. (2012). Discovery of prostamide F2alpha and its role in inflammatory pain and dorsal horn nociceptive neuron hyperexcitability. *PLoS One*, 7(2). e31111. http://dx.doi.org/10.1371/journal.pone.0031111.

Giuffrida, A., & Piomelli, D. (1998). Isotope dilution GC/MS determination of anandamide and other fatty acylethanolamides in rat blood plasma. *FEBS Letters*, *422*(3), 373–376. http://dx.doi.org/10.1016/S0014-5793(98)00046-5 [pii].

Hansen, H. S. (2010). Palmitoylethanolamide and other anandamide congeners. Proposed role in the diseased brain. *Experimental Neurology*, *224*(1), 48–55. http://dx.doi.org/10.1016/j.expneurol.2010.03.022.

Hansen, H. S., & Diep, T. A. (2009). N-Acylethanolamines, anandamide and food intake. *Biochemical Pharmacology*, *78*(6), 553–560. http://dx.doi.org/10.1016/j.bcp.2009.04.024.

Hardison, S., Weintraub, S. T., & Giuffrida, A. (2006). Quantification of endocannabinoids in rat biological samples by GC/MS: Technical and theoretical considerations. *Prostaglandins & Other Lipid Mediators*, *81*(3–4), 106–112. http://dx.doi.org/10.1016/j.prostaglandins.2006.08.002.

Hu, S. S., Bradshaw, H. B., Chen, J. S., Tan, B., & Walker, J. M. (2008). Prostaglandin E2 glycerol ester, an endogenous COX-2 metabolite of 2-arachidonoylglycerol, induces hyperalgesia and modulates NFkappaB activity. *British Journal of Pharmacology*, *153*(7), 1538–1549. http://dx.doi.org/10.1038/bjp.2008.33.

Huang, S. M., Bisogno, T., Petros, T. J., Chang, S. Y., Zavitsanos, P. A., Zipkin, R. E., et al. (2001). Identification of a new class of molecules, the arachidonyl amino acids, and characterization of one member that inhibits pain. *The Journal of Biological Chemistry*, *276*(46), 42639–42644. http://dx.doi.org/10.1074/jbc.M107351200.

Huang, S. M., Bisogno, T., Trevisani, M., Al-Hayani, A., De Petrocellis, L., Fezza, F., et al. (2002). An endogenous capsaicin-like substance with high potency at recombinant and native vanilloid VR1 receptors. *Proceedings of the National Academy of Sciences of the United States of America*, *99*(12), 8400–8405. http://dx.doi.org/10.1073/pnas.122196999.

Huang, S. M., Strangman, N. M., & Walker, J. M. (1999). Liquid chromatographic-mass spectrometric measurement of the endogenous cannabinoid 2-arachidonylglycerol in the spinal cord and peripheral nervous system. *Zhongguo Yao Li Xue Bao*, *20*(12), 1098–1102.

Izzo, A. A., Piscitelli, F., Capasso, R., Marini, P., Cristino, L., Petrosino, S., et al. (2010). Basal and fasting/refeeding-regulated tissue levels of endogenous PPAR-alpha ligands in Zucker rats. *Obesity (Silver Spring)*, *18*(1), 55–62. http://dx.doi.org/10.1038/oby.2009.186 oby2009186 [pii].

Kantae, V., Ogino, S., Noga, M., Harms, A. C., van Dongen, R. M., Onderwater, G. L., et al. (2017). Quantitative profiling of endocannabinoids and related N-acylethanolamines in human CSF using nano LC-MS/MS. *Journal of Lipid Research*, *58*, 615–624. http://dx.doi.org/10.1194/jlr.D070433.

Kempe, K., Hsu, F. F., Bohrer, A., & Turk, J. (1996). Isotope dilution mass spectrometric measurements indicate that arachidonylethanolamide, the proposed endogenous ligand of the cannabinoid receptor, accumulates in rat brain tissue post mortem but is contained at low levels in or is absent from fresh tissue. *The Journal of Biological Chemistry*, *271*(29), 17287–17295.

Kilaru, A., Isaac, G., Tamura, P., Baxter, D., Duncan, S. R., Venables, B. J., et al. (2010). Lipid profiling reveals tissue-specific differences for ethanolamide lipids in mice lacking fatty acid amide hydrolase. *Lipids*, *45*(9), 863–875. http://dx.doi.org/10.1007/s11745-010-3457-5.

Kingsley, P. J., & Marnett, L. J. (2007). LC-MS-MS analysis of neutral eicosanoids. *Methods in Enzymology*, *433*, 91–112. http://dx.doi.org/10.1016/S0076–6879(07)33005-X.

Kirkham, T. C., Williams, C. M., Fezza, F., & Di Marzo, V. (2002). Endocannabinoid levels in rat limbic forebrain and hypothalamus in relation to fasting, feeding and satiation: Stimulation of eating by 2-arachidonoyl glycerol. *British Journal of Pharmacology*, *136*(4), 550–557. http://dx.doi.org/10.1038/sj.bjp.0704767.

Kirkwood, J. S., Broeckling, C. D., Donahue, S., & Prenni, J. E. (2016). A novel microflow LC-MS method for the quantitation of endocannabinoids in serum. *Journal of Chromatography. B, Analytical Technologies in the Biomedical and Life Sciences*, *1033-1034*, 271–277. http://dx.doi.org/10.1016/j.jchromb.2016.08.035.

Kohno, M., Hasegawa, H., Inoue, A., Muraoka, M., Miyazaki, T., Oka, K., et al. (2006). Identification of N-arachidonylglycine as the endogenous ligand for orphan G-protein-coupled receptor GPR18. *Biochemical and Biophysical Research Communications*, *347*(3), 827–832. http://dx.doi.org/10.1016/j.bbrc.2006.06.175.

Kondo, S., Kondo, H., Nakane, S., Kodaka, T., Tokumura, A., Waku, K., et al. (1998). 2-Arachidonoylglycerol, an endogenous cannabinoid receptor agonist: Identification as one of the major species of monoacylglycerols in various rat tissues, and evidence for its generation through CA2+-dependent and -independent mechanisms. *FEBS Letters*, *429*(2), 152–156. http://dx.doi.org/10.1016/S0014-5793(98)00581-X [pii].

Kozak, K. R., & Marnett, L. J. (2002). Oxidative metabolism of endocannabinoids. *Prostaglandins, Leukotrienes, and Essential Fatty Acids*, *66*(2-3), 211–220. http://dx.doi.org/10.1054/plef.2001.0359.

Lam, P. M., Marczylo, T. H., El-Talatini, M., Finney, M., Nallendran, V., Taylor, A. H., et al. (2008). Ultra performance liquid chromatography tandem mass spectrometry method for the measurement of anandamide in human plasma. *Analytical Biochemistry*, *380*(2), 195–201. http://dx.doi.org/10.1016/j.ab.2008.05.033.

Lambert, D. M., & Di Marzo, V. (1999). The palmitoylethanolamide and oleamide enigmas: Are these two fatty acid amides cannabimimetic? *Current Medicinal Chemistry*, *6*(8), 757–773.

Lauckner, J. E., Jensen, J. B., Chen, H. Y., Lu, H. C., Hille, B., & Mackie, K. (2008). GPR55 is a cannabinoid receptor that increases intracellular calcium and inhibits M current. *Proceedings of the National Academy of Sciences of the United States of America*, *105*(7), 2699–2704. http://dx.doi.org/10.1073/pnas.0711278105.

Lehtonen, M., Storvik, M., Malinen, H., Hyytia, P., Lakso, M., Auriola, S., et al. (2011). Determination of endocannabinoids in nematodes and human brain tissue by liquid chromatography electrospray ionization tandem mass spectrometry. *Journal of Chromatography. B, Analytical Technologies in the Biomedical and Life Sciences*, *879*(11-12), 677–694. http://dx.doi.org/10.1016/j.jchromb.2011.02.004.

Leishman, E., Cornett, B., Spork, K., Straiker, A., Mackie, K., & Bradshaw, H. B. (2016). Broad impact of deleting endogenous cannabinoid hydrolyzing enzymes and the CB1 cannabinoid receptor on the endogenous cannabinoid-related lipidome in eight regions of the mouse brain. *Pharmacological Research*, *110*, 159–172. http://dx.doi.org/10.1016/j.phrs.2016.04.020.

Ligresti, A., Bisogno, T., Matias, I., De Petrocellis, L., Cascio, M. G., Cosenza, V., et al. (2003). Possible endocannabinoid control of colorectal cancer growth. *Gastroenterology*, *125*(3), 677–687. http://dx.doi.org/10.1016/S0016-5085(03)00881-3 [pii].

Lin, S., Khanolkar, A. D., Fan, P., Goutopoulos, A., Qin, C., Papahadjis, D., et al. (1998). Novel analogues of arachidonylethanolamide (anandamide): Affinities for the CB1 and CB2 cannabinoid receptors and metabolic stability. *Journal of Medicinal Chemistry*, *41*(27), 5353–5361. http://dx.doi.org/10.1021/jm970257g.

Long, J. Z., LaCava, M., Jin, X., & Cravatt, B. F. (2011). An anatomical and temporal portrait of physiological substrates for fatty acid amide hydrolase. *Journal of Lipid Research*, *52*(2), 337–344. http://dx.doi.org/10.1194/jlr.M012153.

Lucanic, M., Held, J. M., Vantipalli, M. C., Klang, I. M., Graham, J. B., Gibson, B. W., et al. (2011). N-Acylethanolamine signalling mediates the effect of diet on lifespan in Caenorhabditis elegans. *Nature*, *473*(7346), 226–229. http://dx.doi.org/10.1038/nature10007.

Maccarrone, M., Attina, M., Cartoni, A., Bari, M., & Finazzi-Agro, A. (2001). Gas chromatography-mass spectrometry analysis of endogenous cannabinoids in healthy and tumoral human brain and human cells in culture. *Journal of Neurochemistry*, *76*(2), 594–601.

Matias, I., Wang, J. W., Moriello, A. S., Nieves, A., Woodward, D. F., & Di Marzo, V. (2006). Changes in endocannabinoid and palmitoylethanolamide levels in eye tissues of patients with diabetic retinopathy and age-related macular degeneration. *Prostaglandins, Leukotrienes, and Essential Fatty Acids*, *75*(6), 413–418. http://dx.doi.org/10.1016/j.plefa.2006.08.002.

Matsuda, L. A., Lolait, S. J., Brownstein, M. J., Young, A. C., & Bonner, T. I. (1990). Structure of a cannabinoid receptor and functional expression of the cloned cDNA. *Nature*, *346*(6284), 561–564. http://dx.doi.org/10.1038/346561a0.

McHugh, D., Hu, S. S., Rimmerman, N., Juknat, A., Vogel, Z., Walker, J. M., et al. (2010). N-Arachidonoyl glycine, an abundant endogenous lipid, potently drives directed cellular migration through GPR18, the putative abnormal cannabidiol receptor. *BMC Neuroscience*, *11*, 44. http://dx.doi.org/10.1186/1471-2202-11-44.

McHugh, D., Page, J., Dunn, E., & Bradshaw, H. B. (2012). Delta(9) -tetrahydrocannabinol and N-arachidonyl glycine are full agonists at GPR18 receptors and induce migration in human endometrial HEC-1B cells. *British Journal of Pharmacology*, *165*(8), 2414–2424. http://dx.doi.org/10.1111/j.1476-5381.2011.01497.x.

McHugh, D., Roskowski, D., Xie, S., & Bradshaw, H. B. (2014). Delta(9)-THC and N-arachidonoyl glycine regulate BV-2 microglial morphology and cytokine release plasticity: Implications for signaling at GPR18. *Frontiers in Pharmacology*, *4*, 162. http://dx.doi.org/10.3389/fphar.2013.00162.

Mechoulam, R., Ben-Shabat, S., Hanus, L., Ligumsky, M., Kaminski, N. E., Schatz, A. R., et al. (1995). Identification of an endogenous 2-monoglyceride, present in canine gut, that binds to cannabinoid receptors. *Biochemical Pharmacology*, *50*(1), 83–90. http://dx.doi.org/. 10.1016/0006-2952(95)00109-D [pii].

Miller, S., Leishman, E., Oehler, O., Daily, L., Murataeva, N., Wager-Miller, J., et al. (2016). Evidence for a GPR18 role in diurnal regulation of intraocular pressure. *Investigative Ophthalmology & Visual Science*, *57*(14), 6419–6426. http://dx.doi.org/10.1167/iovs.16-19437.

Milman, G., Maor, Y., Abu-Lafi, S., Horowitz, M., Gallily, R., Batkai, S., et al. (2006). N-Arachidonoyl L-serine, an endocannabinoid-like brain constituent with vasodilatory properties. *Proceedings of the National Academy of Sciences of the United States of America*, *103*(7), 2428–2433. http://dx.doi.org/10.1073/pnas.0510676103.

Moreno, E., Andradas, C., Medrano, M., Caffarel, M. M., Perez-Gomez, E., Blasco-Benito, S., et al. (2014). Targeting CB2-GPR55 receptor heteromers modulates cancer cell signaling. *The Journal of Biological Chemistry*, *289*(32), 21960–21972. http://dx.doi.org/10.1074/jbc.M114.561761.

Muccioli, G. G., & Stella, N. (2008). An optimized GC-MS method detects nanomolar amounts of anandamide in mouse brain. *Analytical Biochemistry*, *373*(2), 220–228. http://dx.doi.org/10.1016/j.ab.2007.09.030.

Munro, S., Thomas, K. L., & Abu-Shaar, M. (1993). Molecular characterization of a peripheral receptor for cannabinoids. *Nature*, *365*(6441), 61–65. http://dx.doi.org/10.1038/365061a0.

Murataeva, N., Dhopeshwarkar, A., Yin, D., Mitjavila, J., Bradshaw, H., Straiker, A., et al. (2016). Where's my entourage? The curious case of 2-oleoylglycerol, 2-linolenoylglycerol, and 2-palmitoylglycerol. *Pharmacological Research*, *110*, 173–180. http://dx.doi.org/10.1016/j.phrs.2016.04.015.

Nucci, C., Gasperi, V., Tartaglione, R., Cerulli, A., Terrinoni, A., Bari, M., et al. (2007). Involvement of the endocannabinoid system in retinal damage after high intraocular pressure-induced ischemia in rats. *Investigative Ophthalmology & Visual Science*, *48*(7), 2997–3004. http://dx.doi.org/10.1167/iovs.06-1355.

Obata, T., Sakurai, Y., Kase, Y., Tanifuji, Y., & Horiguchi, T. (2003). Simultaneous determination of endocannabinoids (arachidonylethanolamide and 2-arachidonylglycerol) and isoprostane (8-epiprostaglandin F2alpha) by gas chromatography-mass spectrometry-selected ion monitoring for medical samples. *Journal of Chromatography. B, Analytical Technologies in the Biomedical and Life Sciences*, *792*(1), 131–140. http://dx.doi.org/10.1016/S1570-0232(03)00311-8 [pii]. .

Oh, D. Y., Yoon, J. M., Moon, M. J., Hwang, J. I., Choe, H., Lee, J. Y., et al. (2008). Identification of farnesyl pyrophosphate and N-arachidonylglycine as endogenous ligands for GPR92. *The Journal of Biological Chemistry*, *283*(30), 21054–21064. http://dx.doi.org/10.1074/jbc.M708908200.

Oka, S., Tsuchie, A., Tokumura, A., Muramatsu, M., Suhara, Y., Takayama, H., et al. (2003). Ether-linked analogue of 2-arachidonoylglycerol (noladin ether) was not detected in the brains of various mammalian species. *Journal of Neurochemistry*, *85*(6), 1374–1381. http://dx.doi.org/10.1046/j.1471-4159.2003.01804 [pii]. .

Opitz, C. A., Rimmerman, N., Zhang, Y., Mead, L. E., Yoder, M. C., Ingram, D. A., et al. (2007). Production of the endocannabinoids anandamide and 2-arachidonoylglycerol by endothelial progenitor cells. *FEBS Letters*, *581*(25), 4927–4931. http://dx.doi.org/10.1016/j.febslet.2007.09.032.

Palandra, J., Prusakiewicz, J., Ozer, J. S., Zhang, Y., & Heath, T. G. (2009). Endogenous ethanolamide analysis in human plasma using HPLC tandem MS with electrospray ionization. *Journal of Chromatography. B, Analytical Technologies in the Biomedical and Life Sciences*, *877*(22), 2052–2060. http://dx.doi.org/10.1016/j.jchromb.2009.05.043.

Patel, S., Rademacher, D. J., & Hillard, C. J. (2003). Differential regulation of the endocannabinoids anandamide and 2-arachidonylglycerol within the limbic forebrain by dopamine receptor activity. *The Journal of Pharmacology and Experimental Therapeutics*, *306*(3), 880–888. http://dx.doi.org/10.1124/jpet.103.054270.

Pertwee, R. G. (2007). GPR55: A new member of the cannabinoid receptor clan? *British Journal of Pharmacology*, *152*(7), 984–986. http://dx.doi.org/10.1038/sj.bjp.0707464.

Petrosino, S., Iuvone, T., & Di Marzo, V. (2010). N-palmitoyl-ethanolamine: Biochemistry and new therapeutic opportunities. *Biochimie*, *92*(6), 724–727. http://dx.doi.org/10.1016/j.biochi.2010.01.006.

Piscitelli, F., Carta, G., Bisogno, T., Murru, E., Cordeddu, L., Berge, K., et al. (2011). Effect of dietary krill oil supplementation on the endocannabinoidome of metabolically relevant tissues from high-fat-fed mice. *Nutrition & Metabolism (London)*, *8*(1), 51. http://dx.doi.org/10.1186/1743-7075-8-51.

Raboune, S., Stuart, J. M., Leishman, E., Takacs, S. M., Rhodes, B., Basnet, A., et al. (2014). Novel endogenous N-acyl amides activate TRPV1-4 receptors, BV-2 microglia, and are regulated in brain in an acute model of inflammation. *Frontiers in Cellular Neuroscience*, *8*, 195. http://dx.doi.org/10.3389/fncel.2014.00195.

Richardson, D., Ortori, C. A., Chapman, V., Kendall, D. A., & Barrett, D. A. (2007). Quantitative profiling of endocannabinoids and related compounds in rat brain using

liquid chromatography-tandem electrospray ionization mass spectrometry. *Analytical Biochemistry*, *360*(2), 216–226. http://dx.doi.org/10.1016/j.ab.2006.10.039.
Rimmerman, N., Bradshaw, H. B., Hughes, H. V., Chen, J. S., Hu, S. S., McHugh, D., et al. (2008). N-palmitoyl glycine, a novel endogenous lipid that acts as a modulator of calcium influx and nitric oxide production in sensory neurons. *Molecular Pharmacology*, *74*(1), 213–224. http://dx.doi.org/10.1124/mol.108.045997.
Rovito, D., Giordano, C., Vizza, D., Plastina, P., Barone, I., Casaburi, I., et al. (2013). Omega-3 PUFA ethanolamides DHEA and EPEA induce autophagy through PPARgamma activation in MCF-7 breast cancer cells. *Journal of Cellular Physiology*, *228*(6), 1314–1322. http://dx.doi.org/10.1002/jcp.24288.
Saghatelian, A., & Cravatt, B. F. (2005). Discovery metabolite profiling—Forging functional connections between the proteome and metabolome. *Life Sciences*, 77(14), 1759–1766. http://dx.doi.org/10.1016/j.lfs.2005.05.019.
Saghatelian, A., McKinney, M. K., Bandell, M., Patapoutian, A., & Cravatt, B. F. (2006). A FAAH-regulated class of N-acyl taurines that activates TRP ion channels. *Biochemistry*, *45*(30), 9007–9015. http://dx.doi.org/10.1021/bi0608008.
Saghatelian, A., Trauger, S. A., Want, E. J., Hawkins, E. G., Siuzdak, G., & Cravatt, B. F. (2004). Assignment of endogenous substrates to enzymes by global metabolite profiling. *Biochemistry*, *43*(45), 14332–14339. http://dx.doi.org/10.1021/bi0480335.
Sasso, O., Pontis, S., Armirotti, A., Cardinali, G., Kovacs, D., Migliore, M., et al. (2016). Endogenous N-acyl taurines regulate skin wound healing. *Proceedings of the National Academy of Sciences of the United States of America*, *113*(30), E4397–E4406. http://dx.doi.org/10.1073/pnas.1605578113.
Schmid, P. C., Kuwae, T., Krebsbach, R. J., & Schmid, H. H. (1997). Anandamide and other N-acylethanolamines in mouse peritoneal macrophages. *Chemistry and Physics of Lipids*, *87*(2), 103–110. http://dx.doi.org/10.1016/S0009-3084(97)00032-7 [pii].
Schmid, P. C., Schwartz, K. D., Smith, C. N., Krebsbach, R. J., Berdyshev, E. V., & Schmid, H. H. (2000). A sensitive endocannabinoid assay. The simultaneous analysis of N-acylethanolamines and 2-monoacylglycerols. *Chemistry and Physics of Lipids*, *104*(2), 185–191. http://dx.doi.org/10.1016/S0009-3084(99)00124-3 [pii].
Schreiber, D., Harlfinger, S., Nolden, B. M., Gerth, C. W., Jaehde, U., Schomig, E., et al. (2007). Determination of anandamide and other fatty acyl ethanolamides in human serum by electrospray tandem mass spectrometry. *Analytical Biochemistry*, *361*(2), 162–168. http://dx.doi.org/10.1016/j.ab.2006.11.027.
Sergi, M., Battista, N., Montesano, C., Curini, R., Maccarrone, M., & Compagnone, D. (2013). Determination of the two major endocannabinoids in human plasma by mu-SPE followed by HPLC-MS/MS. *Analytical and Bioanalytical Chemistry*, *405*(2-3), 785–793. http://dx.doi.org/10.1007/s00216-012-6273-3.
Silvestri, C., Paris, D., Martella, A., Melck, D., Guadagnino, I., Cawthorne, M., et al. (2015). Two non-psychoactive cannabinoids reduce intracellular lipid levels and inhibit hepatosteatosis. *Journal of Hepatology*, *62*(6), 1382–1390. http://dx.doi.org/10.1016/j.jhep.2015.01.001.
Smoum, R., Bar, A., Tan, B., Milman, G., Attar-Namdar, M., Ofek, O., et al. (2010). Oleoyl serine, an endogenous N-acyl amide, modulates bone remodeling and mass. *Proceedings of the National Academy of Sciences of the United States of America*, *107*(41), 17710–17715. http://dx.doi.org/10.1073/pnas.0912479107.
Starowicz, K., Cristino, L., & Di Marzo, V. (2008). TRPV1 receptors in the central nervous system: Potential for previously unforeseen therapeutic applications. *Current Pharmaceutical Design*, *14*(1), 42–54.
Stock, K., Kumar, J., Synowitz, M., Petrosino, S., Imperatore, R., Smith, E. S., et al. (2012). Neural precursor cells induce cell death of high-grade astrocytomas through stimulation of TRPV1. *Nature Medicine*, *18*(8), 1232–1238. http://dx.doi.org/10.1038/nm.2827.

Stuart, J. M., Paris, J. J., Frye, C., & Bradshaw, H. B. (2013). Brain levels of prostaglandins, endocannabinoids, and related lipids are affected by mating strategies. *International Journal of Endocrinology*, *2013*, 436252. http://dx.doi.org/10.1155/2013/436252.

Sugiura, T., Kondo, S., Sukagawa, A., Nakane, S., Shinoda, A., Itoh, K., et al. (1995). 2-Arachidonoylglycerol: A possible endogenous cannabinoid receptor ligand in brain. *Biochemical and Biophysical Research Communications*, *215*(1), 89–97. http://dx.doi.org/10.1006/bbrc.1995.2437 [pii].

Tan, B., O'Dell, D. K., Yu, Y. W., Monn, M. F., Hughes, H. V., Burstein, S., et al. (2010). Identification of endogenous acyl amino acids based on a targeted lipidomics approach. *Journal of Lipid Research*, *51*(1), 112–119. http://dx.doi.org/10.1194/jlr.M900198-JLR200.

Tan, B., Yu, Y. W., Monn, M. F., Hughes, H. V., O'Dell, D. K., & Walker, J. M. (2009). Targeted lipidomics approach for endogenous N-acyl amino acids in rat brain tissue. *Journal of Chromatography. B, Analytical Technologies in the Biomedical and Life Sciences*, *877*(26), 2890–2894. http://dx.doi.org/10.1016/j.jchromb.2009.01.002.

Tortoriello, G., Rhodes, B. P., Takacs, S. M., Stuart, J. M., Basnet, A., Raboune, S., et al. (2013). Targeted lipidomics in Drosophila melanogaster identifies novel 2-monoacylglycerols and N-acyl amides. *PLoS One*, *8*(7). e67865. http://dx.doi.org/10.1371/journal.pone.0067865.

Turman, M. V., Kingsley, P. J., Rouzer, C. A., Cravatt, B. F., & Marnett, L. J. (2008). Oxidative metabolism of a fatty acid amide hydrolase-regulated lipid, arachidonoyltaurine. *Biochemistry*, *47*(12), 3917–3925. http://dx.doi.org/10.1021/bi702530z.

Ueda, N., Yamamoto, K., Yamamoto, S., Tokunaga, T., Shirakawa, E., Shinkai, H., et al. (1995). Lipoxygenase-catalyzed oxygenation of arachidonylethanolamide, a cannabinoid receptor agonist. *Biochimica et Biophysica Acta*, *1254*(2), 127–134.

Verhoeckx, K. C., Voortman, T., Balvers, M. G., Hendriks, H. F., Wortelboer, H. M., & Witkamp, R. F. (2011). Presence, formation and putative biological activities of N-acyl serotonins, a novel class of fatty-acid derived mediators, in the intestinal tract. *Biochimica et Biophysica Acta*, *1811*(10), 578–586. http://dx.doi.org/10.1016/j.bbalip.2011.07.008.

Vogeser, M., Hauer, D., Christina Azad, S., Huber, E., Storr, M., & Schelling, G. (2006). Release of anandamide from blood cells. *Clinical Chemistry and Laboratory Medicine*, *44*(4), 488–491. http://dx.doi.org/10.1515/CCLM.2006.065.

Williams, J., Wood, J., Pandarinathan, L., Karanian, D. A., Bahr, B. A., Vouros, P., et al. (2007). Quantitative method for the profiling of the endocannabinoid metabolome by LC-atmospheric pressure chemical ionization-MS. *Analytical Chemistry*, *79*(15), 5582–5593. http://dx.doi.org/10.1021/ac0624086.

Willoughby, K. A., Moore, S. F., Martin, B. R., & Ellis, E. F. (1997). The biodisposition and metabolism of anandamide in mice. *The Journal of Pharmacology and Experimental Therapeutics*, *282*(1), 243–247.

Wolfson, M. L., Correa, F., Leishman, E., Vercelli, C., Cymeryng, C., Blanco, J., et al. (2015). Lipopolysaccharide-induced murine embryonic resorption involves changes in endocannabinoid profiling and alters progesterone secretion and inflammatory response by a CB1-mediated fashion. *Molecular and Cellular Endocrinology*, *411*, 214–222. http://dx.doi.org/10.1016/j.mce.2015.04.032.

Wood, J. T., Williams, J. S., Pandarinathan, L., Courville, A., Keplinger, M. R., Janero, D. R., et al. (2008). Comprehensive profiling of the human circulating endocannabinoid metabolome: Clinical sampling and sample storage parameters. *Clinical Chemistry and Laboratory Medicine*, *46*(9), 1289–1295. http://dx.doi.org/10.1515/CCLM.2008.242.

Woodward, D. F., Carling, R. W., Cornell, C. L., Fliri, H. G., Martos, J. L., Pettit, S. N., et al. (2008). The pharmacology and therapeutic relevance of endocannabinoid derived cyclo-oxygenase (COX)-2 products. *Pharmacology & Therapeutics*, *120*(1), 71–80. http://dx.doi.org/10.1016/j.pharmthera.2008.08.001.

Yang, H. Y., Karoum, F., Felder, C., Badger, H., Wang, T. C., & Markey, S. P. (1999). GC/MS analysis of anandamide and quantification of N-arachidonoylphosphatidylethanolamides in various brain regions, spinal cord, testis, and spleen of the rat. *Journal of Neurochemistry*, *72*(5), 1959–1968.

Yore, M. M., Syed, I., Moraes-Vieira, P. M., Zhang, T., Herman, M. A., Homan, E. A., et al. (2014). Discovery of a class of endogenous mammalian lipids with anti-diabetic and anti-inflammatory effects. *Cell*, *159*(2), 318–332. http://dx.doi.org/10.1016/j.cell.2014.09.035.

Yu, M., Ives, D., & Ramesha, C. S. (1997). Synthesis of prostaglandin E2 ethanolamide from anandamide by cyclooxygenase-2. *The Journal of Biological Chemistry*, *272*(34), 21181–21186.

Zamberletti, E., Piscitelli, F., De Castro, V., Murru, E., Gabaglio, M., Colucci, P., et al. (2017). Lifelong imbalanced linoleic/alpha-linolenic acid intake impairs emotional and cognitive behavior in adult rats via changes in brain endocannabinoid system. *Journal of Lipid Research*, *58*, 301–316. http://dx.doi.org/10.1194/jlr.M068387.

Zoerner, A. A., Batkai, S., Suchy, M. T., Gutzki, F. M., Engeli, S., Jordan, J., et al. (2012). Simultaneous UPLC-MS/MS quantification of the endocannabinoids 2-arachidonoyl glycerol (2AG), 1-arachidonoyl glycerol (1AG), and anandamide in human plasma: Minimization of matrix-effects, 2AG/1AG isomerization and degradation by toluene solvent extraction. *Journal of Chromatography. B, Analytical Technologies in the Biomedical and Life Sciences*, *883-884*, 161–171. http://dx.doi.org/10.1016/j.jchromb.2011.06.025.

Zoerner, A. A., Gutzki, F. M., Batkai, S., May, M., Rakers, C., Engeli, S., et al. (2011). Quantification of endocannabinoids in biological systems by chromatography and mass spectrometry: A comprehensive review from an analytical and biological perspective. *Biochimica et Biophysica Acta*, *1811*(11), 706–723. http://dx.doi.org/10.1016/j.bbalip.2011.08.004.

Zoerner, A. A., Gutzki, F. M., Suchy, M. T., Beckmann, B., Engeli, S., Jordan, J., et al. (2009). Targeted stable-isotope dilution GC-MS/MS analysis of the endocannabinoid anandamide and other fatty acid ethanol amides in human plasma. *Journal of Chromatography. B, Analytical Technologies in the Biomedical and Life Sciences*, 877(26), 2909–2923. http://dx.doi.org/10.1016/j.jchromb.2009.04.016.

Zygmunt, P. M., Ermund, A., Movahed, P., Andersson, D. A., Simonsen, C., Jonsson, B. A., et al. (2013). Monoacylglycerols activate TRPV1—A link between phospholipase C and TRPV1. *PLoS One*, *8*(12). e81618. http://dx.doi.org/10.1371/journal.pone.0081618.

Zygmunt, P. M., Julius, I., Di Marzo, I., & Hogestatt, E. D. (2000). Anandamide—The other side of the coin. *Trends in Pharmacological Sciences*, *21*(2), 43–44.

CHAPTER TWO

Endocannabinoid Turnover

Christopher J. Fowler*, Patrick Doherty†, Stephen P.H. Alexander‡,1
*Umeå University, Umeå, Sweden
†Wolfson Centre for Age-Related Disease, King's College London, London, United Kingdom
‡Life Sciences, University of Nottingham Medical School, Nottingham, United Kingdom
[1]Corresponding author: e-mail address: steve.alexander@nottingham.ac.uk

Contents

Abstract

In this review, we consider the biosynthetic, hydrolytic, and oxidative metabolism of the endocannabinoids anandamide and 2-arachidonoylglycerol. We describe the enzymes associated with these events and their characterization. We identify the inhibitor profile for these enzymes and the status of therapeutic exploitation, which to date has been limited to clinical trials for fatty acid amide hydrolase inhibitors. To bring the review to a close, we consider whether point block of a single enzyme is likely to be the most successful approach for therapeutic exploitation of the endocannabinoid system.

Advances in Pharmacology, Volume 80
ISSN 1054-3589
http://dx.doi.org/10.1016/bs.apha.2017.03.006

ABBREVIATIONS

2-AG 2-arachidonoylglycerol
AA arachidonic acid
ABHD6 αβ hydrolase 6
AEA anandamide, *N*-arachidonoylethanolamine
COX cyclooxygenase
CYP cytochrome P450
DAG diacylglycerol
DAGL diacylglycerol lipase
FAAH fatty acid amide hydrolase
FABP fatty acid-binding protein
LOX lipoxygenase
MAGL monoacylglycerol lipase
NAAA *N*-acylethanolamine acid amidase
NAE *N*-acylethanolamine
NAPE *N*-acylphosphatidylethanolamine
NAPE-PLD *N*-acylphosphatidylethanolamine phospholipase D
OEA *N*-oleoylethanolamine
PEA *N*-palmitoylethanolamine
PG prostaglandin
PLA phospholipase A

1. INTRODUCTION

In this report, we assess the principle routes by which the endocannabinoids anandamide and 2-arachidonoylglycerol (2-AG) are produced in biological systems, and their hydrolysis and biotransformation.

Anandamide (AEA, *N*-arachidonoylethanolamine) and 2-arachidonoyl-*sn*-glycerol (2-AG) are arachidonic acid derivatives which are synthesized and hydrolyzed by independent, parallel pathways (Fig. 1). However, a feature they share with arachidonic acid is the possibility of biotransformation, via oxidative metabolism (Fig. 1). We review the enzymes responsible for endocannabinoid turnover, as well as the potential for therapeutic exploitation.

2. BIOSYNTHESIS OF AEA AND RELATED *N*-ACYLETHANOLAMINE

The synthesis of AEA and *N*-acylethanolamines (NAEs) has been well reviewed elsewhere (Ueda, Tsuboi, & Uyama, 2013) and so will be dealt with briefly here. The pioneering work on NAE synthesis was undertaken by Harald Schmid, Patricia Schmid, and colleagues who delineated the key steps.

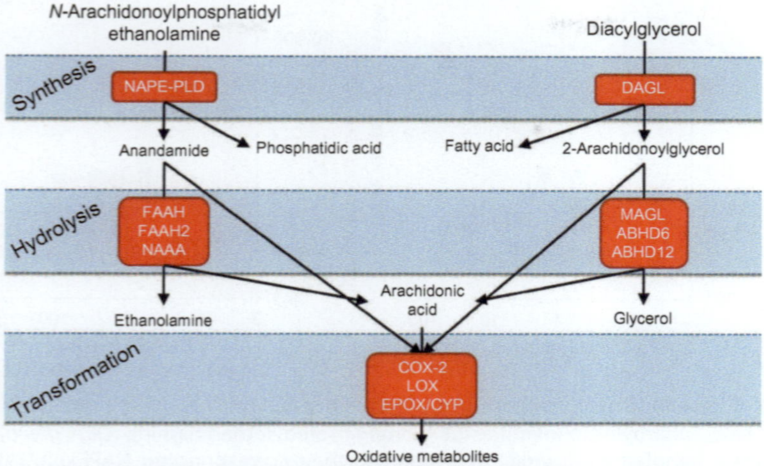

Fig. 1 Parallel and convergent pathways of endocannabinoid metabolism. The graphic illustrates three phases of endocannabinoid turnover: synthesis, hydrolysis, and transformation. For clarity, a number of alternative, apparently minor pathways of endocannabinoid metabolism are not shown.

The first step is the transacylation of membrane phosphatidylethanolamine-containing phospholipids to form *N*-acylphosphatidylethanolamines (NAPEs) by a calcium-dependent *N*-acyltransferase (Natarajan, Reddy, Schmid, & Schmid, 1982; Natarajan, Schmid, Reddy, Zuzarte-Augustin, & Schmid, 1983) that has recently been identified as the cytosolic enzyme PLA2G4E (Ogura, Parsons, Kamat, & Cravatt, 2016). Calcium-independent formation of NAPEs from phospholipids is catalyzed by a family of phospholipase A/acyltransferase (PLA/AT) enzymes, where PLA/AT 1, 2, and 5 have greater *N*-acyltransferase activity than phospholipase 1/2 activity (Uyama et al., 2012). NAPEs are thereafter metabolized to the corresponding NAEs by a variety of pathways, including hydrolysis catalyzed by NAPE-hydrolyzing phospholipase D (Schmid, Reddy, Natarajan, & Schmid, 1983); production and subsequent dephosphorylation of NAE phosphates (Liu et al., 2006; Okamoto, Morishita, Tsuboi, Tonai, & Ueda, 2004); and production and hydrolysis of lyso-NAPE (Sun et al., 2004). Finally, NAEs can be produced from *N*-acylethanolamine plasmalogen (by both *N*-acylphosphatidylethanolamine phospholipase D (NAPE-PLD)-dependent and -independent pathways (Rahman et al., 2016; Tsuboi et al., 2011). Consistent with this multiplicity of pathways, genetic deletion of NAPE-PLD reduces, but does not remove completely, NAE levels in the brain (Leishman, Mackie, Luquet, & Bradshaw, 2016; Leung, Saghatelian,

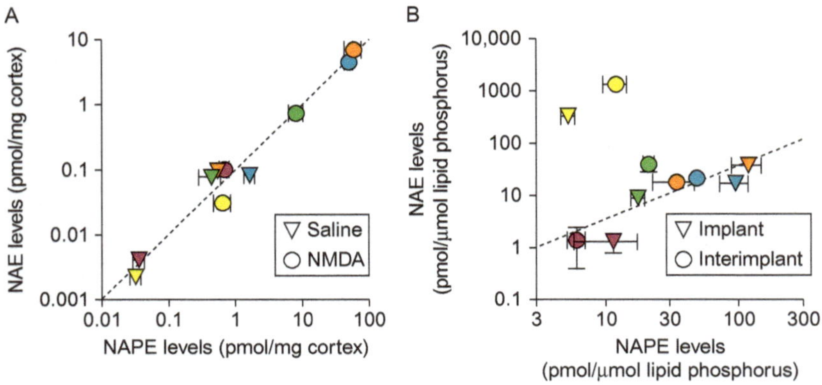

Fig. 2 Regulation of NAE synthesis. (A and B) Levels of AEA (*yellow*), palmitoylethanolamide (PEA, *blue*), stearoylethanolamide (SEA, *orange*), oleoylethanolamide (OEA, *green*), and linoleoylethanolamide (*purple*) in relation to their corresponding NAPEs. In (A), the values (means ± SEM, when not enclosed by the symbols, $N = 3$–6) are for cerebral cortices from rat pups 24 h after intrastriatal injection of either saline or 25 nmol of NMDA and are drawn from the data of Hansen, Ikonomidou, et al. (2001) and Hansen, Schmid, et al. (2001). The regression line was calculated from the mean logged values and has a slope of 0.99 ± 0.06. In panel B, the values (means ± SD, $N = 3$) are for uterine implantation and interimplantation sites for female mice on pregnancy day 7 and are drawn from the data of Schmid et al. (1997). The regression line, calculated from the mean logged values for all NAEs except the two AEA values, has a slope of 1.04 ± 0.34. The highest mean value of AEA (1345 pmol/μmol lipid phosphorous) corresponds to 20 pmol/mg tissue.

Simon, & Cravatt, 2006; Tsuboi et al., 2011). The situation is further complicated by the finding that NAPE-PLD can be allosterically modulated by bile acids (Margheritis et al., 2016; Schmid et al., 1983).

Given the central position of NAPE as a precursor to NAE, it would be expected that the levels of the NAE species match those of NAPE and of the membrane phospholipids. In the brain, this is the case. As an example, data from Hansen and colleagues (Hansen, Ikonomidou, Bittigau, Hansen, & Hansen, 2001; Hansen, Schmid, et al., 2001) investigating levels of these lipids in young rat cerebral cortex are shown in Fig. 2. There is a very good correlation between the levels of the NAPE and corresponding NAE species, with a large increase in both following intrastriatal injection of the glutamatergic excitotoxin *N*-methyl-D-aspartate (NMDA). In all cases, the NAE levels are ~10% of the corresponding NAPE levels. However, there are no rules without exception (a rule in itself!) and the exception in this case is the uterus, where endocannabinoids play a key role in reproductive

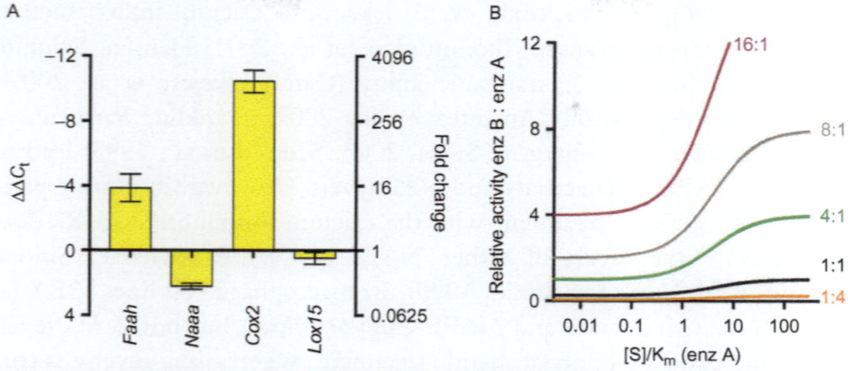

Fig. 3 Relative expression of the AEA catabolic enzymes: regulation and consequences. (A) Changes in the mRNA expression of *Faah*, *Naaa*, *Cox2*, and *Lox15* in RAW264.7 cells following 24h incubation with lipopolysaccharide and interferon-γ. The data are shown as mean ±95% bootstrapped percentile confidence limits of the difference in the ΔC_t values between untreated and treated cells, $N = 7$–16. A $\Delta\Delta C_t$ of x corresponds to a 2^{-x}-fold change, and this is shown on the *right axis*. The bootstrapped percentile confidence limits of the difference were calculated using 100,000 iterations with the package Hmisc for the R computer programme. Panel B shows the relative activities for two enzymes A and B at different relative concentrations (shown as enz B: enz A in the figure) of the two enzymes, calculated assuming both enzymes have the same k_{cat}, while the K_m for enzyme A is four times lower than that for enzyme B. To our knowledge, such kinetic constants for FAAH and COX-2 have not been presented where the enzymes have been assayed under the same conditions (i.e., pH, presence or absence of detergent, etc.). The family of curves demonstrates that the metabolic pathway of the substrate, i.e., via enzyme A or B, clearly depends on the ambient concentration and relative expression of the enzymes. *Drawn from data recalculated from the study of Gabrielsson et al. (2017).*

behavior (review, see Paria, Wang, & Dey, 2002). In this case, the NAEs other than AEA are again roughly 10% of the corresponding NAPE levels, whereas AEA levels are much higher than expected (Fig. 3).

A second observation relates to the calcium sensitivity of PLA2G4E (Ogura et al., 2016) and of NAPE-PLD (Okamoto et al., 2004). Such calcium sensitivity presents an obvious regulation point, whereby extracellular events leading to an increased intracellular calcium will stimulate NAE synthesis. Indeed, NAPE synthesis in cultured cortical neurons is increased following treatment with the calcium ionophore ionomycin in a manner potentiated by treatments increasing cyclic AMP levels in the cells (forskolin, vasoactive intestinal peptide) (Cadas, Gaillet, Beltramo, Venance, &

Piomelli, 1996). In vivo, toxic events leading to calcium influx, such as NMDA treatment (Hansen, Ikonomidou, et al., 2001; Hansen, Schmid, et al., 2001) (see Fig. 2), traumatic injury (Garcia-Ovejero et al., 2009), and oxygen deprivation (Amantea et al., 2007; Franklin, Parmentier-Batteur, Walter, Greenberg, & Stella, 2003; Schmid et al., 1995) lead to increased NAPE-PLD activity and NAE levels. However, in murine peritoneal macrophages, treatment with the calcium ionophore A23187 does not increase the levels of either NAEs or NAPEs (Kuwae, Shiota, Schmid, Krebsbach, & Schmid, 1999). In macrophage cell lines, AEA (as well as *N*-acyltransferase and NAPE-PLD activities) but not 2-AG levels can be increased by lipolysaccharide treatment, whereas the reverse is true when platelet-activating factor is used as a stimulus (Berdyshev, Schmid, Krebsbach, & Schmid, 2001; Liu et al., 2003). This is compounded by different expression levels of the AEA and 2-AG synthetic enzymes in different cells. A nice example of this comes from the work of Freund, Katona, and colleagues who demonstrated that NAPE-PLD is located presynaptically in hippocampal glutamatergic axon terminals (Nyilas et al., 2008), in contrast to the synthetic machinery for 2-AG. Clearly, AEA/NAE and 2-AG syntheses are regulated differentially in a cell- and stimulus-dependent manner.

3. DIACYLGLYCEROL LIPASE-DEPENDENT SYNTHESIS OF 2-AG

2-AG was the second putative endocannabinoid to be identified a few years after AEA, acting as a full agonist at CB_1 and CB_2 receptors (Mechoulam et al., 1995; Sugiura et al., 1995). Interestingly, prior to this, 2-AG was largely studied as an intermediate in a two-step pathway that releases arachidonic acid (AA) from diacylglycerol (DAG) in platelets and other cells. For example, thrombin treatment of human platelets was postulated to stimulate the generation of DAG by a phospholipase C (PLC), followed by the sequential hydrolysis of DAG by a diacylglycerol lipase (DAGL) acting at the *sn*-1 position to generate 2-AG, and a monoacylglycerol lipase (MAGL) acting at the *sn*-2 position to liberate AA (Bell, Kennerly, Stanford, & Majerus, 1979; Prescott & Majerus, 1983). Subsequently other groups went on to confirm the release of AA through a DAGL/MAGL pathway in platelet-derived growth factor-stimulated Swiss 3T3 cells (Hasegawa-Sasaki, 1985) and in dorsal root ganglion neurons (Allen, Gammon, Ousley, McCarthy, & Morell, 1992). Remarkably, the above pathway for AA synthesis is conspicuous by its absence from some sections of the mainstream literature based on the continuing dogma that AA levels are largely governed by phospholipase A_2 (PLA_2) activity (Bazinet & Laye, 2014). We will discuss recent experiments that have provided unequivocal evidence for DAGL regulating the level of AA in the nervous system and some other tissues, and confirm the importance of DAGL activity for 2-AG biosynthesis and endocannabinoid signaling throughout the nervous system.

The first reported biochemical purification of a DAGL was in 1984 (Farooqui, Taylor, & Horrocks, 1984); the authors identified a ~27-kDa enzyme that was not directly activated by calcium, but subsequently reported to be phosphorylated and activated by cAMP-dependent protein kinase (Rosenberger, Farooqui, & Horrocks, 2007). However, it was a bioinformatics strategy that resulted in the cloning and characterization of the first specific DAGLs (Bisogno et al., 2003). A single enzyme is present in lower species such as *Drosophila* and nematodes, but a gene duplication event has resulted in the presence of two very closely related enzymes, namely DAGLα and DAGLβ, in vertebrates and other species. These enzymes are not obviously related to the above 27 kDa DAGL, as both have an N-terminal four transmembrane domains followed an intracellular canonical α/β hydrolase domain resulting in a molecular mass of 70–125 kDa. The presence of a C-terminal tail (~300 amino acids) in DAGLα is the main distinguishing feature between itself and DAGLβ. The transmembrane domain and the C-terminal tail are not required for enzyme activity (Singh et al., 2016) and most likely regulate trafficking and compartmentalization of the enzymes within polarized cells (Reisenberg, Singh, Williams, & Doherty, 2012). Functional evidence suggests differential expression of the two enzymes in the CNS, with DAGLα being present in isolated neurones and DAGLβ expressed in microglia (Viader et al., 2016). The catalytic activity of both enzymes has been characterized in detail; they are *sn*-1 specific DAGLs that can make and release 2-AG from cells in response to calcium stimulation (Bisogno et al., 2003). Interestingly, although the enzymes selectively act at the *sn*-1 position, they show little preference for substrates with differing lipid groups at the *sn*-2 position which can include arachidonic, oleic, linoleic, and stearic acid, suggesting that they can synthesize a range of monoacylglycerols. This makes sense of their expression in species such as *Drosophila* that do not synthesize AA; here, the enzymes are more likely to synthesize lipids such as 2-linoleoyl glycerol (Tortoriello et al., 2013).

4. 2-AG, AA, AND AEA LEVELS IN DAGL KNOCKOUT MICE

The contribution that the cloned DAGLs make to the biosynthesis of 2-AG, and the requirement of this for endocannabinoid signaling, has been directly addressed by the generation of independent lines of knockout mice. Given the importance of endocannabinoid function for behavior, we largely focus our attention on endocannabinoid levels in the adult brain and on the requirement of the cloned DAGLs for synaptic function. Other DAGL-dependent functions, including roles in axonal growth and guidance in the developing brain and the regulation of neurogenesis in the postnatal brain, have recently been reviewed elsewhere (Maccarrone, Guzman, Mackie, Doherty, & Harkany, 2014; Oudin, Hobbs, & Doherty, 2011).

Expression will dictate function and in the first cloning paper DAGLα transcripts were reported to be enriched in the nervous system with protein expression seen at relatively high levels in neuronal dendrites that appose CB_1 positive synaptic terminals (Bisogno et al., 2003). However, DAGLα and DAGLβ are present in neural stem cells in the adult brain (Goncalves et al., 2008) and more recent RNA-sequencing experiments on isolated cell types from the mouse cerebral cortex clearly show DAGLα transcripts to be present in astrocytes, neurons, oligodendrocyte precursor cells, and microglia (Zhang et al., 2014). In contrast, the same database shows that DAGLβ transcripts are found almost exclusively in microglia. Thus, DAGLα is well placed to regulate the 2-AG levels in several cell types in the brain, with DAGLβ perhaps contributing alongside DAGLα in a more restricted manner within neural stem cells and microglia, the "resident macrophages" within the brain.

At the level of the whole brain and spinal cord 75%–80% reductions in 2-AG levels have been observed in DAGLα knockout mice, with ~50% reductions seen in adipose tissue and liver (Gao et al., 2010). Similar reductions of ~80% (or more) have been reported in cerebellum, hippocampus, striatum, whole cortex, prefrontal cortex, and amygdala in three additional DAGLα knockout lines (Jenniches et al., 2016; Shonesy et al., 2014; Tanimura et al., 2010), with a complete loss of stimulus generated 2-AG (Tanimura et al., 2010) and no difference between the sexes (Shonesy et al., 2014). The one anomaly appears to be the forebrain where significant, but less dramatic decreases have been reported (Shonesy et al., 2014). Overall, these data indicate that DAGLα is responsible for maintaining nearly all the basal 2-AG in the nervous system, as well as being required for stimulus induced increases.

Nonetheless, residual 2-AG is found in the nervous system of DAGLα knockout mice implicating DAGLβ and/or other enzymes in the biosynthesis of this lipid. 2-AG levels were variable but not significantly different in the cerebellum, hippocampus, and striatum of one line of DAGLβ knockout mice (Tanimura et al., 2010). However, a 50% decrease in 2-AG at the level of the whole brain has been reported in an independent DAGLβ knockout line (Gao et al., 2010). Thus, it would appear that DAGLα is primarily responsible for the biosynthesis of 2-AG in the brain, but DAGLβ can make a contribution, possibly within a restricted set of cell types (see earlier for details).

As discussed earlier, DAGL activity was first studied in the context of a DAGL/MAGL pathway that generates AA in cells yet much of the mainstream literature remains focused on the notion that the bulk and signaling pools of AA are governed by the activities of the PLA_2 family of enzymes (Bazinet & Laye, 2014). In this context, it was a major surprise to see parallel reductions in AA and 2-AG levels in the brains of DAGLα knockout mice. For example, in the brain and spinal cord, there are 75%–80% reductions in AA in DAGLα knockout mice (Gao et al., 2010). Similar dramatic reductions in AA are seen in the forebrain, prefrontal cortex, amygdala, and striatum in independent lines of DAGLα knockout animals (Jenniches et al., 2016; Shonesy et al., 2014; Tanimura et al., 2010). It follows that the DAGLα/MAGL pathway is responsible for the biosynthesis of most of the 2-AG and AA throughout the brain. Importantly, this pathway also appears to provide the signaling pool of AA that is mobilized to generate eicosanoids in the brain, with up to 80% reductions in the inflammatory prostaglandins PGD_2 and PGE_2 seen in DAGLα knockout mice (Ogasawara et al., 2016). Inhibition of the eicosanoid pathway at the level of MAGL dramatically reduces much of the neurodegeneration seen in animal models of Alzheimer's and Parkinson's disease (Nomura et al., 2011; Piro et al., 2012), with inhibition at the level of DAGL impairing lipopolysaccharide-induced anapyrexia (Ogasawara et al., 2016). Thus it is clear that the DAGL/MAGL pathway can generate prostaglandins that promote neuroinflammation in the brain. Interestingly, in the periphery evidence from knockout and pharmacological studies also show that DAGLβ regulates proinflammatory responses by regulating 2-AG, AA, and eicosanoid levels in a manner that is distinct but complementary with cytosolic PLA_2 (Hsu et al., 2012).

A perhaps even more surprising observation made in the DAGLα knockout mice studies was a reduction in the level of AEA in the brain. In this context, there is a significant 40%–50% reduction of AEA in the whole brain of DAGLα knockout mice (Gao et al., 2010; Ogasawara et al., 2016). The reason for this unexpected cross-talk between the biosynthesis of the two major endocannabinoids does not appear to involve an obviously straightforward biosynthetic pathway (Di Marzo, 2011), but it is clearly a robust finding and on that basis it can be concluded that DAGLα is the key enzyme in a simple pathway that generates the bulk of the 2-AG and AA found in the brain, but it can also contribute in a more complex manner to the steady-state levels of AEA levels in some brain regions. We do not, as yet, know the consequence of knocking out DAGLα and DAGLβ on 2-AG levels in the brain, and it remains possible that a small pool of 2-AG (perhaps 10%–20% of the total) might be maintained by a different biosynthetic pathway. In this context, an enzyme previously characterized as a phospholipase A_1 (and termed DDHD2) has recently been purified from the brain and cloned based on exhibiting DAGL activity with evidence obtained that it can contribute to bulk 2-AG levels following overexpression in CHO cells (Araki et al., 2016). The importance of this enzyme in regulating the bulk levels or stimulus induced signaling pools of 2-AG in cells and tissues remains to be determined.

5. PHARMACOLOGICAL INHIBITION OF THE DAGLs MIMICS THE KNOCKOUT RESULTS

Genetic approaches to study enzyme function need to be interpreted with some caution given that the relatively long-term loss of function in one pathway can lead to alterations in other pathways with these secondary changes influencing the measured endpoints. On the other hand, whereas pharmacological approaches have the advantage of temporal resolution, they can be limited by drug availability and selectivity; for review, see Janssen and van der Stelt (2016). In the case of the DAGLs, the historical pharmacological studies have largely relied on the use of RHC80267 and/or tetrahydrolipstatin (THL), but results obtained with them have sometimes been contentious as although they can inhibit DAGL activity they also inhibit other serine lipases and can show poor tissue penetration (Hoover, Blankman, Niessen, & Cravatt, 2008; Janssen et al., 2015). A set of centrally active DAGL inhibitors has recently been developed that, when used with appropriate controls, has allowed for the analysis of the effects of acute inhibition of DAGL activity on lipid networks in the brain (Ogasawara et al.,

2016). These 1,2,3-triazole urea-based drugs are highly selective across the discernible family of α/β domain serine hydrolases, but show limited selectivity between DAGLα and DAGLβ. Within 2 h administration to animals, these novel inhibitors (DH376 and DO34) fully mimic the reductions in 2-AG (>80%), AA (>80%), and AEA (~50%) measured in parallel studies on DAGLα knockout mice. Concomitant increases in the level of the 2-AG precursor 1-stearoyl-2-arachidonyl-*sn*-glycerol were also seen in the drug treated and knockout animals. Importantly, the levels of the prostaglandins PGD_2 and PGE_2 were also rapidly reduced by ~80% following pharmacological block of DAGL activity, as were the LPS induced increases in these prostaglandins and inflammatory cytokines demonstrating the importance of the DAGLα/MAGL pathway for the rapid generation of inflammatory mediators in the brain. LEI105 represents a distinct chemical class of reversible DAGL-selective inhibitors, based on α-ketoheterocycles (Baggelaar et al., 2015). The use of this compound in electrophysiological experiments reinforced the role of DAGL in short-term plasticity of synaptic activity in the hippocampus.

6. DAGL-DEPENDENT ENDOCANNABINOID SIGNALING REGULATES SYNAPTIC FUNCTION

The above genetic and pharmacological studies have established that DAGLα plays a central role in regulating 2-AG, AA, and prostaglandin synthesis in the brain and other tissues. However, they do not directly address the role of DAGLα or DAGLβ in endocannabinoid signaling pathways. 2-AG has a short half-life (Jarai et al., 2000) and a relatively low affinity for the CB_1/CB_2 receptors (Sugiura & Waku, 2000); thus, it is reasonable to assume that "on-demand" physiological endocannabinoid signaling via the DAGLs will require their close proximity to the cannabinoid receptors.

It has long been recognized that AEA and/or 2-AG serve as retrograde synaptic messengers throughout the nervous system (Alger, 2012). DAGLα is well placed to be the key enzyme in this pathway as its expression in neurons is restricted to dendrites in the adult brain (Bisogno et al., 2003) with high-resolution imaging studies showing enrichment in all postsynaptic sites that juxtapose CB_1-positive synaptic terminals (Katona et al., 2006; Uchigashima et al., 2007; Yoshida et al., 2006, 2011). Live-cell imaging has recently shown DAGLα to be localized to an endosomal compartment that can shuttle the enzyme to and from the surface of the dendritic spine in dynamic manner (Zhou et al., 2016). It follows that 2-AG might be made within endosomes possibly providing a regulated vesicular release mechanism to be considered alongside the current model that posits passive diffusion from the cell membrane. 2-AG mobilization at synapses is established to be triggered by excitatory neurotransmitters (glutamate, acetylcholine, dopamine) acting on their respective postsynaptic receptors and involves a G-protein- and/or calcium-stimulated synthesis of substrate by a PLCβ, however there also appears to be an additional calcium-dependent step operating independently of substrate synthesis (Ohno-Shosaku & Kano, 2014). One possibility is that calcium (and other signals) might stimulate phosphorylation and opening of a regulatory lid on DAGLα to facilitate substrate access to the catalytic site (Reisenberg et al., 2012).

Depolarization-induced suppression of inhibition or excitation (DSI/DSE) is perhaps the best-characterized endocannabinoid function in the adult brain (Ohno-Shosaku & Kano, 2014). Numerous studies on DAGLα knockout mice have identified it as the pivotal enzyme controlling this phasic form of synaptic plasticity throughout the nervous system (Gao et al., 2010; Tanimura et al., 2010; Yoshino et al., 2011). In contrast, there is little if any effect of knocking out DAGLβ on this almost ubiquitous form of synaptic plasticity (Gao et al., 2010; Tanimura et al., 2010). It is now clear that DAGLα generates the signaling pool of 2-AG that acts on presynaptic CB_1 receptors to dampen the release of excitatory and inhibitory neurotransmitters to regulate phasic and tonic forms of synaptic plasticity (Lee et al., 2015; Ramikie et al., 2014; Younts & Castillo, 2014). This in turn impacts on a myriad of fundamental behaviors including appetite, pain, and cognition (Alger & Kim, 2011). Indeed, it is noteworthy that DAGLα and CB_1 receptor KO mice share the same disrupted phenotypes (Powell et al., 2015) implicating 2-AG as the "workhorse" endocannabinoid in the nervous system. The adverse psychiatric consequences of inhibiting CB_1 function in humans revealed in clinical trials for obesity with a CB_1 antagonist (Moreira & Crippa, 2009) are also likely to be consequential to the disruption of 2-AG signaling at synapses as DAGLα KO mice have been used to demonstrate a causative link between synaptic endocannabinoid signaling and anxiety and depressive behaviors (Jenniches et al., 2016; Shonesy et al., 2014). In addition, dysfunction of tonic 2-AG signaling appears to play a key and possible reversible role in autism (Anderson et al., 2015; Busquets-Garcia et al., 2013; Foldy, Malenka, & Sudhof, 2013; Jung et al., 2012; Kerr, Downey, Conboy, Finn, & Roche, 2013). Importantly, pharmacological modulation of 2-AG signaling is being investigated as a treatment for major disorders including depression, pain, obesity, and neurodegeneration (Kohnz & Nomura, 2014).

7. RELEASE AND REUPTAKE OF ENDOCANNABINOIDS

The mechanism(s) by which endocannabinoids are released from cells and subsequently cleared from the extracellular space have been a matter of controversy, the key question being whether or not there exists an as yet unidentified plasma membrane transporter for these lipids (for reviews of the data from proponents and opponents, respectively, of the concept of a plasma endocannabinoid membrane transporter, see Fowler, 2013; Nicolussi & Gertsch, 2015). It is possible that certain cell types may utilize proteins like pannexin-1 for the release of endocannabinoids (Hill, Bialecki, Wellinger, & Thompson, 2015), but more data are needed. What is clear is that endocannabinoids (and NAEs) can be cleared from the extracellular space, and that there are intracellular proteins with other primary functions that can shuttle these lipids, once they have crossed the plasma membrane, to their intracellular locations, be it the TRPV1 receptor (for AEA), PPARα (for palmitoylethanolamide, PEA), or their catabolic enzymes (Kaczocha, Glaser, & Deutsch, 2009; Oddi et al., 2009).

The best characterized of these shuttling proteins with respect to endocannabinoids are fatty acid-binding proteins, FAPB5 and 7. Crystallographic studies have indicated that AEA binds, albeit with a lower affinity than arachidonic acid, to FABP5 with its lipophilic chain forming a loop in the substrate-binding pocket of this protein and with hydrogen bonding between the hydroxyl groups of the ethanolamine to a Tyr^{131} residue. The interaction of FABP5 with 2-AG is largely similar, albeit with looser hydrophobic contacts and more hydrogen bonding (Sanson et al., 2014). Pharmacological inhibition of FABP5/7 reduces uptake of AEA into wild-type HeLa cells and by other FABP5-expressing cell types, but does not inhibit AEA uptake by FABP5 shRNA-expressing HeLa cells (Berger et al., 2012; Bjorklund, Blomqvist, Hedlin, Persson, & Fowler, 2014). Mice-lacking FABP5 and 7 show increased brain levels of AEA, PEA, and *N*-oleoylethanolamide (OEA), but not 2-AG (Kaczocha et al., 2015). A fatty acid amide hydrolase (FAAH)-like transporter protein, derived from processing of the FAAH gene, has also been proposed as an intracellular carrier protein, but its existence has been disputed (Fu et al., 2012; Leung, Elmes, Glaser, Deutsch, & Kaczocha, 2013).

8. ENZYMATIC HYDROLYSIS OF AEA AND RELATED NAEs

The enzymes responsible for the hydrolysis of AEA and related NAEs to their respective long-chain fatty acids are FAAH and *N*-acylethanolamine-hydrolyzing acid amidase (NAAA). FAAH is a membrane-bound homodimer belonging to the serine hydrolase family of enzymes and with a wide substrate selectivity including *N*-acylethanolamines, *N*-acylamides, and *N*-acyltaurines (Bachur & Udenfriend, 1966; Boger et al., 2000; Deutsch & Chin, 1993; McKinney & Cravatt, 2006; Schmid et al., 1995). Molecular dynamics and crystallographic studies have indicated that the substrate enters the active site via a membrane access channel, where a triad of residues (Ser^{241}, Ser^{217}, and Lys^{142}) are necessary for hydrolysis to occur, and where additional residues (Phe^{432} and Trp^{531}) may act as a "dynamic paddle" to ensure correct substrate orientation and localization (Bracey, Hanson, Masuda, Stevens, & Cravatt, 2002; Mileni et al., 2008; Palermo et al., 2015). In the hippocampus, FAAH has a postsynaptic location, consistent with an orthograde release of AEA synthesized presynaptically by NAPE-PLD and in contrast to the retrograde release of 2-AG (Gulyas et al., 2004; Nyilas et al., 2008).

In mammals, but not rodents, a second FAAH (FAAH-2) has been found, with a preferential localization within lipid rafts rather than the endoplasmic reticulum (the location of FAAH) (Kaczocha, Glaser, Chae, Brown, & Deutsch, 2010; Wei, Mikkelsen, McKinney, Lander, & Cravatt, 2006). The two FAAH species have different relative hydrolysis rates for substrates. Thus at pH 9 (in the region of the pH optimum for both FAAH enzymes), the rate of hydrolysis of 100 μM AEA, OEA, PEA, and *N*-oleoyltaurine, respectively, relative to that of oleamide was 1.75, 0.58, 0.22, and 0.77 for human FAAH transfected into COS-7 cells, and 0.055, 0.23, 0.024, and not detected for *N*-terminal FLAG-tagged FAAH-2 transfected into these cells (Wei et al., 2006). The sensitivity of the two enzymes to inhibition is also different, with FAAH-2 being more sensitive than FAAH(-1) to inhibition by the carbamate inhibitor URB597 and the α-ketoheterocycle OL-135, while the reverse is true for the piperazinyl phenyl urea compound JNJ-1661010 and the isoflavone biochanin A (Karbarz et al., 2009; Thors, Burston, et al., 2010; Wei et al., 2006) (Table 1).

In addition to FAAH, NAEs are hydrolyzed by NAAA, an enzyme with a pH optimum around pH 5, and with a preference for the unsaturated substrates over the saturated substrates (PEA > myristoylethanolamide > stearoylethanolamide (SEA) ≃ OEA > linoleoylethanolamide > AEA

Table 1 Pharmacological Tools Used to Investigate Endocannabinoid Turnover

Compound	Comment
DH376	A selective DAGL inhibitor
DO34	A selective DAGL inhibitor
JJKK048	A potent, selective MAGL inhibitor
JNJ-1661010	An irreversible inhibitor with a modest selectivity for FAAH-2
JZL184	A selective MAGL inhibitor, with reduced potency at the rat enzyme compared to human and mouse
KT185	An orally active inhibitor of ABHD6
LEI015	An orally active, reversible DAGL inhibitor
MAFP	A nonselective irreversible inhibitor of many endocannabinoid-metabolizing enzymes, including FAAH, MAGL, ABHD6, and ABHD12
OL-135	A reversible inhibitor with a modest selectivity for FAAH compared to FAAH-2
RHC80267	A DAGL inhibitor, which fails to inhibit ABHD12
Tetrahydrolipstatin	A DAGL inhibitor, which also inhibits ABHD12 and pancreatic lipase
URB597	An irreversible inhibitor with a modest selectivity for FAAH compared to FAAH-2
WWL123	An ABHD6 inhibitor
WWL70	An ABHD6 inhibitor

For further information and the appropriate citations, please refer to the text.

(Ueda, Yamanaka, & Yamamoto, 2001). The enzyme has its highest distribution in the lung where it is localized to the lysosomes of macrophages (Tsuboi et al., 2007; Ueda et al., 2001). NAAA is a glycoprotein with sequence homology to acid ceramidase rather than FAAH (Tsuboi et al., 2005).

9. ENZYMATIC HYDROLYSIS OF 2-AG AND RELATED MONOACYLGLYCEROLS

Multiple enzyme activities have been identified to be capable of hydrolyzing 2-AG in vitro, including MAGL (Dinh, Carpenter, Leslie, et al., 2002), ABHD2 (Miller et al., 2016), αβ hydrolase 6

(ABHD6) (Blankman, Simon, & Cravatt, 2007; Navia-Paldanius, Savinainen, & Laitinen, 2012), ABHD12 (Navia-Paldanius et al., 2012), neuropathy target esterase (van Tienhoven, Atkins, Li, & Glynn, 2002), and carboxylesterase 1 (Xie et al., 2010). However, it is clear that MAGL performs the bulk of 2-AG hydrolysis in most tissues given the impact of gene disruption on 2-AG levels (Pan et al., 2011; Zhong et al., 2011). In addition, a functional, activity-based protein profiling approach using mouse brain membranes indicated that MAGL accounted for the majority of 2-AG hydrolysis (~85%), while ABHD6 and ABHD12 accounted for the remainder (Blankman et al., 2007). Despite this predominance of MAGL, it is quite likely that some of these enzymes have influential roles on 2-AG turnover, albeit in niche locations, both at tissue and cellular levels.

Aside from a common substrate, many of these enzymes have a common structure in that they are α/β hydrolases. These are a large family of enzymes characterized by a primary sequence motif known as an α/β hydrolase fold domain—an extended organization of α-helices and β-sheets—where the most recognizable family member is acetylcholinesterase (Thomas, Brown, & Brown, 2014). This family also includes the diacylglycerol lipases (DAGLα and β), epoxide hydrolases, and lipoprotein and endothelial lipases.

MAGL. MAGL is a 303-aa protein (~33 kDa) serine hydrolase, with a characteristic triad of a charge relay of Asp^{239}-His^{269} around the catalytic nucleophile Ser^{122}. There are no identifiable transmembrane (TM) domains, but the enzyme is found associated with both cytosolic and particulate compartments (Ghafouri et al., 2004). In adipose tissue, MAGL performs the final step in lipolysis, hydrolyzing monoacylglycerols to produce free fatty acid and glycerol; this role was identified over 30 years before a role in endocannabinoid turnover was suggested (Vaughan, Berger, & Steinberg, 1964). In some tissues, such as the brain, it appears that MAGL-evoked arachidonic acid is the predominant route for prostaglandin production (Nomura et al., 2011 and above). MAGL shows hydrolytic preference for 2-AG, but not AEA (Dinh, Carpenter, Leslie, et al., 2002; Dinh, Freund, & Piomelli, 2002), but with little specificity between acylglycerols (Ghafouri et al., 2004; Vandevoorde et al., 2005).

ABHD2. The *ABHD2* gene encodes a 425-aa protein (~48 kDa) serine hydrolase (Ser^{207}-Asp^{345}-His^{376}). A single TM is predicted at 10–30, with an extracellular catalytic domain. Glycosylation is predicted at Asn^{136} and Asn^{410}, while a single nucleotide polymorphism has been described (Arg^{253}Gln). ABHD2 was initially cloned as one of three α/β-hydrolases from mouse lung (Edgar & Polak, 2002). The mRNA was expressed in mouse brain, heart, kidney, liver, lungs, skeletal muscle, and spleen, but was highest in testes (Edgar & Polak, 2002). Gene trap analysis in mice suggested an expression in smooth muscle (vascular and nonvascular), but not skeletal muscle (Miyata et al., 2005). The mice-lacking *abhd2* appeared to have normal vasculature, but explants were more proliferative and cuff placement resulted in greater intimal hyperplasia. A number of links with potential therapeutic indications have been reported, for example, in unstable angina (Miyata et al., 2008), hepatitis B virus propagation (Ding, Yang, Sun, Lou, & Wang, 2008), age-related pulmonary emphysema (Jin et al., 2009), ovarian (Yamanoi et al., 2016), and prostate cancer (Obinata et al., 2016). ABHD2 is reported to have progesterone-dependent MAGL activity and to be inhibited by MAFP (Miller et al., 2016). In addition, ABHD2 appears to be able to hydrolyze triacylglycerols (Naresh Kumar et al., 2016).

ABHD6. ABHD6 is a 337-aa protein (~38 kDa) serine hydrolase (Ser^{148}-Asp^{278}-His^{306}). A single TM is predicted at Phe^{9}-Leu^{29}, with an intracellular catalytic domain. ABHD6 is a monoacylglycerol hydrolase (Navia-Paldanius et al., 2012), with little selectivity for 1- compared to 2-acylglycerols (Thomas et al., 2013), and possibly bis(monoacylglycerol) phosphate hydrolase (Pribasnig et al., 2015). Antisense knockdown of ABHD6 led to accumulation of numerous phospholipids and lysophospholipids in mouse liver implying a role in glycerophospholipid turnover in the liver (Thomas et al., 2013). ABHD6 has been implicated in diabetes/metabolic disorder (Zhao et al., 2016, 2015), inflammation (Alhouayek, Masquelier, Cani, Lambert, & Muccioli, 2013), and epilepsy (Naydenov et al., 2014).

ABHD12. ABHD12 is a 398-aa protein (~45 kDa) serine hydrolase (Ser^{246}-Asp^{333}-His^{372}). A single TM is predicted at 75–95, with an extracellular catalytic domain. ABHD12 is a monoacylglycerol hydrolase (Navia-Paldanius et al., 2012), but may also regulate lysophosphatidylserine levels (Kamat et al., 2015). Loss-of-function mutations in ABHD12 are associated with a disorder known as PHARC (polyneuropathy, hearing loss, ataxia, retinitis pigmentosa, and cataracts) (Fiskerstrand et al., 2010).

10. PHARMACOLOGICAL INHIBITORS OF MONOACYLGLYCEROL HYDROLASE ACTIVITIES

There is a tantalizing indication for potential therapeutic exploitation of these enzymes, but the realization of this potential is absolutely dependent on the provision of new information on the distribution of these enzymes and the identification of their "natural" substrates. In addition, generation of cheap, reproducible high-throughput screening assays will facilitate novel drug discovery to allow future pharmacological investigation, thereby enhancing an understanding of the role/s of these enzymes in pathological circumstances, leading ultimately to their therapeutic exploitation.

MAGL inhibitors. For MAGL activity, a number of useful tools are commercially available. JZL184 is a relatively selective (certainly compared to FAAH) irreversible MAGL inhibitor with a pIC_{50} value of 8.1–8.4 (Chang et al., 2012; Long et al., 2009) in human and mouse. JZL184 is slightly less potent against rat MAGL, with a pIC_{50} value of 6.5–7.1 (Woodhams et al., 2012). In a separate study, a similar discrepancy between mouse and rat potency of JZL184 was also noted, although with slightly lower potencies (Aaltonen et al., 2013). It's likely that these lab-to-lab differences reflect the irreversible nature of the inhibitor, where conditions such as substrate concentration, pH, protein content, and (probably most influential) preincubation period are major sources of variation.

JJKK048 is even more potent and selective as a MAGL inhibitor, with a subnanomolar potency (pIC_{50} value of 9.4–9.7), with essentially equivalent potency at mouse, rat, or human enzymes (Aaltonen et al., 2013). Although substantially less potent (pIC_{50} 6.6), Compound 21 (Hernandez-Torres et al., 2014) represents a reversible MAGL inhibitor, which is active in vivo.

The use of JZL184 in vivo produced effects similar to those obtained using THC or synthetic CB_1 cannabinoid agonists (Long et al., 2009), indicating that there may be psychoactive limiting factors for therapeutic application of MAGL inhibitors. Despite this, there are reports of anxiolysis (Sciolino, Zhou, & Hohmann, 2011), reduction in pain behaviors (Aaltonen et al., 2016; Woodhams et al., 2012), and nausea-like behaviors (Sticht et al., 2012), as well as neuroprotection in a model of Parkinson's disease (Fernandez-Suarez et al., 2014).

ABHD6 inhibitors. WWL70 was the first described selective ABHD6 inhibitor; screening mouse brain membranes using the activity-based protein profiling system generated a pIC_{50} value of ~7.2 (Li, Blankman, & Cravatt, 2007). From the same group, WWL123 is a similarly structured inhibitor with a slightly less potent profile (Bachovchin et al., 2010). In addition, KT185 has been described as an orally active ABHD6-selective inhibitor (Hsu et al., 2013).

In vivo administration of WWL70 was neuroprotective in a mouse model of traumatic brain injury (Tchantchou & Zhang, 2013), and also alleviated symptoms in a model of multiple sclerosis in a manner dependent on

CB_2 cannabinoid receptors (Wen, Ribeiro, Tanaka, & Zhang, 2015). WWL70 also protected mice from the weight gain associated with a high-fat diet (Thomas et al., 2013), in a manner consistent with the involvement of the nuclear hormone receptors PPARs (Zhao et al., 2016; see chapter "The role of nuclear hormone receptors in cannabinoid function" by O'Sullivan and Pistis, this volume). WWL123 has also been shown to be effective in vivo, by reducing seizures in an epilepsy model (Naydenov et al., 2014).

ABHD12 inhibitors. Currently, there is no selective inhibitor that targets ABHD12. However, it is possible to use a process of elimination to identify involvement of ABHD12 in monoacylglycerol hydrolase activity. Thus, ABHD12 is relatively insensitive to the MAGL inhibitors JZL184 or JJKK-048, the ABHD6 inhibitor WWL70 or the DAGL inhibitor RHC80267, but may be inhibited by the nonselective serine hydrolase inhibitor MAFP and THL (more widely known as an inhibitor of DAGL, see earlier, and pancreatic lipase) (Blankman et al., 2007).

11. OXIDATIVE METABOLISM OF ENDOCANNABINOIDS

Given that AEA and 2-AG have an arachidonoyl side-chain, it is not surprising that they share some of the metabolic pathways of arachidonic acid, or that many of the products of these pathways have been shown to have biological actions of their own. The main enzymes involved are summarized below. Aficionados of chemical structures are referred to Urquhart, Nicolaou, and Woodward (2015), where these catabolic pathways are well illustrated.

Cyclooxygenase (COX)-2 pathway. Both AEA and 2-AG are metabolized by COX-2, but not by COX-1 (due to a narrower active site), to yield prostaglandin ethanolamides (PG-EAs) and prostaglandin glyceryl esters (PG-GEs), respectively (Kozak, Rowlinson, & Marnett, 2000; Yu, Ives, & Ramesha, 1997). COX-2 acts as a functional heterodimer, whereby allosteric binding to one site affects the catalytic activity at the other, and crystallographic studies of COX-2 have indicated that 1-AG binds slightly differently to the two sites (Mitchener et al., 2015; Vecchio & Malkowski, 2011). $PGF_{2\alpha}$-EA formation from AEA proceeds via the PGF-EA synthase catalyzed reduction of PGH_2-EA (Moriuchi et al., 2008; Yang, Ni, Woodward, Tang-Liu, & Ling, 2005) and produces its biological effects, including an increased firing of spinal cord nociceptive neurons, as a result of an interaction with a heterodimeric receptor that is not responsive to $PGF_{2\alpha}$ (Gatta et al., 2012; Woodward, Wang, & Poloso, 2013). Most of the work on the properties of PG-GEs have been undertaken using the more stable 1,3-regioisomers, but a picture is emerging whereby both PG-EA and PG-GE compounds can affect inflammation, with both pro- and antiinflammatory effects being reported (review, see Alhouayek & Muccioli, 2014). The stable PG-EA analogue bimatoprost is clinically used for the treatment of glaucoma (see Woodward et al., 2013). Relatively little is known about the metabolism of PG-EAs, but a major metabolic pathway for PG-GEs is hydrolysis to PG catalyzed by several enzymes, lysophospholipase A_2 playing a major role in this respect (Manna et al., 2014).

Lipoxygenase (LOX) pathways. Less work has been undertaken on lipoxygenase (LOX)-catalyzed hydroperoxidation of the endocannabinoids, but both AEA and 2-AG are substrates of 12- and 15-LOX to produce products that are biologically active either at CB receptors or at peroxisome proliferator-active receptor α (Edgemond, Hillard, Falck, Kearn, & Campbell, 1998; Hampson et al., 1995; Kozak et al., 2002; Moody, Kozak, Ji, & Marnett, 2001; Ueda et al., 1995; van der Stelt et al., 2002). In addition, the 15-LOX product of AEA can be metabolized by glutathione transferases to form cysteinyl-containing metabolites ("eoxamides," in analogy with the eoxins produced from arachidonic acid) (Forsell, Brunnstrom, Johannesson, & Claesson, 2012). The biological properties of the eoxamides are not known.

CYP450 pathways. In 1995, Bornheim and colleagues reported that the incubation of AEA with liver microsomes in the presence of NADPH resulted in the production of several compounds, the levels of which could be induced following pretreatment of the mice with CYP450 enzyme inducers (Bornheim, Kim, Chen, & Correia, 1995). Subsequent work mainly by Hollenberg and colleagues have identified CYP3A4-, CYP2D6-, CYP4F2-, and CYP2J2-derived AEA metabolites, and shown that the 5,6-epoxide metabolite of AEA is a reasonably potent and selective CB_2 receptor agonist (McDougle, Kambalyal, Meling, & Das, 2014; Snider, Kornilov, Kent, & Hollenberg, 2007; Snider, Nast, Tesmer, & Hollenberg, 2009; Snider et al., 2008; Walker, Griffin, Hammar, & Hollenberg, 2016). CYP-derived metabolites of 2-AG with activity toward CB receptors have also been described (Chen et al., 2008; McDougle et al., 2014).

12. INTEGRATING THE CATABOLISM OF THE ENDOCANNABINOIDS AND RELATED NAEs IN HEALTH AND DISEASE

From the above, it is clear that there are a multiplicity of synthetic and degradative pathways for the endocannabinoids. At first sight, this would suggest that a "point block" (i.e., a selective inhibition or genetic deletion of one of the metabolic enzymes) would be expected to have a limited effect (since the endocannabinoid would merely find another metabolic route), unless the enzyme in question was predominant. Indeed, under extreme conditions (such as genetic deletion), additional metabolic pathways in addition to those described earlier may come into play (Mulder & Cravatt, 2006). As pointed out previously, deletion of NAPE-PLD reduces, but does not completely block, AEA production in the brain (Leishman et al., 2016; Leung et al., 2006; Tsuboi et al., 2011). In this section, the effects of point blocks of the catabolic enzyme FAAH are considered.

Early studies using FAAH inhibitors and FAAH$^{-/-}$ mice demonstrated that, providing enzyme activity was sufficiently inhibited, brain levels of AEA were dramatically increased (Cravatt et al., 2001; Kathuria et al., 2003). This is not a universal finding: in lipopolysaccharide + interferon-γ-activated macrophages, for example, hydrolysis of exogenous AEA is totally blocked by the FAAH inhibitor URB597, but the endogenous levels of AEA are, at best, only modestly affected (Gouveia-Figueira et al., 2015). Studies investigating the effects of FAAH inhibition and/or genetic deletion on AEA and related NAE levels either in different brain regions or in different parts of the body have been undertaken, but these tend to suffer from statistical issues such as small sample sizes, lack of consideration of unequal variances between groups and, not least, lack of compensation for multiple significance testing. This does not impact upon the large-scale changes reported, but more modest changes may be either over-interpreted or missed completely.

An alternative approach is to look at the organism as a whole. In a study from 2014, a three compartment model (brain, plasma, and rest of body) was used to simulate the changes over time in plasma AEA, PEA, OEA, and linoleoyl ethanolamide levels in humans treated with the FAAH inhibitor PF-04457845. They could simulate the observed data well, but only if the model included an FAAH-independent clearance (Benson et al., 2014). The authors suggested that NAAA may be a suitable candidate for this additional clearance, on the basis that PEA was also encompassed by this finding. Certainly, inhibition of NAAA increases PEA and OEA levels in mouse lungs (Ribeiro et al., 2015), but it is unclear as to whether the more limited organ distribution of this enzyme is sufficient to explain the data.

This somewhat complex system becomes even more convoluted when patients with diseases potentially tractable to treatment with inhibitors of AEA/NAE hydrolysis are considered, such as patients with pain and inflammation (for review for FAAH and pain, see Fowler, 2015; for inflammation and NAAA, see Alhouayek et al., 2015; Solorzano et al., 2009, for examples in experimental animals). In this case, the situation is complicated by the presence and influence of cytokines and other factors that can dramatically affect the relative expression of the catabolic enzymes. Thus, in addition to a large induction in COX-2 activity, cytokines like the interleukins IL-4 and IL-10 increase FAAH activity, while IL-12 and interferon-γ reduce it (Maccarrone, Valensise, et al., 2001; Thors, Bergh, et al., 2010). In unstimulated RAW264.7 macrophages, the mRNA expression of NAAA is about 160-fold higher than that of FAAH. However, upon activation with 24 h of treatment with lipopolysaccharide + interferon-γ, NAAA mRNA is reduced fivefold, while FAAH mRNA is increased fourfold (Gabrielsson, Gouveia-Figueira, Häggström, Alhouayek, & Fowler, 2017) (see Fig. 3). While these changes are less than the 1400-fold induction of COX-2 in the cells, the treatment clearly changes the balance of AEA catabolic enzymes in the cells. Further, changes are likely to be cell specific: in lymphocytes, for example, lipopolysaccharide reduces rather than increases FAAH expression (Maccarrone, De Petrocellis, et al., 2001). Such changes in the relative expression of the catabolic enzymes may provide an explanation for the loss of effect of the FAAH inhibitor URB597 toward increasing hindpaw AEA, OEA, and 2-AG levels in rats with neuropathic pain following spinal nerve ligation (Jhaveri, Richardson, Kendall, Barrett, & Chapman, 2006). This phenomenon could be a contributing factor to the failure in clinical trials of the FAAH inhibitor PF-04457845 in osteoarthritis (Huggins, Smart, Langman, Taylor, & Young, 2012) and of the "peripherally active" FAAH inhibitor ASP3652 in chronic prostatitis/chronic pelvic pain syndrome (Wagenlehner et al., 2017), although it is to be noted for the latter that there was improvement in micturition outcomes. In the osteoarthritis trial using PF-04457845, blood plasma AEA levels were maintained at increased levels by drug treatment; clearly, however, levels at the therapeutically relevant locations are unknown (see the systems biology approach of Benson et al. (2014) addressed earlier). Modeling changes in levels of AEA and other relevant metabolites is by no means easy, but a simple model can be constructed from the known K_m and k_{cat} values for FAAH and COX-2 for given AEA concentrations in the vicinity of the enzymes (Fig. 3). Add to this (a) the ability of endogenous lipids such as cholesterol, phosphatidylcholine, dihydrolipoic acid, and AEA-derived LOX metabolites to influence the activity of FAAH and/or NAAA (Dainese et al., 2014; Tai et al., 2012; van der Stelt et al., 2002) and (b) differences in CYP3A4, 2BC, and 2D6 polymorphisms with respect to their ability to metabolize AEA (Pratt-Hyatt, Zhang, Snider, & Hollenberg, 2010; Sridar, Snider, & Hollenberg, 2011) and it becomes clear that the potential for differences in catabolism of endocannabinoids between cells, organs, individuals, and between healthy volunteers and patients, become considerable.

The aim of this review was to discuss the turnover of endocannabinoids rather than the pharmacology of the system, but it is clear from the above discussion that "point block" may not be optimal in cases where alternative catabolic pathways are present. An interesting alternative is the design of compounds attacking more than one catabolic pathway. One possibility is to target both COX-2 and FAAH. Two approaches have been taken: one is to start from the modest FAAH inhibitory potency of COX inhibitors such as ibuprofen and flurbiprofen, and to optimize the former without compromising the latter. This has led to the identification of (*R*)-2-(2-fluorobiphenyl-4-yl)-*N*-(3-methylpyridin-2-yl)propanamide, a mixed-type reversible inhibitor of FAAH and substrate-selective inhibitor of COX-2 (Gouveia-Figueira et al., 2015; Karlsson et al., 2015). An alternative approach is to link a COX inhibitor (flurbiprofen) to a carbamate FAAH inhibitor with a chemical bridge (Migliore et al., 2016; Sasso et al., 2015). It will be interesting to see whether such compounds prove to be useful in conditions where both COX-2 and FAAH play central roles in AEA catabolism.

13. CONCLUSION

There is an attractive complexity associated with the network of enzymes involved in the synthesis, hydrolysis, and transformation of endocannabinoids. The various genetic models and pharmacological tools are beginning to allow dissection of the patho/physiological roles of these enzymes, which paves the way for future exploitation in a clinical environment.

CONFLICT OF INTEREST

The authors have no conflict of interest to relate.

ACKNOWLEDGMENTS

C.J.F. thanks the Swedish Science Research council (Grant no. 12158) and the Research Funds of the Medical Faculty, Umeå University for research support.

REFERENCES

Aaltonen, N., Kedzierska, E., Orzelska-Gorka, J., Lehtonen, M., Navia-Paldanius, D., Jakupovic, H., et al. (2016). In vivo characterization of the ultrapotent monoacylglycerol lipase inhibitor {4-[bis-(benzo[d][1,3]dioxol-5-yl)methyl]-piperidin-1-yl}(1H-1,2,4-triazol-1-yl)m ethanone (JJKK-048). *The Journal of Pharmacology and Experimental Therapeutics*, *359*, 62–72.

Aaltonen, N., Savinainen, J. R., Ribas, C. R., Ronkko, J., Kuusisto, A., Korhonen, J., et al. (2013). Piperazine and piperidine triazole ureas as ultrapotent and highly selective inhibitors of monoacylglycerol lipase. *Chemistry & Biology*, *20*, 379–390.

Alger, B. E. (2012). Endocannabinoids at the synapse a decade after the dies mirabilis (29 March 2001): What we still do not know. *The Journal of Physiology*, *590*, 2203–2212.

Alger, B. E., & Kim, J. (2011). Supply and demand for endocannabinoids. *Trends in Neurosciences*, *34*, 304–315.

Alhouayek, M., Bottemanne, P., Subramanian, K. V., Lambert, D. M., Makriyannis, A., Cani, P. D., et al. (2015). N-Acylethanolamine-hydrolyzing acid amidase inhibition increases colon N-palmitoylethanolamine levels and counteracts murine colitis. *The FASEB Journal*, *29*, 650–661.

Alhouayek, M., Masquelier, J., Cani, P. D., Lambert, D. M., & Muccioli, G. G. (2013). Implication of the anti-inflammatory bioactive lipid prostaglandin D2-glycerol ester in the control of macrophage activation and inflammation by ABHD6. *Proceedings of the National Academy of Sciences of the United States of America*, *110*, 17558–17563.

Alhouayek, M., & Muccioli, G. G. (2014). COX-2-derived endocannabinoid metabolites as novel inflammatory mediators. *Trends in Pharmacological Sciences*, *35*, 284–292.

Allen, A. C., Gammon, C. M., Ousley, A. H., McCarthy, K. D., & Morell, P. (1992). Bradykinin stimulates arachidonic acid release through the sequential actions of an sn-1 diacylglycerol lipase and a monoacylglycerol lipase. *Journal of Neurochemistry*, *58*, 1130–1139.

Amantea, D., Spagnuolo, P., Bari, M., Fezza, F., Mazzei, C., Tassorelli, C., et al. (2007). Modulation of the endocannabinoid system by focal brain ischemia in the rat is involved in neuroprotection afforded by 17 β-estradiol. *The FEBS Journal*, *274*, 4464–4475.

Anderson, G. R., Aoto, J., Tabuchi, K., Foldy, C., Covy, J., Yee, A. X., et al. (2015). β-Neurexins control neural circuits by regulating synaptic endocannabinoid signaling. *Cell*, *162*, 593–606.

Araki, M., Ohshima, N., Aso, C., Konishi, A., Obinata, H., Tatei, K., et al. (2016). Enzymatic characterization of recombinant rat DDHD2: A soluble diacylglycerol lipase. *Journal of Biochemistry*, *160*, 269–279.

Bachovchin, D. A., Ji, T., Li, W., Simon, G. M., Blankman, J. L., Adibekian, A., et al. (2010). Superfamily-wide portrait of serine hydrolase inhibition achieved by library-versus-library screening. *Proceedings of the National Academy of Sciences of the United States of America*, *107*, 20941–20946.

Bachur, N. R., & Udenfriend, S. (1966). Microsomal synthesis of fatty acid amides. *The Journal of Biological Chemistry*, *241*, 1308–1313.

Baggelaar, M. P., Chameau, P. J., Kantae, V., Hummel, J., Hsu, K. L., Janssen, F., et al. (2015). Highly selective, reversible inhibitor identified by comparative chemoproteomics modulates diacylglycerol lipase activity in neurons. *Journal of the American Chemical Society*, *137*, 8851–8857.

Bazinet, R. P., & Laye, S. (2014). Polyunsaturated fatty acids and their metabolites in brain function and disease. *Nature Reviews. Neuroscience*, *15*, 771–785.

Bell, R. L., Kennerly, D. A., Stanford, N., & Majerus, P. W. (1979). Diglyceride lipase: A pathway for arachidonate release from human platelets. *Proceedings of the National Academy of Sciences of the United States of America*, *76*, 3238–3241.

Benson, N., Metelkin, E., Demin, O., Li, G. L., Nichols, D., & van der Graaf, P. H. (2014). A systems pharmacology perspective on the clinical development of fatty acid amide hydrolase inhibitors for pain. *CPT Pharmacometrics & System Pharmacology*, *3*, e91.

Berdyshev, E. V., Schmid, P. C., Krebsbach, R. J., & Schmid, H. H. (2001). Activation of PAF receptors results in enhanced synthesis of 2-arachidonoylglycerol (2-AG) in immune cells. *The FASEB Journal*, *15*, 2171–2178.

Berger, W. T., Ralph, B. P., Kaczocha, M., Sun, J., Balius, T. E., Rizzo, R. C., et al. (2012). Targeting fatty acid binding protein (FABP) anandamide transporters—A novel strategy for development of anti-inflammatory and anti-nociceptive drugs. *PloS One*, *7*, e50968.

Bisogno, T., Howell, F., Williams, G., Minassi, A., Cascio, M. G., Ligresti, A., et al. (2003). Cloning of the first sn1-DAG lipases points to the spatial and temporal regulation of endocannabinoid signaling in the brain. *The Journal of Cell Biology*, *163*, 463–468.

Bjorklund, E., Blomqvist, A., Hedlin, J., Persson, E., & Fowler, C. J. (2014). Involvement of fatty acid amide hydrolase and fatty acid binding protein 5 in the uptake of anandamide by cell lines with different levels of fatty acid amide hydrolase expression: A pharmacological study. *PloS One*, *9*, e103479.

Blankman, J. L., Simon, G. M., & Cravatt, B. F. (2007). A comprehensive profile of brain enzymes that hydrolyze the endocannabinoid 2-arachidonoylglycerol. *Chemistry & Biology*, *14*, 1347–1356.

Boger, D. L., Fecik, R. A., Patterson, J. E., Miyauchi, H., Patricelli, M. P., & Cravatt, B. F. (2000). Fatty acid amide hydrolase substrate specificity. *Bioorganic & Medicinal Chemistry Letters*, *10*, 2613–2616.

Bornheim, L. M., Kim, K. Y., Chen, B. L., & Correia, M. A. (1995). Microsomal cytochrome P450-mediated liver and brain anandamide metabolism. *Biochemical Pharmacology*, *50*, 677–686.

Bracey, M. H., Hanson, M. A., Masuda, K. R., Stevens, R. C., & Cravatt, B. F. (2002). Structural adaptations in a membrane enzyme that terminates endocannabinoid signaling. *Science*, *298*, 1793–1796.

Busquets-Garcia, A., Gomis-Gonzalez, M., Guegan, T., Agustin-Pavon, C., Pastor, A., Mato, S., et al. (2013). Targeting the endocannabinoid system in the treatment of fragile X syndrome. *Nature Medicine*, *19*, 603–607.

Cadas, H., Gaillet, S., Beltramo, M., Venance, L., & Piomelli, D. (1996). Biosynthesis of an endogenous cannabinoid precursor in neurons and its control by calcium and cAMP. *The Journal of Neuroscience*, *16*, 3934–3942.

Chang, J. W., Niphakis, M. J., Lum, K. M., Cognetta, A. B., III, Wang, C., Matthews, M. L., et al. (2012). Highly selective inhibitors of monoacylglycerol lipase bearing a reactive group that is bioisosteric with endocannabinoid substrates. *Chemistry & Biology*, *19*, 579–588.

Chen, J. K., Chen, J., Imig, J. D., Wei, S., Hachey, D. L., Guthi, J. S., et al. (2008). Identification of novel endogenous cytochrome P450 arachidonate metabolites with high affinity for cannabinoid receptors. *The Journal of Biological Chemistry*, *283*, 24514–24524.

Cravatt, B. F., Demarest, K., Patricelli, M. P., Bracey, M. H., Giang, D. K., Martin, B. R., et al. (2001). Supersensitivity to anandamide and enhanced endogenous cannabinoid signaling in mice lacking fatty acid amide hydrolase. *Proceedings of the National Academy of Sciences of the United States of America*, *98*, 8971–9371.

Dainese, E., De Fabritiis, G., Sabatucci, A., Oddi, S., Angelucci, C. B., Di Pancrazio, C., et al. (2014). Membrane lipids are key modulators of the endocannabinoid-hydrolase FAAH. *The Biochemical Journal*, *457*, 463–472.

Deutsch, D. G., & Chin, S. A. (1993). Enzymatic synthesis and degradation of anandamide, a cannabinoid receptor agonist. *Biochemical Pharmacology*, *46*, 791–796.

Di Marzo, V. (2011). Endocannabinoid signaling in the brain: Biosynthetic mechanisms in the limelight. *Nature Neuroscience*, *14*, 9–15.

Ding, X. R., Yang, J., Sun, D. C., Lou, S. K., & Wang, S. Q. (2008). Whole genome expression profiling of hepatitis B virus-transfected cell line reveals the potential targets of anti-HBV drugs. *The Pharmacogenomics Journal, 8*, 61–70.

Dinh, T. P., Carpenter, D., Leslie, F. M., Freund, T. F., Katona, I., Sensi, S. L., et al. (2002a). Brain monoglyceride lipase participating in endocannabinoid inactivation. *Proceedings of the National Academy of Sciences of the United States of America, 99*, 10819–10824.

Dinh, T. P., Freund, T. F., & Piomelli, D. (2002b). A role for monoglyceride lipase in 2-arachidonoylglycerol inactivation. *Chemistry and Physics of Lipids, 121*, 149–158.

Edgar, A. J., & Polak, J. M. (2002). Cloning and tissue distribution of three murine α/β hydrolase fold protein cDNAs. *Biochemical and Biophysical Research Communications, 292*, 617–625.

Edgemond, W. S., Hillard, C. J., Falck, J. R., Kearn, C. S., & Campbell, W. B. (1998). Human platelets and polymorphonuclear leukocytes synthesize oxygenated derivatives of arachidonylethanolamide (anandamide): Their affinities for cannabinoid receptors and pathways of inactivation. *Molecular Pharmacology, 54*, 180–188.

Farooqui, A. A., Taylor, W. A., & Horrocks, L. A. (1984). Separation of bovine brain mono- and diacylglycerol lipases by heparin sepharose affinity chromatography. *Biochemical and Biophysical Research Communications, 122*, 1241–1246.

Fernandez-Suarez, D., Celorrio, M., Riezu-Boj, J. I., Ugarte, A., Pacheco, R., Gonzalez, H., et al. (2014). The monoacylglycerol lipase inhibitor JZL184 is neuroprotective and alters glial cell phenotype in the chronic MPTP mouse model. *Neurobiology of Aging, 35*, 2603–2616.

Fiskerstrand, T., H'mida-Ben Brahim, D., Johansson, S., M'zahem, A., Haukanes, B. I., Drouot, N., et al. (2010). Mutations in ABHD12 cause the neurodegenerative disease PHARC: An inborn error of endocannabinoid metabolism. *American Journal of Human Genetics, 87*, 410–417.

Foldy, C., Malenka, R. C., & Sudhof, T. C. (2013). Autism-associated neuroligin-3 mutations commonly disrupt tonic endocannabinoid signaling. *Neuron, 78*, 498–509.

Forsell, P. K., Brunnstrom, A., Johannesson, M., & Claesson, H. E. (2012). Metabolism of anandamide into eoxamides by 15-lipoxygenase-1 and glutathione transferases. *Lipids, 47*, 781–791.

Fowler, C. J. (2013). Transport of endocannabinoids across the plasma membrane and within the cell. *The FEBS Journal, 280*, 1895–1904.

Fowler, C. J. (2015). The potential of inhibitors of endocannabinoid metabolism for drug development: A critical review. *Handbook of Experimental Pharmacology, 231*, 95–128.

Franklin, A., Parmentier-Batteur, S., Walter, L., Greenberg, D. A., & Stella, N. (2003). Palmitoylethanolamide increases after focal cerebral ischemia and potentiates microglial cell motility. *The Journal of Neuroscience, 23*, 7767–7775.

Fu, J., Bottegoni, G., Sasso, O., Bertorelli, R., Rocchia, W., Masetti, M., et al. (2012). A catalytically silent FAAH-1 variant drives anandamide transport in neurons. *Nature Neuroscience, 15*, 64–69.

Gabrielsson, L., Gouveia-Figueira, S., Häggström, J., Alhouayek, M., & Fowler, C. J. (2017). The anti-inflammatory compound palmitoylethanolamide inhibits prostaglandin and hydroxyeicosatetraenoic acid production by a macrophage cell line. *Pharmacology Research & Perspectives, 5*, e00300.

Gao, Y., Vasilyev, D. V., Goncalves, M. B., Howell, F. V., Hobbs, C., Reisenberg, M., et al. (2010). Loss of retrograde endocannabinoid signaling and reduced adult neurogenesis in diacylglycerol lipase knock-out mice. *The Journal of Neuroscience, 30*, 2017–2024.

Garcia-Ovejero, D., Arevalo-Martin, A., Petrosino, S., Docagne, F., Hagen, C., Bisogno, T., et al. (2009). The endocannabinoid system is modulated in response to spinal cord injury in rats. *Neurobiology of Disease, 33*, 57–71.

Gatta, L., Piscitelli, F., Giordano, C., Boccella, S., Lichtman, A., Maione, S., et al. (2012). Discovery of prostamide $F_{2\alpha}$ and its role in inflammatory pain and dorsal horn nociceptive neuron hyperexcitability. *PloS One*, *7*, e31111.

Ghafouri, N., Tiger, G., Razdan, R. K., Mahadevan, A., Pertwee, R. G., Martin, B. R., et al. (2004). Inhibition of monoacylglycerol lipase and fatty acid amide hydrolase by analogues of 2-arachidonoylglycerol. *British Journal of Pharmacology*, *143*, 774–784.

Goncalves, M. B., Suetterlin, P., Yip, P., Molina-Holgado, F., Walker, D. J., Oudin, M. J., et al. (2008). A diacylglycerol lipase-CB2 cannabinoid pathway regulates adult subventricular zone neurogenesis in an age-dependent manner. *Molecular and Cellular Neurosciences*, *38*, 526–536.

Gouveia-Figueira, S., Karlsson, J., Deplano, A., Hashemian, S., Svensson, M., Fredriksson, S. M., et al. (2015). Characterisation of (R)-2-(2-fluorobiphenyl-4-yl)-N-(3-methylpyridin-2-yl)propanamide as a dual fatty acid amide hydrolase: Cyclooxygenase inhibitor. *PloS One*, *10*, e0139212.

Gulyas, A. I., Cravatt, B. F., Bracey, M. H., Dinh, T. P., Piomelli, D., Boscia, F., et al. (2004). Segregation of two endocannabinoid-hydrolyzing enzymes into pre- and postsynaptic compartments in the rat hippocampus, cerebellum and amygdala. *The European Journal of Neuroscience*, *20*, 441–458.

Hampson, A. J., Hill, W. A. G., Zanphillips, M., Makriyannis, A., Leung, E., Eglen, R. M., et al. (1995). Anandamide hydroxylation by brain lipoxygenase: Metabolite structures and potencies at the cannabinoid receptor. *Biochimica et Biophysica Acta, Lipids and Lipid Metabolism*, *1259*, 173–179.

Hansen, H. H., Ikonomidou, C., Bittigau, P., Hansen, S. H., & Hansen, H. S. (2001a). Accumulation of the anandamide precursor and other N-acylethanolamine phospholipids in infant rat models of in vivo necrotic and apoptotic neuronal death. *Journal of Neurochemistry*, *76*, 39–46.

Hansen, H. H., Schmid, P. C., Bittigau, P., Lastres-Becker, I., Berrendero, F., Manzanares, J., et al. (2001b). Anandamide, but not 2-arachidonoylglycerol, accumulates during in vivo neurodegeneration. *Journal of Neurochemistry*, *78*, 1415–1427.

Hasegawa-Sasaki, H. (1985). Early changes in inositol lipids and their metabolites induced by platelet-derived growth factor in quiescent Swiss mouse 3T3 cells. *The Biochemical Journal*, *232*, 99–109.

Hernandez-Torres, G., Cipriano, M., Heden, E., Bjorklund, E., Canales, A., Zian, D., et al. (2014). A reversible and selective inhibitor of monoacylglycerol lipase ameliorates multiple sclerosis. *Angewandte Chemie (International Ed. in English)*, *53*, 13765–13770.

Hill MN, Bialecki J, Wellinger NL, Thompson RJ (2015). Pannexin-1 channels permit postsynaptic anandamide transport in hippocampal pyramidal neurons. 25th Annual symposium of the international cannabinoid research society, 34.

Hoover, H. S., Blankman, J. L., Niessen, S., & Cravatt, B. F. (2008). Selectivity of inhibitors of endocannabinoid biosynthesis evaluated by activity-based protein profiling. *Bioorganic & Medicinal Chemistry Letters*, *18*, 5838–5841.

Hsu, K. L., Tsuboi, K., Adibekian, A., Pugh, H., Masuda, K., & Cravatt, B. F. (2012). DAGLβ inhibition perturbs a lipid network involved in macrophage inflammatory responses. *Nature Chemical Biology*, *8*, 999–1007.

Hsu, K. L., Tsuboi, K., Chang, J. W., Whitby, L. R., Speers, A. E., Pugh, H., et al. (2013). Discovery and optimization of Piperidyl-1,2,3-triazole ureas as potent, selective, and in vivo-active inhibitors of α/β-hydrolase domain containing 6 (ABHD6). *Journal of Medicinal Chemistry*, *56*, 8270–8279.

Huggins, J. P., Smart, T. S., Langman, S., Taylor, L., & Young, T. (2012). An efficient randomised, placebo-controlled clinical trial with the irreversible fatty acid amide hydrolase-1 inhibitor PF-04457845, which modulates endocannabinoids but fails to induce effective analgesia in patients with pain due to osteoarthritis of the knee. *Pain, 153*, 1837–1846.

Janssen, F. J., Baggelaar, M. P., Hummel, J. J., Overkleeft, H. S., Cravatt, B. F., Boger, D. L., et al. (2015). Comprehensive analysis of structure activity relationships of α-Ketoheterocycles as *sn*-1-diacylglycerol lipase alpha inhibitors. *Journal of Medicinal Chemistry, 58*, 9742–9753.

Janssen, F. J., & van der Stelt, M. (2016). Inhibitors of diacylglycerol lipases in neurodegenerative and metabolic disorders. *Bioorganic & Medicinal Chemistry Letters, 26*, 3831–3837.

Jarai, Z., Wagner, J. A., Goparaju, S. K., Wang, L., Razdan, R. K., Sugiura, T., et al. (2000). Cardiovascular effects of 2-arachidonoyl glycerol in anesthetized mice. *Hypertension, 35*, 679–684.

Jenniches, I., Ternes, S., Albayram, O., Otte, D. M., Bach, K., Bindila, L., et al. (2016). Anxiety, stress, and fear response in mice with reduced endocannabinoid levels. *Biological Psychiatry, 79*, 858–868.

Jhaveri, M. D., Richardson, D., Kendall, D. A., Barrett, D. A., & Chapman, V. (2006). Analgesic effects of fatty acid amide hydrolase inhibition in a rat model of neuropathic pain. *The Journal of Neuroscience, 26*, 13318–13327.

Jin, S., Zhao, G., Li, Z., Nishimoto, Y., Isohama, Y., Shen, J., et al. (2009). Age-related pulmonary emphysema in mice lacking α/β hydrolase domain containing 2 gene. *Biochemical and Biophysical Research Communications, 380*, 419–424.

Jung, K. M., Sepers, M., Henstridge, C. M., Lassalle, O., Neuhofer, D., Martin, H., et al. (2012). Uncoupling of the endocannabinoid signalling complex in a mouse model of fragile X syndrome. *Nature Communications, 3*, 1080.

Kaczocha, M., Glaser, S. T., Chae, J., Brown, D. A., & Deutsch, D. G. (2010). Lipid droplets are novel sites of *N*-acylethanolamine inactivation by fatty acid amide hydrolase-2. *The Journal of Biological Chemistry, 285*, 2795–2806.

Kaczocha, M., Glaser, S. T., & Deutsch, D. G. (2009). Identification of intracellular carriers for the endocannabinoid anandamide. *Proceedings of the National Academy of Sciences of the United States of America, 106*, 6375–6380.

Kaczocha, M., Glaser, S. T., Maher, T., Clavin, B., Hamilton, J., O'Rourke, J., et al. (2015). Fatty acid binding protein deletion suppresses inflammatory pain through endocannabinoid/*N*-acylethanolamine-dependent mechanisms. *Molecular Pain, 11*, 52.

Kamat, S. S., Camara, K., Parsons, W. H., Chen, D. H., Dix, M. M., Bird, T. D., et al. (2015). Immunomodulatory lysophosphatidylserines are regulated by ABHD16A and ABHD12 interplay. *Nature Chemical Biology, 11*, 164–171.

Karbarz, M. J., Luo, L., Chang, L., Tham, C. S., Palmer, J. A., Wilson, S. J., et al. (2009). Biochemical and biological properties of 4-(3-phenyl-[1,2,4] thiadiazol-5-yl)-piperazine-1-carboxylic acid phenylamide, a mechanism-based inhibitor of fatty acid amide hydrolase. *Anesthesia and Analgesia, 108*, 316–329.

Karlsson, J., Morgillo, C. M., Deplano, A., Smaldone, G., Pedone, E., Luque, F. J., et al. (2015). Interaction of the N-(3-methylpyridin-2-yl) amide derivatives of flurbiprofen and ibuprofen with FAAH: Enantiomeric selectivity and binding mode. *PloS One, 10*, e0142711.

Kathuria, S., Gaetani, S., Fegley, D., Valino, F., Duranti, A., Tontini, A., et al. (2003). Modulation of anxiety through blockade of anandamide hydrolysis. *Nature Medicine, 9*, 76–81.

Katona, I., Urban, G. M., Wallace, M., Ledent, C., Jung, K. M., Piomelli, D., et al. (2006). Molecular composition of the endocannabinoid system at glutamatergic synapses. *The Journal of Neuroscience, 26*, 5628–5637.

Kerr, D. M., Downey, L., Conboy, M., Finn, D. P., & Roche, M. (2013). Alterations in the endocannabinoid system in the rat valproic acid model of autism. *Behavioural Brain Research, 249*, 124–132.

Kohnz, R. A., & Nomura, D. K. (2014). Chemical approaches to therapeutically target the metabolism and signaling of the endocannabinoid 2-AG and eicosanoids. *Chemical Society Reviews, 43*, 6859–6869.

Kozak, K. R., Gupta, R. A., Moody, J. S., Ji, C., Boeglin, W. E., DuBois, R. N., et al. (2002). 15-Lipoxygenase metabolism of 2-arachidonylglycerol: Generation of a peroxisome proliferator-activated receptor α agonist. *The Journal of Biological Chemistry*, *277*, 23278–23286.

Kozak, K. R., Rowlinson, S. W., & Marnett, L. J. (2000). Oxygenation of the endocannabinoid, 2-arachidonylglycerol, to glyceryl prostaglandins by cyclooxygenase-2. *The Journal of Biological Chemistry*, *275*, 33744–33749.

Kuwae, T., Shiota, Y., Schmid, P. C., Krebsbach, R., & Schmid, H. H. O. (1999). Biosynthesis and turnover of anandamide and other N-acylethanolamines in peritoneal macrophages. *FEBS Letters*, *459*, 123–127.

Lee, S. H., Ledri, M., Toth, B., Marchionni, I., Henstridge, C. M., Dudok, B., et al. (2015). Multiple forms of endocannabinoid and endovanilloid signaling regulate the tonic control of GABA release. *The Journal of Neuroscience*, *35*, 10039–10057.

Leishman, E., Mackie, K., Luquet, S., & Bradshaw, H. B. (2016). Lipidomics profile of a NAPE-PLD KO mouse provides evidence of a broader role of this enzyme in lipid metabolism in the brain. *Biochimica et Biophysica Acta*, *1861*, 491–500.

Leung, K., Elmes, M. W., Glaser, S. T., Deutsch, D. G., & Kaczocha, M. (2013). Role of FAAH-like anandamide transporter in anandamide inactivation. *PloS One*, *8*, e79355.

Leung, D., Saghatelian, A., Simon, G. M., & Cravatt, B. F. (2006). Inactivation of *N*-acyl phosphatidylethanolamine phospholipase D reveals multiple mechanisms for the biosynthesis of endocannabinoids. *Biochemistry*, *45*, 4720–4726.

Li, W., Blankman, J. L., & Cravatt, B. F. (2007). A functional proteomic strategy to discover inhibitors for uncharacterized hydrolases. *Journal of the American Chemical Society*, *129*, 9594–9595.

Liu, J., Batkai, S., Pacher, P., Harvey-White, J., Wagner, J. A., Cravatt, B. F., et al. (2003). Lipopolysaccharide induces anandamide synthesis in macrophages via CD14/MAPK/phosphoinositide 3-kinase/NF-κB independently of platelet activating factor. *The Journal of Biological Chemistry*, *278*, 45034–45039.

Liu, J., Wang, L., Harvey-White, J., Osei-Hyiaman, D., Razdan, R., Gong, Q., et al. (2006). A biosynthetic pathway for anandamide. *Proceedings of the National Academy of Sciences of the United States of America*, *103*, 13345–13350.

Long, J. Z., Li, W., Booker, L., Burston, J. J., Kinsey, S. G., Schlosburg, J. E., et al. (2009). Selective blockade of 2-arachidonoylglycerol hydrolysis produces cannabinoid behavioral effects. *Nature Chemical Biology*, *5*, 37–44.

Maccarrone, M., De Petrocellis, L., Bari, M., Fezza, F., Salvati, S., Di Marzo, V., et al. (2001a). Lipopolysaccharide downregulates fatty acid amide hydrolase expression and increases anandamide levels in human peripheral lymphocytes. *Archives of Biochemistry and Biophysics*, *393*, 321–328.

Maccarrone, M., Guzman, M., Mackie, K., Doherty, P., & Harkany, T. (2014). Programming of neural cells by (endo)cannabinoids: From physiological rules to emerging therapies. *Nature Reviews. Neuroscience*, *15*, 786–801.

Maccarrone, M., Valensise, H., Bari, M., Lazzarin, N., Romanini, C., & Finazzi-Agro, A. (2001b). Progesterone up-regulates anandamide hydrolase in human lymphocytes: Role of cytokines and implications for fertility. *Journal of Immunology*, *166*, 7183–7189.

Manna, J. D., Wepy, J. A., Hsu, K., Chang, J. W., Cravatt, B. F., & Marnett, L. J. (2014). Identification of the major prostaglandin glycerol Ester hydrolase in human cancer cells. *The Journal of Biological Chemistry*, *289*, 33741–33753.

Margheritis, E., Castellani, B., Magotti, P., Peruzzi, S., Romeo, E., Natali, F., et al. (2016). Bile acid recognition by NAPE-PLD. *ACS Chemical Biology*, *11*, 2908–2914.

McDougle, D. R., Kambalyal, A., Meling, D. D., & Das, A. (2014). Endocannabinoids anandamide and 2-arachidonoylglycerol are substrates for human CYP2J2 epoxygenase. *The Journal of Pharmacology and Experimental Therapeutics*, *351*, 616–627.

McKinney, M. K., & Cravatt, B. F. (2006). Structure-based design of a FAAH variant that discriminates between the *N*-acyl ethanolamine and taurine families of signaling lipids. *Biochemistry*, *45*, 9016–9022.

Mechoulam, R., Benshabat, S., Hanus, L., Ligumsky, M., Kaminski, N. E., Schatz, A. R., et al. (1995). Identification of an endogenous 2-monoglyceride, present in canine gut, that binds to cannabinoid receptors. *Biochemical Pharmacology*, *50*, 83–90.

Migliore, M., Pontis, S., Fuentes de Arriba, A. L., Realini, N., Torrente, E., Armirotti, A., et al. (2016). Second-generation non-covalent NAAA inhibitors are protective in a model of multiple sclerosis. *Angewandte Chemie (International Ed. in English)*, *55*, 11193–11197.

Mileni, M., Johnson, D. S., Wang, Z., Everdeen, D. S., Liimatta, M., Pabst, B., et al. (2008). Structure-guided inhibitor design for human FAAH by interspecies active site conversion. *Proceedings of the National Academy of Sciences of the United States of America*, *105*, 12820–12824.

Miller, M. R., Mannowetz, N., Iavarone, A. T., Safavi, R., Gracheva, E. O., Smith, J. F., et al. (2016). Unconventional endocannabinoid signaling governs sperm activation via the sex hormone progesterone. *Science*, *352*, 555–559.

Mitchener, M. M., Hermanson, D. J., Shockley, E. M., Brown, H. A., Lindsley, C. W., Reese, J., et al. (2015). Competition and allostery govern substrate selectivity of cyclooxygenase-2. *Proceedings of the National Academy of Sciences of the United States of America*, *112*, 12366–12371.

Miyata, K., Nakayama, M., Mizuta, S., Hokimoto, S., Sugamura, K., Oshima, S., et al. (2008). Elevated mature macrophage expression of human ABHD2 gene in vulnerable plaque. *Biochemical and Biophysical Research Communications*, *365*, 207–213.

Miyata, K., Oike, Y., Hoshii, T., Maekawa, H., Ogawa, H., Suda, T., et al. (2005). Increase of smooth muscle cell migration and of intimal hyperplasia in mice lacking the α/β hydrolase domain containing 2 gene. *Biochemical and Biophysical Research Communications*, *329*, 296–304.

Moody, J. S., Kozak, K. R., Ji, C., & Marnett, L. J. (2001). Selective oxygenation of the endocannabinoid 2-arachidonylglycerol by leukocyte-type 12-lipoxygenase. *Biochemistry*, *40*, 861–866.

Moreira, F. A., & Crippa, J. A. (2009). The psychiatric side-effects of rimonabant. *Revista Brasileira de Psiquiatria*, *31*, 145–153.

Moriuchi, H., Koda, N., Okuda-Ashitaka, E., Daiyasu, H., Ogasawara, K., Toh, H., et al. (2008). Molecular characterization of a novel type of prostamide/prostaglandin F synthase, belonging to the thioredoxin-like superfamily. *The Journal of Biological Chemistry*, *283*, 792–801.

Mulder, A. M., & Cravatt, B. F. (2006). Endocannabinoid metabolism in the absence of fatty acid amide hydrolase (FAAH): Discovery of phosphorylcholine derivatives of *N*-acyl ethanolamines. *Biochemistry*, *45*, 11267–11277.

Naresh Kumar, M., Thunuguntla, V. B., Veeramachaneni, G. K., Chandra Sekhar, B., Guntupalli, S., & Bondili, J. S. (2016). Molecular characterization of human ABHD2 as TAG lipase and ester hydrolase. *Bioscience Reports*, *36*, e00358.

Natarajan, V., Reddy, P. V., Schmid, P. C., & Schmid, H. H. O. (1982). *N*-acylation of ethanolamine phospholipids in canine myocardium. *Biochimica et Biophysica Acta*, *712*, 342–355.

Natarajan, V., Schmid, P. C., Reddy, P. V., Zuzarte-Augustin, M. L., & Schmid, H. H. (1983). Biosynthesis of N-acylethanolamine phospholipids by dog brain preparations. *Journal of Neurochemistry*, *41*, 1303–1312.

Navia-Paldanius, D., Savinainen, J. R., & Laitinen, J. T. (2012). Biochemical and pharmacological characterization of human α/β-hydrolase domain containing 6 (ABHD6) and 12 (ABHD12). *Journal of Lipid Research*, *53*, 2413–2424.

Naydenov, A. V., Horne, E. A., Cheah, C. S., Swinney, K., Hsu, K. L., Cao, J. K., et al. (2014). ABHD6 blockade exerts antiepileptic activity in PTZ-induced seizures and in spontaneous seizures in R6/2 mice. *Neuron, 83*, 361–371.

Nicolussi, S., & Gertsch, J. (2015). Endocannabinoid transport revisited. *Vitamins and Hormones, 98*, 441–485.

Nomura, D. K., Morrison, B. E., Blankman, J. L., Long, J. Z., Kinsey, S. G., Marcondes, M. C., et al. (2011). Endocannabinoid hydrolysis generates brain prostaglandins that promote neuroinflammation. *Science, 334*, 809–813.

Nyilas, R., Dudok, B., Urban, G. M., Mackie, K., Watanabe, M., Cravatt, B. F., et al. (2008). Enzymatic machinery for endocannabinoid biosynthesis associated with calcium stores in glutamatergic axon terminals. *The Journal of Neuroscience, 28*, 1058–1063.

Obinata, D., Takada, S., Takayama, K. I., Urano, T., Ito, A., Ashikari, D., et al. (2016). Abhydrolase domain containing 2, an androgen target gene, promotes prostate cancer cell proliferation and migration. *European Journal of Cancer, 57*, 39–49.

Oddi, S., Fezza, F., Pasquariello, N., D'Agostino, A., Catanzaro, G., De Simone, C., et al. (2009). Molecular identification of albumin and Hsp70 as cytosolic anandamide-binding proteins. *Chemistry & Biology, 16*, 624–632.

Ogasawara, D., Deng, H., Viader, A., Baggelaar, M. P., Breman, A., den Dulk, H., et al. (2016). Rapid and profound rewiring of brain lipid signaling networks by acute diacylglycerol lipase inhibition. *Proceedings of the National Academy of Sciences of the United States of America, 113*, 26–33.

Ogura, Y., Parsons, W. H., Kamat, S. S., & Cravatt, B. F. (2016). A calcium-dependent acyltransferase that produces *N*-acyl phosphatidylethanolamines. *Nature Chemical Biology, 12*, 669–671.

Ohno-Shosaku, T., & Kano, M. (2014). Endocannabinoid-mediated retrograde modulation of synaptic transmission. *Current Opinion in Neurobiology, 29C*, 1–8.

Okamoto, Y., Morishita, J., Tsuboi, K., Tonai, T., & Ueda, N. (2004). Molecular characterization of a phospholipase D generating anandamide and its congeners. *The Journal of Biological Chemistry, 279*, 5298–5305.

Oudin, M. J., Hobbs, C., & Doherty, P. (2011). DAGL-dependent endocannabinoid signalling: Roles in axonal pathfinding, synaptic plasticity and adult neurogenesis. *The European Journal of Neuroscience, 34*, 1634–1646.

Palermo, G., Bauer, I., Campomanes, P., Cavalli, A., Armirotti, A., Girotto, S., et al. (2015). Keys to lipid selection in fatty acid amide hydrolase catalysis: Structural flexibility, gating residues and multiple binding pockets. *PLoS Computational Biology, 11*, e1004231.

Pan, B., Wang, W., Zhong, P., Blankman, J. L., Cravatt, B. F., & Liu, Q. S. (2011). Alterations of endocannabinoid signaling, synaptic plasticity, learning, and memory in monoacylglycerol lipase knock-out mice. *The Journal of Neuroscience, 31*, 13420–13430.

Paria, B. C., Wang, H., & Dey, S. K. (2002). Endocannabinoid signaling in synchronizing embryo development and uterine receptivity for implantation. *Chemistry and Physics of Lipids, 121*, 201–210.

Piro, J. R., Benjamin, D. I., Duerr, J. M., Pi, Y., Gonzales, C., Wood, K. M., et al. (2012). A dysregulated endocannabinoid-eicosanoid network supports pathogenesis in a mouse model of Alzheimer's disease. *Cell Reports, 1*, 617–623.

Powell, D. R., Gay, J. P., Wilganowski, N., Doree, D., Savelieva, K. V., Lanthorn, T. H., et al. (2015). Diacylglycerol lipase α knockout mice demonstrate metabolic and behavioral phenotypes similar to those of cannabinoid. Receptor 1 knockout mice. *Frontiers in Endocrinology (Lausanne), 6*, 86.

Pratt-Hyatt, M., Zhang, H., Snider, N. T., & Hollenberg, P. F. (2010). Effects of a commonly occurring genetic polymorphism of human CYP3A4 (I118V) on the metabolism of anandamide. *Drug Metabolism and Disposition, 38*, 2075–2082.

Prescott, S. M., & Majerus, P. W. (1983). Characterization of 1,2-diacylglycerol hydrolysis in human platelets. Demonstration of an arachidonoyl-monoacylglycerol intermediate. *The Journal of Biological Chemistry*, *258*, 764–769.

Pribasnig, M. A., Mrak, I., Grabner, G. F., Taschler, U., Knittelfelder, O., Scherz, B., et al. (2015). α/β Hydrolase domain-containing 6 (ABHD6) degrades the late endosomal/lysosomal lipid Bis (monoacylglycero)phosphate. *The Journal of Biological Chemistry*, *290*, 29869–29881.

Rahman, I. A., Tsuboi, K., Hussain, Z., Yamashita, R., Okamoto, Y., Uyama, T., et al. (2016). Calcium-dependent generation of N-acylethanolamines and lysophosphatidic acids by glycerophosphodiesterase GDE7. *Biochimica et Biophysica Acta*, *1861*, 1881–1892.

Ramikie, T. S., Nyilas, R., Bluett, R. J., Gamble-George, J. C., Hartley, N. D., Mackie, K., et al. (2014). Multiple mechanistically distinct modes of endocannabinoid mobilization at central amygdala glutamatergic synapses. *Neuron*, *81*, 1111–1125.

Reisenberg, M., Singh, P. K., Williams, G., & Doherty, P. (2012). The diacylglycerol lipases: Structure, regulation and roles in and beyond endocannabinoid signalling. *Philosophical Transactions of the Royal Society of London. Series B, Biological Sciences*, *367*, 3264–3275.

Ribeiro, A., Pontis, S., Mengatto, L., Armirotti, A., Chiurchiu, V., Capurro, V., et al. (2015). A potent systemically active N-Acylethanolamine acid amidase inhibitor that suppresses inflammation and human macrophage activation. *ACS Chemical Biology*, *10*, 1838–1846.

Rosenberger, T. A., Farooqui, A. A., & Horrocks, L. A. (2007). Bovine brain diacylglycerol lipase: Substrate specificity and activation by cyclic AMP-dependent protein kinase. *Lipids*, *42*, 187–195.

Sanson, B., Wang, T., Sun, J., Wang, L., Kaczocha, M., Ojima, I., et al. (2014). Crystallographic study of FABP5 as an intracellular endocannabinoid transporter. *Acta Crystallographica. Section D, Biological Crystallography*, *70*, 290–298.

Sasso, O., Migliore, M., Habrant, D., Armirotti, A., Albani, C., Summa, M., et al. (2015). Multitarget fatty acid amide hydrolase/cyclooxygenase blockade suppresses intestinal inflammation and protects against nonsteroidal anti-inflammatory drug-dependent gastrointestinal damage. *The FASEB Journal*, *29*, 2616–2627.

Schmid, P. C., Krebsbach, R. J., Perry, S. R., Dettmer, T. M., Maasson, J. L., & Schmid, H. H. O. (1995). Occurrence and postmortem generation of anandamide and other long chain *N*-acylethanolamines in mammalian brain. *FEBS Letters*, *375*, 117–120.

Schmid, P. C., Reddy, P. V., Natarajan, V., & Schmid, H. H. O. (1983). Metabolism of N-acylethanolamine phospholipids by a mammalian phosphodiesterase of the phospholipase D type. *The Journal of Biological Chemistry*, *258*, 9302–9306.

Sciolino, N. R., Zhou, W., & Hohmann, A. G. (2011). Enhancement of endocannabinoid signaling with JZL184, an inhibitor of the 2-arachidonoylglycerol hydrolyzing enzyme monoacylglycerol lipase, produces anxiolytic effects under conditions of high environmental aversiveness in rats. *Pharmacological Research*, *64*, 226–234.

Shonesy, B. C., Bluett, R. J., Ramikie, T. S., Baldi, R., Hermanson, D. J., Kingsley, P. J., et al. (2014). Genetic disruption of 2-arachidonoylglycerol synthesis reveals a key role for endocannabinoid signaling in anxiety modulation. *Cell Reports*, *9*, 1644–1653.

Singh, P. K., Markwick, R., Lu, L., Howell, F. V., Williams, G., & Doherty, P. (2016). Assay and inhibition of the purified catalytic domain of diacylglycerol lipase beta. *Biochemistry*, *55*, 2713–2721.

Snider, N. T., Kornilov, A. M., Kent, U. M., & Hollenberg, P. F. (2007). Anandamide metabolism by human liver and kidney microsomal cytochrome P450 enzymes to form hydroxyeicosatetraenoic and epoxyeicosatrienoic acid ethanolamides. *The Journal of Pharmacology and Experimental Therapeutics*, *321*, 590–597.

Snider, N. T., Nast, J. A., Tesmer, L. A., & Hollenberg, P. F. (2009). A cytochrome P450-derived epoxygenated metabolite of anandamide is a potent cannabinoid. Receptor 2-selective agonist. *Molecular Pharmacology*, *75*, 965–972.

Snider, N. T., Sikora, M. J., Sridar, C., Feuerstein, T. J., Rae, J. M., & Hollenberg, P. F. (2008). The endocannabinoid anandamide is a substrate for the human polymorphic cytochrome P450 2D6. *The Journal of Pharmacology and Experimental Therapeutics*, *327*, 538–545.

Solorzano, C., Zhu, C., Battista, N., Astarita, G., Lodola, A., Rivara, S., et al. (2009). Selective *N*-acylethanolamine-hydrolyzing acid amidase inhibition reveals a key role for endogenous palmitoylethanolamide in inflammation. *Proceedings of the National Academy of Sciences of the United States of America*, *106*, 20966–20971.

Sridar, C., Snider, N. T., & Hollenberg, P. F. (2011). Anandamide oxidation by wild-type and polymorphically expressed CYP2B6 and CYP2D6. *Drug Metabolism and Disposition*, *39*, 782–788.

Sticht, M. A., Long, J. Z., Rock, E. M., Limebeer, C. L., Mechoulam, R., Cravatt, B. F., et al. (2012). Inhibition of monoacylglycerol lipase attenuates vomiting in *Suncus murinus* and 2-arachidonoyl glycerol attenuates nausea in rats. *British Journal of Pharmacology*, *165*, 2425–2435.

Sugiura, T., Kondo, S., Sukagawa, A., Nakane, S., Shinoda, A., Itoh, K., et al. (1995). 2-Arachidonoylgylcerol: A possible endogenous cannabinoid receptor ligand in brain. *Biochemical and Biophysical Research Communications*, *215*, 89–97.

Sugiura, T., & Waku, K. (2000). 2-Arachidonoylglycerol and the cannabinoid receptors. *Chemistry and Physics of Lipids*, *108*, 89–106.

Sun, Y. X., Tsuboi, K., Okamoto, Y., Tonai, T., Murakami, M., Kudo, I., et al. (2004). Biosynthesis of anandamide and *N*-palmitoylethanolamine by sequential actions of phospholipase A_2 and lysophospholipase D. *The Biochemical Journal*, *380*, 749–756.

Tai, T., Tsuboi, K., Uyama, T., Masuda, K., Cravatt, B. F., Houchi, H., et al. (2012). Endogenous molecules stimulating N-acylethanolamine-hydrolyzing acid amidase (NAAA). *ACS Chemical Neuroscience*, *3*, 379–385.

Tanimura, A., Yamazaki, M., Hashimotodani, Y., Uchigashima, M., Kawata, S., Abe, M., et al. (2010). The endocannabinoid 2-arachidonoylglycerol produced by diacylglycerol lipase alpha mediates retrograde suppression of synaptic transmission. *Neuron*, *65*, 320–327.

Tchantchou, F., & Zhang, Y. (2013). Selective inhibition of alpha/beta-hydrolase domain 6 attenuates neurodegeneration, alleviates blood brain barrier breakdown and improves functional recovery in a mouse model of traumatic brain injury. *Journal of Neurotrauma*, *30*, 565–579.

Thomas, G., Betters, J. L., Lord, C. C., Brown, A. L., Marshall, S., Ferguson, D., et al. (2013). The serine hydrolase ABHD6 is a critical regulator of the metabolic syndrome. *Cell Reports*, *5*, 508–520.

Thomas, G., Brown, A. L., & Brown, J. M. (2014). *In vivo* metabolite profiling as a means to identify uncharacterized lipase function: Recent success stories within the alpha beta hydrolase domain (ABHD) enzyme family. *Biochimica et Biophysica Acta*, *1841*, 1097–1101.

Thors, L., Bergh, A., Persson, E., Hammarsten, P., Stattin, P., Egevad, L., et al. (2010a). Fatty acid amide hydrolase in prostate cancer: Association with disease severity and outcome, CB1 receptor expression and regulation by IL-4. *PloS One*, *5*, e12275.

Thors, L., Burston, J. J., Alter, B. J., McKinney, M. K., Cravatt, B. F., Ross, R. A., et al. (2010b). Biochanin a, a naturally occurring inhibitor of fatty acid amide hydrolase. *British Journal of Pharmacology*, *160*, 549–560.

Tortoriello, G., Rhodes, B. P., Takacs, S. M., Stuart, J. M., Basnet, A., Raboune, S., et al. (2013). Targeted Lipidomics in *Drosophila melanogaster* identifies novel 2-monoacylglycerols and N-acyl amides. *PloS One*, *8*, e67865.

Tsuboi, K., Okamoto, Y., Ikematsu, N., Inoue, M., Shimizu, Y., Uyama, T., et al. (2011). Enzymatic formation of N-acylethanolamines from N-acylethanolamine plasmalogen through N-acylphosphatidylethanolamine-hydrolyzing phospholipase D-dependent and -independent pathways. *Biochimica et Biophysica Acta, 1811*, 565–577.

Tsuboi, K., Sun, Y. X., Okamoto, Y., Araki, N., Tonai, T., & Ueda, N. (2005). Molecular characterization of N-acylethanolamine-hydrolyzing acid amidase, a novel member of the choloylglycine hydrolase family with structural and functional similarity to acid ceramidase. *The Journal of Biological Chemistry, 280*, 11082–11092.

Tsuboi, K., Zhao, L. Y., Okamoto, Y., Araki, N., Ueno, M., Sakamoto, H., et al. (2007). Predominant expression of lysosomal N-acylethanolamine-hydrolyzing acid amidase in macrophages revealed by immunochemical studies. *Biochimica et Biophysica Acta, Lipids and Lipid Metabolism, 1771*, 623–632.

Uchigashima, M., Narushima, M., Fukaya, M., Katona, I., Kano, M., & Watanabe, M. (2007). Subcellular arrangement of molecules for 2-arachidonoyl-glycerol-mediated retrograde signaling and its physiological contribution to synaptic modulation in the striatum. *The Journal of Neuroscience, 27*, 3663–3676.

Ueda, N., Tsuboi, K., & Uyama, T. (2013). Metabolism of endocannabinoids and related N-acylethanolamines: Canonical and alternative pathways. *The FEBS Journal, 280*, 1874–1894.

Ueda, N., Yamamoto, K., Yamamoto, S., Tokunaga, T., Shirakawa, E., Shinkai, H., et al. (1995). Lipoxygenase-catalyzed oxygenation of arachidonylethanolamide, a cannabinoid receptor agonist. *Biochimica et Biophysica Acta, Lipids and Lipid Metabolism, 1254*, 127–134.

Ueda, N., Yamanaka, K., & Yamamoto, S. (2001). Purification and characterization of an acid amidase selective for *N*-palmitoylethanolamine, a putative endogenous anti-inflammatory substance. *The Journal of Biological Chemistry, 276*, 35552–35557.

Urquhart, P., Nicolaou, A., & Woodward, D. F. (2015). Endocannabinoids and their oxygenation by cyclo-oxygenases, lipoxygenases and other oxygenases. *Biochimica et Biophysica Acta, 1851*, 366–376, PM:25543004.

Uyama, T., Ikematsu, N., Inoue, M., Shinohara, N., Jin, X. H., Tsuboi, K., et al. (2012). Generation of N-acylphosphatidylethanolamine by members of the phospholipase a/acyltransferase (PLA/AT) family. *The Journal of Biological Chemistry, 287*, 31905–31919.

van der Stelt, M., van Kuik, J. A., Bari, M., Van Zadelhoff, G., Leeflang, B. R., Veldink, G. A., et al. (2002). Oxygenated metabolites of anandamide and 2-arachidonoylglycerol: Conformational analysis and interaction with cannabinoid receptors, membrane transporter, and fatty acid amide hydrolase. *Journal of Medicinal Chemistry, 45*, 3709–3720.

van Tienhoven, M., Atkins, J., Li, Y., & Glynn, P. (2002). Human neuropathy target esterase catalyzes hydrolysis of membrane lipids. *The Journal of Biological Chemistry, 277*, 20942–20948.

Vandevoorde, S., Saha, B., Mahadevan, A., Razdan, R. K., Pertwee, R. G., Martin, B. R., et al. (2005). Influence of the degree of unsaturation of the acyl side chain upon the interaction of analogues of 1-arachidonoylglycerol with monoacylglycerol lipase and fatty acid amide hydrolase. *Biochemical and Biophysical Research Communications, 337*, 104–109.

Vaughan, M., Berger, J. E., & Steinberg, D. (1964). Hormone-sensitive lipase and monoglyceride lipase activities in adipose tissue. *The Journal of Biological Chemistry, 239*, 401–409.

Vecchio, A. J., & Malkowski, M. G. (2011). The structural basis of endocannabinoid oxygenation by cyclooxygenase-2. *The Journal of Biological Chemistry, 286*, 20736–20745.

Viader, A., Ogasawara, D., Joslyn, C. M., Sanchez-Alavez, M., Mori, S., Nguyen, W., et al. (2016). A chemical proteomic atlas of brain serine hydrolases identifies cell type-specific pathways regulating neuroinflammation. *eLife, 5*, e12345.

Wagenlehner, F. M., Van Till, J. W., Houbiers, J. G., Martina, R. V., Cerneus, D. P., Melis, J. H., et al. (2017). Fatty acid amide hydrolase inhibitor treatment in men with chronic prostatitis/chronic pelvic pain syndrome, an adaptive double-blind

randomized controlled trial. *Urology*, in press. http://dx.doi.org/10.1016/j.urology.2017.02.09.
Walker, V. J., Griffin, A. P., Hammar, D. K., & Hollenberg, P. F. (2016). Metabolism of anandamide by human cytochrome P450 2J2 in the reconstituted system and human intestinal Microsomes. *The Journal of Pharmacology and Experimental Therapeutics*, *357*, 537–544.
Wei, B. Q., Mikkelsen, T. S., McKinney, M. K., Lander, E. S., & Cravatt, B. F. (2006). A second fatty acid amide hydrolase with variable distribution among placental mammals. *The Journal of Biological Chemistry*, *281*, 36569–36578.
Wen, J., Ribeiro, R., Tanaka, M., & Zhang, Y. (2015). Activation of CB2 receptor is required for the therapeutic effect of ABHD6 inhibition in experimental autoimmune encephalomyelitis. *Neuropharmacology*, *99*, 196–209.
Woodhams, S. G., Wong, A., Barrett, D. A., Bennett, A. J., Chapman, V., & Alexander, S. P. H. (2012). Spinal administration of the monoacylglycerol lipase inhibitor JZL184 produces robust inhibitory effects on nociceptive processing and the development of central sensitization in the rat. *British Journal of Pharmacology*, *167*, 1609–1619.
Woodward, D. F., Wang, J. W., & Poloso, N. J. (2013). Recent progress in prostaglandin f2alpha ethanolamide (prostamide f2alpha) research and therapeutics. *Pharmacological Reviews*, *65*, 1135–1147.
Xie, S. Q., Borazjani, A., Hatfield, M. J., Edwards, C. C., Potter, P. M., & Ross, M. K. (2010). Inactivation of lipid glyceryl ester metabolism in human THP1 monocytes/macrophages by activated organophosphorus insecticides: Role of carboxylesterases 1 and 2. *Chemical Research in Toxicology*, *23*, 1890–1904.
Yamanoi, K., Matsumura, N., Murphy, S. K., Baba, T., Abiko, K., Hamanishi, J., et al. (2016). Suppression of ABHD2, identified through a functional genomics screen, causes anoikis resistance, chemoresistance and poor prognosis in ovarian cancer. *Oncotarget*, 7, 47620–47636.
Yang, W., Ni, J. S., Woodward, D. F., Tang-Liu, D. D. S., & Ling, K. H. J. (2005). Enzymatic formation of prostamide $F_{2\alpha}$ from anandamide involves a newly identified intermediate metabolite, prostamide H_2. *Journal of Lipid Research*, *46*, 2745–2751.
Yoshida, T., Fukaya, M., Uchigashima, M., Miura, E., Kamiya, H., Kano, M., et al. (2006). Localization of diacylglycerol lipase-α around postsynaptic spine suggests close proximity between production site of an endocannabinoid, 2-arachidonoyl-glycerol, and presynaptic cannabinoid CB1 receptor. *The Journal of Neuroscience*, *26*, 4740–4751.
Yoshida, T., Uchigashima, M., Yamasaki, M., Katona, I., Yamazaki, M., Sakimura, K., et al. (2011). Unique inhibitory synapse with particularly rich endocannabinoid signaling machinery on pyramidal neurons in basal amygdaloid nucleus. *Proceedings of the National Academy of Sciences of the United States of America*, *108*, 3059–3064.
Yoshino, H., Miyamae, T., Hansen, G., Zambrowicz, B., Flynn, M., Pedicord, D., et al. (2011). Postsynaptic diacylglycerol lipase mediates retrograde endocannabinoid suppression of inhibition in mouse prefrontal cortex. *The Journal of Physiology*, *589*, 4857–4884.
Younts, T. J., & Castillo, P. E. (2014). Endogenous cannabinoid signaling at inhibitory interneurons. *Current Opinion in Neurobiology*, *26*, 42–50.
Yu, M., Ives, D., & Ramesha, C. S. (1997). Synthesis of prostaglandin E_2 ethanolamide from anandamide by cyclooxygenase-2. *The Journal of Biological Chemistry*, *272*, 21181–21186.
Zhang, Y., Chen, K., Sloan, S. A., Bennett, M. L., Scholze, A. R., O'Keeffe, S., et al. (2014). An RNA-sequencing transcriptome and splicing database of glia, neurons, and vascular cells of the cerebral cortex. *The Journal of Neuroscience*, *34*, 11929–11947.
Zhao, S., Mugabo, Y., Ballentine, G., Attane, C., Iglesias, J., Poursharifi, P., et al. (2016). α/β-Hydrolase domain 6 deletion induces adipose browning and prevents obesity and type 2 diabetes. *Cell Reports*, *14*, 2872–2888.
Zhao, S., Poursharifi, P., Mugabo, Y., Levens, E. J., Vivot, K., Attane, C., et al. (2015). α/β-Hydrolase domain-6 and saturated long chain monoacylglycerol regulate insulin secretion promoted by both fuel and non-fuel stimuli. *Molecular Metabolism*, *4*, 940–950.

Zhong, P., Pan, B., Gao, X. P., Blankman, J. L., Cravatt, B. F., & Liu, Q. S. (2011). Genetic deletion of monoacylglycerol lipase alters endocannabinoid-mediated retrograde synaptic depression in the cerebellum. *The Journal of Physiology*, *589*, 4847–4855.

Zhou, Y., Howell, F. V., Glebov, O. O., Albrecht, D., Williams, G., & Doherty, P. (2016). Regulated endosomal trafficking of diacylglycerol lipase alpha (DAGLalpha) generates distinct cellular pools; implications for endocannabinoid signaling. *Molecular and Cellular Neurosciences*, *76*, 76–86.

CHAPTER THREE

Cannabis Pharmacology: The Usual Suspects and a Few Promising Leads

Ethan B. Russo*,[1], Jahan Marcu†
*PHYTECS, Los Angeles, CA, United States
†Americans for Safe Access, Patient Focused Certification, Washington, DC, United States
[1]Corresponding author: e-mail address: erusso@phytecs.com

Contents

Advances in Pharmacology, Volume 80
ISSN 1054-3589
http://dx.doi.org/10.1016/bs.apha.2017.03.004

Abstract

The golden age of cannabis pharmacology began in the 1960s as Raphael Mechoulam and his colleagues in Israel isolated and synthesized cannabidiol, tetrahydrocannabinol, and other phytocannabinoids. Initially, THC garnered most research interest with sporadic attention to cannabidiol, which has only rekindled in the last 15 years through a demonstration of its remarkably versatile pharmacology and synergy with THC. Gradually a cognizance of the potential of other phytocannabinoids has developed. Contemporaneous assessment of cannabis pharmacology must be even far more inclusive. Medical and recreational consumers alike have long believed in unique attributes of certain cannabis chemovars despite their similarity in cannabinoid profiles. This has focused additional research on the pharmacological contributions of mono- and sesquiterpenoids to the effects of cannabis flower preparations. Investigation reveals these aromatic compounds to contribute modulatory and therapeutic roles in the cannabis entourage far beyond expectations considering their modest concentrations in the plant. Synergistic relationships of the terpenoids to cannabinoids will be highlighted and include many complementary roles to boost therapeutic efficacy in treatment of pain, psychiatric disorders, cancer, and numerous other areas. Additional parts of the cannabis plant provide a wide and distinct variety of other compounds of pharmacological interest, including the triterpenoid friedelin from the roots, canniprene from the fan leaves, cannabisin from seed coats, and cannflavin A from seed sprouts. This chapter will explore the unique attributes of these agents and demonstrate how cannabis may yet fulfil its potential as Mechoulam's professed "pharmacological treasure trove."

ABBREVIATIONS

BCP beta-caryophyllene
CB_1 cannabinoid type 1 receptor
CB_2 cannabinoid type 2 receptor
DEA Drug Enforcement Agency
DEET *N*,*N*-dimethyl-toluamide
ECS endocannabinoid system
EO essential oil
FEMA Flavor and Extract Manufacturers' Association
GRAS Generally Recognized As Safe
GVHD graft-vs-host-disease
MAGL monoacylglycerol lipase
MRSA methicillin-resistant *Staphylococcus aureus*
NAAA *N*-acylethanolamine-hydrolyzing acid amidase
PPARγ peroxisome proliferator-activated receptor gamma
TRP transient receptor potential
TRPA1 TRP ankyrin-type 1

1. INTRODUCTION

Mammals and plants are exposed to cannabinoids and related compounds that notably modulate their growth and physiology. The human species in the Old World grew up around the >70 million-year-old cannabis plant, giving us a natural affinity to cannabinoids (Clarke & Merlin, 2012). This plant has been documented as a provider of food, clothing, textiles, and medicine for millennia. For thousands of years, the plant has been associated with relieving symptoms of disease and has demonstrated numerous therapeutic properties (Russo, 2007, 2011).

In this century, we are finally beginning to understand the precise pharmacological mechanisms underlying the effects of cannabis and related preparations, most of which can be explained through the endocannabinoid system (ECS). As perhaps the most significant human biological scientific discovery in the last 30 years, the ECS is only now being integrated into medical school curricula.

Analytical chemistry has revealed a rich and abundant "pharmacological treasure trove" in the plant. Compounds that may affect the pharmacology of cannabinoids are abundant in nature, and so we may dangerously and mistakenly consider their presence to be trivial. If so, this could cause us to lose sight of the subtlety and efficiency of their design when applied in combination. There are some 100 clinical studies and thousands of articles on the pharmacology and pharmacodynamics of cannabis and its influence on how humans eat, sleep, heal, and learn.

In this review, we hope to demystify some of the wonder of cannabis as a medicine by providing a concise overview of the pharmacological mechanisms of cannabis compounds, which will hopefully guide medical school curricula, advances in therapies, and lead to changes in public health approaches both nationally and internationally. As government information sources are updated with cannabis research conducted in the current century, the future of cannabis in society will depend strongly on how well we understand this plant, of which our access to for research and medicine currently floats on the winds of politics (Fig. 1).

2. CANNABIS PHYTOCANNABINOIDS (FIG. 2)

2.1 Tetrahydrocannabinol

The pharmacology of tetrahydrocannabinol (THC) is perhaps the most well studied of any scheduled substance, having well over 100 published clinical studies of medical cannabis and related products which contain THC (Ben Amar, 2006; Hazekamp & Grotenhermen, 2010; Kowal, Hazekamp, & Grotenhermen, 2016; Marcu, 2016; Pertwee & Cascio, 2014; Russo & Hohmann, 2012). THC, among a pantheon of over 100 (Hanus, Meyer, Munoz, Taglialatela-Scafati, & Appendino, 2016), is the most common phytocannabinoid in cannabis drug chemotypes, and is produced in the plant via an allele codominant with CBD (de Meijer et al., 2003). THC displays both cannabinoid receptor-dependent and -independent mechanisms.

THC interacts efficiently with CB_1 ($K_i = 5.05$–80.3 nM) and CB_2 receptors ($K_i = 1.73$–75.3 nM), which underlies its activities in modulating pain, spasticity, sedation, appetite, and mood (Russo, 2011). Additionally, it is a bronchodilator (Williams, Hartley, & Graham, 1976), neuroprotective antioxidant (Hampson, Grimaldi, Axelrod, & Wink, 1998), antipruritic agent in cholestatic jaundice (Neff et al., 2002) and has 20 times the antiinflammatory power of aspirin and twice that of hydrocortisone (Evans, 1991). THC is likely to avoid potential pitfalls of either COX-1

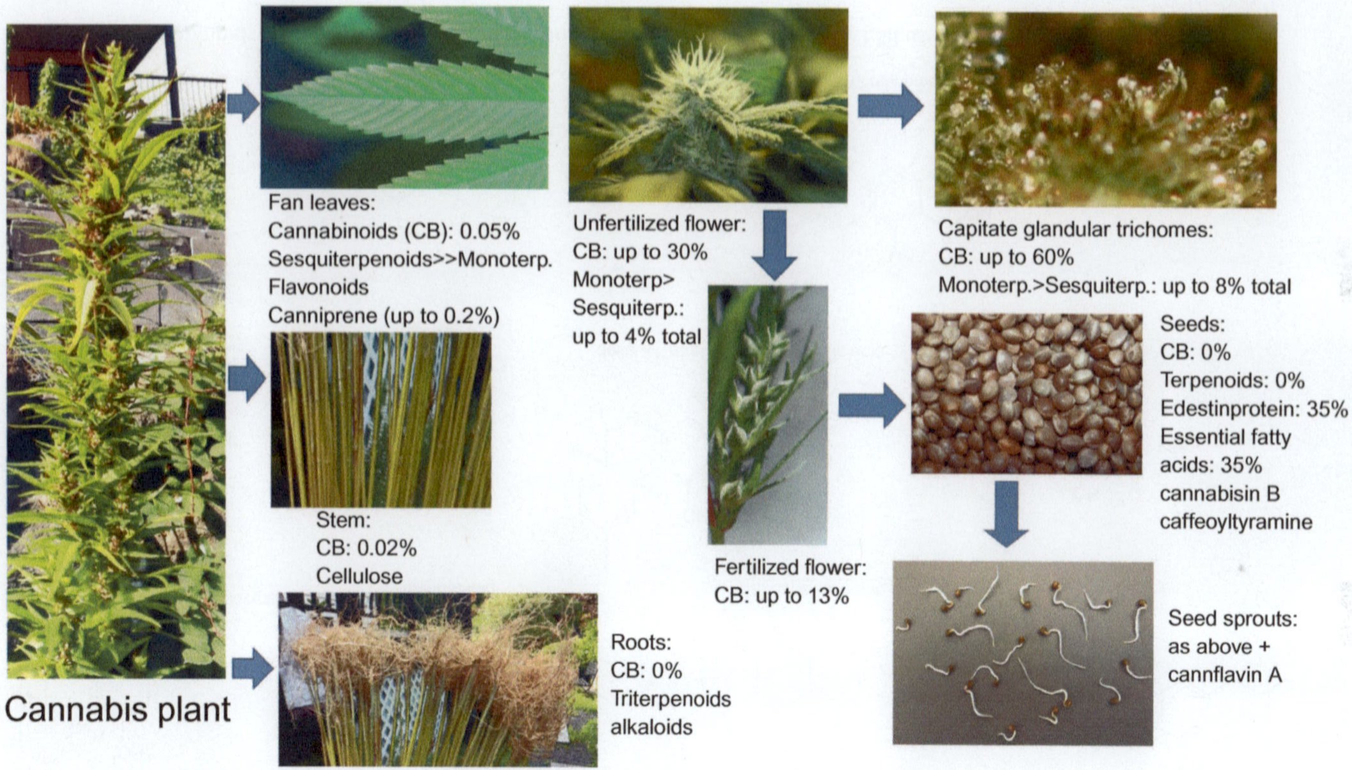
Cannabis plant
Fan leaves:
Cannabinoids (CB): 0.05%
Sesquiterpenoids>>Monoterp.
Flavonoids
Canniprene (up to 0.2%)
Stem:
CB: 0.02%
Cellulose
Roots:
CB: 0%
Triterpenoids
alkaloids
Unfertilized flower:
CB: up to 30%
Monoterp>
Sesquiterp.:
up to 4% total
Fertilized flower:
CB: up to 13%
Capitate glandular trichomes:
CB: up to 60%
Monoterp.>Sesquiterp.: up to 8% total
Seeds:
CB: 0%
Terpenoids: 0%
Edestinprotein: 35%
Essential fatty
acids: 35%
cannabisin B
caffeoyltyramine
Seed sprouts:
as above +
cannflavin A

Fig. 1 The cannabis plant, its parts, and their phytochemical components. Component percentages are based on information from Callaway (2004), (Meier & Mediavilla, 1998) and Potter (2009) (all photos by EBR).

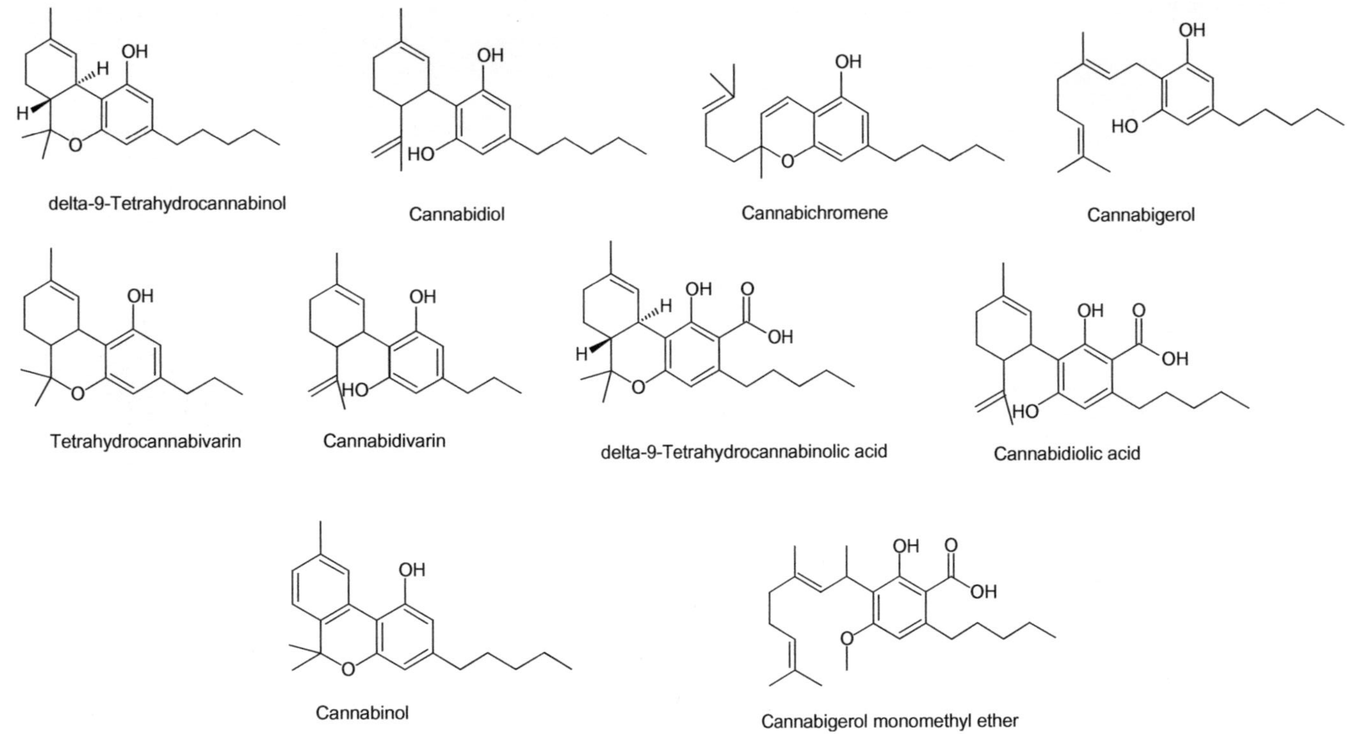

Fig. 2 Phytocannabinoids commonly encountered in cannabis (all structures drawn by EBR using ChemSketch 2015.2.5).

or COX-2 inhibition, as such activity is only noted at concentrations far above those attained therapeutically (Stott, Guy, Wright, & Whittle, 2005).

While THC stimulates both CB_1 and CB_2 receptors, the role and distribution of these two proteins is distinct. Stimulation of CB_1 receptors by THC can lead to a tetrad of effects in assays with laboratory animals; these effects include: suppression of locomotor activity, hypothermia, catalepsy (ring test), and antinociceptive effects in the tail flick test (Martin et al., 1991). CB_2 receptor stimulation is associated with pain relief and antiinflammatory activities (Pacher & Mechoulam, 2011), but it is not associated with other CB_1 effects such as appetite stimulation.

2.1.1 THC Mechanisms at CB_1 and CB_2

THC-mediated CB_1 receptor stimulation inhibits forskolin-stimulated adenylate cyclase (AC) and leads to the inhibition N-, Q-, L-type calcium channels. Ion channels can be modulated from CB_1 receptor stimulation. For example, CB_1 receptor stimulation releases G proteins to activate inwardly rectifying potassium channels, which may be induced by a variety of CB_1 partial agonists (Console-Bram, Marcu, & Abood, 2012). This receptor signaling also stimulates the activity of MAP kinases. MAP kinase pathways are often activated by GPCRs and can alter the activity of ERK1/2, c-Jun N-terminal kinase (JNK), p38 MAP kinase, and/or ERK5 proteins. The stimulation of their activity can control cell growth and their metabolism.

CB_1 localization is widespread, and the distribution parallels the known pharmacological actions of THC; the locations of CB_1 receptors make them a good therapeutic target (Herkenham et al., 1990; Pacher, 2006; Russo, 2016a). CB_1 has particularly high expression in neuronal tissue, specifically in pre- and postsynaptic neurons in the central nervous system (CNS). CB_1 protein is found in the nucleus of solitary tract (i.e., antiemetic effects), hypothalamus, motor systems, motor cortex, basal ganglia, cerebellum, spinal cord (motor neurons in spinal cord), eye, sympathetic ganglia (also enteric nervous system), immune system (bone marrow, thymus, spleen, tonsils), breast cancer cell lines, and other peripheral sites such as the heart, lungs, adrenals, kidneys, liver, colon, prostrate pancreas, testes, ovaries, and placenta.

THC-mediated CB_2 receptor stimulation leads to inhibition of forskolin-stimulated AC activation and stimulating MAP kinases but lack the effects on ion channels of CB_1. CB_2 is localized mainly in cells of the immune system, such as bone marrow, thymus, spleen, tonsils, T and B lymphocytes, monocytes, NK cells, PMN, and mast cells. The levels of CB_2 expression increase during activation/differentiation of immune cells. During inflammation or injury, the number of CB_2 receptors available for stimulation increases significantly. CB_2 is also found in tissue of the uterus, lung, bone (osteoclasts, osteoblasts, osteocytes), microglia, and brainstem neurons. CB_2 DNA mutations or polymorphisms are associated with osteoporosis in human populations, and strains of mice that are engineered without CB_2 can have accelerated age-related trabecular bone loss.

The maximal effect of THC at the CB receptor proteins is well below that of synthetic cannabinoids (i.e., nabilone, HU-210, JWH-018, etc.). Hence, THC, as well as anandamide, are classified as partial agonists because other ligands or cannabinoids exist, which are much more potent at cannabinoid receptors (Matsuda, Lolait, Brownstein, Young, & Bonner, 1990; Pacher, 2006). For example, 11-hydroxy metabolites of THC that are generated by the liver from oral administration of THC interact more efficiently at CB_1 receptors. It should also be noted that cannabinoid drugs with equal (i.e., Marinol®) or greater (i.e., nabilone) potency than THC, have been approved and available by prescription for decades, but no significant black market exists for these expensive and hard to obtain standardized preparations nor has addiction treatment been a significant issue for these cannabis-based medicines (Calhoun, Galloway, & Smith, 1998; Robson, 2011).

2.1.2 THC Activity Independent of CB_1 and CB_2

THC has been reported to interact with a wide variety of proteins including various receptors, channels, and enzymes. These pharmacological actions of THC are well documented in biochemical and mammalian research studies. Findings and research demonstrating actions of THC above 10 μM concentration are beyond the scope of this chapter as beyond this concentration, the results become difficult to interpret as far as what the physiological significance could be.

2.1.3 Receptors and Channels

At <1 μM THC can activate GPR18, GPR55, peroxisome proliferator-activated receptor gamma (PPARγ) nuclear receptors, as well as TRPA1 and TRPV2 cation channels, while enhancing the activity of non-CB receptors on sensory neurons mediating the release of calcitonin gene-related peptide (an effector in migraine attacks) and potentiating glycine-ligated ion channels (important for pain relief) (Hong & Liu, 2017). Conversely, THC blocks or antagonizes the activity of $5\text{-}HT_{3A}$ ligand-gated ion and TRPM8 cation channel at <1 μM.

Between 1 and 10 μM, THC can activate the PPARγ nuclear receptor, TRPV3 and TRPV4 cation channels, and potentiate the activity of β-adrenoceptors. THC can either block or activate GPR55 at these concentrations, depending on experimental conditions. Perhaps most relevant to current clinic and public health issues is the ability of THC to displace opiates from the μ-opioid receptor, as well as allosterically modulate the μ- and δ-opioid receptor to inhibit their activity between 1 and 10 μM (Lichtman, Sheikh, Loh, & Martin, 2001; Pertwee et al., 2010). This perhaps underlies the potential of cannabis as part of a viable solution to the opiate crisis in terms of treating addiction, withdrawal, and harnessing the benefits of cannabinoid-opiate coadministration in the clinic (Americans for Safe Access, 2016). When THC and morphine are coadministered, ¼ the dose of morphine is required to reach significant reductions in pain (Naef et al., 2003).

Conversely, THC inhibits T-type calcium (Cav3) voltage-gated ion channels, potassium Kv1.2 voltage-gated ion channels, conductance in Na^+ voltage-gated ion channels (−), and conductance in gap junctions between cells at concentrations between 1 and 10 μM. THC can also interact with a variety of enzymes such as phosphlipases, lysophosphatidylcholine acyl transferase, lipoxygenase, Na^+-K^+-ATPase, Mg^{2+}-ATPase, CYP1A1, CYP1A2, CYP1B1, CYP2B6, CYP2C9, and monoamine oxidase activity (Evans, 1991; Pertwee, 1988; Pertwee & Cascio, 2014; Yamaori et al., 2012; Yamaori, Kushihara, Yamamoto, & Watanabe, 2010; Yamaori, Okamoto, Yamamoto, & Watanabe, 2011). The synaptic conversion of tyrosine to noradrenaline and dopamine (DA) is increased by THC while norepinephrine-induced melatonin biosynthesis is inhibited.

Recently, THC has shown significant benefits in helping to reduce complications during organ transplant and in graft-vs-host-disease (GVHD) in mammals. The research on THC in GVHD and transplant has already affected public policy in California, where cannabis use no longer constitutes grounds for being dismissed from transplant waiting list. The perceived pharmacological effects of THC may also be dependent on diet of the mammal (Balvers et al., 2012; Lafourcade et al., 2011; Lowette, Roosen, Tack, & Berghe, 2015), due to the fact that anandamide and endocannabinoids are derived in vivo from omega-3 and -6 fatty acid intake and their dietary deficiency could lead to uncoupling of G protein-coupled receptors.

2.2 Cannabidiol

The main nonintoxicating phytocannabinoids are cannabidiol (CBD) and its acidic precursor cannabidiolic acid. These are the most abundant phytocannabinoids in European hemp (Upton et al., 2013). CBD has a very low affinity for CB receptors but may have significant CB_1- and

CB_2-independent mechanisms of action and possess the unique ability to antagonize CB_1 at very low concentrations when in the presence of THC (Thomas et al., 2007). This observed antagonism may be related to CBD's ability to act as a negative allosteric modulator at CB_1 receptors (Laprairie, Bagher, Kelly, & Denovan-Wright, 2015).

CBD is reported to be an agonist at TRPV1 (Bisogno et al., 2001) and 5-HT_{1A} receptors (Russo, Burnett, Hall, & Parker, 2005) and to enhance adenosine receptor signaling (Carrier, Auchampach, & Hillard, 2006). Exceptional tolerability of CBD in humans has been demonstrated (Mechoulam, Parker, & Gallily, 2002). CBD can produce a wide range of pharmacological activity including anticonvulsive, antiinflammatory, antioxidant, and antipsychotic effects. These effects underlie the neuroprotective properties of CBD and support its role in the treatment of a number of neurological and neurodegenerative disorders, including epilepsy, Parkinson disease, amyotrophic lateral sclerosis, Huntington disease, Alzheimer disease, and multiple sclerosis (de Lago & Fernández-Ruiz, 2007; Hofmann & Frazier, 2013; Martin-Moreno et al., 2011; Scuderi et al., 2009).

CBD possesses the unique ability to counteract the intoxicating and adverse effects of cannabis, such as anxiety, tachycardia, hunger, and sedation in rats and humans (Murillo-Rodriguez, Millan-Aldaco, Palomero-Rivero, Mechoulam, & Drucker-Colin, 2006; Nicholson, Turner, Stone, & Robson, 2004; Russo, 2011; Russo & Guy, 2006). The benefits of CBD include reducing the unwanted side effects of THC, a dynamic pharmacological effect that has been fairly well studied in clinical trials. CBD is included in a specific ratio of 1:1 in the medicinal cannabis preparation and licensed pharmaceutical known as Sativex®, which has been studied in numerous properly controlled clinical trials representing thousands of patient/years of data (Flachenecker, Henze, & Zettl, 2014; Rog, Nurmiko, Friede, & Young, 2005; Sastre-Garriga, Vila, Clissold, & Montalban, 2011; Wade, Collin, Stott, & Duncombe, 2010).

Recently, CBD demonstrated its strong antiinflammatory and immunosuppressive properties in a phase II study on GVHD (Yeshurun et al., 2015). CBD (300 mg/day) starting a week before the procedure was associated with less mortality and complications.

There is recent report that CBD isomerizes to THC under acidic conditions in vitro, but there is no evidence that directly supports that this is actually occurring in humans (Deiana et al., 2012; Grotenhermen, Russo, & Zuardi, 2017; Russo, 2017).

2.3 Cannabigerol

This compound was purified from cannabis the same year as THC (Gaoni & Mechoulam, 1964), but cannabigerol (CBG) lacks its psychotropic effects (Grunfeld & Gresty, 1998; Grunfeld & Edery, 1969). Normally, CBG appears as a relatively low concentration intermediate in the plant, but recent breeding work has yielded cannabis chemotypes lacking in downstream enzymes that express 100% of their phytocannabinoid content as CBG (de Meijer & Hammond, 2005; de Meijer, Hammond, & Micheler, 2009). CBG, the parent phytocannabinoid compound, has a relatively weak partial agonistic effect at CB_1 (K_i 440 nM) and CB_2 (K_i 337 nM) (Gauson et al., 2007).

CBG may stimulate a range of receptors important for pain, inflammation, and heat sensitization. This compound can antagonize TRPV8 receptors and stimulates TRPV1, TRPV2, TRPA1, TRPV3, TRPV4, and α2-adrenoceptor activity (Cascio, Gauson, Stevenson, Ross, & Pertwee, 2010; De Petrocellis & Di Marzo, 2010; De Petrocellis et al., 2011). It is a relatively potent TRPM8 antagonist for possible application in prostate cancer and detrusor overactivity and bladder pain (De Petrocellis & Di Marzo, 2010; Mukerji et al., 2006). CBG can also antagonize the stimulation of serotonin 5-HT_{1A} and CB_1 receptors with significant efficiency. Older work supports gamma aminobutyric acid (GABA) uptake inhibition greater than THC or CBD that could suggest muscle relaxant properties (Banerjee, Snyder, & Mechoulam, 1975).

Analgesic and antierythemic effects and the ability to block lipooxygenase were said to surpass those of THC (Evans, 1991). CBG demonstrated modest antifungal effects (ElSohly, Turner, Clark, & Eisohly, 1982). CBG has remarkable anticancer properties in basic research models, it has proved to be an effective cytotoxic in high dosage on human epithelioid carcinoma and is one of the more effective phytocannabinoids against breast cancer (Baek et al., 1998; Ligresti et al., 2006). CBG has significant antidepressant effects in the rodent tail suspension model and is a mildly antihypertensive agent (Maor, Gallily, & Mechoulam, 2006; Musty & Deyo, 2006). Additionally, CBG inhibits keratinocyte proliferation suggesting utility in psoriasis (Wilkinson & Williamson, 2007).

CBG is a strong AEA uptake inhibitor and a powerful agent against MRSA (methicillin-resistant *Staphylococcus aureus*) (Appendino et al., 2008; De Petrocellis et al., 2011). Finally, CBG behaves as a potent α2-adrenoreceptor agonist, supporting analgesic effects previously noted, and moderate 5-HT_{1A} antagonist suggesting antidepressant properties (Cascio et al., 2010; Formukong, Evans, & Evans, 1988).

2.4 Cannabichromene

Cannabichromene (CBC) was first reported to be isolated by two groups, using either a hexane/florisil extraction method from hashish or a benzene percolation of hemp (Claussen, Von Spulak, & Korte, 1966; Gaoni & Mechoulam, 1966). This cannabinoid represents ~0.3% of constituents from confiscated cannabis, and it is important to note that varieties and preparations exist in the commercial and medical markets with significantly higher content (de Meijer & Limited, 2011; Mehmedic et al., 2010; Meijer, Hammond, & Micheler, 2008; Swift, Wong, Li, Arnold, & McGregor, 2013). CBC-rich cannabis strains are the result of selecting for the inheritance of a recessive gene, achievable through extensive cross-breeding. CBC or CBC-like derivatives have also been found in *Rhododendron anthopogonoides*, at the time of this writing, this species and its extracts are not listed under the list of scheduled drugs by the DEA (Iwata & Kitanaka, 2011).

CBC can interact with transient receptor potential (TRP) cation channels that inhibit endocannabinoid inactivation, and stimulate CB_2 receptors ($K_i \sim 100$ nm), but it does not have significant activity at CB_1 receptors ($K_i > 1$ μM) (De Petrocellis et al., 2011, 2012, 2008; Shinjyo & Di Marzo, 2013). TRP channels and the ECS are involved in inflammation and have a role in pain. In mice, CBC can relieve pain, potentiate the analgesic effects of THC, ameliorate-induced colonic inflammation, and paw edema by demonstrably inhibiting macrophage and MAGL activity (Cascio & Pertwee, 2014; Davis & Hatoum, 1983; Maione et al., 2011).

The mechanism underlying CBC's observed effects in mammals is supported by pharmacodynamic studies (De Petrocellis et al., 2008; Ligresti et al., 2006; Romano et al., 2013). These have shown that CBC can stimulate TRP ankyrin-type 1 (TRPA1) cation channels ($EC_{50} = 90$ nM), and desensitize these channels ($IC_{50} = 370$ nM). Further evidence for the role of CBC in inflammation includes the compounds ability to interact with TRPV4 and TRPV3 cation channels ($EC_{50} = 600$ nM and 1.9 μM, respectively), and desensitize TRPV2 and TRPV4 ($IC_{50} = 6.5$ and 9.9 μM, respectively) (Cascio & Pertwee, 2014; De Petrocellis et al., 2012). Beyond inflammation and pain, CBC may have a positive effect on the viability of mammalian adult neural stem cell progenitor cells, which are an essential component of brain function in health and disease (Shinjyo & Di Marzo, 2013).

In summary, CBC can be one of the most abundant nonintoxicating CBs found in cannabis, due to a recessive gene (Brown & Harvey, 1990; Holley, Hadley, & Turner, 1975). CBC can cause strong antiinflammatory effects in animal models of edema through non-CB receptor mechanisms (DeLong, Wolf, Poklis, & Lichtman, 2010). CBC has been shown to significantly interact with TRP cation channels, including TRPA1, TRPV1–4, and TRPV8 (Pertwee & Cascio, 2014). CBC can also produce behavioral activity of the cannabinoid tetrad. The effects of CBC, particularly nociception in animal models, can be augmented for additive results when THC is co-administered.

2.5 Cannabinol

Cannabinol (CBN) is the nonenzymatic oxidation byproduct of THC and is most commonly an artifact found after prolonged storage, especially at higher temperatures. CBN was the first cannabinoid to be identified and isolated from cannabis (Wood, Spivey, & Easterfield, 1899). This discovery was most likely due to rampant degradation of THC to CBN due to poor quality control, the transportation and storage conditions related to the 19th century; challenges that are still difficult to overcome in existing cannabis products (Upton et al., 2013).

Relative to THC, CBN maintains about ¼ the potency (K_i at $CB_1=211.2$ nM, $CB_2=126.4$ nM) (Rhee et al., 1997). CBN can be sedative, anticonvulsant in animal and human studies, and has demonstrated significant properties related to antiinflammatory, antibiotic, and anti-MRSA activity (minimum inhibitory concentration (MIC) 11 μg/mL) (Appendino et al., 2008; Evans, 2007; McPartland & Russo, 2001; Musty, Karniol, Shirikawa, Takahashi, & Knobel, 1976; Turner, Elsohly, & Boeren, 1980).

CBN has potential as a component in topical applications, inhibiting keratinocyte proliferation (low micromolar) via CBR-independent mechanisms, suggesting utility in psoriasis (Wilkinson & Williamson, 2007). Beyond cannabinoid proteins, the compound has TRPV2 (high-threshold thermosensor) agonistic effects (EC_{50} 77.7 μM), which are of interest in possible topical applications in treating burns (Qin et al., 2008; Russo, 2014). A review of phytocannabinoids summarized the ability of CBN to inhibit the activity of a number of enzymes, including cyclooxygenase, lipoxygenase, and a host of cytochrome P450 (CYP) enzymes (e.g., CYP1A1, CYP1A2, CYP2B6, CYP2C9, CYP3A4, CYP3A5, CYP2A6, CYP2D6, CYP1B1, and CYP3A7) (Pertwee & Cascio, 2014). CBN may also stimulate the activity of phospholipases. CBN additionally stimulates recruitment of quiescent mesenchymal stem cells in marrow (10 μM) promoting bone formation (Scutt & Williamson, 2007) and can affect breast cancer resistance proteins (IC_{50} approximately 145 μM) (Holland, Allen, & Arnold, 2008).

2.6 Tetrahydrocannabivarin

Tetrahydrocannabivarin (THCV) is a propyl analogue of THC most often encountered in low concentration in dried plant material, but in THCV-rich plants up to 16% THCV by dry weight has been recorded (Meijer & Hammond, 2005). Mechanistically speaking, THCV can behave as both an agonist and an antagonist at CB_1 receptors depending on the concentration (Pertwee, 2008). THCV produces weight loss, and decreases body fat and serum leptin concentrations with increased energy expenditure in obese mice (Cawthorne, Wargent, Zaibi, Stott, & Wright, 2007; Riedel et al., 2009). THCV also demonstrates prominent anticonvulsant properties in rodent cerebellum and pyriform cortex (Hill et al., 2010). THCV appears as a fractional component of many southern African cannabis chemotypes, although plants highly predominant in this agent have been produced (de Meijer et al., 2003; de Meijer & Hammond, 2016). THCV has the CB_2-based ability to suppress carageenan-induced hyperalgesia and inflammation, and both phases of formalin-induced pain behavior via CB_1 and CB_2 in mice (Bolognini et al., 2010).

Antagonizing CB_1 receptors can suppress appetite and the intoxicating effects of THC. However, caution must be emphasized when developing CB_1 receptor antagonists. Clinical studies in human populations studying the antagonists of CB_1 receptors with the drug rimonabant (SR141716A) led to depressive episodes and potentially worsened neurodegenerative disease outcomes, and ultimately this drug was withdrawn from the market (McLaughlin, 2012). Despite this setback, SR141716A remains a very important research tool for unlocking potential medical treatments targeting the CB receptors and deepening the understanding of the ECS. Importantly, the neutral antagonism mechanism of action of THCV seems to be free of the adverse events associated with the CB_1 inverse agonists (McPartland, Duncan, Di Marzo, & Pertwee, 2015).

2.7 Tetrahydrocannabinolic Acid

Cannabinoid acids are found as primary metabolites in cannabis plants. For example, tetrahydrocannabinol acid (THCA-A) is synthesized in glandular trichomes of the cannabis plant and forms THC after the parent compound is decarboxylated by UV exposure, prolonged storage, or heat (Moreno-Sanz, 2016). THCA-A can represent up to 90% of total THC content in the plant, it has about 70% conversion rate into THC when smoked (Dussy, Hamberg, Luginbuhl, Schwerzmann, & Briellmann, 2005): decarboxylation of THCA to THC is incomplete even at high temperatures in gas chromatography. Additionally, THCA can be detected in serum, urine, and oral fluid of cannabis consumers up to 8 h after smoking (Jung, Kempf, Mahler, & Weinmann, 2007). The cannabinoid acids do not produce any significant or documented psychotropic effects. THCA-A is the immediate natural precursors of THC. THCA-A is one the primary phytocannabinoid metabolites and can cause apoptosis of insect cells (Sirikantaramas et al., 2004).

THCA-A is reported to be a weak agonist of CB_1 and CB_2 receptors compared with THC (K_i CB1 = 630 vs 3.5 nM; K_i CB_2 = 890 vs 3.2 nM) (Verhoeckx et al., 2006). In other laboratories, THCA-A effectively bound to both cannabinoid receptors, displaying a higher affinity for CB_1, with K_i values of 23.51–3.5 and 56.13–8.2 nM, respectively. In fact, THCA-A (log $IC_{50} = 1.793 \pm 0.00$) and THC (log $IC_{50} = 1.941–0.01$) displaced CP-55,940 from CB_1 in a similar range of concentrations (Rosenthaler et al., 2014).

THCA-A attenuated nausea-induced gaping in rats and vomiting in shrews through a mechanism that required CB_1 activation, which is reversible with a CB_1 receptor antagonist (Rock, Kopstick, Limebeer, & Parker, 2013). The authors provide additional evidence that this observed effect of THCA-A is not due to the conversion of THCA-A to THC. The effects of THCA-A appear to be partially mediated through cannabinoid receptors, without any reported psychotropic effects associated with THC. The evidence suggests that THCA-A is restricted to the periphery with limited access to the CNS through the blood brain barrier (BBB). This is probably due the presence of a carboxylic acid on THCA-A; such polar residues decrease CNS penetration through the ATP-binding cassette family of transporters (Moreno-Sanz et al., 2013). In fact, brain disposition has been reported for several cannabinoids, but not THCA-A (Alozie, Martin, Harris, & Dewey, 1980; Deiana et al., 2012).

THCA-A can inhibit the release of tumor necrosis factor-alpha (TNF-α) (Verhoeckx et al., 2006), can efficiently interact with TRPM8 channels and can stimulate or desensitize a range of other TRP cation channels. THCA-A has been found to inhibit enzymes responsible for the breakdown of endocannabinoids, as well as COX-1 and -2, thus stimulating the ECS by increasing levels of endogenous cannabinoids. In a basic model of Parkinson's disease, THCA-A (10 μM) increased cell survival and significantly ameliorated altered neurite morphology (Moldzio et al., 2012). THCA-A reduces cell viability of various cancer cell lines when administered in vitro (Moreno-Sanz, 2016). Basic research has conclusively shown that THCA-A can have immunomodulatory, antiinflammatory, neuroprotective and antineoplastic activity.

2.8 Cannabidivarin

Cannabidivarin (CBDV) was probably first reported in a benzene extract from a Thai cannabis variety referred to as "Meao" (Shoyama, Hirano, Makino, Umekita, & Nishioka, 1977). Oral CBDV (60 mg/kg) administered to rats can cross the BBB (Deiana et al., 2012). CBDV is capable of activating and blocking, depending on experimental conditions, a diverse number of cation channels. At less than <1 μM TRPA1, TRPM8, and TRPV4 are influenced by CBDV, while around 1–10 μM affects the activity of TRVP1, TRVP2, and TRVP3 cation channels. In addition to cationic influences, this propyl analogue of CBD engages the ECS by inhibiting endocannabinoid degradation at 10 μM through modulating the rate of diacylglycerol lipase activity and *N*-acylethanolamine-hydrolyzing acid amidase (NAAA), the effects of which could magnified with CBDV's ability to inhibit the cellular uptake of anandamide (Pertwee & Cascio, 2014). CBDV also possess the potential for the treatment of nausea and vomiting (Rock, Sticht, & Parker, 2014). There is strong evidence that CBDV has significant anticonvulsant properties, which may rival CBD's therapeutic potential in treating epilepsy, particularly seizures of partial onset (focal seizures) (Williams, Jones, & Whalley, 2014).

2.9 Cannabidiolic Acid

Cannabidiolic acid (CBDA) is the natural precursor or CBD, and this acidic phytocannabinoid can target GPR55, TRPA1, TRPV1, and TRPM8 at concentrations between 1 and 10 μM. At higher concentrations, the compound can inhibit ECS degradation enzymes. CBDA can inhibit by COX-1 and COX-2 (Takeda, Misawa, Yamamoto, & Watanabe, 2008). CBDA also shares CBD's ability to enhance 5-HT_{1A} receptor activation but the acidic compound does not interact efficiency with CB_1 receptors as either an agonist or antagonist (Bolognini et al., 2013; McPartland et al., 2015). The affinity at 5-HT_{1A} for CBDA is greater than an order of magnitude higher compared to CBD. Evidence from animals demonstrates significant antiemetic effects from CBDA (10 or 200 mg/kg ip) (Moreno-Sanz, 2016; Rock & Parker, 2015).

2.10 Cannabigerol Monomethyl Ether

This phytocannabinoid is commonly encountered in cannabis, but has not been researched for pharmacological activity. It is included here to highlight that its presence with relative frequency supports its investigation as a research priority.

3. CANNABIS TERPENOIDS

Terpenoids are aromatic compounds that fulfill unique ecological roles for plants in protection from predation, attraction of pollinators, and myriad other roles (Elzinga, Fischedick, Podkolinski, & Raber, 2015; Fischedick, Hazekamp, Erkelens, Choi & Verpoorte, 2010; McPartland & Russo, 2001, 2014; Russo, 2011). Two excellent general references are Baser and Buchbauer (2016) and Langenheim (1994). They are typically produced in dedicated structures, which in the case of cannabis are the glandular trichomes, the same source of phytocannabinoid production (Potter, 2009). Typically, many are produced by a given plant and form its essential oil (EO). In cannabis, the biochemical diversity of these components is remarkable, with as many as 200 described, although some are artifacts of steam distillation (Lawless, 1995). The biochemical profile of terpenoids in a given plant is more genetically than environmentally determined (Franz & Novak, 2010).

Whereas, the biosynthetic enzymes for phytocannabinoids have been identified for several years, it was only recently that several terpenoid synthases were analyzed in cannabis (Booth, Page & Bohlmann, 2017). Regulation of terpenoid and cannabinoid production in the plant remain important research priorities.

A great deal of debate has surrounded the relative importance, or lack thereof, of cannabis terpenoids to the pharmacological effects of the plant. Despite existing at seemingly low concentrations in a preparation, they have proven to be potent: small amounts in ambient air produce marked behavioral effects to increase or decrease activity levels in rodents, even when observed serum levels are low or negligible (Buchbauer, Jirovetz, Jager, Plank & Dietrich, 1993). Their physiological mechanisms are protean particularly in the CNS, attributable to their lipophilicity, and include effects on ion channels, neurotransmitter, odorant, and tastant receptors, among others (Buchbauer, 2010). Terpenoids, particularly monoterpenoids, are highly bioavailable via inhalation (Falk, Hagberg, Lof, Wigaeus-Hjelm, & Wang, 1990; Falk, Lof, Hagberg, Hjelm, & Wang, 1991; Falk-Filipsson, Lof, Hagberg, Hjelm, & Wang, 1993).

Terpenoid concentrations in cannabis flowers were previously commonly reported in the 1% range, but up to 10% within trichomes (Potter, 2009), but this situation has changed due to selective breeding, such that flower concentrations of 3.5% (Fischedick, Hazekamp, et al., 2010) or even higher in modern chemovars are now encountered.

Many have argued that cannabis is primarily a botanical delivery device for THC, while others have espoused a more holistic assessment (see McPartland, Guy, & Di Marzo, 2014; Russo, 2011 for a broader discussion). Certainly, medical consumers must fall into the latter group, as sales figures for herbal cannabis overwhelm those for THC (Marinol®) as a pure compound. Sativex®, a standardized oromucosal whole cannabis extract that is now approved as a prescription in 29 countries, was purposely designed to incorporate terpenoids, which comprise 6%–7% of total cannabinoid (Guy & Stott, 2005).

While controlled double-blind trials exploring cannabinoid–terpenoid interactions have yet to take place and are sorely required, observational information has been offered: limonene added to THC enhanced the experience to be more "cerebral and euphoric," while myrcene rendered THC more "physical, mellow, sleepy." The three together were considered more "cannabimimetic" than THC alone (Name Withheld, 2006), THC taken in isolation being more dysphoric than euphoric (Calhoun et al., 1998), and displaying a much narrower therapeutic index than whole cannabis (Russo, 2011; Sellers et al., 2013). Clinical trial data comparing rates of adverse events also favor cannabis extracts over THC (Russo, 2013).

While the following will summarize prior publications, emphasis will be placed on newer findings and agents not previously examined in relation to cannabis pharmacology. Unless otherwise indicated, all the agents are Generally Recognized As Safe (GRAS) by the US Food and Drug Administration (FDA) and/or are approved as food additives by the Flavor and Extract Manufacturers' Association (FEMA). According to a recent publication (Giese, Lewis, Giese, & Smith, 2015), 50 cannabis terpenes are routinely encountered in North American chemovars, but 17 are most common, all of which are discussed herein. Of these, several predominate to form eight "Terpene Super Classes": myrcene, terpinolene, ocimene, limonene, α-pinene, humulene, linalool, and β-caryophyllene (BCP).

Similarly, Fischedick (2017) analyzed cannabis samples from a single California cannabis dispensary over the course of a year, and identified five terpenoid groups based on predominant content: myrcene, terpinolene, myrcene/limonene, caryophyllene, and bisabolol.

4. CANNABIS MONOTERPENOIDS (FIG. 3)

4.1 β-Myrcene

β-Myrcene is the most prevalent terpene in modern cannabis chemovars in the United States (Giese et al., 2015) and in Europe (Hazekamp, Tejkalová, & Papadimitriou, 2016), and is likely most responsible for

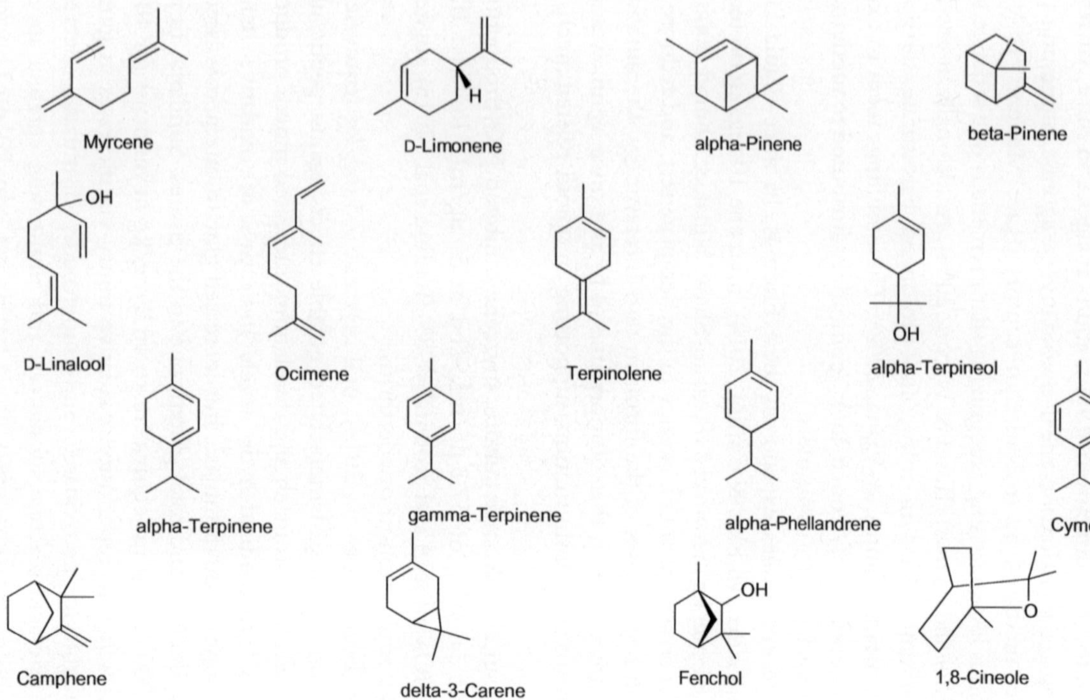

Fig. 3 Monoterpenoids commonly encountered in cannabis (all structures drawn by EBR using ChemSketch 2015.2.5).

sedative effects of many of the common preparations in commerce. As previously reviewed (Russo, 2011), myrcene is antiinflammatory via prostaglandin E-2 (PGE-2) (Lorenzetti, Souza, Sarti, Santos Filho, & Ferreira, 1991), blocks carcinogenic effects of aflatoxin in the liver (De-Oliveira, Ribeiro-Pinto, & Paumgartten, 1997), and is analgesic in mice, an activity that is abrogated by naloxone, the μ-opioid inverse agonist, suggesting a narcotic effect mediated by α-2 adrenoreceptors (Rao, Menezes, & Viana, 1990). This is less surprising recognizing that myrcene is one sedative agent of hops (*Humulus lupulus*) (Bisset & Wichtl, 2004). Additionally, it produces muscle relaxant effects in mice, and prolonged barbiturate sleep time (do Vale, Furtado, Santos, & Viana, 2002). These findings seem to explain the phenomenology of "couch-lock" commonly attributed to modern cannabis chemovars by its consumers.

More recent studies expand on these findings. In mice (Paula-Freire, Andersen, Gama, Molska, & Carlini, 2014), myrcene 10 mg/kg po (equivalent to 0.81 mg/kg in humans) (Reagan-Shaw, Nihal, & Ahmad, 2008) significantly increased paw lick latency in the hot-plate test, and reduced pain behavior in both phases of the formalin test. Interestingly, the duration of analgesic effect exceeds that of morphine (4 h) and once again, was abrogated by naloxone administration, supporting an opioid-related mechanism of action.

In human chondrocyte culture, myrcene inhibited NO production by IL-1β with an IC_{50} of 37.3 μg/mL, and at 50 μg/mL, lowered IL-1β-induced iNOS mRNA and protein by 78% (Rufino et al., 2015), suggesting therapeutic application in osteoarthritis.

In rats (Bonamin et al., 2014), oral myrcene 7.5 mg/kg (equivalent to 1.2 mg/kg in humans) demonstrated notable effects against peptic ulcers: decreased lesions in stomach and duodenum, increased mucus production, and mucosal malondialdehyde levels indicative of oxidative damage, decreased superoxide dismutase, but increased glutathione peroxidase, glutathione reductase, and total glutathione in the tissues. Similarly, in mice, myrcene 200 mg/kg ip (equivalent to 16.2 mg/kg in humans) for 10 days prevented ischemic/reperfusion oxidative injury via increases in glutathione, glutathione peroxidase, and superoxide dismutase, decreasing thiobarbituric acid reactive substances, and eliminating cerebral apoptosis and other histological changes (Ciftci, Oztanir, & Cetin, 2014). This activity suggests the possibility of synergistic benefits with the neuroprotective antioxidant effects of THC and CBD (Hampson et al., 1998; Lafuente et al., 2011).

4.2 D-Limonene

Limonene is a cyclic monoterpene common to citrus rinds and is common in nature, though more sporadically encountered in contemporary cannabis. It displays high bioavailability with 70% absorption after human pulmonary administration (Falk-Filipsson et al., 1993), is rapidly metabolized (Falk-Filipsson et al., 1993), but accumulates in adipose tissues and the brain, with an estimated human lethal dose of 0.5–5 g/kg. It is nonsensitizing (Von Burg, 1995).

Limonene is the parent compound to the entire family of monoterpenoids in the plant, and its biosynthetic enzyme, limonene synthase and others in cannabis are promiscuous in their substrates with various terpenoid end-products (Booth et al., 2017), via regulatory mechanisms that remain to be elucidated. Experiments in mice confirm limonene to be strongly anxiolytic, boosting serotonin levels in prefrontal cortex, and dopamine in hippocampus mediated via 5-HT_{1A} receptors (Carvalho-Freitas & Costa, 2002; Komiya, Takeuchi, & Harada, 2006; Pultrini Ade, Galindo, & Costa, 2006). Orange terpenes, primarily limonene, boosted mouse motility after inhalation by 35.25%, while decreasing activity after caffeine 33.19% (Buchbauer et al., 1993). Human clinical work supports these activities, as a study in Japan (Komori, Fujiwara, Tanida, Nomura, & Yokoyama, 1995), demonstrated that depressed patients exposed to citrus scent experienced normalization of Hamilton Depression Scores (HADS), allowing discontinuation of antidepressants in 9/12 hospitalized patients. Additionally, immune stimulation (CD4/8 ratio normalization) was documented. Limonene has an impressively supportive history as an "antidote" to excessive psychoactive adverse events produced by THC (Russo, 2011).

Limonene demonstrated prominent antibiotic effects vs *S. aureus* and *Pseudomonas aeruginosa* (Onawunmi, Yisak, & Ogunlana, 1984). Recently, concentrations of 400 μg/mL inhibited biofilm formation of the pathogen *Streptococcus pyogenes* SF370 and *S. nutans*, which produces dental caries, downregulating various genes mediating surface-associated proteins (Subramenium, Vijayakumar, & Pandian, 2015). Considering that cannabinoids also interfere with quorum-sensing in biofilm formation (Soni, Smoum, Breuer, Mechoulam, & Steinberg, 2015), cannabinoid/terpenoid synergy in this mechanism of action is certainly likely.

Citrus EOs were an effective treatment against dermatophytes (Sanguinetti et al., 2007; Singh et al., 2010), and display radical scavenging abilities (Choi, Song, Ukeda, & Sawamura, 2000). Two citrus EOs also suppressed *Propionibacterium acnes*, the pathogen in acne (MIC 0.31 μL/mL), more powerfully than triclosan (Kim et al., 2008), while simultaneously lowering TNF-α production.

Limonene also demonstrates chemotherapeutic properties, inducing apoptosis of breast cancer cells among others. It was utilized in high doses in Phase II RCTs (Vigushin et al., 1998), with good safety, but less impressive efficacy. A more recent study in humans demonstrated that, in women with preoperative breast cancer, an oral intake of 2 g of D-limonene a day produced a mean concentration of 41.3 μg/g of biopsy breast tissue, and reduced cyclin D1 expression that could lead to cell-cycle arrest and decreased proliferation (Miller et al., 2013).

A blood orange (*Citrus sinensis*) volatile emulsion that was 95.35% D-limonene at 100 ppm induced apoptosis in Bcl-2 human colon cancer cells, activating p38 and inhibiting Akt, and inhibited the angiogenesis marker, vascular endothelial growth factor 80%, decreased cell migration, downregulated MMP-9 expression, and reduced tube formation (Chidambara Murthy, Jayaprakasha, & Patil, 2012). Limonene's primary metabolite, perillic acid, also has cytotoxic effects, and additionally produces antianxiety effects in rat brain (Fukumoto et al., 2008).

A patent has been filed based on the ability of limonene to ameliorate gastro-esophageal reflux (Harris, 2010) and a commercial capsule preparation is available.

Limonene 10 mg/kg po reduced hyperalgesia in mice induced by intrathecal administration of HIV glycoprotein toxin gp120, as well as prevented increases in IL-1β and IL-10 levels (Piccinelli et al., 2017). Mechanical sensitivity induced by TNF-α, was prevented, as was IL-1β cold sensitivity.

Limonene 10 mg/kg po reduced inflammation scores, weight loss, and TNF-α in ibuprofen-induced rat colitis, as well as decreased peripheral IL-6 inflammatory marker in elderly humans receiving a daily supplement that was 95% limonene for 56 days (d'Alessio et al., 2013).

At high concentrations, limonene prevented oxidative damage in human lens epithelial cells via regulation of caspase-3 and -9, Bax, and Bcl-2, as well as inhibition of p38 MAPK phosphorylation (Bai, Zheng, Wang, & Liu, 2016), suggesting therapeutic use to prevent cataracts.

Limonene is an agonist at A_{2A} adenosine receptors (Park, Lee, Yaoyao, Jun, & Lee, 2011) and could synergize activity with both THC (direct activator) and CBD (uptake inhibitor via competition for the nucleotide binding site of the ENT1 transporter) (Carrier et al., 2006), a relationship that is now the subject of active research.

Limonene 50 μM increased mitochondrial biogenesis, activated the AMPK energy regulator, increased brown adipocyte markers PGC-1α

UCP1, and induced "browning" of 3T3-L1 adipocytes by activating β-3-AR and ERK signaling pathway (Lone & Yun, 2016), suggesting a putative role in obesity treatment. Certainly, interesting synergies are possible with the anorexic effects of CBD and THCV (McPartland et al., 2015), and modulatory effects of THC on weight and microbiome balance (Cluny, Keenan, Reimer, Le Foll, & Sharkey, 2015).

4.3 β-Ocimene

Ocimene is one of the most common monoterpenes found in nature. In the field of botanical medicine, there is an association of β-ocimene in EOs with anticonvulsant activity, antifungal activity, antitumor activity, and pest resistance (Bomfim et al., 2016; Cascone et al., 2015; Sayyah, Nadjafnia, & Kamalinejad, 2004). Ocimene is also a volatile pheromone important for the social regulation of honeybee colonies. The commercial applications of exploiting that attraction to produce "cannabis honey" have not been missed by the cannabis industry emerging in the United States, and subsequently by law enforcement agencies to detect illicit drugs by "trained honeybees," which were proposed to replace sniffer dogs in 2015 (Kennell, 2016; Maisonnasse, Lenoir, Beslay, Crauser, & Le Conte, 2010; Schott, Klein, & Vilcinskas, 2015).

Significant ocimene content is being reported by medical cannabis laboratories in California and Washington State (Elzinga et al., 2015). Ocimene is also a major component of the EO of cannabis varieties developed by the international medical cannabis producer, Bedrocan, which supplies standardized cannabis to pharmacies in Europe (Fischedick, Van Der Kooy, & Verpoorte, 2010). The effects and associations of cannabinoid and ocimene co-administration remain unclear but warrant further attention.

4.4 γ-Terpinene

This cyclic monoterpene is common to *Eucalyptus* spp., and to EO of cumin (*Cuminum cyminum*, 32%), whereas it is a minor component in cannabis. In mice, oral pretreatment with of 25–50 mg/kg (equivalent to 2–4 mg/kg human) inhibited extravasation of fluid in an acetic acid microvascular permeability model, reduced peritonitis after carageenan, neutrophil migration, and production of interleukin-1β and TNF-α vs controls, as well as lung inflammation after acute injury, thus demonstrating broad antiinflammatory effects (Ramalho, Pacheco de Oliveira, Lima, Bezerra-Santos, & Piuvezam, 2015). γ-Terpinene demonstrated little antioxidant or antiproliferative activity in a recent experiment (Fitsiou et al., 2016).

4.5 α-Terpinene

A major component of tea tree oil (*Melaleuca alternifolia*, 13%) it is found in low concentrations in cannabis. It inhibited oxidation of LDL and linoleic acid and was potent as a scavenger of DPPH radicals (Tisserand & Young, 2014). It demonstrated modest activity as a synergist to diminazene aceturate in treatment of *Trypanasoma evansi*, a protozoal pathogen of horses and other animals (Baldissera et al., 2016).

4.6 α-Terpineol

Terpineol is a cyclic monoterpenoid alcohol (Bhatia, Letizia, & Api, 2008). Its inhalation diminished mouse motility 45% (Buchbauer et al., 1993). It displayed dose-dependent antibiotic efficacy vs *S. aureus*, *S. epidermidis*, and *P. acnes* (Raman, Weir, & Bloomfield, 1995), among others, particularly in its customary vehicle of tea tree oil (*M. alternifolia*) (Carson & Riley, 1995). An MIC of 0.78 μL/mL was noted on *Escherichia coli*, with observed cell wall and membrane rupture (Li et al., 2014). α-Terpineol 100 μg/disk produced significant zones of inhibition in culture of four drug-resistant *Helicobacter pylori* cultures (Miyamoto, Okimoto, & Kuwano, 2014). Moderate effects against two strains of *Plasmodium falciparum* malaria were noted in an EO with major terpineol component (Campbell, Gammon, Smith, Abrahams, & Purves, 1997).

The small cell lung cancer cell line NCI-H69 was sensitive to α-terpineol at a high dose (IC_{50} approximately 260 μM) via suppression of NF-κB signaling (Hassan, Gali-Muhtasib, Goransson, & Larsson, 2010). In a U937 leukemia cell line, α-terpineol reduced LPS-induced cytokine production of IL-1β, IL-6, and IL-10, but not TNF-α (Nogueira, Aquino, Rossa Junior, & Spolidorio, 2014).

Nociceptive behavior in mice was significantly reduced by doses of 25 mg/kg ip and above on early and late paw licking post formalin, writhing after ip acetic acid, and after paw injections of glutamate or capsaicin, without motor impairment (Quintans-Junior et al., 2011). Similarly, 50–100 mg/kg ip dosing in mice inhibited hyperalgesia postcarageenan or TNF-α, PGE2, or DA administration, and neutrophil migration in a pleurisy model (de Oliveira et al., 2012).

It was reported that fatty liver was produced in mice after daily injections of 10 or 500 mg/kg ip of α-terpineol for 2 weeks (Choi, Sim, Choi, Lee, & Lee, 2013), an exposure level likely never attainable with a cannabis-based medicine.

Two recent studies from Iran are of interest. Pretreatment with α-terpineol 5–20 mg/kg ip significantly reduced jumping behavior typical of withdrawal effect in mice rendered morphine-dependent (Parvardeh, Moghimi, Eslami, & Masoudi, 2016), while 20–40 mg/kg ip doses reduced the development of tolerance to morphine analgesia. These results suggest possible synergy of this ingredient with other cannabis components attenuating addiction: CBD and BCP (Russo, 2011).

Higher doses of α-terpineol (50–200 mg/kg ip) in rats subjected to cerebral ischemia improved spatial learning in a water maze vs controls, restored hippocampal long-term potentiation, and lowered malondialdehyde levels indicative of lipid peroxidation (Moghimi, Parvardeh, Zanjani, & Ghafghazi, 2016). This activity certainly suggests the possibility of synergistic benefit in conjunction with benefits ascribed to CBD in similar experiments in newborn pigs (Lafuente et al., 2011).

4.7 α-Pinene

α-Pinene, a bicyclic monoterpene, is the most widely distributed terpenoid in Nature (Noma & Asakawa, 2010), but this versatile therapeutic agent is unfortunately represented in lower concentration in modern cannabis chemovars, although it is reportedly relatively abundant in the "Blue Dream" chemovar in Southern California (Backes, 2014). It has high bioavailability via inhalation (60%) with rapid metabolism and redistribution (Falk et al., 1990).

Its pharmacological effects are legion: antiinflammatory via PGE-1 (Gil, Jimenez, Ocete, Zarzuelo, & Cabo, 1989), bronchodilator in humans at low exposure levels (Falk et al., 1990), antibiotic in EO that was equally effective as vancomycin against MRSA and other resistant bacteria (Kose, Deniz, Sarikurkcu, Aktas, & Yavuz, 2010) (MIC 125 μg/mL) in an EO of *Salvia rosifolia* composed of 34.8% pinene, and was the most potent compound in a tea tree EO vs *P. acnes* and *Staph* spp. (Raman et al., 1995). Efficacy was also noted for α-pinene for MRSA, *Cryptococcus neoformans* and *Candida albicans* biofilms (Rivas da Silva et al., 2012). α-Pinene dramatically increased antibiotic efficacy by lowering the MIC of ciprofloxacin, erythromycin, and triclosan against the gastroenteritis pathogen, *Campylobacter jejuni*, by promoting *cmeABC* and *Cj1687* antimicrobial efflux genes, decreasing bacterial membrane integrity, and disrupting heat-shock responses (Kovac et al., 2015). It was also beneficial against *Leishmania amazonensis* promastigotes (IC_{50} 19.7 μg/mL) and axenic and intracellular amastigote forms (IC_{50} 43.9 and 38.1 μg/mL) (Rodrigues et al., 2015). α-Pinene demonstrated larvicidal activity against *Anopholes subpictus*, vector of malaria (LC_{50} [lethal concentration] 32.09 μg/mL), *Aedes albopictus*, vector of dengue (LC_{50} 34.09 μg/mL), and

Culex tritaeniorhynchus, vector of Japanese encephalitis (LC_{50} 36.75 μg/mL) (Govindarajan, Rajeswary, Hoti, Bhattacharyya, & Benelli, 2016).

Pinene increased mouse motility after inhalation 13.77% (Buchbauer et al., 1993). Its greatest therapeutic value may derive from its acetylcholinesterase inhibition (Perry, Houghton, Theobald, Jenner, & Perry, 2000), producing an IC_{50} of 0.44 mM (Miyazawa & Yamafuji, 2005), which serves to reduce or eliminate one of the primary adverse events associated with THC, that of short-term memory impairment. This ability may also serve admirably in treatment of dementia, a syndrome in which THC has already produced benefits in counteracting agitation (Russo, Guy, & Robson, 2007; Volicer, Stelly, Morris, McLaughlin, & Volicer, 1997).

Inhalation of α-pinene in mice at 10 μL/L concentration produced an anxiolytic effect in the elevated plus maze, with general brain distribution and increase in tyrosine hydroxylase mRNA in the midbrain (Kasuya et al., 2015). In chronic inhalation over 5 days, anxiolytic effects were maintained (Satou, Kasuya, Maeda, & Koike, 2014).

α-Pinene has also been suggested as a modulator of THC overdose events (Russo, 2011), with historical anecdotes supporting its use as an antidote to cannabis intoxication. α-Pinene at a concentration of 2 μg/mL produced 69% protection in rat astrocytes against H_2O_2-induced cell death (Elmann et al., 2009).

Chronic pinene exposure led to decreased melanoma growth in mice at 180 ng/L (1 ppm) in ambient air, a dose too low to directly affect tumor (Kusuhara et al., 2012). This mental health-promoting effect attributed here to pinene exposure, is known in Japan as "Shinrin-yoku" or "forest bathing." In contrast, a direct synergistic and isobolographic benefit was observed with α-pinene in combination with paclitaxel vs nonsmall-cell A549 lung carcinoma cells with evidence of apoptosis (Zhang et al., 2015). α-Pinene inhibited BEL-7402 human hepatoma cell growth 79.3%, both time and dose dependently over 3 days at 8 mg/L concentration (Chen et al., 2015), causing cycle arrest in G2/M phase, a decrease in tumor xenografts vs control ($P < 0.01$), and equivalent to that from 5-flurouracil, an increase in Chk1 and -2 expression, indicative of DNA damage leading to cell death.

4.8 β-Pinene

A bicyclic monoterpene isomer, β-pinene is commonly encountered in conjunction with α-pinene. It proved to have equal antibiotic efficacy to α-pinene against *S. aureus* (MRSA), and *C. neoformans* and *C. albicans* biofilms (Rivas da Silva et al., 2012). Like its isomer, β-pinene demonstrated the ability to synergize with paclitaxel vs nonsmall-cell A549 lung carcinoma cells with evidence of apoptosis (Zhang et al., 2015), but unlike α-pinene, it failed to prevent astrocyte damage by H_2O_2 (Elmann et al., 2009). Little additional pharmacological research has been evident otherwise on the pure compound, particularly with regard to its psychopharmacology.

4.9 Linalool

Linalool is a noncyclic monoterpenoid that is commonly extracted from lavender (*Lavandula* spp.), rose (Rosa spp.), basil (*Ocimum basilicum*), and neroli oil (*Citrus aurantium*). The psychotropic anxiolytic activity has been reviewed in detail (Russo, 2001, 2011). Linalool has established sedative, antidepressant, anxiolytic, and immune potentiating effects and can represent a significant portion (<6%) of the EO of cannabis (McPartland & Russo, 2001). This terpene can also have analgesic and anticonvulsant effects (Batista et al., 2010; Leal-Cardoso et al., 2010; Peana et al., 2006; Russo, 2011). It is also antinociceptive at high doses in mice via ionotropic glutamate receptors (Batista et al., 2008). Linalool demonstrated anticonvulsant and antiglutamatergic activity, and reduced seizures as part of *O. basilicum* EO after exposure to pentylenetetrazole, picrotoxin, and strychnine (Elisabetsky, Marschner, & Souza, 1995; Ismail, 2006). Furthermore, linalool decreased K^+-stimulated glutamate release and uptake in mouse synaptosomes (Silva Brum, Emanuelli, Souza, & Elisabetsky, 2001). Recent reports support the possibility that small concentrations found in certain cannabis chemovars may exert anticonvulsant benefits in human patients (Russo, 2016b; Sulak, Saneto, & Goldstein, 2017).

Linalool alone demonstrated an MIC of 0.625 μL/mL on *P. acnes* (Kim et al., 2008). Linalool in ambient air decreased mouse motility 73%, confirming its potent sedative effects (Buchbauer et al., 1993). In traditional aromatherapy, linalool is the likely suspect in the remarkable therapeutic capabilities of lavender EO to alleviate skin burns without scarring (Gattefosse, 1993). Pertinent to this, the local anesthetic effects of linalool are equal to those of procaine and menthol (Ghelardini, Galeotti, Salvatore, & Mazzanti, 1999; Re et al., 2000). Another explanation would be its ability to produce hot-plate analgesia in mice ($P<0.001$) that was reduced by administration of an adenosine A_{2A} antagonist (Peana et al., 2006). This terpene can also influence CYP enzymes in rat liver, suggesting that it can alter the pharmacokinetics of cannabis administration (Noskova, Dovrtelova, Zendulka, Řemínek, & Jurica, 2016).

Linalool displays powerful antileishmanial activity, and as a presumed lavender EO component, decreased morphine opioid usage after inhalation vs placebo ($P=0.04$) in gastric banding in morbidly obese surgical patients (do Socorro et al., 2003; Kim et al., 2007). Linalool incorporated nanoparticles are being explored as a novel anticancer agent (Han et al., 2016).

4.10 Camphene

Camphene is a cyclic monoterpene common to conifers, especially Douglas fir (*Pseudotsuga menziesii*), and is present in many cannabis chemovars in low titer. In an ointment with menthol and other EOs, camphene reduced experimentally induced bronchospasm in animals, suggesting application in human chronic obstructive pulmonary disease (Schafer & Schafer, 1981).

Camphene administered to hyperlipidemic rats at 30 μg/g (equivalent to 4.87 mg/kg in humans) led to a 54.5% decrease in total cholesterol, 54% in LDL-cholesterol, and 34.5% in triglycerides (all $P<0.001$) (Vallianou, Peroulis, Pantazis, & Hadzopoulou-Cladaras, 2011). Reductions in cholesterol in HepG2 cells paralleled those attained with mevinolin, but in contrast, camphene seemingly worked independently of HMG-CoA reductase inhibition. Synergy of camphene with other components of Chios mastic gum (*Pistacia lentiscus*) was also observed. In subsequent work (Vallianou & Hadzopoulou-Cladaras, 2016), camphene inhibited cholesterol production 39% at 100 μM in HepG2 cells, while also decreasing triglycerides 34% and increasing apolipoprotein AI expression, likely mediated via SREBP-1 upregulation and MTP inhibition.

Camphene displayed weak antinociceptive effects on acetic acid-induced writhing in mice at 200 mg/kg (Quintans-Junior et al., 2013), but prevented AAPH-induced lipoperoxidation at 0.01 μg/mL, and demonstrated antioxidant activity and superoxide radical inhibition at the same concentration.

Camphene supplemented to the high-fat diet of mice at the high dose of 200 mg/kg/day (corresponding to 16 mg/kg/day in humans) reduced 17% body weight reduction vs controls (Kim, Choi, Choi, Choi, & Park, 2014), and increased adiponectin levels and receptor mRNA expression in liver.

Camphene induced apoptosis in a variety of cancer cell lines, notably B16F10-Nex2 melanoma with an IC_{50} of 71.2 μg/mL (Girola et al., 2015) and produced chromatin condensation, shrinkage of cells, apoptotic body formation, fragmentation of nucleus and activation of caspase-3. It was also active against grafted tumor with peritumoral injection (10 mg/mL) in mice.

Camphene was utilized as a porogen for the production of nano/macroporous polycaprolactone microspheres for injectable cell delivery (Kim, Hwang, & Shin, 2016).

4.11 Terpinolene

Terpinolene is a cyclic monoterpene, common to *Pinus* spp., but richest in parsnip EO (*Pastinaca sativa* 69%) (Tisserand & Young, 2014). It is a common component of some commercial cannabis chemovars (Giese et al., 2015), its presence is said to be characteristic of "sativa" types (Hazekamp et al., 2016).

Terpinolene has been demonstrated to prevent LDL oxidation, of interest in treatment of atherogenesis and coronary artery disease (Grassmann, Hippeli, Spitzenberger, & Elstner, 2005).

It was sedative in mice at 0.1 mg, reducing motor activity to 67.8% (Ito & Ito, 2013), whereas subjective reports in humans suggest greater stimulation in terpinolene-rich cannabis chemovars (data on file, Napro Research 2016), possibly attributable to cholinesterase inhibition effects in the presence of THC, a pharmacological effect measured with IC_{50} at 156.4 μg/mL (Bonesi et al., 2010).

At a concentration of 0.05%, terpinolene markedly reduced AKT1 expression in K562 human CML cells and significantly stimulated apoptosis (Okumura, Yoshida, Nishimura, Kitagishi, & Matsuda, 2012). At extreme dosing (>50 mg/L), terpinolene demonstrated marginally greater antiproliferative effects against neuroblastoma as compared to neuronal cell lines (Aydin, Turkez, & Tasdemir, 2013). Over a similar dosage range, it showed antioxidant effects in human lymphocytes (Turkez, Aydin, Geyikoglu, & Cetin, 2015).

Terpinolene is reportedly also antifungal and larvicidal (Aydin et al., 2013). A subactive antinociceptive and antiinflammatory dosage of 3.125 mg/kg po in rats synergized with diclofenac, and reduced hyperalgesia, an effect blocked by ketanserin, suggesting mediation via 5-HT_{2A} receptors (Macedo et al., 2016).

4.12 α-Phellandrene

A cyclic monoterpene, α-phellandrene is widespread in nature, but rich in frankincense (*Boswellia sacra*), comprising 42% of the EO (Tisserand & Young, 2014). It produced cholinesterase inhibition with an IC_{50} of 120.2 μg/mL (Bonesi et al., 2010). Multiple assays in mice (Lima et al., 2012) demonstrated antinociceptive effects: acetic acid-induced abdominal writhing (3.125 mg/kg/po or 0.25 mg/kg human equivalent), both phases of the formalin test (50 mg/kg/po, or 0.54 mg/kg human), capsaicin injection (3.125 mg/kg/po, or 0.25 mg/kg human equivalent), glutamate injection (12.5 mg/kg/po, or 1 mg/kg human) and carageenan injection (only at 3 h at 25 mg/kg/po, or 2 mg/kg human). Effects were blocked by multiple agents, suggesting mediation by glutamatergic, opioid, nitrergic, cholinergic, and adrenergic mechanisms.

In rats, phellandrene at 10 mg/kg/d po (1.6 mg/kg human equivalent) prevented spared nerve injury-induced mechanical and cold hyperalgesia, while also demonstrating an antidepressant effect in reducing immobility in the forced swim test 85%, but without decreasing locomotor activity in the open field (Piccinelli et al., 2015).

While not demonstrating antimicrobial effects per se, phellandrene mildly stimulated macrophage proliferation in mice via Mac-3 and promoted function in vivo (Lin et al., 2013), suggesting ability to suppress intracellular bacterial growth.

Subsequent work demonstrated a wide variety of effects on gene expression affecting DNA repair, cell cycle, and apoptosis in WEHI-3 murine leukemia cells (Lin et al., 2015, 2014).

At 30 μM concentration with 24 h of exposure, 15.8% of human liver tumor J5 cells became necrotic, possibly due to depletion of ATP (Hsieh et al., 2014). Subsequently, findings were attributed to multiple pathways: regulation of mTOR, LC-3II expression, p53 signaling and NF-κB activation (Hsieh et al., 2015).

In carageenan injections in rodents, phellandrene 50 mg/kg po pretreatment induced neutrophil migration inhibition, and TNF-α release (both $P<0.001$) (Siqueira et al., 2016) and decreased mast cell degranulation ($P<0.05$), suggesting possible applications in arthritic and allergic conditions.

4.13 γ-Cadinene

A bicyclic sesquiterpene, while more common in other EOs, it is found at low concentration in current cannabis chemovars tested (Hazekamp et al., 2016). Cadinene demonstrated larvicidal activity against *Anopholes stephensi*, vector of malaria (LC_{50} [lethal concentration] 8.23 μg/mL), *Aedes aegypti*, vector of dengue (LC_{50} 9.03 μg/mL), and *Culex quinquefaciatus*, vector of filariasis (LC_{50} 9.86 μg/mL) (Govindarajan, Rajeswary, & Benelli, 2016). Little additional pharmacological data is available on the isolated compound.

4.14 Δ^3-Carene

A bicyclic monoterpenoid alkene most associated with turpentine from conifers, it is also prevalent in white pepper (*Piper nigrum*, 25%) (Tisserand & Young, 2014), but is found in low concentration in cannabis.

Studies from Scandinavia in sawmills have documented high-exposure human irritancy reactions in skin and lungs, with pulmonary intake and slight increased airway resistance at 450 mg/m^3 exposure (Falk et al., 1991), with rapid metabolism and high adipose tissue affinity. The occupational exposure limit recommendation in Sweden for it or other turpentine components is 150 mg/m^3 (Kasanen et al., 1999). Carene hydroperoxide was noted to be an allergen (Edman et al., 2003), and skin sensitization in guinea pigs at very high concentrations increased airway reactivity (Lastbom, Boman, Johnsson, Camner, & Ryrfeldt, 2003). Carene concentrations, along with limonene and pinene, are common volatile organic compounds elevated in new home construction (Krol, Namiesnik, & Zabiegala, 2014).

Carene was rapidly absorbed, distributed, and metabolized in human volunteers after oral administration (Schmidt, Belov, & Goen, 2015). A low concentration (5 μM) stimulated mineralization in mouse osteoblastic cells by increasing protein expression; activation of MAP kinases; and expression of osteoblast genes, osteopontin, and type I collagen (Jeong, Kim, Min, & Kim, 2008), suggesting a possible therapeutic role in osteoporosis treatment.

Carene demonstrated larvicidal activity against *Anopholes stephensi*, vector of malaria (LC_{50} [lethal concentration] 16.37 μg/mL), *A. aegypti*, vector of dengue (LC_{50} 17.91 μg/mL), and *C. quinquefaciatus*, vector of filariasis (LC_{50} 19.5 μg/mL) (Govindarajan, Rajeswary, Hoti, et al., 2016; Govindarajan, Rajeswary, et al., 2016).

Carene content was judged to be a marker of "sativa" cannabis chemovars (Hazekamp et al., 2016).

4.15 ρ-Cymene

A cyclic monoterpene, common to thyme (*Thymus vulgaris*) (27.4%), but a minor component in cannabis, ρ-cymene was active against *Bacteroides fragilis*, *C. albicans*, and *Clostridium perfringens* (Carson & Riley, 1995). It was sedative in mice at 0.04 mg in air, reducing motor activity to 47.3% of baseline (Ito & Ito, 2013). Additionally, it statistically significantly reduced acetic acid-induced writhing and both phases of formalin-induced pain in mice at 50 mg/kg (Quintans-Junior et al., 2013). It showed little antioxidant or antiproliferative effects in a recent study (Fitsiou et al., 2016).

4.16 Fenchol

A bicyclic monoterpenoid, fenchol (or fenchyl alcohol) is an FDA-approved flavor additive and rated GRAS by FEMA (Bhatia, McGinty, Letizia, & Api, 2008). Oral doses above 2 g/kg were fatal in rats, demonstrating lethargy, ataxia, flaccidity, and coma, whereas a 4% cutaneous application in humans was nonsensitizing. It is common to basil (*O. basilicum*), and to California cannabis chemovars (Giese et al., 2015), but in low concentrations, such that the noted toxicity would be unlikely a factor even in concentrates.

4.17 1,8-Cineole (Eucalyptol)

This bicyclic monoterpenoid ether is a major component of *Eucalyptus* spp. EOs, and is largely responsible for their pharmacology (Barbosa, Filomeno, & Teixeira, 2016). A prior review (McPartland & Russo, 2001) noted its myriad activities including increasing cerebral blood flow after inhalation, increasing rat locomotion, and as an antiinflammatory, analgesic, antibiotic, antifungal, and antiviral against *Herpes simplex 2*, but it is barely present in modern cannabis chemovars (Hazekamp et al., 2016).

5. CANNABIS SESQUITERPENOIDS (FIG. 4)

5.1 β-Caryophyllene

BCP, a bicyclic sesquiterpenes alkene, is the most common terpenoid in cannabis extracts, and is nearly ubiquitous in food in the food supply. The extensive potent and various pharmacological activities for BCP summarized below, are rarely noted for any individual compound that also has a wide therapeutic index, safety, and low toxicity. BCP acts as a selective full agonist at CB_2 with strong potency (100 nM), and its antiinflammatory effects are reduced in CB_2 knockout mice (Gertsch, 2008). BCP activity at CB_2 has been confirmed in rodent models of nociception and pain (Katsuyama et al., 2013; Paula-Freire et al., 2014), colitis (Bento et al., 2011), and nephrotoxicity (Horváth, Mukhopadhyay, Haskó, & Pacher, 2012). Russo (2011) proposes mechanisms whereby BCP synergizes with THC to impart antipruritic effects and gastric cytoprotection, and with CBD to impart antiinflammatory benefits. CB_2 agonists (likely including caryophyllene) have been shown to reduce drug administration (cocaine) and improve scores of depression and anxiety in animal models (Bahi et al., 2014; Onaivi et al., 2008; Xi et al., 2011). BCP demonstrated larvicidal activity against *A. subpictus*, vector of malaria (LC_{50} [lethal concentration]

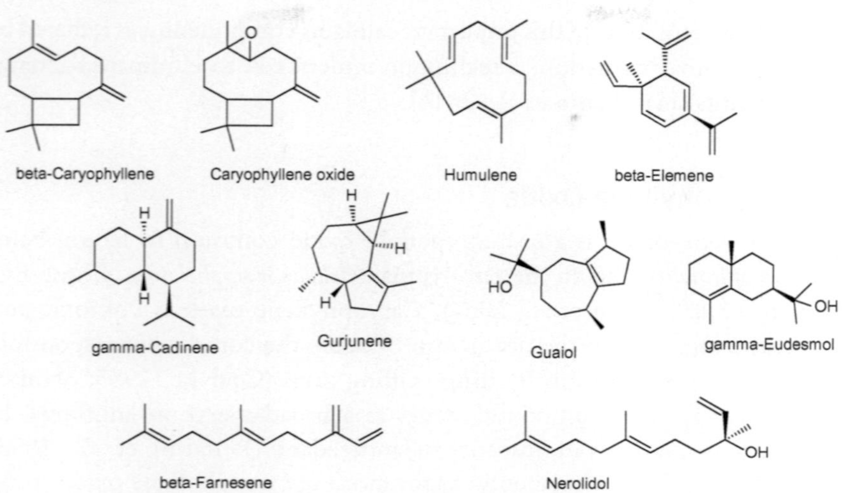

Fig. 4 Sesquiterpenoids commonly encountered in cannabis (all structures drawn by EBR using ChemSketch 2015.2.5).

41.66 μg/mL), *A. albopictus*, vector of dengue (LC_{50} 44.77 μg/mL), and *C. tritaeniorhynchus*, vector of Japanese encephalitis (LC_{50} 48.17 μg/mL) (Govindarajan, Rajeswary, Hoti, et al., 2016; Govindarajan, Rajeswary, et al., 2016). As a monotherapeutic agent, BCP provides many other benefits, reviewed by Fidyt, Fiedorowicz, and Strządała (2016).

According to an exhaustive review, BCP activates peroxisome proliferated activator receptors (PPARs) isoforms, inhibits pathways triggered by the activation of toll-like receptor complexes (i.e., CD14/TLR4/MD2), reduces immunoinflammatory processes, and exhibits synergy with μ-opioid receptor pathways (Sharma et al., 2016). Additionally, BCP is a potent antagonist of homomeric nicotinic acetylcholine receptors (7-nAChRs) and devoid of effects mediated by serotonergic and GABAergic receptors. BCP modulates numerous molecular targets by altering their gene expression, signaling pathways, or through direct interaction. Basic experiments have demonstrated strong evidence for cardioprotective, hepatoprotective, gastroprotective, neuroprotective, nephroprotective, antioxidant, antiinflammatory, antimicrobial, and immunemodulator activities. Thus, it has shown potent therapeutic promise in neuropathic pain, neurodegenerative, and metabolic diseases. A recent publication extends its therapeutic potential to protection from alcoholic steatohepatitis via antiinflammatory effects and alleviation of metabolic disturbances (Varga et al., 2017).

The concentration of this important cannabis component was reduced to 10% by gamma-irradiation, a technique undertaken to eliminate bacterial contaminants (Hazekamp et al., 2016).

5.2 Caryophyllene Oxide

Caryophyllene oxide is a sesquiterpenoid oxide common to lemon balm (*Melissa officinalis*), and to the eucalyptus, *Melaleuca stypheloides*, whose EO contains 43.8% (Farag et al., 2004). Caryophyllene oxide is nontoxic and nonsensitizing, and has the distinction of being the component responsible for cannabis identification by drug-sniffing dogs (Opdyke, 1983; Stahl & Kunde, 1973). This compound serves as a broad-spectrum antifungal in plant defense and as an insecticidal/antifeedant (Bettarini et al., 1993; Langenheim, 1994). Therapeutic applications of caryophyllene oxide could exploit the antifungal efficacy observed in clinical study of onychomycosis compared to ciclopiroxalamine and sulconazole, with an 8% concentration affecting eradication in 15 days (Yang, Michel, Chaumont, & Millet-Clerc, 1999). This agent also demonstrates antiplatelet aggregation properties in vitro (Lin et al., 2003).

5.3 Humulene (α-Caryophyllene)

Humulene provides some defense to plants and their products, as this compound can inhibit fruit fly mating (Shelly & Nishimoto, 2015). Humulene at a concentration of 1.5 μg/mL produced 50% protection in rat astrocytes against H_2O_2-induced cell death, and was concentrated seven-fold in those cells (Elmann et al., 2009). The potentiating effect of BCP on the anticancer activity of α-humulene, isocaryophyllene, and paclitaxel against MCF-7, DLD-1, and L-929 human tumor cell lines has been evaluated (Legault & Pichette, 2007). A noncytotoxic concentration of BCP significantly increased the anticancer activity of α-humulene and isocaryophyllene on MCF-7 cells: α-humulene or isocaryophyllene alone (32 μg/mL) inhibited cell growth by about 50% and 69%, respectively, compared with 75% and 90% when combined with 10 μg/mL BCP. Little additional pharmacology, particularly psychopharmacology of the compound has been evident; a recent major review of *H. lupulus* (hops), of which it is a major EO component, merely mentioned its presence without additional commentary (Zanoli & Zavatti, 2008).

5.4 β-Elemene

Elemene is a monocyclic sesquiterpenoid polyalkene reported from some cannabis chemovars, and common to myrrh (*Commiphora myrrha*, 9%) and other similar resins (Tisserand & Young, 2014). Elemene via injection has been approved by the regulatory authority in China since 1993 for treatment of cancer. However, a 2006 Cochrane-style review or 127 RCTs showed poor adherence to CONSORT recommendations and very low Jadad scale scoring in available studies (Peng et al., 2006). A subsequent study in rats at 80 mg/kg IV (equivalent to 13 mg/kg in humans) showed good passage through the blood–brain barrier and attainment of high brain tissue levels, as well as noteworthy tumor inhibition and life extension (Wu et al., 2009). A more recent meta-analysis of studies in malignancy (Xu, Zheng, Li, Xu, & Fu, 2013) examined clinical studies up to 2011, examining claims of efficacy in 38 relevant trials. Overall response rate of elemene with chemotherapy was favorable in lung cancer ($P<0.00001$), hepatic carcinoma ($P=0.002$), metastatic brain cancer ($P=0.02$), and leukemia ($P=0.0004$), but not in gastric carcinoma. Clinical benefit was also seen in combination therapy vs chemotherapy alone in 13 lung cancer trials, 5 with hepatic carcinoma, 7 with gastric carcinoma, and 5 with leukemia, out of 30 examined. Similar comparison failed to show improved 1-year survival in lung cancer or liver cancer, or 2-year survival in lung cancer. Higher degrees of leukopenia were significantly lower ($P=0.0007$) in the elemene plus chemotherapy groups.

Various subsequent studies have examined mechanisms of action of elemene in malignancy. Elemene 100 μM increased cytotoxicity significantly in various cell lines overexpressing the ABCB1 transporter of paclitaxel, colchicine, and vinblastine by inhibiting it efflux activity. Elemene significantly diminished mRNA transcription and P-gp and BCRP gene expression, as well as CD44 and 24-/low cell and CBRP^{+} cell rates and serum-free cell sphere forming in breast cancer stem cells (Dong et al., 2015). It also dose dependently inhibited survival and proliferation of glioblastoma multiforme cell lines when combined with temozolomide or radiation (Liu et al., 2015) by inhibiting DNA repair via effects on ATM, AKT, and ERK signaling. In A549 human basal cells, elemene increased radiosensitivity through upregulation of p53 and downregulation of Bcl-2-producing apoptosis, and downregulation of DNA-PKcs inhibiting DSB repair (K. Zou, Liu, Zhang, & Zou, 2015). Radiosensitivity of gastric cancer was also enhanced by diminished Pak1 activation (Liu et al., 2015). Elemene was the first drug reported to inhibit TOPO I and IIα simultaneously, as demonstrated in

HepG-2 human hepatic carcinoma, producing cell arrest in S phase and apoptosis (Gong et al., 2015). Elemene mediated multidrug resistance or various genes in exosomes in MCF-7 human breast cancer cells, sensitizing them to docetaxel and adriacin (Zhang et al., 2015). In ECA-109 esophageal carcinoma cells, elemene reduced proliferation significantly via regulation of inhibition of hTERT expression by IncRNA CDKN2B-AS1 (Hu et al., 2015). In U87 glioblastoma cells, elemene reduced proliferation, increase apoptosis, reduced invasiveness, and mouse xenograft growth (Zhu et al., 2015), while downregulating stemness markers CD133 and ATP-binding cassette subfamily G member 2 and N-cadherin and β-catenin mesenchymal markers. In a review of molecular mechanisms (Jiang et al., 2016), elemene was noted to inhibit cancer growth via multiple mechanisms of proliferative signaling suppression: MAPK and PI3K/Akt/mTOR pathways, upregulation of growth suppressors, promotion of apoptosis, diminishing invasion and metastasis, affecting cell immortality, and reducing angiogenesis. While concentrations of elemene employed would likely never be attained with cannabis extracts, the distinct possibility of synergy or elemene with chemotherapeutic phytocannabinoids should certainly be explored. Combination with THC, CBD (Marcu et al., 2010), and temozolomide (Torres et al., 2011) for treatment of glioblastoma multiforme would be especially worthy of investigation.

A 0.5% elemene emulsion injection proved effective as a sclerosing agent in 23 consecutive patients treated for chylothorax with good reported safety (Jianjun, Song, Yin, Jia, & Donglei, 2008).

Elemene prevented human umbilical vein endothelial cell (HUVEC) damage by hydrogen peroxide in vitro, inhibited smooth muscle proliferation and migration, and neointima formation after vessel injury in rats (Wu, Wang, Tang, Long, & Yin, 2011). In subsequent work (Liu et al., 2015), elemene also decreased reactive oxygen species (ROS) and mitogen-activated protein kinase signaling in HUVECs, and suggesting utility in atherosclerosis treatment.

In a rat model of hepatic fibrosis, elemene downregulated plasma endotoxins, serum TNF-α, and expression of CD14, the coreceptor for bacterial lipopolysaccharide detection (Liu et al., 2011).

Elemene 12.5–50 μg/mL inhibited osteogenic differentiation from cultured human hip joint capsule fibroblasts via inhibition of the BMP/SMADs pathway, suggesting its ability to reduce ectopic ossification in ankylosing spondylitis (Zhou et al., 2015).

Elemene 10–200 μg/mL also reduced viability and increased apoptosis of rheumatoid arthritis fibroblast-like synoviocytes via induction of ROS and p38 MAPK activation, implying therapeutic potential in that disorder (Zou et al., 2016).

Elemene presence was said to be characteristic of "indica" chemovars of cannabis (Hazekamp et al., 2016). Although its concentrations in most cannabis chemovars are low, emphasis is placed here due to its versatility as a potential anticancer agent worthy of selective breeding to increase its titer, and possibly synergize with chemotherapeutic phytocannabinoids (Ligresti et al., 2006).

5.5 Guaiol

According to Lawless (1995), guaiol, a bicyclic sesquiterpenoid alkene alcohol, is a major component (42%–72%) of the EO of guaiacwood from the species *Bulnesia sarmienti*, a tree of Paraguay and Argentina, with a pleasant rose-like aroma, and is nontoxic, nonirritating, and nonsensitizing. It has been employed in aromatherapy to treat arthritis, rheumatoid arthritis, and gout. Reported actions of the EO are antiinflammatory, antioxidant, antirheumatic, antiseptic, diaphoretic, diuretic, and laxative. The EO of another species in which guaiol was a component displayed antibiotic properties (de Moura et al., 2002). A report (Parker, 2003) has also shown guaiol to have weak 5-alpha reductase inhibitory effects, and this could be helpful in benign prostatic hyperplasia, or even in treatment of male-pattern baldness, a benefit of cannabis reported independently in the Arabic and Chinese literature.

Guaiol inhibited nonsmall-cell lung cancer cells in vitro, and in vivo in nude mice (as effectively as cisplatin at the same 8 mg/kg dose) (Yang et al., 2016) with mitotic arrest in S phase in A549 and H1299 cells, downregulation of RAD51 homologous recombination repair factor and inducing apoptosis.

Guaiol showed contact toxicity for two moth species and efficacy as a fumigant for *Musca domestica* houseflies with LC_{50} of 16.9 μL/L (Liu, Wang, Xie, & Mu, 2013). It also demonstrated bite-deterrence index (BDI) against *A. aegypti* of 0.82, and vs *Anopholes quadrimaculatus* a BDI of 0.82, comparable to *N,N*-dimethyl-toluamide (DEET) at a concentration of 25 nM/cm^3, but was ineffective against larvae (Ali et al., 2015).

Guaiol was said to be a distinguishing factor in Afghan cannabis chemovars (Hillig & Mahlberg, 2004), with similar claim for "indica" chemovars (Hazekamp et al., 2016). As a sesquiterpenoid alcohol, it would be expected to produce sedative effects (Schnaubelt, 1998), often attributed to Afghan genetics.

5.6 Eudesmol Isomers

These isomers are bicyclic sesquiterpenoid alkene alcohols. Presence of both β- and γ-eudesmol isomers was judged to be characteristic of Afghani cannabis (Hillig & Mahlberg, 2004), or "indica" chemovars (Hazekamp et al., 2016).

Alpha-eudesmol inhibits calcium channels and was shown to attenuate neurogenic vasodilation, decrease dural extravasation, inhibit depolarization-evoked CGRP and substance P release from sensory nerve terminals without cardiovascular effects (Asakura et al., 2000), suggesting clinical application in migraine.

β-Eudesmol has been reported to be hepatoprotective against carbon-tetrachloride and galactosoamine-induced cytotoxicity in cultured rat hepatocytes (Kiso, Tohkin, & Hikino, 1983), and to inhibit electroshock-induced seizures in mice, additive to phenytoin (Chiou, Ling, & Chang, 1997). Other older reports (summarized in Li et al., 2013) note its ability to block nicotinic receptors at the neuromuscular junctions, display antiinflammatory effects, and antagonize toxicity related to organophosphate poisoning.

Recent investigation of β-eudesmol indicates its ability in mice to stimulate gastric emptying and intestinal motility via inhibition of dopamine D_2 and serotonin 5-HT_2 receptors in a dose-dependent fashion (25–100 mg/kg) (Kimura & Sumiyoshi, 2012).

Several reports document efficacy in cancer: β-eudesmol produced apoptosis in human leukemia HL60 cell culture, producing apoptosis via effects on JNK signaling in mitochondria (Li et al., 2013); both α- and β-eudesmol produced cytotoxic effects in low μg/mL concentrations in human hepatocellular carcinoma HepG2 cells with increase in caspase-3 activation, loss of mitochondrial membrane potential and apoptosis (D. S. Bomfim et al., 2013); β-eudesmol reduced human cholangiocarcinoma xenograft tumors in nude mice 91.6% at a dose of 100 mg/kg with prolongation of survival by 64.4% (Plengsuriyakarn, Karbwang, & Na-Bangchang, 2015); and it also inhibited proliferation of human lung A549 and colon HT29 and Caco-2 cells, superoxide synthesis in A549, and cell adhesion and migration in A549 and HT29 lines at high concentrations (100 μM) (Ben Sghaier et al., 2016). While it is unlikely that such concentrations would be attainable in herbal cannabis or concentrates, these results suggest possibilities for synergy with other cannabis components.

β-Eudesmol demonstrated BDI against *A. aegypti* of 0.81, and *A. quadrimaculatus* mosquitoes with BDI of 0.82, comparable to DEET at a concentration of 25 nM/cm^3, but was ineffective against larvae (Ali et al., 2015).

Additionally, β-eudesmol in low micromolar concentrations inhibited activity of histidine decarboxylase and mast cell degranulation in a human cell line, HMC-1 (Han et al., 2017), suggesting its possible application in treatment of allergies.

5.7 Nerolidol

Nerolidol, previously reviewed (Russo, 2011), is a noncyclic sesquiterpene alkene alcohol with sedative properties (Binet, Binet, Miocque, Roux, & Bernier, 1972; Lapczynski, Bhatia, Letizia, & Api, 2008), common to citrus peels. It reduced colon adenoma formation in rats (Wattenberg, 1991). It enhanced skin penetration of 5-fluorouracil (Cornwell & Barry, 1994), and it produced growth inhibition of dermophytes (Langenheim, 1994). Unlike some conventional cutaneous preparations, nerolidol is nontoxic and non-sensitizing (Lapczynski, Letizia, & Api, 2008). Potent antimalarial (Lopes et al., 1999; Rodrigues Goulart et al., 2004) and antileishmanial effects (Arruda, D'Alexandri, Katzin, & Uliana, 2005) have been noted, including an IC_{50} of 7.0 μM in a recent experiment (Camargos et al., 2014). Although present in Sativex®, it seems to exist at only minimal concentration in Californian chemovars (Giese et al., 2015).

5.8 Gurjunene

Gurjunene, a tricyclic sesquiterpene alkene, has also been reported in cannabis, but it is difficult to distinguish it analytically from nerolidol (Hazekamp et al., 2016). Gurjunene is common to EO of agarwood (*Aquilaria agallocha*) (Takemoto, Ito, Shiraki, Yagura, & Honda, 2008), and when administered as a vapor to mice it produced a biphasic dose-response, effectively reducing locomotor activity at 1.5%, but stimulating activity at 15% concentration.

5.9 γ-Cadinene

A bicyclic sesquiterpene, while more common in other EOs, cadinene is found in low concentration in current cannabis chemovars tested (Hazekamp et al., 2016). Cadinene demonstrated larvicidal activity against the *Anopholes stephensi*, vector of malaria (LC_{50} [lethal concentration] 8.23 μg/mL), *A. aegypti*, vector of dengue (LC_{50} 9.03 μg/mL), and *C. quinquefaciatus*, vector of filariasis (LC_{50} 9.86 μg/mL) (Govindarajan, Rajeswary, Hoti, et al., 2016; Govindarajan, Rajeswary, et al., 2016). Little pharmacology of the isolated compound is available, otherwise.

5.10 β-Farnesene

Trans-β-farnesene, an acyclic sesquiterpenes alkene, common to green apple and its scent, and some higher animals, is present in trace amounts in some cannabis chemovars, and was considered characteristic of "sativa" types (Hazekamp et al., 2016). Said to possess DPPH free radical scavenging, anticarcinogenic, antibacterial, and antifungal activity (Turkez et al., 2014), β-farnesene also demonstrated dose-related neuroprotective effects on cultured rat primary cortical neurons, blocking H_2O_2-induced intracellular LDH release and reduced DNA damage 47.8%, suggesting application in neurodegenerative diseases.

6. CANNABIS ODDS AND ENDS: ROOT TRITERPENOIDS AND ALKALOIDS, LEAF FLAVONOIDS, SEED COATS, AND SPROUTS (FIG. 5)

While it is clear that the unfertilized female flowering tops with their capitate glandular trichomes are the preeminent phytotherapeutic factory in cannabis, other parts of the plant produce distinctive chemistries of their own, and offer synergistic possibilities in cannabis combinations from this "pharmacological treasure trove" (Mechoulam, 2005). Considering that many parts of the plant are commonly discarded, these "extraneous" materials deserve much closer scrutiny and consideration.

6.1 Friedelin

While cannabis roots contain no phytocannabinoids (Potter, 2009), mono- or sesquiterpenoids, they do produce triterpenoids, the 30-carbon molecules that are the most diverse phytochemicals in nature, derived by cyclization of squalene. They display a wide spectrum of antiinflammatory, antipyretic,

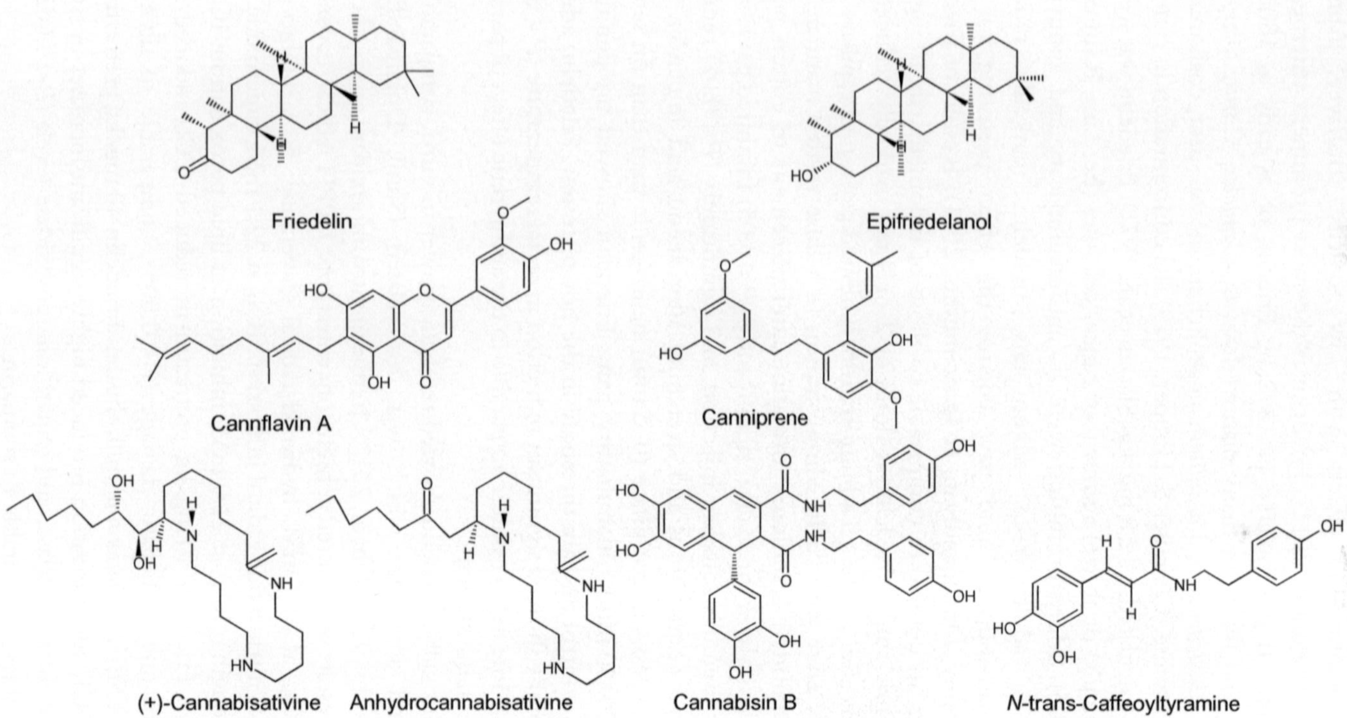

Fig. 5 Cannabis odds and ends: triterpenoids, alkaloids, flavonoids, bibenzyls, etc. (all structures drawn by EBR using ChemSketch 2015.2.5).

and anticarcinogenic effects with low toxicity (Bishayee, Ahmed, Brankov, & Perloff, 2011). Friedelin is the most prominent triterpenoid in cannabis. It was isolated in 1892 by Friedel, or as early as 1805, as "cerine" and found in many plants (*Aesculus, Cannabis, Citrus, Diospyros, Quercus, Rhododendron, Vaccinium*), algae, lichen, mosses, peat, coal, mineral wax, and swine (Chandler & Hooper, 1979). Its concentration in cannabis root was calculated as 12.8 mg/kg (Slatkin et al., 1971). Friedelin was weakly active (35 μM or above) against four cancer cell lines (Ee, Lim, Rahmat, & Lee, 2005). More promising were its antiinflammatory and antipyretic effects. In adult Wistar albino rats, friedelin markedly reduced carrageenan-induced hind paw edema, the effect persisting for 6 h (Antonisamy, Duraipandiyan, & Ignacimuthu, 2011). Results of friedelin at 40 mg/kg dose were comparable to those of indomethacin 10 mg/kg. In the same study, friedelin at doses of 2 or 4 mg markedly reduced rat ear edema after croton oil administration, inhibited peritoneal capillary permeability after acetic acid administration in a dose-related manner. Friedelin inhibited granuloma formation after placement of cotton pellets subcutaneously in the axillae, significantly ($P<0.05$) inhibited paw swelling after Freund's adjuvant injection, and significantly ($P<0.05$) reduced abdominal constrictions and stretching after acetic acid injection. The effect was less on first phase (0–5 min) neurogenic pain than on second phase (20–30 min) inflammatory pain. Friedelin showed no significant effect vs control on pain threshold in the hot-plate test. Friedelin administered orally showed significant reduction in rectal temperature ($P<0.05$) after yeast injection, results comparable to the antipyretic effect of paracetamol (acetaminophen).

Additionally, friedelin showed reducing power in vitro, comparable to BHT and ascorbate, which was dose-related (Sunil, Duraipandiyan, Ignacimuthu, & Al-Dhabi, 2013). In five in vitro antioxidant assays, the following results were noted at high concentrations: DPPH radical scavenging effect: IC_{50} at 21.1 mM, hydroxyl radical scavenging: 50% inhibition at 19.8 mM, nitric oxide radical inhibition: IC_{50} at 22.1 mM, superoxide radical scavenging: IC_{50} at 21.9 mM, inhibition of lipid peroxidation: IC_{50} at 18.1 mM. Friedelin 40 mg/kg pretreatment reduced CCl_4-induced LFT elevations due to hepatic damage ($P<0.005$), comparable to silymarin extract of *Silybum marianum* (milk thistle). Friedelin 40 mg/kg pretreatment before CCl_4 administration produced highly significant increases in superoxide dismutase, catalase, and glutathione peroxidase levels ($P<0.005$) to normal values, comparable to silymarin.

Friedelin demonstrated antimycobacterial activity against three non-pathogenic species at a MIC of 800 μg/mL and merited mention as a natural African antituberculosis agent (Chinsembu, 2016). Interestingly, this usage parallels that of cannabis leaf macerated in warm water and taken as a treatment for TB by the Bapedi healers of Limpopo Province, South Africa (Semenya, Potgieter, Tshisikhawe, Shava, & Maroyi, 2012), and certainly, friedelin may be contributing to any therapeutic benefit.

Friedelin was also effective in protecting against ethanol-induced gastric ulceration in rats (Antonisamy et al., 2015). Oral treatment at 35 mg/kg reduced gross and histological effects, increased mucosal PGE2 level 5.1-fold and NO 2.55-fold, as well as significantly reducing microvascular permeability. Friedelin increased gastric mucus content 3.12-fold and pH 4.03-fold vs control animals, also reducing DNA fragmentation and caspase-3 activity. Overall, the level of gastroprotection with friedelin scored 88.21% as compared to the standard drug, omeprazole, at 90.82%. Synergy of friedelin as a preventive of gastrointestinal ulcers would certainly be possible with reports of similar benefits attributed to THC (Douthwaite, 1947) and caryophyllene (Tambe, Tsujiuchi, Honda, Ikeshiro, & Tanaka, 1996).

6.2 Epifriedelanol

This closely related triterpenoid molecule had a measured concentration in cannabis root of 21.3 mg/kg (Slatkin et al., 1971). It was utilized to assess adriamycin-induced cell senescence in human fibroblasts (HDF) and HUVECs (Yang, Son, Jung, Zheng, & Kim, 2011), wherein epifriedelanol was especially active, and also decreased SA-β-gl activity, p53 protein, and ROS. The authors stated, "This compound [epifriedelanol] may be a promising candidate for developing dietary supplements or cosmetics to modulate tissue aging-associated diseases".

6.3 Cannabis Root Alkaloids: Cannabisativine and Anhydrocannabisativine

Cannabisativine was isolated from cannabis root (Lotter & Abraham, 1975; Slatkin, Knapp, Schiff, Turner, & Mole, 1975) with calculated concentrations of 2.5 mg/kg (Turner, Hsu, Knapp, Schiff, & Slatkin, 1976) or 0.0004% (Mechoulam et al., 1988). Anhydrocannabisativine was isolated from cannabis roots and leaves (Elsohly et al., 1978), at calculated concentrations of 0.3 mg/kg or 0.00046% (Mechoulam et al., 1988). No pharmacological information is available on either substance: "They are present in miniscule amounts and are presumably not relevant to any cannabis biological activity" (Raphael, Personal comm. to EBR 2013).

6.4 Other Root Components

Slatkin (Slatkin et al., 1975) isolated additional compounds from cannabis root with methanol: sitosterol (calculated content 1.5%), campestrol (0.78%), stigmasterol (0.56%), choline, and neurine. The same author (Slatkin et al., 1971) isolated *N*(*p*-hydroxy-β-phenylethyl)-*p*-hydroxyl-*trans*-cinnamamide (1.6 mg/kg), with analgesic activity in the mouse tail flick test at 25, 50, and 100 mg/kg sc.

6.5 Cannabis Seeds

Cannabis or hemp seeds are possibly the single most nutritionally complete food on earth, and reportedly harbor powerful antiinflammatory effects. They contain 35% protein as the digestible edestin, and all essential amino acids. The seeds also contain 35% oil, rich in essential fatty acids in what is considered the ideal nutritional 3:1 ω6:ω3 ratio:75% linoleic acid (LA, ω-6), 25% linolenic acid (LNA, ω-3), and 9% gamma-linolenic acid (GLA, ω-6) (Callaway, 2004).

Hemp hulls, often discarded during manufacture of nutritional products, also contain interesting pharmacology. Two compounds were isolated from Chinese varieties (Chen et al., 2012). Antioxidant activity against DPPH radical revealed IC_{50} 9.42 μg/mL for *N*-*trans*-caffeoyltyramine and 11.17 μ/mL for cannabisin B, both higher than ariciresinol diglucoside (SDG) and soybean isoflones (ISO). Both compounds also showed prominent activity in inhibiting human LDL oxidation. In subsequent work (Chen et al., 2013), cannabisin B produced antiproliferative effects in HepG2 human hepatocarcinoma cells (dose dependently up to 500 μM) via arrest in the S phase, and induction of autophagic cell death via regulation of the AKT/mTOR pathway.

6.6 Cannabis Flavonoids

Cannflavin A (CFA) is a flavone unique to cannabis (aerial parts), but is very difficult to isolate and purify via crystallization from its isomer, cannflavin B. It inhibits PGE_2 30 times more powerfully than ASA and displays an antiinflammatory potency intermediate to that of aspirin and dexamethasone (Barrett, Scutt, & Evans, 1986). It remained little studied beyond this for many years, when it was noted to be produced in hemp seed sprouts of certain cultivars (Werz et al., 2014). CFA suppressed PGE_2, the primary mediator of inflammation, and directly inhibited mPGES-1 (at 1.8 μM), a target in inflammation and cancer. Cannflavin A did not significantly inhibit COX-1 nor COX-2, thus potentially avoiding adverse events such as gastrointestinal bleeding, myocardial infarctions, and cerebrovascular accidents associated with the latter agents. The authors indicated that dual inhibition of mPGES-1 and 5-LO is considered the ideal profile to treat inflammatory conditions with fewest side effects.

Cannabis leaves contain about 1% total flavonoids, especially apigenin and quercetin (see McPartland & Russo, 2001 for additional review).

6.7 Cannabis Bibenzyl Compounds

Canniprene is an isoprenylated bibenzyl unique to cannabis (Allegrone et al., 2017), that can be vaporized and is potentially present in smoke. Potential antiinflammatory activity was demonstrated via inhibition of 5-LO (IC_{50} 0.4 μM) and COX/mPGES pathway (IC_{50} 10.1 μM). Related compounds, cannabispiranol and cannabispirenone, were seeming inactive. Canniprene concentration in 160 chemovars ranged trace amounts to more than 0.2% in cannabis leaves. While its concentration did not correlate with phytocannabinoid content or developmental stage of the cannabis plant, it did have a reciprocal relationship with cannflavin A. It will be fascinating to explore the ecological roles that these substances play, and the implications that they might harbor for therapeutic application.

7. CONCLUSION

This review has examined the complex and varied pharmacology of cannabis, a plant that should no longer be considered merely a vehicle for THC, but rather, a potential botanical drug mixture of great therapeutic value in consideration of its genetic plasticity and the promise of its many components. Clinical trials that examine synergistic effects of cannabis components are sorely needed, particularly in the area of phytocannabinoid–terpenoid interactions and to assess salient differences between cannabis chemovars attributable to their relative concentrations of entourage compounds.

CONFLICT OF INTEREST

Ethan Russo is Medical Director of PHYTECS, a biomedical research organization with an interest in therapeutic application of substances discussed in this publication.

Jahan Marcu is Chief Science Officer for Americans for Safe Access, a member-based organization working to ensure safe and legal access to cannabis therapeutic uses and research.

ACKNOWLEDGMENTS

The authors would like to thank John McPartland, whose guidance in planning, and selection of cannabis compounds was essential to this effort. Debbie Churgai, technical editor, Americans for Safe Access, kindly provided assistance in editing the manuscript.

REFERENCES

Ali, A., Tabanca, N., Demirci, B., Blythe, E. K., Ali, Z., Baser, K. H., et al. (2015). Chemical composition and biological activity of four salvia essential oils and individual compounds against two species of mosquitoes. *Journal of Agricultural and Food Chemistry*, *63*(2), 447–456. http://doi.org/10.1021/jf504976f.

Allegrone, G., Pollastro, F., Magagnini, G., Taglialatela-Scafati, O., Seegers, J., Koeberle, A., et al. (2017). The bibenzyl canniprene inhibit the production of pro-inflammatory eicosanoids and selectively accumulates in some cannabis strains. *Journal of Natural Products*, *80*(3), 731–734. http://dx.doi.org/10.1021/acs.jnatprod.6b01126.

Alozie, S. O., Martin, B. R., Harris, L. S., & Dewey, W. L. (1980). 3H-Δ9-tetrahydrocannabinol, 3H-cannabinol and 3H-cannabidiol: Penetration and regional distribution in rat brain. *Pharmacology, Biochemistry, and Behavior*, *12*(2), 217–221. http://doi.org/10.1016/0091-3057(80)90359-7.

Americans for Safe Access. (2016). *Medical access to cannabis for pain treatment.* Retrieved January 3, 2017, from http://www.safeaccessnow.org/medical_cannabis_access_for_pain_treatment.

Antonisamy, P., Duraipandiyan, V., Aravinthan, A., Al-Dhabi, N. A., Ignacimuthu, S., Choi, K. C., et al. (2015). Protective effects of friedelin isolated from Azima tetracantha Lam. against ethanol-induced gastric ulcer in rats and possible underlying mechanisms. *European Journal of Pharmacology*, *750*, 167–175. http://doi.org/10.1016/j.ejphar.2015.01.015.

Antonisamy, P., Duraipandiyan, V., & Ignacimuthu, S. (2011). Anti-inflammatory, analgesic and antipyretic effects of friedelin isolated from Azima tetracantha Lam. in mouse and rat models. *Journal of Pharmacy and Pharmacology*, *63*(8), 1070–1077. http://doi.org/10.1111/j.2042-7158.2011.01300.x.

Appendino, G., Gibbons, S., Giana, A., Pagani, A., Grassi, G., Stavri, M., et al. (2008). Antibacterial cannabinoids from cannabis sativa: A structure–activity study. *Journal of Natural Products*, *71*(8), 1427–1430. http://doi.org/10.1021/np8002673.

Arruda, D. C., D'Alexandri, F. L., Katzin, A. M., & Uliana, S. R. (2005). Antileishmanial activity of the terpene nerolidol. *Antimicrobial Agents and Chemotherapy*, *49*(5), 1679–1687.

Asakura, K., Kanemasa, T., Minagawa, K., Kagawa, K., Yagami, T., Nakajima, M., et al. (2000). alpha-eudesmol, a P/Q-type Ca(2+) channel blocker, inhibits neurogenic vasodilation and extravasation following electrical stimulation of trigeminal ganglion. *Brain Research*, *873*(1), 94–101.

Aydin, E., Turkez, H., & Tasdemir, S. (2013). Anticancer and antioxidant properties of terpinolene in rat brain cells. *Arhiv za Higijenu Rada i Toksikologiju*, *64*(3), 415–424. http://doi.org/10.2478/10004-1254-64-2013-2365.

Backes, M. (2014). *Cannabis pharmacy: The practical guide to medical marijuana.* New York: Black Dog & Leventhal.

Baek, S., Kim, Y. O., Kwag, J. S., Choi, K. E., Jung, W. Y., & Han, D. S. (1998). Boron trifluoride etherate on silica-A modified Lewis acid reagent (VII). Antitumor activity of cannabigerol against human oral epitheloid carcinoma cells. *Archives of Pharmacal Research*, *21*(3), 353–356.

Bahi, A., Al Mansouri, S., Al Memari, E., Al Ameri, M., Nurulain, S. M., & Ojha, S. (2014). β-Caryophyllene, a CB2 receptor agonist produces multiple behavioral changes relevant to anxiety and depression in mice. *Physiology & Behavior*, *135C*, 119–124. http://doi.org/10.1016/j.physbeh.2014.06.003.

Bai, J., Zheng, Y., Wang, G., & Liu, P. (2016). Protective effect of D-limonene against oxidative stress-induced cell damage in human lens epithelial cells via the p38 pathway. *Oxidative Medicine and Cellular Longevity*, *2016*, 5962832. http://doi.org/10.1155/2016/5962832.

Baldissera, M. D., Grando, T. H., Souza, C. F., Gressler, L. T., Stefani, L. M., da Silva, A. S., et al. (2016). In vitro and in vivo action of terpinen-4-ol, gamma-terpinene, and alpha-terpinene against Trypanosoma evansi. *Experimental Parasitology*, *162*, 43–48. http://doi.org/10.1016/j.exppara.2016.01.004.

Balvers, M. G. J., Verhoeckx, K. C. M., Bijlsma, S., Rubingh, C. M., Meijerink, J., Wortelboer, H. M., et al. (2012). Fish oil and inflammatory status alter the n-3 to n-6 balance of the endocannabinoid and oxylipin metabolomes in mouse plasma and tissues. *Metabolomics: Official Journal of the Metabolomic Society*, *8*(6), 1130–1147. http://doi.org/10.1007/s11306-012-0421-9.

Banerjee, S. P., Snyder, S. H., & Mechoulam, R. (1975). Cannabinoids: Influence on neurotransmitter uptake in rat brain synaptosomes. *Journal of Pharmacology and Experimental Therapeutics*, *194*(1), 74–81.

Barbosa, L. C., Filomeno, C. A., & Teixeira, R. R. (2016). Chemical variability and biological activities of Eucalyptus spp. essential oils. *Molecules (Basel, Switzerland)*, *21*(12), 33. http://doi.org/10.3390/molecules21121671.

Barrett, M. L., Scutt, A. M., & Evans, F. J. (1986). Cannflavin A and B, prenylated flavones from Cannabis sativa L. *Experientia*, *42*(4), 452–453.

Baser, K. H. C., & Buchbauer, G. (2016). *Handbook of essential oils: Science, technology, and applications* (2nd ed.). Boca Raton, FL: CRC Press.

Batista, P. A., de Paula Werner, M. F., Oliveira, E. C., Burgos, L., Pereira, P., da Silva Brum, L. F., et al. (2010). The antinociceptive effect of (-)-linalool in models of chronic inflammatory and neuropathic hypersensitivity in mice. *The Journal of Pain*, *11*(11), 1222–1229. http://doi.org/10.1016/j.jpain.2010.02.022.

Batista, P. A., Werner, M. F., Oliveira, E. C., Burgos, L., Pereira, P., Brum, L. F., et al. (2008). Evidence for the involvement of ionotropic glutamatergic receptors on the antinociceptive effect of (-)-linalool in mice. *Neuroscience Letters*, *440*(3), 299–303. http://doi.org/10.1016/j.neulet.2008.05.092.

Ben Amar, M. (2006). Cannabinoids in medicine: A review of their therapeutic potential. *Journal of Ethnopharmacology*, *105*(1–2), 1–25. http://doi.org/10.1016/j.jep.2006.02.001.

Ben Sghaier, M., Mousslim, M., Pagano, A., Ammari, Y., Luis, J., & Kovacic, H. (2016). beta-Eudesmol, a sesquiterpene from Teucrium ramosissimum, inhibits superoxide production, proliferation, adhesion and migration of human tumor cell. *Environmental Toxicology and Pharmacology*, *46*, 227–233. http://doi.org/10.1016/j.etap.2016.07.019.

Bento, A. F., Marcon, R., Dutra, R. C., Claudino, R. F., Cola, M., Leite, D. F. P., et al. (2011). β-Caryophyllene inhibits dextran sulfate sodium-induced colitis in mice through CB2 receptor activation and PPARγ pathway. *The American Journal of Pathology*, *178*(3), 1153–1166. http://doi.org/10.1016/j.ajpath.2010.11.052.

Bettarini, F., Borgonovi, G. E., Fiorani, T., Gagliardi, I., Caprioli, V., Massardo, P., et al. (1993). Antiparasitic compounds from East African plants: Isolation and biological activity of anonaine, matricarianol, canthin-6-one, and caryophyllene oxide. *Insect Science and Its Application*, *14*(1), 93–99.

Bhatia, S. P., Letizia, C. S., & Api, A. M. (2008). Fragrance material review on alpha-terpineol. *Food Chem Toxicol*, *46*(Suppl. 11), S280–S285. http://doi.org/10.1016/j.fct.2008.06.027.

Bhatia, S. P., McGinty, D., Letizia, C. S., & Api, A. M. (2008). Fragrance material review on fenchyl alcohol. *Food Chem Toxicol*, *46*(Suppl 11), S157–159. http://dx.doi.org/10.1016/j.fct.2008.06.047.

Binet, L., Binet, P., Miocque, M., Roux, M., & Bernier, A. (1972). Recherches sur les proprietes pharmcodynamiques (action sedative et action spasmolytique) de quelques alcools terpeniques aliphatiques. *Annales Pharmaceutiques Françaises*, *30*(9), 611–616.

Bishayee, A., Ahmed, S., Brankov, N., & Perloff, M. (2011). Triterpenoids as potential agents for the chemoprevention and therapy of breast cancer. *Frontiers in Bioscience (Landmark Edition)*, *16*, 980–996.

Bisogno, T., Hanus, L., De Petrocellis, L., Tchilibon, S., Ponde, D. E., Brandi, I., et al. (2001). Molecular targets for cannabidiol and its synthetic analogues: Effect on vanilloid VR1 receptors and on the cellular uptake and enzymatic hydrolysis of anandamide. *The British Journal of Pharmacology*, *134*(4), 845–852.

Bisset, N. G., & Wichtl, M. (2004). *Herbal drugs and phytopharmaceuticals: A handbook for practice on a scientific basis* (3rd ed.). Stuttgart, Boca Raton: Medpharm Scientific Publishers; CRC Press.

Bolognini, D., Costa, B., Maione, S., Comelli, F., Marini, P., Di Marzo, V., et al. (2010). The plant cannabinoid Delta9-tetrahydrocannabivarin can decrease signs of inflammation and inflammatory pain in mice. *British Journal of Pharmacology*, *160*(3), 677–687. http://doi.org/10.1111/j.1476-5381.2010.00756.x.

Bolognini, D., Rock, E. M., Cluny, N. L., Cascio, M. G., Limebeer, C. L., Duncan, M., et al. (2013). Cannabidiolic acid prevents vomiting in Suncus murinus and nausea-induced behaviour in rats by enhancing 5-HT1A receptor activation. *British Journal of Pharmacology*, *168*(6), 1456–1470. http://doi.org/10.1111/bph.12043.

Bomfim, D. S., Ferraz, R. P., Carvalho, N. C., Soares, M. B., Pinheiro, M. L., Costa, E. V., et al. (2013). Eudesmol isomers induce caspase-mediated apoptosis in human hepatocellular carcinoma HepG2 cells. *Basic & Clinical Pharmacology & Toxicology*, *113*(5), 300–306. http://doi.org/10.1111/bcpt.12097.

Bomfim, L. M., Menezes, L. R. A., Rodrigues, A. C. B. C., Dias, R. B., Rocha, C. A. G., Soares, M. B. P., et al. (2016). Antitumour activity of the microencapsulation of Annona vepretorum essential oil. *Basic & Clinical Pharmacology & Toxicology*, *118*(3), 208–213. http://doi.org/10.1111/bcpt.12488.

Bonamin, F., Moraes, T. M., Dos Santos, R. C., Kushima, H., Faria, F. M., Silva, M. A., et al. (2014). The effect of a minor constituent of essential oil from Citrus aurantium: The role of β-myrcene in preventing peptic ulcer disease. *Chemico-Biological Interactions*, *212*, 11–19. http://doi.org/10.1016/j.cbi.2014.01.009.

Bonesi, M., Menichini, F., Tundis, R., Loizzo, M. R., Conforti, F., Passalacqua, N. G., et al. (2010). Acetylcholinesterase and butyrylcholinesterase inhibitory activity of Pinus species essential oils and their constituents. *Journal of Enzyme Inhibition and Medicinal Chemistry*, *25*(5), 622–628. http://doi.org/10.3109/14756360903389856.

Booth, J. K., Page, J. E., & Bohlmann, J. (2017). Terpene synthases from Cannabis sativa. *PLoS ONE*, *12*(3), e0173911. http://dx.doi.org/10.1371/journal.pone.0173911.

Buchbauer, G. (2010). Biological activities of essential oils. In K. H. C. Baser & G. Buchbauer (Eds.), *Handbook of essential oils: Science, technology, and applications* (pp. 235–280). Boca Raton, FL: CRC Press.

Buchbauer, G., Jirovetz, L., Jager, W., Plank, C., & Dietrich, H. (1993). Fragrance compounds and essential oils with sedative effects upon inhalation. *Journal of Pharmaceutical Sciences*, *82*(6), 660–664.

Brown, N. K., & Harvey, D. J. (1990). In vitro metabolism of cannabichromene in seven common laboratory animals. *Drug Metabolism and Disposition*, *18*(6), 1065–1070.

Calhoun, S. R., Galloway, G. P., & Smith, D. E. (1998). Abuse potential of dronabinol (Marinol). *Journal of Psychoactive Drugs*, *30*(2), 187–196. http://doi.org/10.1080/02791072.1998.10399689.

Callaway, J. C. (2004). Hempseed as a nutritional resource: An overview. *Euphytica, 140*, 65–72.

Camargos, H. S., Moreira, R. A., Mendanha, S. A., Fernandes, K. S., Dorta, M. L., & Alonso, A. (2014). Terpenes increase the lipid dynamics in the Leishmania plasma membrane at concentrations similar to their IC50 values. *PloS One, 9*(8). e104429. http://doi.org/10.1371/journal.pone.0104429.

Campbell, W. E., Gammon, D. W., Smith, P., Abrahams, M., & Purves, T. D. (1997). Composition and antimalarial activity in vitro of the essential oil of Tetradenia riparia. *Planta Medica, 63*(3), 270–272.

Carrier, E. J., Auchampach, J. A., & Hillard, C. J. (2006). Inhibition of an equilibrative nucleoside transporter by cannabidiol: A mechanism of cannabinoid immunosuppression. *Proceedings of the National Academy of Sciences of the United States of America, 103*(20), 7895–7900.

Carson, C. F., & Riley, T. V. (1995). Antimicrobial activity of the major components of the essential oil of Melaleuca alternifolia. *The Journal of Applied Bacteriology, 78*(3), 264–269.

Carvalho-Freitas, M. I., & Costa, M. (2002). Anxiolytic and sedative effects of extracts and essential oil from Citrus aurantium L. *Biological & Pharmaceutical Bulletin, 25*(12), 1629–1633.

Cascio, M. G., Gauson, L. A., Stevenson, L. A., Ross, R. A., & Pertwee, R. G. (2010). Evidence that the plant cannabinoid cannabigerol is a highly potent α2-adrenoceptor agonist and moderately potent 5HT1A receptor antagonist. *British Journal of Pharmacology, 159*(1), 129–141. http://doi.org/10.1111/j.1476-5381.2009.00515.x.

Cascio, M. G., & Pertwee, R. G. (2014). Known pharmacological actions of nine nonpsychotropic phytocannabinoids. In R. G. Pertwee (Ed.), *Handbook of cannabis* (pp. 137–156). Oxford, UK: Oxford University Press. http://doi.org/10.1093/acprof:oso/9780199662685.003.0007.

Cascone, P., Iodice, L., Maffei, M. E., Bossi, S., Arimura, G.-I., & Guerrieri, E. (2015). Tobacco overexpressing β-ocimene induces direct and indirect responses against aphids in receiver tomato plants. *Journal of Plant Physiology, 173*, 28–32. http://doi.org/10.1016/j.jplph.2014.08.011.

Cawthorne, M. A., Wargent, E., Zaibi, M., Stott, C., & Wright, S. (2007). The CB1 antagonist, delta-9-tetrahydrocannabivarin (THCV) has anti-obesity activity in dietary-induced obese (DIO) mice. In *Presented at the 17th annual symposium on the cannabinoids, Saint-Sauveur, Quebec* (p. 141). Canada: International Cannabinoid Research Society.

Chandler, R. F., & Hooper, S. N. (1979). Friedelin and associated triterpenoids. *Phytochemistry, 18*, 711–724.

Chen, T., Hao, J., He, J., Zhang, J., Li, Y., Liu, R., et al. (2013). Cannabisin B induces autophagic cell death by inhibiting the AKT/mTOR pathway and S phase cell cycle arrest in HepG2 cells. *Food Chemistry, 138*(2–3), 1034–1041. http://doi.org/10.1016/j.foodchem.2012.11.102.

Chen, W., Liu, Y., Li, M., Mao, J., Zhang, L., Huang, R., et al. (2015). Anti-tumor effect of alpha-pinene on human hepatoma cell lines through inducing G2/M cell cycle arrest. *Journal of Pharmacological Sciences, 127*(3), 332–338. http://doi.org/10.1016/j.jphs.2015.01.008.

Chen, T., Wu, Y., Zhang, Y., Wang, B., Hu, Y., Wang, C., et al. (2012). Archaeobotanical study of ancient food and cereal remains at the Astana cemeteries, Xinxiang, China. *PloS One*, 7(9), e45137. http://doi.org/10.1371/journal.pone.0045137.

Chidambara Murthy, K. N., Jayaprakasha, G. K., & Patil, B. S. (2012). D-limonene rich volatile oil from blood oranges inhibits angiogenesis, metastasis and cell death in human colon cancer cells. *Life Sciences, 91*(11–12), 429–439. http://doi.org/10.1016/j.lfs.2012.08.016.

Chinsembu, K. C. (2016). Tuberculosis and nature's pharmacy of putative anti-tuberculosis agents. *Acta Tropica, 153*, 46–56. http://doi.org/10.1016/j.actatropica.2015.10.004.

Chiou, L. C., Ling, J. Y., & Chang, C. C. (1997). Chinese herb constituent beta-eudesmol alleviated the electroshock seizures in mice and electrographic seizures in rat hippocampal slices. *Neuroscience Letters, 231*(3), 171–174.

Choi, Y. J., Sim, W. C., Choi, H. K., Lee, S. H., & Lee, B. H. (2013). Alpha-Terpineol induces fatty liver in mice mediated by the AMP-activated kinase and sterol response element binding protein pathway. *Food and Chemical Toxicology*, *55*, 129–136. http://doi.org/10.1016/j.fct.2012.12.025.

Choi, H. S., Song, H. S., Ukeda, H., & Sawamura, M. (2000). Radical-scavenging activities of citrus essential oils and their components: Detection using 1,1-diphenyl-2-picrylhydrazyl. *Journal of Agricultural and Food Chemistry*, *48*(9), 4156–4161.

Ciftci, O., Oztanir, M. N., & Cetin, A. (2014). Neuroprotective effects of β-myrcene following global cerebral ischemia/reperfusion-mediated oxidative and neuronal damage in a C57BL/J6 mouse. *Neurochemical Research*, *39*(9), 1717–1723. http://doi.org/10.1007/s11064-014-1365-4.

Clarke, R. C., & Merlin, M. D. (2012). *Cannabis: Evolution and ethnobotany*. Berkeley: University of California Press.

Claussen, U., Von Spulak, F., & Korte, F. (1966). Zur chemischen klassifizierung von pflanzen—XXXI, haschisch—X: Cannabichromen, ein neuer haschisch-inhalts-stoff. *Tetrahedron*, *22*(4), 1477–1479. http://doi.org/10.1016/S0040-4020(01)99445-1.

Cluny, N. L., Keenan, C. M., Reimer, R. A., Le Foll, B., & Sharkey, K. A. (2015). Prevention of diet-induced obesity effects on body weight and gut microbiota in mice treated chronically with delta9-tetrahydrocannabinol. *PloS One*, *10*(12), e0144270. http://doi.org/10.1371/journal.pone.0144270.

Console-Bram, L., Marcu, J., & Abood, M. E. (2012). Cannabinoid receptors: Nomenclature and pharmacological principles. *Progress in Neuro-Psychopharmacology & Biological Psychiatry*, *38*(1), 4–15. http://doi.org/10.1016/j.pnpbp.2012.02.009.

Cornwell, P. A., & Barry, B. W. (1994). Sesquiterpene components of volatile oils as skin penetration enhancers for the hydrophilic permeant 5-fluorouracil. *The Journal of Pharmacy and Pharmacology*, *46*(4), 261–269.

d'Alessio, P. A., Ostan, R., Bisson, J. F., Schulzke, J. D., Ursini, M. V., & Bene, M. C. (2013). Oral administration of d-limonene controls inflammation in rat colitis and displays anti-inflammatory properties as diet supplementation in humans. *Life Sciences*, *92*(24–26), 1151–1156. http://doi.org/10.1016/j.lfs.2013.04.013.

Davis, W. M., & Hatoum, N. S. (1983). Neurobehavioral actions of cannabichromene and interactions with Δ9-tetrahydrocannabinol. *General Pharmacology: The Vascular System*, *14*(2), 247–252. http://doi.org/10.1016/0306-3623(83)90004-6.

DeLong, G. T., Wolf, C. E., Poklis, A., & Lichtman, A. H. (2010). Pharmacological evaluation of the natural constituent of Cannabis sativa, cannabichromene and its modulation by Δ(9)-tetrahydrocannabinol. *Drug and Alcohol Dependence*, *112*(1–2), 126–133. http://doi.org/10.1016/j.drugalcdep.2010.05.019.

de Meijer, E. P. M., Bagatta, M., Carboni, A., Crucitti, P., Moliterni, V. M. C., Ranalli, P., et al. (2003). The inheritance of chemical phenotype in Cannabis sativa L. *Genetics*, *163*(1), 335–346.

de Meijer, E. P. M., & Hammond, K. M. (2005). The inheritance of chemical phenotype in Cannabis sativa L. (II): Cannabigerol predominant plants. *Euphytica*, *145*, 189–198.

de Meijer, E. P. M., & Hammond, K. M. (2016). The inheritance of chemical phenotype in Cannabis sativa L. (V): Regulation of the propyl-/pentyl cannabinoid ratio, completion of a genetic model. *Euphytica*, *210*(2), 291–307. http://doi.org/10.1007/s10681-016-1721-3.

de Meijer, E. P. M., Hammond, K. M., & Micheler, M. (2009). The inheritance of chemical phenotype in Cannabis sativa L. (III): Variation in cannabichromene proportion. *Euphytica*, *165*, 293–311.

de Meijer, E., & Limited, G. P. (2011). Cannabis sativa plants rich in cannabichromene and its acid, extracts thereof and methods of obtaining extracts there from (12/936,947).

de Moura, N. F., Simionatto, E., Porto, C., Hoelzel, S. C., Dessoy, E. C., Zanatta, N., et al. (2002). Quinoline alkaloids, coumarins and volatile constituents of Helietta longifoliata. *Planta Medica*, *68*(7), 631–634.

de Oliveira, M. G., Marques, R. B., de Santana, M. F., Santos, A. B., Brito, F. A., Barreto, E. O., et al. (2012). Alpha-terpineol reduces mechanical hypernociception and inflammatory response. *Basic & Clinical Pharmacology & Toxicology*, *111*(2), 120–125. http://doi.org/10.1111/j.1742-7843.2012.00875.x.

De Petrocellis, L., & Di Marzo, V. (2010). Non-CB1, non-CB2 receptors for endocannabinoids, plant cannabinoids, and synthetic cannabimimetics: Focus on G-protein-coupled receptors and transient receptor potential channels. *Journal of Neuroimmune Pharmacology*, *5*(1), 103–121. http://doi.org/10.1007/s11481-009-9177-z.

De Petrocellis, L., Ligresti, A., Moriello, A. S., Allara, M., Bisogno, T., Petrosino, S., et al. (2011). Effects of cannabinoids and cannabinoid-enriched Cannabis extracts on TRP channels and endocannabinoid metabolic enzymes. *British Journal of Pharmacology*, *163*(7), 1479–1494. http://dx.doi.org/10.1111/j.1476-5381.2010.01166.x.

De Petrocellis, L., Orlando, P., Moriello, A. S., Aviello, G., Stott, C., Izzo, A. A., et al. (2012). Cannabinoid actions at TRPV channels: Effects on TRPV3 and TRPV4 and their potential relevance to gastrointestinal inflammation. *Acta Physiologica*, *204*(2), 255–266. http://doi.org/10.1111/j.1748-1716.2011.02338.x.

De Petrocellis, L., Vellani, V., Schiano-Moriello, A., Marini, P., Magherini, P. C., Orlando, P., et al. (2008). Plant-derived cannabinoids modulate the activity of transient receptor potential channels of ankyrin type-1 and melastatin type-8. *The Journal of Pharmacology and Experimental Therapeutics*, *325*(3), 1007–1015. http://doi.org/10.1124/jpet.107.134809.

Deiana, S., Watanabe, A., Yamasaki, Y., Amada, N., Arthur, M., Fleming, S., et al. (2012). Plasma and brain pharmacokinetic profile of cannabidiol (CBD), cannabidivarine (CBDV), Delta(9)-tetrahydrocannabivarin (THCV) and cannabigerol (CBG) in rats and mice following oral and intraperitoneal administration and CBD action on obsessive-compulsive behaviour. *Psychopharmacology (Berl)*, *219*(3), 859–873. http://dx.doi.org/10.1007/s00213-011-2415-0.

de Lago, E., & Fernández-Ruiz, J. (2007). Cannabinoids and neuroprotection in motor-related disorders. *CNS & Neurological Disorders Drug Targets*, *6*(6), 377–387. http://doi.org/10.2174/187152707783399210.

De-Oliveira, A. C., Ribeiro-Pinto, L. F., & Paumgartten, J. R. (1997). In vitro inhibition of CYP2B1 monooxygenase by beta-myrcene and other monoterpenoid compounds. *Toxicology Letters*, *92*(1), 39–46. http://doi.org/10.1016/S0378-4274(97)00034-9, S0378427497000349 [pii].

do Socorro, S. R. M. S., Mendonca-Filho, R. R., Bizzo, H. R., de Almeida Rodrigues, I., Soares, R. M., Souto-Padron, T., et al. (2003). Antileishmanial activity of a linalool-rich essential oil from Croton cajucara. *Antimicrobial Agents and Chemotherapy*, *47*(6), 1895–1901.

do Vale, T. G., Furtado, E. C., Santos, J. G., Jr., & Viana, G. S. (2002). Central effects of citral, myrcene and limonene, constituents of essential oil chemotypes from Lippia alba (Mill.) n.e. Brown. *Phytomedicine*, *9*(8), 709–714.

Dong, Y., Li, L., Wang, L., Zhou, T., Liu, J. W., & Gao, Y. J. (2015). Preliminary study of the effects of beta-elemene on MCF-7/ADM breast cancer stem cells. *Genetics and Molecular Research*, *14*(1), 2347–2355. http://doi.org/10.4238/2015.March.27.20.

Douthwaite, A. H. (1947). Choice of drugs in the treatment of duodenal ulcer. *British Medical Journal*, *2*(4514), 43–47.

Dussy, F. E., Hamberg, C., Luginbuhl, M., Schwerzmann, T., & Briellmann, T. A. (2005). Isolation of Delta9-THCA-A from hemp and analytical aspects concerning the determination of Delta9-THC in cannabis products. *Forensic Science International*, *149*(1), 3–10.

Edman, K., Lofstedt, H., Berg, P., Eriksson, K., Axelsson, S., Bryngelsson, I., et al. (2003). Exposure assessment to alpha- and beta-pinene, delta(3)-carene and wood dust in industrial production of wood pellets. *The Annals of Occupational Hygiene, 47*(3), 219–226.

Ee, G. C., Lim, C. K., Rahmat, A., & Lee, H. L. (2005). Cytotoxic activities of chemical constituents from Mesua daphnifolia. *Tropical Biomedicine, 22*(2), 99–102.

Elisabetsky, E., Marschner, J., & Souza, D. O. (1995). Effects of linalool on glutamatergic system in the rat cerebral cortex. *Neurochemical Research, 20*(4), 461–465.

Elmann, A., Mordechay, S., Rindner, M., Larkov, O., Elkabetz, M., & Ravid, U. (2009). Protective effects of the essential oil of Salvia fruticosa and its constituents on astrocytic susceptibility to hydrogen peroxide-induced cell death. *Journal of Agricultural and Food Chemistry, 57*(15), 6636–6641. http://doi.org/10.1021/jf901162f.

ElSohly, H. N., Turner, C. E., Clark, A. M., & Eisohly, M. A. (1982). Synthesis and antimicrobial activities of certain cannabichromene and cannabigerol related compounds. *Journal of Pharmaceutical Sciences, 71*(12), 1319–1323.

Elsohly, M. A., Turner, C. E., Phoebe, C. H. J., Knapp, J. E., Schiff, P. L. J., & Slatkin, D. J. (1978). Anhydrocannabisativine, a new alkaloid from Cannabis sativa L. *Journal of Pharmaceutical Sciences, 67*(1), 124.

Elzinga, S., Fischedick, J., Podkolinski, R., & Raber, J. C. (2015). Cannabinoid and terpenes as chemotaxonomic markers in cannabis. *Natural Products Chemistry & Research, 3*(4), 1–9.

Evans, F. J. (1991). Cannabinoids: The separation of central from peripheral effects on a structural basis. *Planta Medica, 57*(7), S60–S67.

Evans, F. J. (2007). Cannabinoids: The separation of central from peripheral effects on a structural basis. *Planta Medica, 57*(S 1), S60–S67. http://doi.org/10.1055/s-2006-960231.

Falk, A. A., Hagberg, M. T., Lof, A. E., Wigaeus-Hjelm, E. M., & Wang, Z. P. (1990). Uptake, distribution and elimination of alpha-pinene in man after exposure by inhalation. *Scandinavian Journal of Work, Environment and Health, 16*(5), 372–378.

Falk, A., Lof, A., Hagberg, M., Hjelm, E. W., & Wang, Z. (1991). Human exposure to 3-carene by inhalation: Toxicokinetics, effects on pulmonary function and occurrence of irritative and CNS symptoms. *Toxicology and Applied Pharmacology, 110*(2), 198–205.

Falk-Filipsson, A., Lof, A., Hagberg, M., Hjelm, E. W., & Wang, Z. (1993). d-limonene exposure to humans by inhalation: Uptake, distribution, elimination, and effects on the pulmonary function. *Journal of Toxicology and Environmental Health, 38*(1), 77–88.

Farag, R. S., Shalaby, A. S., El-Baroty, G. A., Ibrahim, N. A., Ali, M. A., & Hassan, E. M. (2004). Chemical and biological evaluation of the essential oils of different Melaleuca species. *Phytotherapy Research, 18*(1), 30–35.

Fidyt, K., Fiedorowicz, A., & Strządała, L. (2016). β-caryophyllene and β-caryophyllene oxide—Natural compounds of anticancer and analgesic properties. *Cancer Medicine, 5*(10), 3007–3017.

Fischedick, J. (2017). Indentification of terpenoid chemotypes among high (-)-*trans*-Δ^9-tetrahydrocannabinol-producing Cannabis sativa L. cultivars. *Cannabis and Cannabinoid Research, 2.1*, 34–47. http://dx.doi.org/10.1089/can.2016.0040.

Fischedick, J. T., Hazekamp, A., Erkelens, T., Choi, Y. H., & Verpoorte, R. (2010). Metabolic fingerprinting of Cannabis sativa L., cannabinoids and terpenoids for chemotaxonomic and drug standardization purposes. *Phytochemistry, 71*(17–18), 2058–2073. http://doi.org/10.1016/j.phytochem.2010.10.001.

Fischedick, J., Van Der Kooy, F., & Verpoorte, R. (2010). Cannabinoid receptor 1 binding activity and quantitative analysis of Cannabis sativa L. smoke and vapor. *Chemical & Pharmaceutical Bulletin, 58*(2), 201–207.

Fitsiou, E., Anestopoulos, I., Chlichlia, K., Galanis, A., Kourkoutas, I., Panayiotidis, M. I., et al. (2016). Antioxidant and antiproliferative properties of the essential oils of Satureja thymbra and Satureja parnassica and their major constituents. *Anticancer Research, 36*(11), 5757–5763. http://dx.doi.org/10.21873/anticanres.11159.

Flachenecker, P., Henze, T., & Zettl, U. K. (2014). Nabiximols (THC/CBD oromucosal spray, Sativex®) in clinical practice—Results of a multicenter, non-interventional study (MOVE 2) in patients with multiple sclerosis spasticity. *European Neurology*, *71*(5–6), 271–279. http://dx.doi.org/10.1159/000357427.

Formukong, E. A., Evans, A. T., & Evans, F. J. (1988). Analgesic and antiinflammatory activity of constituents of Cannabis sativa L. *Inflammation*, *12*(4), 361–371.

Franz, C., & Novak, J. (2010). Sources of essential oils. In K. H. C. Baser & G. Buchbauer (Eds.), *Handbook of essential oils: Science, technology, and applications* (pp. 39–82). Boca Raton, FL: CRC Press.

Fukumoto, S., Morishita, A., Furutachi, K., Terashima, T., Nakayama, T., & Yokogoshi, H. (2008). Effect of flavour components in lemon essential oil on physical or psychological stress. *Stress and Health*, *24*, 3–12.

Gaoni, Y., & Mechoulam, R. (1964). The structure and function of cannabigerol, a new hashish constituent. *Proceedings of the Chemical Society*, *1*, 82.

Gaoni, Y., & Mechoulam, R. (1966). Cannabichromene, a new active principle in hashish. *Chemical Communications (London)*, *1*, 20–21. http://doi.org/10.1039/C19660000020.

Gattefosse, R.-M. (1993). Gatefosse's aromatherapy (R. W. Tisserand, Trans.). Essex: C.W. Daniel.

Gauson, L. A., Stevenson, L. A., Thomas, A., Baillie, G. L., Ross, R. A., & Pertwee, R. G. (2007). Cannabigerol behaves as a partial agonist at both CB1 and CB2 receptors. In *Presented at the 17th annual symposium on the cannabinoids, Saint-Sauveur, Quebec* (p. 206). Canada: International Cannabinoid Research Society.

Gertsch, J. (2008). Anti-inflammatory cannabinoids in diet: Towards a better understanding of CB(2) receptor action? *Communicative & Integrative Biology*, *1*(1), 26–28.

Ghelardini, C., Galeotti, N., Salvatore, G., & Mazzanti, G. (1999). Local anaesthetic activity of the essential oil of Lavandula angustifolia. *Planta Medica*, *65*(8), 700–703. http://doi.org/10.1055/s-1999-14045.

Giese, M. W., Lewis, M. A., Giese, L., & Smith, K. M. (2015). Development and validation of a reliable and robust method for the analysis of cannabinoids and terpenes in cannabis. *Journal of AOAC International*, *98*(6), 1503–1522. http://doi.org/10.5740/jaoacint.15-116.

Gil, M. L., Jimenez, J., Ocete, M. A., Zarzuelo, A., & Cabo, M. M. (1989). Comparative study of different essential oils of Bupleurum gibraltaricum Lamarck. *Pharmazie*, *44*(4), 284–287.

Girola, N., Figueiredo, C. R., Farias, C. F., Azevedo, R. A., Ferreira, A. K., Teixeira, S. F., et al. (2015). Camphene isolated from essential oil of Piper cernuum (Piperaceae) induces intrinsic apoptosis in melanoma cells and displays antitumor activity in vivo. *Biochemical and Biophysical Research Communications*, *467*(4), 928–934. http://doi.org/10.1016/j.bbrc.2015.10.041.

Gong, M., Liu, Y., Zhang, J., Gao, Y. J., Zhai, P. P., Su, X., et al. (2015). beta-Elemene inhibits cell proliferation by regulating the expression and activity of topoisomerases I and IIalpha in human hepatocarcinoma HepG-2 cells. *BioMed Research International*, *2015*, 153987. http://doi.org/10.1155/2015/153987.

Govindarajan, M., Rajeswary, M., & Benelli, G. (2016). Delta-Cadinene, Calarene and delta-4-Carene from Kadsura heteroclita essential oil as novel larvicides against malaria, dengue and filariasis mosquitoes. *Combinatorial Chemistry & High Throughput Screening*, *19*(7), 565–571.

Govindarajan, M., Rajeswary, M., Hoti, S. L., Bhattacharyya, A., & Benelli, G. (2016). Eugenol, alpha-pinene and beta-caryophyllene from Plectranthus barbatus essential oil as eco-friendly larvicides against malaria, dengue and Japanese encephalitis mosquito vectors. *Parasitology Research*, *115*(2), 807–815. http://dx.doi.org/10.1007/s00436-015-4809-0.

Grassmann, J., Hippeli, S., Spitzenberger, R., & Elstner, E. F. (2005). The monoterpene terpinolene from the oil of Pinus mugo L. in concert with alpha-tocopherol and beta-carotene effectively prevents oxidation of LDL. *Phytomedicine, 12*(6–7), 416–423.

Grotenhermen, F., Russo, E. B., & Zuardi, A. W. (2017). Even high doses of oral cannabidiol do not cause THC-like effects in humans. *Cannabis and Cannabinoid Research, 2.1*, 1–4. http://dx.doi.org/10.1089/can.2016.0036.

Grunfeld, Y., & Edery, H. (1969). Psychopharmacological activity of the active constituents of hashish and some related cannabinoids. *Psychopharmacologia, 14*(3), 200–210.

Grunfeld, E., & Gresty, M. A. (1998). Relationship between motion sickness, migraine and menstruation in crew members of a "round the world" yacht race. *Brain Research Bulletin, 47*(5), 433–436.

Guy, G. W., & Stott, C. G. (2005). The development of Sativex- a natural cannabis-based medicine. In R. Mechoulam (Ed.), *Cannabinoids as therapeutics* (pp. 231–263). Basel, Switzerland: Birkhäuser Verlag.

Hampson, A. J., Grimaldi, M., Axelrod, J., & Wink, D. (1998). Cannabidiol and (-)Delta9-tetrahydrocannabinol are neuroprotective antioxidants. *Proceedings of the National Academy of Sciences of the United States of America, 95*(14), 8268–8273.

Han, H. D., Cho, Y.-J., Cho, S. K., Byeon, Y., Jeon, H. N., Kim, H.-S., et al. (2016). Linalool-incorporated nanoparticles as a novel anticancer agent for epithelial ovarian carcinoma. *Molecular Cancer Therapeutics, 15*(4), 618–627. http://doi.org/10.1158/1535-7163.MCT-15-0733-T.

Han, N. R., Moon, P. D., Ryu, K. J., Jang, J. B., Kim, H. M., & Jeong, H. J. (2017). Beta-eudesmol suppresses allergic reactions via inhibiting mast cell degranulation. *Clinical and Experimental Pharmacology and Physiology, 44*(2), 257–265. http://dx.doi.org/10.1111/1440-1681.12698.

Hanus, L. O., Meyer, S. M., Munoz, E., Taglialatela-Scafati, O., & Appendino, G. (2016). Phytocannabinoids: A unified critical inventory. *Natural Product Reports, 33*(12), 1357–1392. http://dx.doi.org/10.1039/c6np00074f.

Harris, B. (2010). Phytotherapeutic uses of essential oils. In K. H. C. Baser & G. Buchbauer (Eds.), *Handbook of essential oils: Science, technology, and applications* (pp. 315–352). Boca Raton: CRC Press.

Hassan, S. B., Gali-Muhtasib, H., Goransson, H., & Larsson, R. (2010). Alpha terpineol: A potential anticancer agent which acts through suppressing NF-kappaB signalling. *Anticancer Research, 30*(6), 1911–1919.

Hazekamp, A., & Grotenhermen, F. (2010). Review on clinical studies with cannabis and cannabinoids 2005-2009. *Cannabinoids, 5*(Special), 1–21.

Hazekamp, A., Tejkalová, K., & Papadimitriou, S. (2016). Cannabis: From cultivar to chemovar II—A metabolomics approach to cannabis classification. *Cannabis and Cannabinoid Research, 1*(1), 202–215. http://doi.org/10.1089/can.2016.0017.

Herkenham, M., Lynn, A. B., Little, M. D., Johnson, M. R., Melvin, L. S., de Costa, B. R., et al. (1990). Cannabinoid receptor localization in brain. *Proceedings of the National Academy of Sciences of the United States of America, 87*(5), 1932–1936.

Hill, A. J., Weston, S. E., Jones, N. A., Smith, I., Bevan, S. A., Williamson, E. M., et al. (2010). Delta-Tetrahydrocannabivarin suppresses in vitro epileptiform and in vivo seizure activity in adult rats. *Epilepsia, 51*(8), 1522–1532. http://doi.org/10.1111/j.1528-1167.2010.02523.x.

Hillig, K. W., & Mahlberg, P. G. (2004). A chemotaxonomic analysis of cannabinoid variation in Cannabis (Cannabaceae). *American Journal of Botany, 91*(6), 966–975. http://doi.org/10.3732/ajb.91.6.966.

Hofmann, M. E., & Frazier, C. J. (2013). Marijuana, endocannabinoids, and epilepsy: Potential and challenges for improved therapeutic intervention. *Experimental Neurology, 244*, 43–50. http://doi.org/10.1016/j.expneurol.2011.11.047.

Holley, J. H., Hadley, K. W., & Turner, C. E. (1975). Constituents of *Cannabis sativa* L. XI: Cannabidiol and cannabichromene in samples of known geographical origin. *Journal of Pharmaceutical Sciences*, *64*(5), 892–894.

Holland, M. L., Allen, J. D., & Arnold, J. C. (2008). Interaction of plant cannabinoids with the multidrug transporter ABCC1 (MRP1). *European Journal of Pharmacology*, *591*(1–3), 128–131. http://doi.org/10.1016/j.ejphar.2008.06.079.

Hong, P., & Liu, Y. (2017). Calcitonin gene-related peptide antagonism for acute treatment of migraine: A meta-analysis. *The International Journal of Neuroscience*, *127*(1), 20–27. http://doi.org/10.3109/00207454.2015.1137915.

Horváth, B., Mukhopadhyay, P., Haskó, G., & Pacher, P. (2012). The endocannabinoid system and plant-derived cannabinoids in diabetes and diabetic complications. *The American Journal of Pathology*, *180*(2), 432–442. http://doi.org/10.1016/j.ajpath.2011.11.003.

Hsieh, L. C., Hsieh, S. L., Chen, C. T., Chung, J. G., Wang, J. J., & Wu, C. C. (2015). Induction of alpha-phellandrene on autophagy in human liver tumor cells. *The American Journal of Chinese Medicine*, *43*(1), 121–136. http://doi.org/10.1142/S0192415X15500081.

Hsieh, S. L., Li, Y. C., Chang, W. C., Chung, J. G., Hsieh, L. C., & Wu, C. C. (2014). Induction of necrosis in human liver tumor cells by alpha-phellandrene. *Nutrition and Cancer*, *66*(6), 970–979. http://doi.org/10.1080/01635581.2014.936946.

Hu, Z., Wu, H., Li, Y., Hou, Q., Wang, Y., Li, S., et al. (2015). Beta-elemene inhibits the proliferation of esophageal squamous cell carcinoma by regulating long noncoding RNA-mediated inhibition of hTERT expression. *Anti-Cancer Drugs*, *26*(5), 531–539. http://doi.org/10.1097/CAD.0000000000000216.

Ismail, M. (2006). Central properties and chemical composition of Ocimum basilicum essential oil. *Pharmaceutical Biology*, *44*(8), 619–626.

Ito, K., & Ito, M. (2013). The sedative effect of inhaled terpinolene in mice and its structure-activity relationships. *Journal of Natural Medicines*, *67*(4), 833–837. http://doi.org/10.1007/s11418-012-0732-1.

Iwata, N., & Kitanaka, S. (2011). New cannabinoid-like chromane and chromene derivatives from Rhododendron anthopogonoides. *Chemical & Pharmaceutical Bulletin*, *59*(11), 1409–1412.

Jeong, J. G., Kim, Y. S., Min, Y. K., & Kim, S. H. (2008). Low concentration of 3-carene stimulates the differentiation of mouse osteoblastic MC3T3-E1 subclone 4 cells. *Phytotherapy Research*, *22*(1), 18–22. http://doi.org/10.1002/ptr.2247.

Jiang, S., Ling, C., Li, W., Jiang, H., Zhi, Q., & Jiang, M. (2016). Molecular mechanisms of anti-cancer activities of β-elemene: Targeting hallmarks of cancer. *Anti-Cancer Agents in Medicinal Chemistry*, *16*(11), 1426–1434.

Jianjun, Q., Song, Z., Yin, L., Jia, Z., & Donglei, L. (2008). Treatment of chylothorax with elemene. *The Thoracic and Cardiovascular Surgeon*, *56*(2), 103–105. http://doi.org/10.1055/s-2007-965708.

Jung, J., Kempf, J., Mahler, H., & Weinmann, W. (2007). Detection of Delta9-tetrahydrocannabinolic acid A in human urine and blood serum by LC-MS/MS. *Journal of Mass Spectrometry*, *42*(3), 354–360. http://doi.org/10.1002/jms.1167.

Kasanen, J. P., Pasanen, A. L., Pasanen, P., Liesivuori, J., Kosma, V. M., & Alarie, Y. (1999). Evaluation of sensory irritation of delta3-carene and turpentine, and acceptable levels of monoterpenes in occupational and indoor environment. *Journal of Toxicology and Environmental Health. Part A*, *57*(2), 89–114.

Kasuya, H., Okada, N., Kubohara, M., Satou, T., Masuo, Y., & Koike, K. (2015). Expression of BDNF and TH mRNA in the brain following inhaled administration of alpha-pinene. *Phytotherapy Research*, *29*(1), 43–47. http://doi.org/10.1002/ptr.5224.

Katsuyama, S., Mizoguchi, H., Kuwahata, H., Komatsu, T., Nagaoka, K., Nakamura, H., et al. (2013). Involvement of peripheral cannabinoid and opioid receptors in beta-caryophyllene-induced antinociception. *European Journal of Pain (London, England)*, *17*(5), 664–675. http://doi.org/10.1002/j.1532-2149.2012.00242.x.

Kennell, J. (2016). *A beekeeper has trained bees to make honey from cannabis resin*. Retrieved January 22, 2017, from http://thescienceexplorer.com/nature/beekeeper-has-trained-bees-make-honey-cannabis-resin.
Kim, S. S., Baik, J. S., Oh, T. H., Yoon, W. J., Lee, N. H., & Hyun, C. G. (2008). Biological activities of Korean Citrus obovoides and Citrus natsudaidai essential oils against acne-inducing bacteria. *Bioscience, Biotechnology, and Biochemistry*, *72*(10), 2507–2513.
Kim, S., Choi, Y., Choi, S., Choi, Y., & Park, T. (2014). Dietary camphene attenuates hepatic steatosis and insulin resistance in mice. *Obesity (Silver Spring)*, *22*(2), 408–417. http://doi.org/10.1002/oby.20554.
Kim, S. Y., Hwang, J. Y., & Shin, U. S. (2016). Preparation of nano/macroporous polycaprolactone microspheres for an injectable cell delivery system using room temperature ionic liquid and camphene. *Journal of Colloid and Interface Science*, *465*, 18–25. http://doi.org/10.1016/j.jcis.2015.11.055.
Kim, J. T., Ren, C. J., Fielding, G. A., Pitti, A., Kasumi, T., Wajda, M., et al. (2007). Treatment with lavender aromatherapy in the post-anesthesia care unit reduces opioid requirements of morbidly obese patients undergoing laparoscopic adjustable gastric banding. *Obesity Surgery*, *17*(7), 920–925.
Kimura, Y., & Sumiyoshi, M. (2012). Effects of an Atractylodes lancea rhizome extract and a volatile component beta-eudesmol on gastrointestinal motility in mice. *Journal of Ethnopharmacology*, *141*(1), 530–536. http://doi.org/10.1016/j.jep.2012.02.031.
Kiso, Y., Tohkin, M., & Hikino, H. (1983). Antihepatotoxic principles of Atractylodes rhizomes. *Journal of Natural Products*, *46*(5), 651–654.
Komiya, M., Takeuchi, T., & Harada, E. (2006). Lemon oil vapor causes an anti-stress effect via modulating the 5-HT and DA activities in mice. *Behavioural Brain Research*, *172*(2), 240–249. http://doi.org/10.1016/j.bbr.2006.05.006.
Komori, T., Fujiwara, R., Tanida, M., Nomura, J., & Yokoyama, M. M. (1995). Effects of citrus fragrance on immune function and depressive states. *Neuroimmunomodulation*, *2*(3), 174–180.
Kose, E. O., Deniz, I. G., Sarikurkcu, C., Aktas, O., & Yavuz, M. (2010). Chemical composition, antimicrobial and antioxidant activities of the essential oils of Sideritis erythrantha Boiss. and Heldr. (var. erythrantha and var. cedretorum P.H. Davis) endemic in Turkey. *Food and Chemical Toxicology*, *48*(10), 2960–2965. http://dx.doi.org/10.1016/j.fct.2010.07.033.
Kovac, J., Simunovic, K., Wu, Z., Klancnik, A., Bucar, F., Zhang, Q., et al. (2015). Antibiotic resistance modulation and modes of action of (-)-alpha-pinene in Campylobacter jejuni. *PloS One*, *10*(4), e0122871. http://doi.org/10.1371/journal.pone.0122871.
Kowal, M. A., Hazekamp, A., & Grotenhermen, F. (2016). Review on clinical studies with cannabis and cannabinoids 2010-2014. *Cannabinoids*, *11*(Special), 1–18.
Krol, S., Namiesnik, J., & Zabiegala, B. (2014). alpha-Pinene, 3-carene and d-limonene in indoor air of Polish apartments: The impact on air quality and human exposure. *The Science of the Total Environment*, *468–469*, 985–995. http://doi.org/10.1016/j.scitotenv.2013.08.099.
Kusuhara, M., Urakami, K., Masuda, Y., Zangiacomi, V., Ishii, H., Tai, S., et al. (2012). Fragrant environment with alpha-pinene decreases tumor growth in mice. *Biomedical Research*, *33*(1), 57–61.
Lafourcade, M., Larrieu, T., Mato, S., Duffaud, A., Sepers, M., Matias, I., et al. (2011). Nutritional omega-3 deficiency abolishes endocannabinoid-mediated neuronal functions. *Nature Neuroscience*, *14*(3), 345–350. http://doi.org/10.1038/nn.2736.
Lafuente, H., Alvarez, F. J., Pazos, M. R., Alvarez, A., Rey-Santano, M. C., Mielgo, V., et al. (2011). Cannabidiol reduces brain damage and improves functional recovery after acute hypoxia-ischemia in newborn pigs. *Pediatric Research*, *70*(3), 272–277. http://doi.org/10.1203/PDR.0b013e3182276b11.

Langenheim, J. H. (1994). Higher plant terpenoids: A phytocentric overview of their ecological roles. *Journal of Chemical Ecology, 20*(6), 1223–1279.

Lapczynski, A., Bhatia, S. P., Letizia, C. S., & Api, A. M. (2008). Fragrance material review on nerolidol (isomer unspecified). *Food Chem Toxicol, 46*(Suppl. 11), S247–S250. http://dx.doi.org/10.1016/j.fct.2008.06.063. S0278-6915(08)00355-4 [pii].

Lapczynski, A., Letizia, C. S., & Api, A. M. (2008). Addendum to Fragrance material review on linalool. *Food and Chemical Toxicology, 46*(Suppl. 11), S190–S192.

Laprairie, R. B., Bagher, A. M., Kelly, M. E. M., & Denovan-Wright, E. M. (2015). Cannabidiol is a negative allosteric modulator of the type 1 cannabinoid receptor. *British Journal of Pharmacology, 172*(20), 4790–4805. http://doi.org/10.1111/bph.13250.

Lastbom, L., Boman, A., Johnsson, S., Camner, P., & Ryrfeldt, A. (2003). Increased airway responsiveness of a common fragrance component, 3-carene, after skin sensitisation—A study in isolated guinea pig lungs. *Toxicology Letters, 145*(2), 189–196.

Lawless, J. (1995). *The illustrated encyclopedia of essential oils: The complete guide to the use of oils in aromatherapy and herbalism.* Shaftesbury, Dorset, [England]; Rockport, Mass: Element.

Leal-Cardoso, J. H., da Silva-Alves, K. S., Ferreira-da-Silva, F. W., dos Santos-Nascimento, T., Joca, H. C., de Macedo, F. H. P., et al. (2010). Linalool blocks excitability in peripheral nerves and voltage-dependent Na+ current in dissociated dorsal root ganglia neurons. *European Journal of Pharmacology, 645*(1–3), 86–93.

Legault, J., & Pichette, A. (2007). Potentiating effect of β-caryophyllene on anticancer activity of α-humulene, isocaryophyllene and paclitaxel. *Journal of Pharmacy and Pharmacology, 59*(12), 1643–1647. http://doi.org/10.1211/jpp.59.12.0005.

Li, Q., Li, L., Wang, F., CHEN, J., Zhao, Y., Wang, P., et al. (2013). Dietary capsaicin prevents nonalcoholic fatty liver disease through transient receptor potential vanilloid 1-mediated peroxisome proliferator-activated receptor delta activation. *Pflügers Archiv: European Journal of Physiology, 465*(9), 1303–1316. http://doi.org/10.1007/s00424-013-1274-4.

Li, L., Shi, C., Yin, Z., Jia, R., Peng, L., Kang, S., et al. (2014). Antibacterial activity of alpha-terpineol may induce morphostructural alterations in Escherichia coli. *Brazilian Journal of Microbiology, 45*(4), 1409–1413.

Lichtman, A. H., Sheikh, S. M., Loh, H. H., & Martin, B. R. (2001). Opioid and cannabinoid modulation of precipitated withdrawal in delta(9)-tetrahydrocannabinol and morphine-dependent mice. *Journal of Pharmacology and Experimental Therapeutics, 298*(3), 1007–1014.

Ligresti, A., Moriello, A. S., Starowicz, K., Matias, I., Pisanti, S., De Petrocellis, L., et al. (2006). Antitumor activity of plant cannabinoids with emphasis on the effect of cannabidiol on human breast carcinoma. *Journal of Pharmacology and Experimental Therapeutics, 318*(3), 1375–1387. http://doi.org/10.1124/jpet.106.105247.

Lima, D. F., Brandao, M. S., Moura, J. B., Leitao, J. M., Carvalho, F. A., Miura, L. M., et al. (2012). Antinociceptive activity of the monoterpene alpha-phellandrene in rodents: Possible mechanisms of action. *Journal of Pharmacy and Pharmacology, 64*(2), 283–292. http://doi.org/10.1111/j.2042-7158.2011.01401.x.

Lin, W. Y., Kuo, Y. H., Chang, Y. L., Teng, C. M., Wang, E. C., Ishikawa, T., et al. (2003). Anti-platelet aggregation and chemical constituents from the rhizome of Gynura japonica. *Planta Medica, 69*(8), 757–764.

Lin, J. J., Lin, J. H., Hsu, S. C., Weng, S. W., Huang, Y. P., Tang, N. Y., et al. (2013). Alpha-phellandrene promotes immune responses in normal mice through enhancing macrophage phagocytosis and natural killer cell activities. *In Vivo, 27*(6), 809–814.

Lin, J. J., Wu, C. C., Hsu, S. C., Weng, S. W., Ma, Y. S., Huang, Y. P., et al. (2015). Alpha-phellandrene-induced DNA damage and affect DNA repair protein expression in WEHI-3 murine leukemia cells in vitro. *Environmental Toxicology, 30*(11), 1322–1330. http://doi.org/10.1002/tox.22003.

Lin, J. J., Yu, C. C., Lu, K. W., Chang, S. J., Yu, F. S., Liao, C. L., et al. (2014). alpha-Phellandrene alters expression of genes associated with DNA damage, cell cycle, and apoptosis in murine leukemia WEHI-3 cells. *Anticancer Research*, *34*(8), 4161–4180.

Liu, J. S., Che, X. M., Chang, S., Qiu, G. L., He, S. C., Fan, L., et al. (2015). beta-elemene enhances the radiosensitivity of gastric cancer cells by inhibiting Pak1 activation. *World Journal of Gastroenterology*, *21*(34), 9945–9956. http://doi.org/10.3748/wjg.v21.i34.9945.

Liu, T., Wang, C. J., Xie, H. Q., & Mu, Q. (2013). Guaiol–a naturally occurring insecticidal sesquiterpene. *Natural Product Communications*, *8*(10), 1353–1354.

Liu, J., Zhang, Z., Gao, J., Xie, J., Yang, L., & Hu, S. (2011). Downregulation effects of beta-elemene on the levels of plasma endotoxin, serum TNF-alpha, and hepatic CD14 expression in rats with liver fibrosis. *Frontiers in Medicine*, *5*(1), 101–105. http://doi.org/10.1007/s11684-011-0111-4.

Lone, J., & Yun, J. W. (2016). Monoterpene limonene induces brown fat-like phenotype in 3T3-L1 white adipocytes. *Life Sciences*, *153*, 198–206. http://doi.org/10.1016/j.lfs.2016.04.010.

Lopes, N. P., Kato, M. J., Andrade, E. H., Maia, J. G., Yoshida, M., Planchart, A. R., et al. (1999). Antimalarial use of volatile oil from leaves of Virola surinamensis (Rol.) Warb. by Waiapi Amazon Indians. *Journal of Ethnopharmacology*, *67*(3), 313–319.

Lorenzetti, B. B., Souza, G. E., Sarti, S. J., Santos Filho, D., & Ferreira, S. H. (1991). Myrcene mimics the peripheral analgesic activity of lemongrass tea. *Journal of Ethnopharmacology*, *34*(1), 43–48.

Lotter, H. L., & Abraham, D. J. (1975). Cannabisativine, a new alkaloid from Cannabis sativa L. root. *Tetrahedron Letters*, *16*(33), 2815–2818.

Lowette, K., Roosen, L., Tack, J., & Berghe, P. V. (2015). Effects of high-fructose diets on central appetite signaling and cognitive function. *Frontiers in Nutrition*, *2*, 1–5. http://doi.org/10.3389/fnut.2015.00005/abstract.

Macedo, E. M., Santos, W. C., Sousa, B. P. N., Lopes, E. M., Piauilino, C. A., Cunha, F. V., et al. (2016). Association of terpinolene and diclofenac presents antinociceptive and anti-inflammatory synergistic effects in a model of chronic inflammation. *Brazilian Journal of Medical and Biological Research = Revista Brasileira De Pesquisas Médicas E Biológicas/Sociedade Brasileira De Biofísica ... [Et Al.]*, *49*(7), 10. http://doi.org/10.1590/1414-431X20165103.

Maione, S., Piscitelli, F., Gatta, L., Vita, D., De Petrocellis, L., Palazzo, E., et al. (2011). Non-psychoactive cannabinoids modulate the descending pathway of antinociception in anaesthetized rats through several mechanisms of action. *British Journal of Pharmacology*, *162*(3), 584–596. http://doi.org/10.1111/j.1476-5381.2010.01063.x.

Maisonnasse, A., Lenoir, J.-C., Beslay, D., Crauser, D., & Le Conte, Y. (2010). E-β-ocimene, a volatile brood pheromone involved in social regulation in the honey bee colony (Apis mellifera). *PloS One*, *5*(10), e13531. http://doi.org/10.1371/journal.pone.0013531.

Maor, Y., Gallily, R., & Mechoulam, R. (2006). The relevance of the steric factor in the biological activity of CBD derivatives-a tool in identifying novel molecular target for cannabinoids. In *Presented at the symposium on the cannabinoids, Tihany* (p. 1). Hungary: International Cannabinoid Research Society.

Marcu, J. P. (2016). An overview of major and minor phytocannabinoids. In V. R. Preedy (Ed.), Neuropathology of drug addictions and substance misuse (pp. 672–678). Elsevier Academic Press: Amsterdam; Boston, MA. http://doi.org/10.1016/B978-0-12-800213-1.00062-6.

Marcu, J. P., Christian, R. T., Lau, D., Zielinski, A. J., Horowitz, M. P., Lee, J., et al. (2010). Cannabidiol enhances the inhibitory effects of 9-tetrahydrocannabinol on human glioblastoma cell proliferation and survival. *Molecular Cancer Therapeutics*, *9*(1), 180–189. http://doi.org/10.1158/1535-7163.MCT-09-0407.

Martin, B. R., Compton, D. R., Thomas, B. F., Prescott, W. R., Little, P. J., Razdan, R. K., et al. (1991). Behavioral, biochemical, and molecular modeling evaluations of cannabinoid analogs. *Pharmacology, Biochemistry, and Behavior, 40*(3), 471–478. http://doi.org/10.1016/0091-3057(91)90349-7.

Martin-Moreno, A. M., Reigada, D., Ramirez, B. G., Mechoulam, R., Innamorato, N., Cuadrado, A., et al. (2011). Cannabidiol and other cannabinoids reduce microglial activation in vitro and in vivo: Relevance to Alzheimer's disease. *Molecular Pharmacology, 79*(6), 964–973. http://doi.org/10.1124/mol.111.071290.

Matsuda, L. A., Lolait, S. J., Brownstein, M. J., Young, A. C., & Bonner, T. I. (1990). Structure of a cannabinoid receptor and functional expression of the cloned cDNA. *Nature, 346*(6284), 561–564. http://doi.org/10.1038/346561a0.

McLaughlin, P. J. (2012). Reports of the death of CB1 antagonists have been greatly exaggerated. *Behavioural Pharmacology, 23*(5–6), 537–550. http://doi.org/10.1097/FBP.0b013e3283566a8c.

McPartland, J. M., Duncan, M., Di Marzo, V., & Pertwee, R. G. (2015). Are cannabidiol and Delta(9)-tetrahydrocannabivarin negative modulators of the endocannabinoid system? A systematic review. *British Journal of Pharmacology, 172*(3), 737–753. http://doi.org/10.1111/bph.12944.

McPartland, J. M., Guy, G. W., & Di Marzo, V. (2014). Care and feeding of the endocannabinoid system: A systematic review of potential clinical interventions that upregulate the endocannabinoid system. *PloS One, 9*(3), e89566. http://doi.org/10.1371/journal.pone.0089566.

McPartland, J. M., & Russo, E. B. (2001). Cannabis and cannabis extracts: Greater than the sum of their parts? *Journal of Cannabis Therapeutics, 1*(3–4), 103–132. http://doi.org/10.1300/J175v01n03_08.

McPartland, J. M., & Russo, E. B. (2014). Non-phytocannabinoid constituents of cannabis and herbal synergy. *Handbook of cannabis*.

Mechoulam, R. (2005). Plant cannabinoids: A neglected pharmacological treasure trove. *British Journal of Pharmacology, 146*(7), 913–915. http://doi.org/10.1038/sj.bjp.0706415.

Mechoulam, R., Feigenbaum, J. J., Lander, N., Segal, M., Järbe, T. U., Hiltunen, A. J., et al. (1988). Enantiomeric cannabinoids: Stereospecificity of psychotropic activity. *Experientia, 44*(9), 762–764.

Mechoulam, R., Parker, L. A., & Gallily, R. (2002). Cannabidiol: An overview of some pharmacological aspects. *The Journal of Clinical Pharmacology, 42*(11 Suppl.), 11S–19S.

Mehmedic, Z., Chandra, S., Slade, D., Denham, H., Foster, S., Patel, A. S., et al. (2010). Potency trends of Δ9-THC and other cannabinoids in confiscated cannabis preparations from 1993 to 2008*. *Journal of Forensic Sciences, 55*(5), 1209–1217. http://doi.org/10.1111/j.1556-4029.2010.01441.x.

Meier, C., & Mediavilla, V. (1998). Factors influencing the yield and the quality of hemp *(Cannabis sativa* L.) essential oil. *Journal of the International Hemp Association, 5*(1), 16–20.

Meijer, E. P. M., & Hammond, K. M. (2005). The inheritance of chemical phenotype in Cannabis sativa L. (II): Cannabigerol predominant plants. *Euphytica, 145*(1–2), 189–198. http://doi.org/10.1007/s10681-005-1164-8.

Meijer, E. P. M., Hammond, K. M., & Micheler, M. (2008). The inheritance of chemical phenotype in Cannabis sativa L. (III): Variation in cannabichromene proportion. *Euphytica, 165*(2), 293–311. http://doi.org/10.1007/s10681-008-9787-1.

Miller, J. A., Lang, J. E., Ley, M., Nagle, R., Hsu, C. H., Thompson, P. A., et al. (2013). Human breast tissue disposition and bioactivity of limonene in women with early-stage breast cancer. *Cancer Prevention Research (Philadelphia, Pa.), 6*(6), 577–584. http://doi.org/10.1158/1940-6207.CAPR-12-0452.

Miyamoto, T., Okimoto, T., & Kuwano, M. (2014). Chemical composition of the essential oil of mastic gum and their antibacterial activity against drug-resistant Helicobacter pylori. *Natural Products and Bioprospecting, 4*(4), 227–231. http://doi.org/10.1007/s13659-014-0033-3.

Miyazawa, M., & Yamafuji, C. (2005). Inhibition of acetylcholinesterase activity by bicyclic monoterpenoids. *Journal of Agricultural and Food Chemistry*, *53*(5), 1765–1768. http://dx.doi.org/10.1021/jf040019b.

Moghimi, M., Parvardeh, S., Zanjani, T. M., & Ghafghazi, S. (2016). Protective effect of alpha-terpineol against impairment of hippocampal synaptic plasticity and spatial memory following transient cerebral ischemia in rats. *The Iranian Journal of Basic Medical Sciences*, *19*(9), 960–969.

Moldzio, R., Pacher, T., Krewenka, C., Kranner, B., Novak, J., Duvigneau, J. C., et al. (2012). Effects of cannabinoids Δ(9)-tetrahydrocannabinol, Δ(9)-tetrahydrocannabinolic acid and cannabidiol in MPP+ affected murine mesencephalic cultures. *Phytomedicine*, *19*(8–9), 819–824. http://doi.org/10.1016/j.phymed.2012.04.002.

Moreno-Sanz, G. (2016). Can you pass the acid test? Critical review and novel therapeutic perspectives of Δ 9-tetrahydrocannabinolic acid A. *Cannabis and Cannabinoid Research*, *1*(1), 124–130. http://doi.org/10.1089/can.2016.0008.

Moreno-Sanz, G., Duranti, A., Melzig, L., Fiorelli, C., Ruda, G. F., Colombano, G., et al. (2013). Synthesis and structure–activity relationship studies of O-biphenyl-3-yl carbamates as peripherally restricted fatty acid amide hydrolase inhibitors. *Journal of Medicinal Chemistry*, *56*(14), 5917–5930.

Mukerji, G., Yiangou, Y., Corcoran, S. L., Selmer, I. S., Smith, G. D., Benham, C. D., et al. (2006). Cool and menthol receptor TRPM8 in human urinary bladder disorders and clinical correlations. *BMC Urology*, *6*, 6. http://doi.org/10.1186/1471-2490-6-6.

Murillo-Rodriguez, E., Millan-Aldaco, D., Palomero-Rivero, M., Mechoulam, R., & Drucker-Colin, R. (2006). Cannabidiol, a constituent of Cannabis sativa, modulates sleep in rats. *FEBS Letters*, *580*(18), 4337–4345.

Musty, R. E., & Deyo, R. A. (2006). A cannabigerol extract alters behavioral despair in an animal model of depression. In *Presented at the symposium on the cannabinoids, Tihany* (p. 32). Hungary: International Cannabinoid Research Society.

Musty, R. E., Karniol, I. G., Shirikawa, I., Takahashi, R. N., & Knobel, E. (1976). Interactions of delta-9-tetrahydrocannabinol and cannabinol in man. *The Pharmacology of Marihuana*, *2*, 559–563.

Naef, M., Curatolo, M., Petersen-Felix, S., Arendt-Nielsen, L., Zbinden, A., & Brenneisen, R. (2003). The analgesic effect of oral delta-9-tetrahydrocannabinol (THC), morphine, and a THC-morphine combination in healthy subjects under experimental pain conditions. *Pain*, *105*(1–2), 79–88.

Name Withheld. (2006). Studying the effects of terpenes. *O'Shaughnessy's* (Spring 2006), 2.

Neff, G. W., O'Brien, C. B., Reddy, K. R., Bergasa, N. V., Regev, A., Molina, E., et al. (2002). Preliminary observation with dronabinol in patients with intractable pruritus secondary to cholestatic liver disease. *The American Journal of Gastroenterology*, *97*(8), 2117–2119.

Nicholson, A. N., Turner, C., Stone, B. M., & Robson, P. J. (2004). Effect of delta-9-tetrahydrocannabinol and cannabidiol on nocturnal sleep and early-morning behavior in young adults. *Journal of Clinical Psychopharmacology*, *24*(3), 305–313.

Nogueira, M. N., Aquino, S. G., Rossa Junior, C., & Spolidorio, D. M. (2014). Terpinen-4-ol and alpha-terpineol (tea tree oil components) inhibit the production of IL-1beta, IL-6 and IL-10 on human macrophages. *Inflammation Research*, *63*(9), 769–778. http://doi.org/10.1007/s00011-014-0749-x.

Noma, Y., & Asakawa, Y. (2010). Biotransformation of monoterpenoids by microorganisms, insects, and mammals. In K. H. C. Baser & G. Buchbauer (Eds.), *Handbook of essential oils: Science, technology, and applications* (pp. 585–736). Boca Raton, FL: CRC Press.

Noskova, K., Dovrtelova, G., Zendulka, O., Řemínek, R., & Jurica, J. (2016). The effect of (-)-linalool on the metabolic activity of liver CYP enzymes in rats. *Physiological Research/Academia Scientiarum Bohemoslovaca*, *65*(Suppl. 4), S499–S504.

Okumura, N., Yoshida, H., Nishimura, Y., Kitagishi, Y., & Matsuda, S. (2012). Terpinolene, a component of herbal sage, downregulates AKT1 expression in K562 cells. *Oncology Letters*, *3*(2), 321–324. http://doi.org/10.3892/ol.2011.491.

Onaivi, E. S., Ishiguro, H., Gong, J.-P., Patel, S., Meozzi, P. A., Myers, L., et al. (2008). Brain neuronal CB2 cannabinoid receptors in drug abuse and depression: From mice to human subjects. *PloS One*, *3*(2), e1640. http://doi.org/10.1371/journal.pone.0001640.

Onawunmi, G. O., Yisak, W. A., & Ogunlana, E. O. (1984). Antibacterial constituents in the essential oil of Cymbopogon citratus (DC.) Stapf. *Journal of Ethnopharmacology*, *12*(3), 279–286.

Opdyke, D. L. J. (1983). Caryophyllene oxide. *Food and Chemical Toxicology*, *21*(5), 661–662.

Pacher, P. (2006). The endocannabinoid system as an emerging target of pharmacotherapy. *Pharmacological Reviews*, *58*(3), 389–462. http://doi.org/10.1124/pr.58.3.2.

Pacher, P., & Mechoulam, R. (2011). Is lipid signaling through cannabinoid 2 receptors part of a protective system? *Progress in Lipid Research*, *50*(2), 193–211. http://doi.org/10.1016/j.plipres.2011.01.001.

Park, H. M., Lee, J. H., Yaoyao, J., Jun, H. J., & Lee, S. J. (2011). Limonene, a natural cyclic terpene, is an agonistic ligand for adenosine A(2A) receptors. *Biochemical and Biophysical Research Communications*, *404*(1), 345–348. http://doi.org/10.1016/j.bbrc.2010.11.121.

Parker, L. A. (2003). Taste avoidance and taste aversion: Evidence for two different processes. *Animal Learning & Behavior*, *31*(2), 165–172.

Parvardeh, S., Moghimi, M., Eslami, P., & Masoudi, A. (2016). Alpha-Terpineol attenuates morphine-induced physical dependence and tolerance in mice: Role of nitric oxide. *The Iranian Journal of Basic Medical Sciences*, *19*(2), 201–208.

Paula-Freire, L. I., Andersen, M. L., Gama, V. S., Molska, G. R., & Carlini, E. L. (2014). The oral administration of trans-caryophyllene attenuates acute and chronic pain in mice. *Phytomedicine*, *21*(3), 356–362. http://doi.org/10.1016/j.phymed.2013.08.006.

Peana, A. T., Rubattu, P., Piga, G. G., Fumagalli, S., Boatto, G., Pippia, P., et al. (2006). Involvement of adenosine A1 and A2A receptors in (-)-linalool-induced antinociception. *Life Sciences*, *78*(21), 2471–2474. http://doi.org/10.1016/j.lfs.2005.10.025.

Peng, X., Zhao, Y., Liang, X., Wu, L., Cui, S., Guo, A., et al. (2006). Assessing the quality of RCTs on the effect of beta-elemene, one ingredient of a Chinese herb, against malignant tumors. *Contemporary Clinical Trials*, *27*(1), 70–82. http://doi.org/10.1016/j.cct.2005.07.002.

Perry, N. S., Houghton, P. J., Theobald, A., Jenner, P., & Perry, E. K. (2000). In-vitro inhibition of human erythrocyte acetylcholinesterase by salvia lavandulaefolia essential oil and constituent terpenes. *Journal of Pharmacy and Pharmacology*, *52*(7), 895–902.

Pertwee, R. G. (1988). The central neuropharmcology of psychotropic cannabinoids. *Pharmacology and Therapeutics*, *36*(2–3), 189–261. http://doi.org/10.1016/0163-7258(88)90106-4.

Pertwee, R. G. (2008). The diverse CB1 and CB2 receptor pharmacology of three plant cannabinoids: Delta9-tetrahydrocannabinol, cannabidiol and delta9-tetrahydrocannabivarin. *British Journal of Pharmacology*, *153*(2), 199–215. http://doi.org/10.1038/sj.bjp.0707442.

Pertwee, R. G., & Cascio, M. G. (2014). Known pharmacological actions of delta-9-tetrahydrocannabinol and of four other chemical constituents of cannabis that activate cannabinoid receptors. In R. G. Pertwee (Ed.), *Handbook of cannabis* (pp. 115–136). Oxford, UK: Oxford University Press. http://doi.org/10.1093/acprof:oso/9780199662685.003.0006.

Pertwee, R. G., Howlett, A. C., Abood, M. E., Alexander, S. P. H., Di Marzo, V., Elphick, M. R., et al. (2010). International Union of Basic and Clinical Pharmacology. LXXIX. Cannabinoid receptors and their ligands: beyond CB_1 and CB_2. *Pharmacological Reviews*, *62*(4), 588–631. http://doi.org/10.1124/pr.110.003004.

Piccinelli, A. C., Morato, P. N., Dos Santos Barbosa, M., Croda, J., Sampson, J., Kong, X., et al. (2017). Limonene reduces hyperalgesia induced by gp120 and cytokines by modulation of IL-1 beta and protein expression in spinal cord of mice. *Life Sciences*, *174*, 28–34. http://doi.org/10.1016/j.lfs.2016.11.017.

Piccinelli, A. C., Santos, J. A., Konkiewitz, E. C., Oesterreich, S. A., Formagio, A. S., Croda, J., et al. (2015). Antihyperalgesic and antidepressive actions of (R)-(+)-limonene, alpha-phellandrene, and essential oil from Schinus terebinthifolius fruits in a neuropathic pain model. *Nutritional Neuroscience*, *18*(5), 217–224. http://doi.org/10.1179/1476830514Y.0000000119.

Plengsuriyakarn, T., Karbwang, J., & Na-Bangchang, K. (2015). Anticancer activity using positron emission tomography-computed tomography and pharmacokinetics of beta-eudesmol in human cholangiocarcinoma xenografted nude mouse model. *Clinical and Experimental Pharmacology and Physiology*, *42*(3), 293–304. http://doi.org/10.1111/1440-1681.12354.

Potter, D. J. (2009). *The propagation, characterisation and optimisation of Cannabis sativa L. as a phytopharmaceutical. Pharmaceutical Sciences* (p.224). London: King's College.

Pultrini Ade, M., Galindo, L. A., & Costa, M. (2006). Effects of the essential oil from Citrus aurantium L. in experimental anxiety models in mice. *Life Sciences*, *78*(15), 1720–1725. http://doi.org/10.1016/j.lfs.2005.08.004.

Qin, N., Neeper, M. P., Liu, Y., Hutchinson, T. L., Lubin, M. L., & Flores, C. M. (2008). TRPV2 is activated by cannabidiol and mediates CGRP release in cultured rat dorsal root ganglion neurons. *The Journal of Neuroscience: The Official Journal of the Society for Neuroscience*, *28*(24), 6231–6238. http://dx.doi.org/10.1523/JNEUROSCI.0504-08.2008. 28/24/6231 [pii].

Quintans-Junior, L., Moreira, J. C., Pasquali, M. A., Rabie, S. M., Pires, A. S., Schroder, R., et al. (2013). Antinociceptive activity and redox profile of the monoterpenes (+)-camphene, p-cymene, and geranyl acetate in experimental models. *ISRN Toxicology*, *2013*, 459530. http://doi.org/10.1155/2013/459530.

Quintans-Junior, L. J., Oliveira, M. G., Santana, M. F., Santana, M. T., Guimaraes, A. G., Siqueira, J. S., et al. (2011). Alpha-terpineol reduces nociceptive behavior in mice. *Pharmaceutical Biology*, *49*(6), 583–586. http://doi.org/10.3109/13880209.2010.529616.

Ramalho, T. R., Pacheco de Oliveira, M. T., Lima, A. L., Bezerra-Santos, C. R., & Piuvezam, M. R. (2015). Gamma-terpinene modulates acute inflammatory response in mice. *Planta Medica*, *81*(14), 1248–1254. http://doi.org/10.1055/s-0035-1557790.

Raman, A., Weir, U., & Bloomfield, S. F. (1995). Antimicrobial effects of tea-tree oil and its major components on Staphylococcus aureus, Staph. epidermidis and Propionibacterium acnes. *Letters in Applied Microbiology*, *21*(4), 242–245.

Rao, V. S., Menezes, A. M., & Viana, G. S. (1990). Effect of myrcene on nociception in mice. *The Journal of Pharmacy and Pharmacology*, *42*(12), 877–878.

Re, L., Barocci, S., Sonnino, S., Mencarelli, A., Vivani, C., Paolucci, G., et al. (2000). Linalool modifies the nicotinic receptor–ion channel kinetics at the mouse neuromuscular junction. *Pharmacological Research*, *42*(2), 177–181. http://doi.org/10.1006/phrs.2000.0671.

Reagan-Shaw, S., Nihal, M., & Ahmad, N. (2008). Dose translation from animal to human studies revisited. *The FASEB Journal*, *22*(3), 659–661. http://doi.org/10.1096/fj.07-9574LSF.

Rhee, Man-Hee, Vogel, Zvi, Barg, Jacob, Bayewitch, Michael, Levy, Rivka, Hanuš, Lumir, et al. (1997). Cannabinol derivatives: Binding to cannabinoid receptors and inhibition of adenylylcyclase. *Journal of Medicinal Chemistry*, *40*(20), 3228–3233. http://doi.org/10.1021/jm970126f.

Riedel, G., Fadda, P., McKillop-Smith, S., Pertwee, R. G., Platt, B., & Robinson, L. (2009). Synthetic and plant-derived cannabinoid receptor antagonists show hypophagic properties in fasted and non-fasted mice. *British Journal of Pharmacology*, *156*(7), 1154–1166. http://doi.org/10.1111/j.1476-5381.2008.00107.x.

Rivas da Silva, A. C., Lopes, P. M., Barros de Azevedo, M. M., Costa, D. C., Alviano, C. S., & Alviano, D. S. (2012). Biological activities of alpha-pinene and beta-pinene enantiomers. *Molecules (Basel, Switzerland)*, *17*(6), 6305–6316. http://doi.org/10.3390/molecules17066305.

Robson, P. (2011). Abuse potential and psychoactive effects of delta-9-tetrahydrocannabinol and cannabidiol oromucosal spray (Sativex), a new cannabinoid medicine. *Expert Opinion on Drug Safety*, *10*(5), 675–685. http://dx.doi.org/10.1517/14740338.2011.575778.

Rock, E. M., Kopstick, R. L., Limebeer, C. L., & Parker, L. A. (2013). Tetrahydrocannabinolic acid reduces nausea-induced conditioned gaping in rats and vomiting in Suncus murinus. *British Journal of Pharmacology*, *170*(3), 641–648. http://doi.org/10.1111/bph.12316.

Rock, E. M., & Parker, L. A. (2015). Synergy between cannabidiol, cannabidiolic acid, and Δ^9-tetrahydrocannabinol in the regulation of emesis in the Suncus murinus (house musk shrew). *Behavioral Neuroscience*, *129*(3), 368–370. http://doi.org/10.1037/bne0000057.

Rock, E. M., Sticht, M. A., & Parker, L. A. (2014). Effect of phytocannabinoids on nausea and vomiting. In R. G. Pertwee (Ed.), *Handbook of cannabis* (pp. 435–454). Oxford, UK: Oxford University Press. http://doi.org/10.1093/acprof:oso/9780199662685.003.0023.

Rodrigues Goulart, H., Kimura, E. A., Peres, V. J., Couto, A. S., Aquino Duarte, F. A., & Katzin, A. M. (2004). Terpenes arrest parasite development and inhibit biosynthesis of isoprenoids in Plasmodium falciparum. *Antimicrobial Agents and Chemotherapy*, *48*(7), 2502–2509.

Rodrigues, K. A., Amorim, L. V., Dias, C. N., Moraes, D. F., Carneiro, S. M., & Carvalho, F. A. (2015). Syzygium cumini (L.) Skeels essential oil and its major constituent alpha-pinene exhibit anti-Leishmania activity through immunomodulation in vitro. *Journal of Ethnopharmacology*, *160*, 32–40. http://doi.org/10.1016/j.jep.2014.11.024.

Rog, D. J., Nurmiko, T., Friede, T., & Young, C. (2005). Randomized controlled trial of cannabis based medicine in central neuropathic pain due to multiple sclerosis. *Neurology*, *65*(6), 812–819.

Romano, B., Borrelli, F., Fasolino, I., Capasso, R., Piscitelli, F., Cascio, M., et al. (2013). The cannabinoid TRPA1 agonist cannabichromene inhibits nitric oxide production in macrophages and ameliorates murine colitis. *British Journal of Pharmacology*, *169*(1), 213–229. http://doi.org/10.1111/bph.12120.

Rosenthaler, S., Pöhn, B., Kolmanz, C., Huu, C. N., Krewenka, C., Huber, A., et al. (2014). Differences in receptor binding affinity of several phytocannabinoids do not explain their effects on neural cell cultures. *Neurotoxicology and Teratology*, *46*, 49–56. http://doi.org/10.1016/j.ntt.2014.09.003.

Rufino, A. T., Ribeiro, M., Sousa, C., Judas, F., Salgueiro, L., Cavaleiro, C., et al. (2015). Evaluation of the anti-inflammatory, anti-catabolic and pro-anabolic effects of E-caryophyllene, myrcene and limonene in a cell model of osteoarthritis. *European Journal of Pharmacology*, *750*, 141–150. http://doi.org/10.1016/j.ejphar.2015.01.018.

Russo, E. B. (2001). *Handbook of psychotropic herbs: A scientific analysis of herbal remedies for psychiatric conditions*. Binghamton, NY: Haworth Press.

Russo, E. B. (2007). History of cannabis and its preparations in saga, science, and sobriquet. *Chemistry & Biodiversity*, *4*(8), 1614–1648.

Russo, E. B. (2011). Taming THC: Potential cannabis synergy and phytocannabinoid-terpenoid entourage effects. *British Journal of Pharmacology*, *163*(7), 1344–1364. http://doi.org/10.1111/j.1476-5381.2011.01238.x.

Russo, E. B. (2013). *Cannabis strains: Do cannabis strains differ?* Retrieved January 18, 2017, from http://www.cannabis-med.org/index.php?tpl=faq&red=faqlist&id=278&lng=en.

Russo, E. B. (2014). The pharmacological history of Cannabis. In R. Pertwee (Ed.), *Handbook of Cannabinoids*. (pp. 23–43). Oxford, United Kingdom: Oxford University Press.

Russo, E. B. (2016a). Beyond cannabis: Plants and the endocannabinoid system. *Trends in Pharmacological Sciences*, *37*(7), 594–605. http://dx.doi.org/10.1016/j.tips.2016.04.005.

Russo, E. B. (2016b). Cannabis and epilepsy: An ancient treatment returns to the fore. *Epilepsy and Behavior*. http://dx.doi.org/10.1016/j.yebeh.2016.09.040.

Russo, E. B. (2017). Cannabis and epilepsy: An ancient treatment returns to the fore. *Epilepsy Behav*, *70*(Pt B), 292–297. http://dx.doi.org/10.1016/j.yebeh.2016.09.040.

Russo, E. B., Burnett, A., Hall, B., & Parker, K. K. (2005). Agonistic properties of cannabidiol at 5-HT-1a receptors. *Neurochemical Research*, *30*(8), 1037–1043.

Russo, E. B., & Guy, G. W. (2006). A tale of two cannabinoids: The therapeutic rationale for combining tetrahydrocannabinol and cannabidiol. *Medical Hypotheses*, *66*(2), 234–246. http://dx.doi.org/10.1016/j.mehy.2005.08.026.

Russo, E. B., Guy, G. W., & Robson, P. J. (2007). Cannabis, pain, and sleep: Lessons from therapeutic clinical trials of Sativex, a cannabis-based medicine. *Chemistry & Biodiversity*, *4*(8), 1729–1743. http://doi.org/10.1002/cbdv.200790150.

Russo, E. B., & Hohmann, A. G. (2012). *Role of cannabinoids in pain management. In Comprehensive treatment of chronic pain by medical, interventional, and integrative approaches* (pp. 181–197). New York, NY: Springer New York. http://doi.org/10.1007/978-1-4614-1560-2_18.

Sastre-Garriga, J., Vila, C., Clissold, S., & Montalban, X. (2011). THC and CBD oromucosal spray (Sativex®) in the management of spasticity associated with multiple sclerosis. *Expert Review of Neurotherapeutics*, *11*(5), 627–637. http://dx.doi.org/10.1586/ern.11.47.

Sanguinetti, M., Posteraro, B., Romano, L., Battaglia, F., Lopizzo, T., De Carolis, E., et al. (2007). In vitro activity of Citrus bergamia (bergamot) oil against clinical isolates of dermatophytes. *The Journal of Antimicrobial Chemotherapy*, *59*(2), 305–308. http://doi.org/10.1093/jac/dkl473.

Satou, T., Kasuya, H., Maeda, K., & Koike, K. (2014). Daily inhalation of alpha-pinene in mice: Effects on behavior and organ accumulation. *Phytotherapy Research*, *28*(9), 1284–1287.

Sayyah, M., Nadjafnia, L., & Kamalinejad, M. (2004). Anticonvulsant activity and chemical composition of Artemisia dracunculus L. essential oil. *Journal of Ethnopharmacology*, *94*(2–3), 283–287.

Scuderi, C., De Filippis, D., Iuvone, T., Blasio, A., Steardo, A., & Esposito, G. (2009). Cannabidiol in medicine: A review of its therapeutic potential in CNS disorders. *Phytotherapy Research*, *23*(5), 597–602. http://doi.org/10.1002/ptr.2625.

Schafer, D., & Schafer, W. (1981). Pharmacological studies with an ointment containing menthol, camphene and essential oils for broncholytic and secretolytic effects. *Arzneimittel-Forschung*, *31*(1), 82–86.

Schmidt, L., Belov, V. N., & Goen, T. (2015). Human metabolism of Delta3-carene and renal elimination of Delta3-caren-10-carboxylic acid (chaminic acid) after oral administration. *Archives of Toxicology*, *89*(3), 381–392. http://doi.org/10.1007/s00204-014-1251-5.

Schnaubelt, K. (1998). *Advanced aromatherapy: The science of essential oil therapy* (1st ed.). Rochester, VT: Healing Arts Press.

Schott, M., Klein, B., & Vilcinskas, A. (2015). Detection of illicit drugs by trained honeybees (Apis mellifera). *PloS One*, *10*(6), e0128528. http://doi.org/10.1371/journal.pone.0128528.

Scutt, A., & Williamson, E. M. (2007). Cannabinoids stimulate fibroblastic colony formation by bone marrow cells indirectly via CB2 receptors. *Calcified Tissue International*, *80*(1), 50–59. http://doi.org/10.1007/s00223-006-0171-7.

Sellers, E. M., Schoedel, K., Bartlett, C., Romach, M., Russo, E. B., Stott, C. G., et al. (2013). A multiple-dose, randomized, double-blind, placebo-controlled, parallel-group QT/QTc study to evaluate the electrophysiologic effects of THC/CBD spray. *Clinical Pharmacology in Drug Development*, *2*(3), 285–294. http://doi.org/10.1002/cpdd.36.

Semenya, S., Potgieter, M., Tshisikhawe, M., Shava, S., & Maroyi, A. (2012). Medicinal utilization of exotic plants by Bapedi traditional healers to treat human ailments in Limpopo province, South Africa. *Journal of Ethnopharmacology*, *144*(3), 646–655. http://doi.org/10.1016/j.jep.2012.10.005.

Sharma, C., Al Kaabi, J. M., Nurulain, S. M., Goyal, S. N., Kamal, M. A., & Ojha, S. (2016). Polypharmacological properties and therapeutic potential of β-caryophyllene: A dietary phytocannabinoid of pharmaceutical promise. *Current Pharmaceutical Design*, *22*(21), 3237–3264.

Shelly, T. E., & Nishimoto, J. I. (2015). Exposure to the plant compound {alpha} -humulene reduces mating success in male Mediterranean fruit flies (Diptera: Tephritidae). *Annals of the Entomological Society of America*, *108*(3), 215–221. http://doi.org/10.1093/aesa/sav008.

Shinjyo, N., & Di Marzo, V. (2013). The effect of cannabichromene on adult neural stem/progenitor cells. *Neurochemistry International*, *63*(5), 432–437. http://doi.org/10.1016/j.neuint.2013.08.002.

Shoyama, Y., Hirano, H., Makino, H., Umekita, N., & Nishioka, I. (1977). Cannabis. X. The isolation and structures of four new propyl cannabinoid acids, tetrahydrocannabivarinic acid, cannabidivarinic acid, cannabichromevarinic acid and cannabigerovarinic acid, from Thai Cannabis, 'Meao variant'. *Chemical & Pharmaceutical Bulletin*, *25*(9), 2306–2311. http://doi.org/10.1248/cpb.25.2306.

Silva Brum, L. F., Emanuelli, T., Souza, D. O., & Elisabetsky, E. (2001). Effects of linalool on glutamate release and uptake in mouse cortical synaptosomes. *Neurochemical Research*, *26*(3), 191–194.

Singh, P., Shukla, R., Prakash, B., Kumar, A., Singh, S., Mishra, P. K., et al. (2010). Chemical profile, antifungal, antiaflatoxigenic and antioxidant activity of Citrus maxima Burm. and Citrus sinensis (L.) Osbeck essential oils and their cyclic monoterpene, DL-limonene. *Food and Chemical Toxicology*, *48*(6), 1734–1740. http://doi.org/10.1016/j.fct.2010.04.001.

Siqueira, H. D., Neto, B. S., Sousa, D. P., Gomes, B. S., da Silva, F. V., Cunha, F. V., et al. (2016). alpha-Phellandrene, a cyclic monoterpene, attenuates inflammatory response through neutrophil migration inhibition and mast cell degranulation. *Life Sciences*, *160*, 27–33. http://doi.org/10.1016/j.lfs.2016.07.008.

Sirikantaramas, S., Morimoto, S., Shoyama, Y., Ishikawa, Y., Wada, Y., Shoyama, Y., et al. (2004). The gene controlling marijuana psychoactivity: Molecular cloning and heterologous expression of delta1-tetrahydrocannabinolic acid synthase from Cannabis sativa L. *The Journal of Biological Chemistry*, *279*(38), 39767–39774.

Slatkin, D. J., Doorenbos, N. J., Harris, L. S., Masoud, A. N., Quimby, M. W., & Schiff, P. L. J. (1971). Chemical constituents of Cannabis sativa L. root. *Journal of Pharmaceutical Sciences*, *60*(12), 1891–1892.

Slatkin, D. J., Knapp, J. E., Schiff, P. L. J., Turner, C. E., & Mole, L. M. J. (1975). Steroids of Cannabis sativa root. *Phytochemistry*, *14*, 580–581.

Soni, D., Smoum, R., Breuer, A., Mechoulam, R., & Steinberg, D. (2015). Effect of the synthetic cannabinoid HU-210 on quorum sensing and on the production of quorum sensing-mediated virulence factors by Vibrio harveyi. *BMC Microbiology*, *15*, 159. http://doi.org/10.1186/s12866-015-0499-0.

Stahl, E., & Kunde, R. (1973). Die Leitsubstanzen der Haschisch-Suchhunde. *Kriminalistik: Zeitschrift Für Die Gesamte Kriminalistische Wissenschaft Und Praxis*, *27*(9), 385–389.

Stott, C. G., Guy, G. W., Wright, S., & Whittle, B. A. (2005). The effects of cannabis extracts Tetranabinex and Nabidiolex on human cytochrome P450-mediated metabolism. In *Presented at the symposium on the cannabinoids* (p. 163). Clearwater, FL: International Cannabinoid Research Association.

Subramenium, G. A., Vijayakumar, K., & Pandian, S. K. (2015). Limonene inhibits streptococcal biofilm formation by targeting surface-associated virulence factors. *Journal of Medical Microbiology*, *64*(8), 879–890. http://doi.org/10.1099/jmm.0.000105.

Sulak, D., Saneto, R., & Goldstein, B. (2017). The current status of artisanal cannabis for the treatment of epilepsy in the United States. *Epilepsy Behav*, *70*(Pt B), 328–333. http://dx.doi.org/10.1016/j.yebeh.2016.12.032.

Sunil, C., Duraipandiyan, V., Ignacimuthu, S., & Al-Dhabi, N. A. (2013). Antioxidant, free radical scavenging and liver protective effects of friedelin isolated from Azima tetracantha Lam. leaves. *Food Chemistry*, *139*(1–4), 860–865. http://doi.org/10.1016/j.foodchem.2012.12.041.

Swift, W., Wong, A., Li, K. M., Arnold, J. C., & McGregor, I. S. (2013). Analysis of cannabis seizures in NSW, Australia: Cannabis potency and cannabinoid profile. *PloS One*, *8*(7), e70052. http://doi.org/10.1371/journal.pone.0070052.

Takeda, S., Misawa, K., Yamamoto, I., & Watanabe, K. (2008). Cannabidiolic acid as a selective cyclooxygenase-2 inhibitory component in cannabis. *Drug Metabolism and Disposition*, *36*(9), 1917–1921. http://doi.org/10.1124/dmd.108.020909.

Takemoto, H., Ito, M., Shiraki, T., Yagura, T., & Honda, G. (2008). Sedative effects of vapor inhalation of agarwood oil and spikenard extract and identification of their active components. *Journal of Natural Medicines*, *62*(1), 41–46. http://doi.org/10.1007/s11418-007-0177-0.

Tambe, Y., Tsujiuchi, H., Honda, G., Ikeshiro, Y., & Tanaka, S. (1996). Gastric cytoprotection of the non-steroidal anti-inflammatory sesquiterpene, beta-caryophyllene. *Planta Medica*, *62*(5), 469–470.

Thomas, A., Baillie, G. L., Phillips, A. M., Razdan, R. K., Ross, R. A., & Pertwee, R. G. (2007). Cannabidiol displays unexpectedly high potency as an antagonist of CB1 and CB2 receptor agonists in vitro. *British Journal of Pharmacology*, *150*(5), 613–623. http://doi.org/10.1038/sj.bjp.0707133.

Tisserand, R., & Young, R. (2014). *Essential oil safety* (2nd ed.). Edinburgh, UK: Churchill Livingstone Elsevier.

Torres, S., Lorente, M., Rodriguez-Fornes, F., Hernandez-Tiedra, S., Salazar, M., Garcia-Taboada, E., et al. (2011). A combined preclinical therapy of cannabinoids and temozolomide against glioma. *Molecular Cancer Therapeutics*, *10*(1), 90–103. http://doi.org/10.1158/1535-7163.MCT-10-0688.

Turkez, H., Aydin, E., Geyikoglu, F., & Cetin, D. (2015). Genotoxic and oxidative damage potentials in human lymphocytes after exposure to terpinolene in vitro. *Cytotechnology*, *67*(3), 409–418. http://doi.org/10.1007/s10616-014-9698-z.

Turkez, H., Sozio, P., Geyikoglu, F., Tatar, A., Hacimuftuoglu, A., & Di Stefano, A. (2014). Neuroprotective effects of farnesene against hydrogen peroxide-induced neurotoxicity in vitro. *Cellular and Molecular Neurobiology*, *34*(1), 101–111. http://doi.org/10.1007/s10571-013-9991-y.

Turner, C. E., Elsohly, M. A., & Boeren, E. G. (1980). Constituents of Cannabis sativa L. XVII. A review of the natural constituents. *Journal of Natural Products*, *43*(2), 169–234.

Turner, C. E., Hsu, M. H., Knapp, J. E., Schiff, P. L. J., & Slatkin, D. J. (1976). Isolation of cannabisativine, an alkaloid, from Cannabis sativa L. root. *Journal of Pharmaceutical Sciences*, *65*(7), 1084–1085.

Upton, R., Craker, L., ElSohly, M., Romm, A., Russo, E., & Sexton, M. (2013). Cannabis inflorescence: Cannabis spp.: Standards of identity, analysis and quality control. In R. Upton (Ed.), Scotts Valley, CA, USA: American Herbal Pharmacopoeia.

Vallianou, I., & Hadzopoulou-Cladaras, M. (2016). Camphene, a plant derived monoterpene, exerts its hypolipidemic action by affecting SREBP-1 and MTP expression. *PloS One*, *11*(1), e0147117. http://doi.org/10.1371/journal.pone.0147117.

Vallianou, I., Peroulis, N., Pantazis, P., & Hadzopoulou-Cladaras, M. (2011). Camphene, a plant-derived monoterpene, reduces plasma cholesterol and triglycerides in hyperlipidemic rats independently of HMG-CoA reductase activity. *PloS One*, *6*(11), e20516. http://doi.org/10.1371/journal.pone.0020516.

Varga, Z. V., Matyas, C., Erdelyi, K., Cinar, R., Nieri, D., Chicca, A., et al. (2017). Beta-caryophyllene protects against alcoholic steatohepatitis by attenuating inflammation and metabolic dysregulation in mice. *British Journal of Pharmacology*. http://dx.doi.org/10.1111/bph.13722.

Verhoeckx, K. C., Korthout, H. A., van Meeteren-Kreikamp, A. P., Ehlert, K. A., Wang, M., van der Greef, J., et al. (2006). Unheated Cannabis sativa extracts and its major compound THC-acid have potential immuno-modulating properties not mediated by CB1 and CB2 receptor coupled pathways. *International Immunopharmacology*, *6*(4), 656–665. http://doi.org/10.1016/j.intimp.2005.10.002.

Vigushin, D. M., Poon, G. K., Boddy, A., English, J., Halbert, G. W., Pagonis, C., et al. (1998). Phase I and pharmacokinetic study of D-limonene in patients with advanced cancer. Cancer Research Campaign Phase I/II Clinical Trials Committee. *Cancer Chemotherapy and Pharmacology*, *42*(2), 111–117.

Volicer, L., Stelly, M., Morris, J., McLaughlin, J., & Volicer, B. J. (1997). Effects of dronabinol on anorexia and disturbed behavior in patients with Alzheimer's disease. *International Journal of Geriatric Psychiatry*, *12*(9), 913–919.

Von Burg, R. (1995). Toxicology update. Limonene. *Journal of Applied Toxicology*, *15*(6), 495–499.

Wattenberg, L. W. (1991). Inhibition of azoxymethane-induced neoplasia of the large bowel by 3-hydroxy-3,7,11-trimethyl-1,6,10-dodecatriene (nerolidol). *Carcinogenesis*, *12*(1), 151–152.

Wade, D. T., Collin, C., Stott, C., & Duncombe, P. (2010). Meta-analysis of the efficacy and safety of Sativex (nabiximols), on spasticity in people with multiple sclerosis. *Multiple Sclerosis*, *16*(6), 707–714. http://dx.doi.org/10.1177/1352458510367462, 16/6/707 [pii].

Werz, O., Seegers, J., Schaible, A. M., Weinigel, C., Barz, D., Koeberle, A., et al. (2014). Cannflavins from hemp sprouts, a novel cannabinoid-free hemp food product, target microsomal prostaglandin E2 synthase-1 and 5-lipoxygenase. *Pharma Nutrition*, *2*(3), 53–60. http://doi.org/10.1016/j.phanu.2014.05.001.

Wilkinson, J. D., & Williamson, E. M. (2007). Cannabinoids inhibit human keratinocyte proliferation through a non-CB1/CB2 mechanism and have a potential therapeutic value in the treatment of psoriasis. *Journal of Dermatological Science*, *45*(2), 87–92.

Williams, S. J., Hartley, J. P., & Graham, J. D. (1976). Bronchodilator effect of delta1-tetrahydrocannabinol administered by aerosol of asthmatic patients. *Thorax*, *31*(6), 720–723.

Williams, C. M., Jones, N. A., & Whalley, B. J. (2014). *Cannabis and epilepsy. In Handbook of cannabis* (pp. 547–563). Oxford, UK: Oxford University Press. http://doi.org/10.1093/acprof:oso/9780199662685.003.0030.

Wood, T. B., Spivey, W. T. N., & Easterfield, T. H. (1899). III.—Cannabinol. Part I. *Journal of the Chemical Society, Transactions*, *75*, 20–36. http://doi.org/10.1039/CT8997500020.

Wu, L., Wang, G., Tang, S., Long, G., & Yin, T. (2011). Protection of endothelial cells, inhibition of neointimal hyperplasia by beta-elemene in an injured artery. *Cardiovascular Drugs and Therapy*, *25*(3), 233–242. http://doi.org/10.1007/s10557-011-6305-9.

Wu, X. S., Xie, T., Lin, J., Fan, H. Z., Huang-Fu, H. J., Ni, L. F., et al. (2009). An investigation of the ability of elemene to pass through the blood-brain barrier and its effect on brain carcinomas. *Journal of Pharmacy and Pharmacology*, *61*(12), 1653–1656. http://doi.org/10.1211/jpp/61.12.0010.

Xi, Z.-X., Peng, X.-Q., Li, X., Song, R., Zhang, H.-Y., Liu, Q.-R., et al. (2011). Brain cannabinoid CB2 receptors modulate cocaine's actions in mice. *Nature Neuroscience*, *14*(9), 1160–1166. http://doi.org/10.1038/nn.2874.

Xu, H. B., Zheng, L. P., Li, L., Xu, L. Z., & Fu, J. (2013). Elemene, one ingredient of a Chinese herb, against malignant tumors: A literature-based meta-analysis. *Cancer Investigation*, *31*(2), 156–166. http://doi.org/10.3109/07357907.2012.756108.

Yamaori, S., Koeda, K., Kushihara, M., Hada, Y., Yamamoto, I., & Watanabe, K. (2012). Comparison in the in vitro inhibitory effects of major phytocannabinoids and polycyclic aromatic hydrocarbons contained in marijuana smoke on cytochrome P450 2C9 activity. *Drug Metabolism and Pharmacokinetics*, *27*(3), 294–300. http://doi.org/10.2133/dmpk.DMPK-11-RG-107.

Yamaori, S., Kushihara, M., Yamamoto, I., & Watanabe, K. (2010). Characterization of major phytocannabinoids, cannabidiol and cannabinol, as isoform-selective and potent inhibitors of human CYP1 enzymes. *Biochemical Pharmacology*, *79*(11), 1691–1698. http://doi.org/10.1016/j.bcp.2010.01.028.

Yamaori, S., Okamoto, Y., Yamamoto, I., & Watanabe, K. (2011). Cannabidiol, a major phytocannabinoid, as a potent atypical inhibitor for CYP2D6. *Drug Metabolism and Disposition*, *39*(11), 2049–2056. http://doi.org/10.1124/dmd.111.041384.

Yang, D., Michel, L., Chaumont, J. P., & Millet-Clerc, J. (1999). Use of caryophyllene oxide as an antifungal agent in an in vitro experimental model of onychomycosis. *Mycopathologia*, *148*(2), 79–82.

Yang, H. H., Son, J. K., Jung, B., Zheng, M., & Kim, J. R. (2011). Epifriedelanol from the root bark of Ulmus davidiana inhibits cellular senescence in human primary cells. *Planta Medica*, 77(5), 441–449. http://doi.org/10.1055/s-0030-1250458.

Yang, Q., Wu, J., Luo, Y., Huang, N., Zhen, N., Zhou, Y., et al. (2016). (-)-Guaiol regulates RAD51 stability via autophagy to induce cell apoptosis in non-small cell lung cancer. *Oncotarget*, 7(38), 62585–62597. http://doi.org/10.18632/oncotarget.11540.

Yeshurun, M., Shpilberg, O., Herscovici, C., Shargian, L., Dreyer, J., Peck, A., et al. (2015). Cannabidiol for the prevention of graft-versus-host-disease after allogeneic hematopoietic cell transplantation: Results of a phase II study. *Biology of Blood and Marrow Transplantation: Journal of the American Society for Blood and Marrow Transplantation*, *21*(10), 1770–1775. http://doi.org/10.1016/j.bbmt.2015.05.018.

Zanoli, P., & Zavatti, M. (2008). Pharmacognostic and pharmacological profile of Humulus lupulus L. *Journal of Ethnopharmacology*, *116*(3), 383–396. http://doi.org/10.1016/j.jep.2008.01.011.

Zhang, J., Zhang, H. D., Yao, Y. F., Zhong, S. L., Zhao, J. H., & Tang, J. H. (2015). beta-elemene reverses chemoresistance of breast cancer cells by reducing resistance transmission via exosomes. *Cellular Physiology and Biochemistry*, *36*(6), 2274–2286. http://doi.org/10.1159/000430191.

Zhou, Y. Y., Liu, H. X., Jiang, N., Feng, X. H., Feng, X. Y., Zhang, H. Q., et al. (2015). Elemene, the essential oil of Curcuma wenyujin, inhibits osteogenic differentiation in ankylosing spondylitis. *Joint, Bone, Spine*, *82*(2), 100–103. http://doi.org/10.1016/j.jbspin.2014.05.004.

Zhu, T., Li, X., Luo, L., Wang, X., Li, Z., Xie, P., et al. (2015). Reversion of malignant phenotypes of human glioblastoma cells by beta-elemene through beta-catenin-mediated regulation of stemness-, differentiation- and epithelial-to-mesenchymal transition-related molecules. *Journal of Translational Medicine*, *13*, 356. http://doi.org/10.1186/s12967-015-0727-2.

Zou, K., Liu, C., Zhang, Z., & Zou, L. (2015). The effect of elemene on lung adenocarcinoma A549 cell radiosensitivity and elucidation of its mechanism. *Clinics (São Paulo, Brazil)*, *70*(8), 556–562. http://doi.org/10.6061/clinics/2015(08)05.

Zou, S., Wang, C., Cui, Z., Guo, P., Meng, Q., Shi, X., et al. (2016). Beta-elemene induces apoptosis of human rheumatoid arthritis fibroblast-like synoviocytes via reactive oxygen species-dependent activation of p38 mitogen-activated protein kinase. *Pharmacological Reports*, *68*(1), 7–11. http://doi.org/10.1016/j.pharep.2015.06.004.

CHAPTER FOUR

Spicing Up Pharmacology: A Review of Synthetic Cannabinoids From Structure to Adverse Events

Colin Davidson*, Jolanta Opacka-Juffry†, Angel Arevalo-Martin‡, Daniel Garcia-Ovejero‡, Eduardo Molina-Holgado‡, Francisco Molina-Holgado†,1

*School of Pharmacy and Biomedical Sciences, University of Central Lancashire, Preston, United Kingdom
†Health Science Research Centre, University of Roehampton, London, United Kingdom
‡Laboratory of Neuroinflammation, Hospital Nacional de Parapléjicos (SESCAM), Toledo, Spain
[1]Corresponding author: e-mail address: f.molina-holgado@roehampton.ac.uk

Contents

Advances in Pharmacology, Volume 80
ISSN 1054-3589
http://dx.doi.org/10.1016/bs.apha.2017.05.001

Abstract

Recreational use of synthetic cannabinoids (SCB), a class of novel psychoactive substances is an increasing public health problem specifically in Western societies, with teenagers, young adults, and the prison population being the most affected. Some of these SCB are analogs of tetrahydrocannabinol, aminoalkylindoles, and other phytocannabinoid analogs have been detected in herbal preparations generically called "Spice." Spice, "K2" or "fake cannabis" is a general term used for variable herbal mixtures of unknown ingredients or chemical composition. SCB are highly potent CB_1 cannabinoid receptor agonists falsely marketed and sold as safe and legal drugs. Here, we present an overview of the endocannabinoid system, CB, and SCB chemical structures and activity at CB receptors. Finally, we highlight the psychological effects of SCB, particularly on learning and memory, and adverse clinical effects including on the cardiovascular system, kidneys, and CNS, including psychosis. Taken together, it is clear that many SCB are extremely dangerous and a major public health problem.

1. THE CANNABINOID SYSTEM, PHYTOCANNABINOIDS, ENDOCANNABINOIDS, AND SYNTHETIC CANNABINOIDS

The plant *Cannabis sativa* produces more than 100 chemical compounds that are named cannabinoids or, more specifically, phytocannabinoids (Andre, Hausman, & Guerriero, 2016; Ligresti, De Petrocellis, & Di Marzo, 2016; Verrotti, Castagnino, Maccarrone, & Fezza, 2016). These terpenophenolic compounds have different relative abundance depending on the cannabis variety, but among them, Δ9-tetrahydrocannabinolic acid (THCA), cannabidiol acid (CBDA), and cannabinolic acid (CBNA) are relatively elevated, followed by cannabigerolic acid (CBGA), cannabichromenic acid (CBCA), cannabinodiolic acid (CBNDA), Δ9-tetrahydrocannabivarin (Δ9-THCV), and cannabidivarin (CBDV) (Andre et al., 2016; Izzo, Borrelli, Capasso, Di Marzo, & Mechoulam, 2009). THCA is the major cannabinoid in the drug-type *Cannabis*, while CBDA predominates in fiber-type hemps. Both THCA and CBDA slowly lose their acidic function (decarboxylate) in the plant on heating and become tetrahydrocannabinol (THC) and cannabidiol, acquiring psychoactive properties, in the case of THC.

Phytocannabinoids are described in detail elsewhere (see chapter "Cannabis Pharmacology: The Usual Suspects and a Few Promising Leads" by Russo and Marcu in this book). Among them, Δ9-THC accounts for most of the psychoactive effects of *Cannabis*. This compound was isolated, described and later synthesized in the 1960s (Mechoulam & Hanus, 2000) opening the door to the identification of the specific receptors for this substance in animals in the 1980s and 1990s (Devane, Dysarz, Johnson, Melvin, & Howlett, 1988; Matsuda, Lolait, Brownstein, Young, & Bonner, 1990; Munro, Thomas, & Abu-Shaar, 1993). It has been demonstrated that THC binds to G coupled-protein receptors at cell membranes. These receptors, named CB_1 and CB_2, are widely distributed throughout the body, CB_1 being predominately expressed in the central nervous system and CB_2 in the immune system. As such, the CB_1 receptor is responsible for the psychoactive effects of THC, while the CB_2 receptor is involved in immune function (Pacher & Kunos, 2013; Pertwee et al., 2010). A more detailed review on the pharmacology of CB_1 and CB_2 receptors can be found in the chapter "CB_1 and CB_2 Receptor Pharmacology" by Howlett and Abood.

The description of cannabinoid receptors led to the finding of their endogenous ligands, termed endocannabinoids, among which two have been more widely studied: *N*-arachidonoylethanolamine (anandamide) and 2-arachidonoylglycerol (2-AG). Both endocannabinoids are formed on demand from membrane lipid precursors by specific synthesizing enzymes. For a wider description on the turnover of endocannabinoids, please see the chapter "Endocannabinoid Turnover" by Fowler et al.

The ensemble of cannabinoid receptors, their endogenous ligands (endocannabinoids), and their enzymatic machinery form the core of what is called the endocannabinoid system (ECS). It must be taken into consideration, however, that this definition of the ECS is currently under debate and may only reflect the axis of a more complex structure. In a wider sense, the ECS may also include other members structurally related to anandamide and 2-AG, but that do not bind to CB_1 or CB_2 receptors with high affinity. These compounds (for example, palmitoylethanolamine, oleamide, or *n*-arachidonoyl dopamine) may behave as allosteric modulators of CB_1/CB_2 receptors, or modulate synthesis, degradation, or uptake of anandamide or 2-AG (Di Marzo & Piscitelli, 2015; Ligresti et al., 2016). Both phytocannabinoids and endocannabinoids may also activate receptors other than CB_1 and CB_2, as with the transient receptor potential cation channels—TRP or GPR55 (Di Marzo & Piscitelli, 2015; Ligresti et al., 2016). These receptors and their natural ligands are also considered related to the wider endocannabinoid family.

The description of cannabinoid receptors and enzymatic machinery triggered the development of whole families of synthetic compounds in the search for new pharmacological tools and new potential therapeutic drugs. Among these synthetic compounds developed are (1) new CB_1/CB_2 receptor agonists and antagonists; (2) inhibitors of the hydrolase enzymes (FAAH and MAGL) or of endocannabinoid transport and uptake, in order to potentiate EC signaling; (3) silent allosteric modulators of CB_1/CB_2 receptors. A detailed description of the current status of all these compounds may be found in other chapters of the current book (see chapter "CB_1 and CB_2 Receptor Pharmacology" by Howlett and Abood, chapter "Functional Selectivity at Cannabinoid Receptors" by Priestley et al., and chapter "Endocannabinoid Turnover" by Fowler et al.).

Some of these synthetic compounds (analogs of Δ9-THC, aminoalkylindoles, and other cannabinoid analogs) have been detected in preparations of the new type of drug generically called "Spice." Spice or "fake cannabis" is a general term used for various herbal mixtures of unknown exact ingredients or chemical composition (Seely, Lapoint, Moran, & Fattore, 2012; Vemuri & Makriyannis, 2015). Product testing of Spice formulations shows that cannabinoid constituents and dosages can vary greatly between products, lots, and even within the same package (Seely et al., 2012). Some of the synthetic cannabinoids (SCB) detected in Spice belong to the "JWH" series initially synthesized by Huffman and Padgett (2005), such as JWH-018 (1-pentyl-3-(1-napthoyl)indole). JWH-018 can be easily synthesized and shows high efficacy at CB_1 receptors (Huffman & Padgett, 2005). Other compounds detected in Spice include HU-210, developed at the Hebrew University in the 1960s, and the cyclohexylphenol (CP) cannabinoids developed by Pfizer in the 1970s (Seely et al., 2012), both of which have some structural similarities to Δ9-THC but are more potent, full agonists at CB_1 receptors. Compounds first synthesized by Alexandros Makriyannis (AM compounds) have also been detected in Spice (Hudson & Ramsey, 2011). Different preparations of Spice have highly variable content including compounds like JWH-018, JWH-073, CP-47,497, JWH-081, JWH-122, JWH-210, and AM-2201. In addition, endocannabinoid-like molecules such as *N*-palmitoylethanolamine (PEA, endogenously synthesized by the same enzyme as anandamide, NAPE-PLD), have been identified in Spice preparations (Seely et al., 2012).

2. SIGNALING PATHWAYS ASSOCIATED TO SCB

While the cannabinoid CB_1 receptor is one of the most abundant G protein-coupled receptors present in the central nervous system (Matsuda et al., 1990), the CB_2 receptor is located predominantly in the immune system (Munro et al., 1993) and is barely found in the CNS. Both CB_1 and CB_2 receptors are preferentially coupled to pertussis toxin-sensitive

Gi/o proteins to inhibit adenylate cyclase and cyclic AMP–protein kinase A (PKA) signaling (Howlett, Johnson, Melvin, & Milne, 1988). However, coupling to Gs or Gq/11 of CB_1 receptors has also been reported (Glass & Felder, 1997; Lauckner, Hille, & Mackie, 2005).

The signaling pathways triggered by natural-, synthetic-, and *endo*-cannabinoids, through CB_1 receptors, have been the focus of extensive research efforts. Upon receptor engagement, cannabinoids activate, among other cascades, phosphatidylinositol 3-kinase/Akt (PI3K/Akt) and mitogen-activated protein kinases (MAPK) such as extracellular signal-regulated kinase (ERK1/2), p38 MAPKs, and JUN N-terminal kinases (JNKs) involved in cell proliferation and survival (Piomelli, 2003). Activation of CB_1 receptors in the neuronal presynaptic terminal inhibits L, N, and P/Q type voltage-activated calcium channels and stimulates inwardly rectifying potassium channels to reduce neurotransmitter release (Kano, Ohno-Shosaku, Hashimotodani, Uchigashima, & Watanabe, 2009). Thus, depolarization of a postsynaptic neuron induces short-term depression of GABA release from axon terminals innervating the same postsynaptic neuron. Further, antagonists of CB_1 receptors block this depolarization-induced suppression of inhibition (DSI) at hippocampal GABAergic synapses, suggesting that an endocannabinoid was the retrograde messenger involved in this synaptic plasticity (Katona & Freund, 2012). In addition, CB_1 receptors also signal from glial cells to neurons to modulate neurotransmission. In fact, in hippocampal astrocytes CB_1 receptors are activated by SCB ligands as well as by endocannabinoids released by neurons (Navarrete & Araque, 2008). This activation increased astrocyte calcium levels from internal stores and the intracellular signaling pathway underlying this effect exhibited specific characteristics. In contrast to the canonical coupling to Gi/o proteins, the calcium elevations are mediated by CB_1 receptors coupled to Gq/11 proteins that activate phospholipase C and produce inositol triphosphate (Navarrete, Díez, & Araque, 2014).

Cannabinoids promote ERK phosphorylation in the hippocampus, CB_1-transfected CHO cells, and human astrocytoma cells (Galve-Roperh, Rueda, Gómez del Pulgar, Velasco, & Guzmán, 2002). In primary cortical neurons, the CB_1 receptor agonist methanandamide evoked a biphasic model of ERK activation and required activation of Gq/11 (PLC/PKC) and Gi (Src, Fyn), the magnitude and duration of ERK activation have been causally linked to specific cellular responses in neurons and neural cells such as the induction of cell proliferation and neuronal maturation (Asimaki & Mangoura, 2011).

The SCB agonists WIN 55,212-2 and HU-210 protect primary astrocytes from ceramide-induced apoptosis via activation of the PI3K/Akt pathway, this prosurvival effect also depends on the modulation of the ERK pathway (Gomez del Pulgar, de Ceballos, Guzman, & Velasco, 2002). Whereas in N1E-115 mouse neuroblastoma cells ERK activation by WIN 55,212-2 is mediated by CB_1 receptor signaling, but required several basally activated pathways including PI3-kinase, Src, and protein phosphatases, but receptor-stimulated inhibition of adenylate cyclase/PKA is absolutely required for ERK activation (Davis, Ronesi, & Lovinger, 2003). In oligodendrocytes, a role for the ERK/MAPK cascade in endocannabinoid-induced oligodendrocyte maturation has been proposed (Gomez et al., 2010), while the synthetic agonists ACEA, JW133, and HU-210 accelerated oligodendrocyte progenitor differentiation through a mechanism dependent on the activation of the PI3K/Akt and mTOR signaling pathways (Gomez et al., 2011). Moreover, the proliferative action of the PI3K/Akt cascade has been investigated in detail in neural stem cells. In cerebellar granule cell precursors HU-210-induced proliferation requires PI3K/Akt/GSK3β signaling. CB_1 receptor activation phosphorylates and inhibits GSK3β thus β-catenin is stabilized and translocates to the nucleus, modulating the expression of genes such as cyclin D1, which is involved in the regulation of cell proliferation (Trazzi, Steger, Mitrugno, Bartesaghi, & Ciani, 2010).

Finally, receptor desensitization has been proposed as a mechanism that terminates cannabinoid agonist signaling and requires phosphorylation by a G protein-coupled receptor kinase and interaction of the phosphorylated receptor with β-arrestins. However, recent reports indicate that β-arrestins, while hindering G-protein signaling, act as scaffold proteins for the endocytic machinery and signaling molecules such as the MAP family of kinases and initiate a second wave of signaling at the cell surface (Nogueras-Ortiz & Yudowski, 2016). In addition, a final wave emerges from receptors localized at intracellular compartments, such as endosomes and lysosomes (Rozenfeld & Devi, 2008).

3. STRUCTURAL CLASSIFICATION OF SCB

Synthetic cannabinoids (SC) have gone through numerous iterations of modification to their chemical structures making their forensic detection and identification difficult (Presley, Gurney, Scott, Kacinko, & Logan, 2016). In

2008, the European Monitoring Centre for Drugs and Drug Abuse (EMCDD; http://www.emcdda.europa.eu/publications/drug-profiles/synthetic-cannabinoids) formally monitored these SCB products in order to control the synthesis, trade, distribution, and human consumption of these substances due to their detrimental health effects (Castaneto et al., 2014; EMCDDA, 2009). To date, novel psychoactive substances (NPS) have been detected in over 100 countries/territories (Schifano, Orsolini, Duccio Papanti, & Corkery, 2015), with a specific high impact in the European teenage population (over 5% of 19–24 years old) (EMCDDA, 2014). At present, the EMCDD and the United Nations Office on Drugs and Crime (UNODC) monitor over 450 NPS of which over 160 substances are SCB (EMCDDA, 2015; Scocard, Benyamina, Coscas, & Karila, 2017; Zawilska & Wojcieszak, 2014). Over 10 recognizable chemical families of SCB are known. Forensic/toxicological analysis, identification, and characterization of the new and/or relatively unknown SCB is performed by using advanced analytical tools such as nuclear magnetic resonance (NMR), bioinformatics, computational chemistry, electrospray ionization, and high-resolution liquid-chromatography tandem mass-spectrometry (HR-LC–MS/MS) tools (Adamowicz & Tokarczyk, 2016; Dunne & Rosengren-Holmberg, 2016; Ford & Berg, 2016; Sahai et al., 2016).

The use of in silico and chemical biochemistry approaches are essential in predicting and identifying the metabolites of SCB and drug subclasses that continue to appear (Presley et al., 2016; Strano-Rossi et al., 2014). A chemoinformatic approach permit a broad screening of SCB to manage and unify analytical data from multiple techniques and instruments, and combine it with chemical and structural information (Lobo Vicente et al., 2016; Sahai et al., 2016).

The compound CP47497 and other indoles were first used as analgesics, in different medicinal chemistry programmes from Sterling Winthrop and Charles Pfizer (CP) company (now Pfizier Inc.) in the 1970s–1980s. The fact that many of these compounds bind to cannabinoid receptors was discovered subsequently (Seely, Prather, James, & Moran, 2011) but have only recently found their way into Spice blends (Calles, 2013).

As described earlier, the synthesis of structurally distinct molecules that bind with high affinity to cannabinoid receptors is a relatively recent phenomena that started with the synthesis of the CB_1 full agonist naphtoyindole JWH-018 (1-pentyl-3-(1-naphtoyl)indole) (Huffman, Dai, Martin, & Compton, 1994; Huffman and Padgett, 2005).

In March 2011, the Drug Enforcement Agency (DEA, USA) classified as schedule class I, five SCB: JWH-018, JWH-073, JWH-200, CP-47,497, and Cannabicyclohexanol (Drug Enforcement Administration, 2010).

As the synthesis of novel SCB is an area in constant development, it is difficult to establish a clear structural classification. Moreover, to date, SCB can be classified into several major structural groups as shown later, depending on their structural evolution as described in Table 1 (Figs. 1–6).

Furthermore, there are several analytical difficulties posed by the task of identifying SCB (i.e., forensic data are limited) because these SCB are not controlled substances in most EU Member States (EMCDDA, 2009). In the United Kingdom, the Physchoactive Substances Act (2016) effectively banned the production, sale, and possession of so-called legal highs including SCB.

A common structural feature of the SCB is a side-chain, where optimal activity for binding CB_1 cannabinoid receptors for psychotropic activity requires more than four and up to nine saturated carbon atoms (see Pertwee et al., 2010, for review). An interesting on-line resource from the EMCDDA, *Interactive* can be found at the following link: (http://www.emcdda.europa.eu/topics/pods/synthetic-cannabinoids). The resource is helpful in facilitating understanding of the chemistry of the SCB and explains the chemical make-up of these compounds.

The structure of the majority of SCB can be divided into four key parts: the core (indole or indazole core) and substituents, the link section (amide, ketone, or ester linker), the ring (naphthyl, quinolinyl, adamantyl, or tetramethylcyclopropyl ring) and substituents, and the tail section.

Table 1 Structural Classification of Synthetic Cannabinoids

1. *Naphthoylindoles, Naphthylmethylindoles, Naphthoylpyrroles, Naphthylmethylindenes*: JWH-007, JWH-018, JWH-073, JWH-200, JWH-398, AM-1221, AM-2201 (*Fluoroalkyl* derivative from JWH018), AM-694, Win-55,212-2
2. *Phenylacetylindoles* (i.e., *benzoylindoles*): JWH-250, RCS-8
3. *Cyclohexylphenols*: CP-47947, CP-55940
4. *Tetramethylcyclopropylindoles*: UR-144, XLR-11 (*Fluoroalkyl* derivative from UR-144)
5. *Adamantoylindoles*: 5F-AKB-48, STS-135
6. *Indazole carboxamides*: AB-PINACA, AB-FUBINACA
7. *Quinolinyl ester*: PB-22

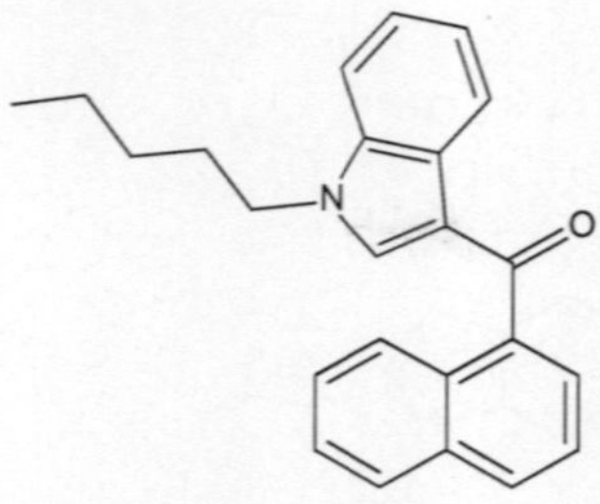

JWH-018

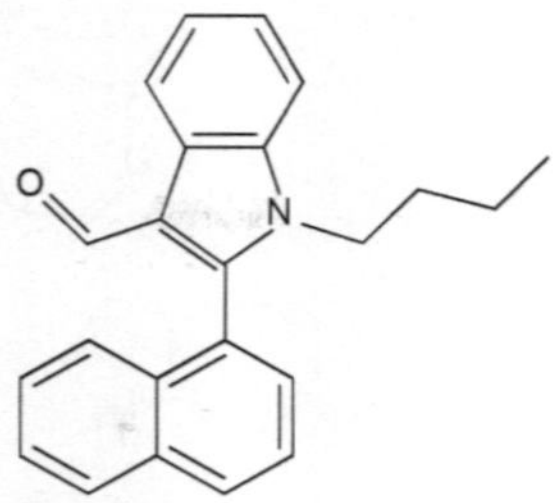

JWH-073

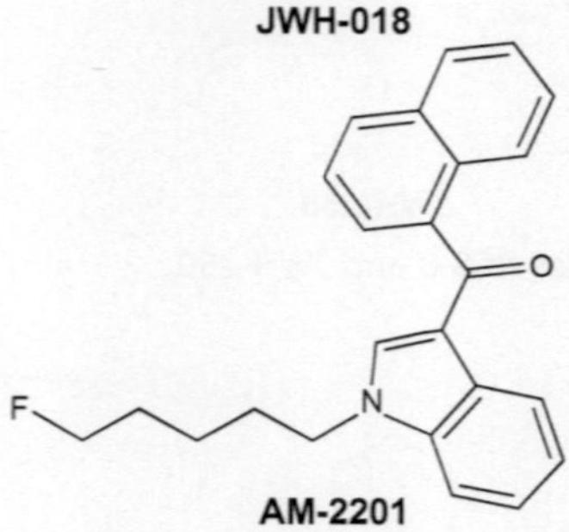

AM-2201

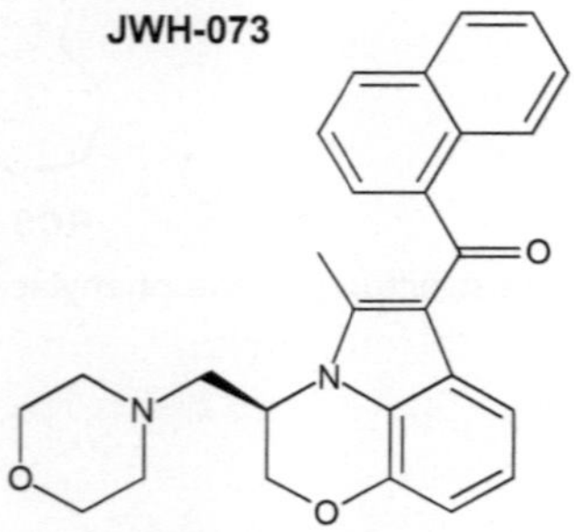

Win 55,212-2

Fig. 1 The structures of four naphthoylindoles with varying degrees of functional selectivity for CB_1 and CB_2 cannabinoid receptors: JWH-018, JWH-073, AM2201, and Win 55,212-2.

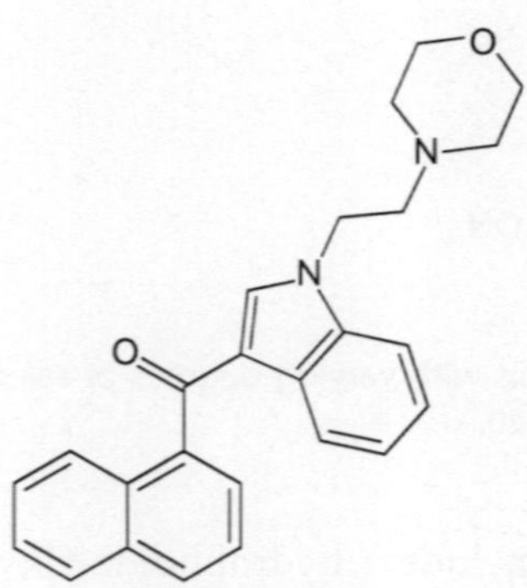

JWH-200

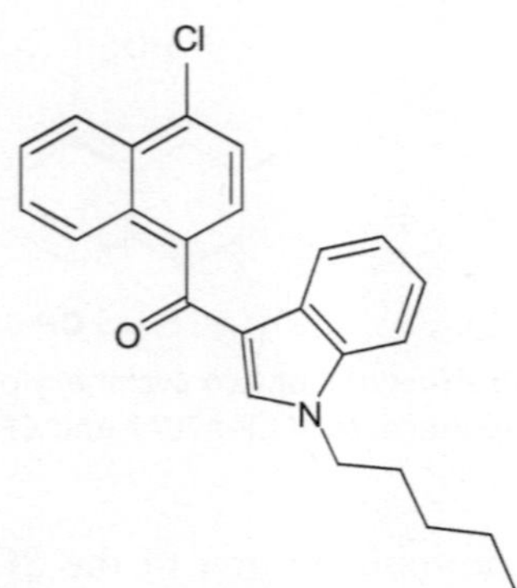

JWH-398

Fig. 2 The structures of the aminoalkylindole JWH-200 and the synthetic cannabinoid JWH-398.

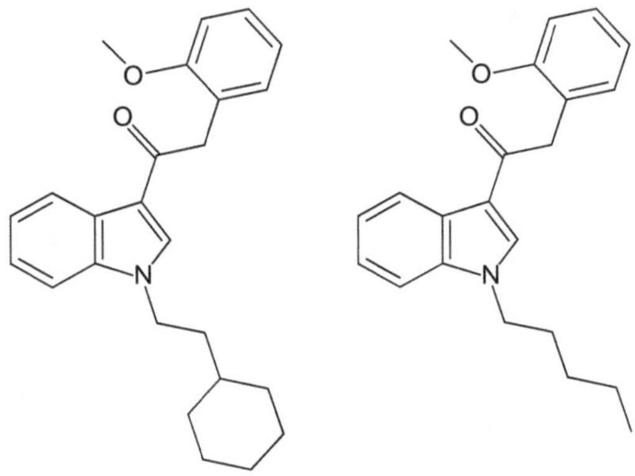

RCS-8 **JWH-250**

Fig. 3 The structures of the phenylacetylindoles RCS-8 and JWH-250.

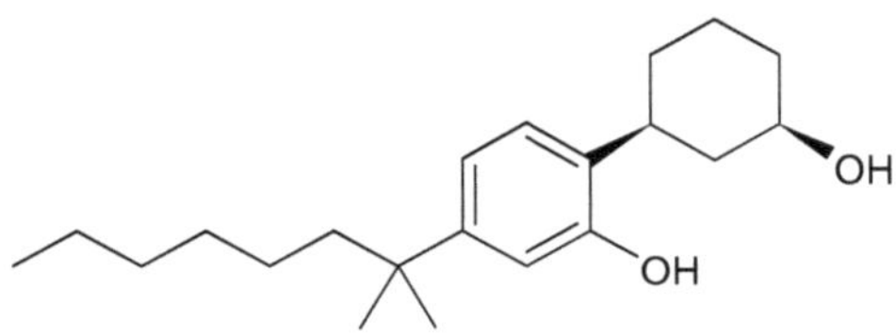

CP-47947

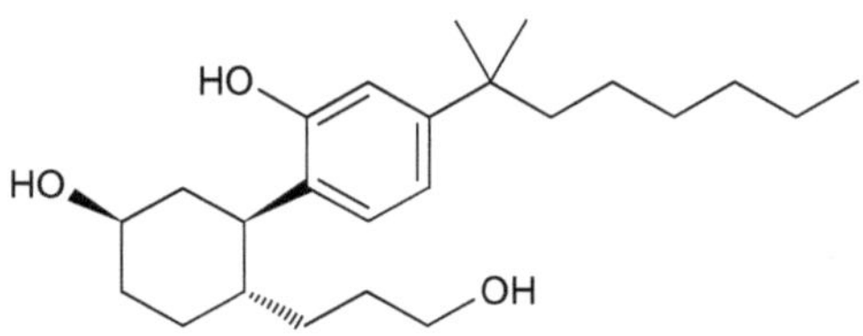

CP-55940

Fig. 4 The structures of two cyclohexylphenols with varying degrees of selectivity for cannabinoid receptors: CP-47947 and CP-55940.

Other common features of the SCB include a hydrophobic alkyl group attached to the indole or indazole ring (Ford, Tai, Fantegrossi, & Prather, 2017).

Adamantyl-cannabinoids are currently the most frequently used class of SCB in the United Kingdom, particularly AKB-48, 5F-AKB-48, and STS-135 (McIlroy, Ford, & Khan, 2016).

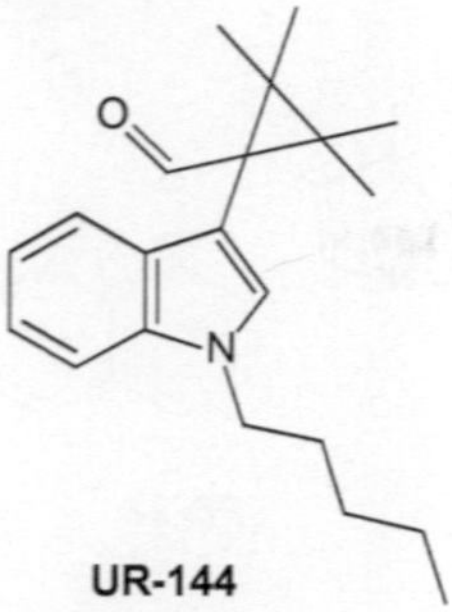

UR-144

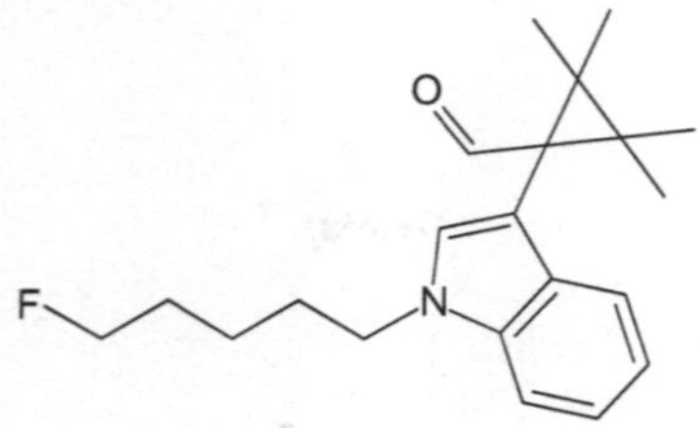

XLR-11

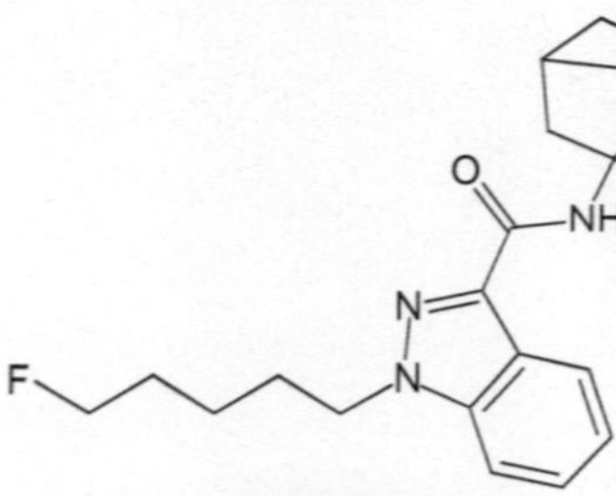

5F-AKB-48

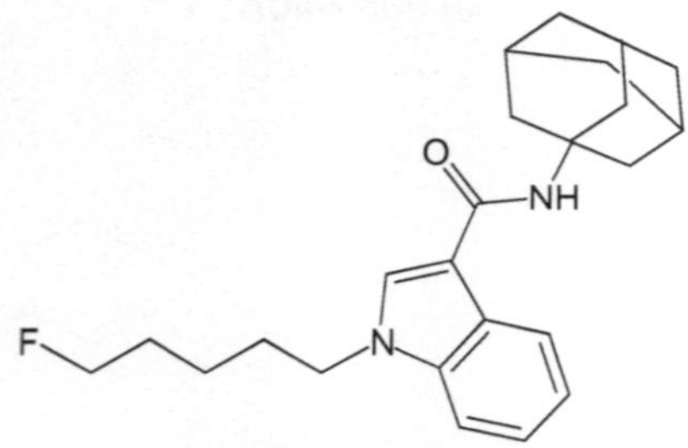

STS-135

Fig. 5 The structures of two tetramethylcyclopropylindoles (UR-144 and XLR-11) and two adamantoylindoles (5F-AKB-48 and STS-135) with varying degrees of selectivity for cannabinoid receptors.

4. CANNABINOID/CB$_1$ RECEPTORS INVOLVEMENT IN MEMORY REGULATION AND PSYCHOSIS

4.1 CB$_1$ Receptor Role in the Regulation of Memory and the Effects of Exogenous Cannabinoids

Endocannabinoids (endocannabinoid) and their central CB$_1$ receptors are richly present within the brain, including the basal ganglia subregions, hippocampus, amygdala, and cerebellum, which is indicative of the wide-ranging roles for endocannabinoid and CB$_1$ receptors in animals and humans (e.g., Herkenham et al., 1991; Mackie, 2008). The distribution of CB$_1$ receptors is consistent with their regulatory roles in the brain, as CB$_1$ receptors are involved in a range of important physiological functions such as movement control, pain processing, brain development and maturation, and learning and memory (Mackie, 2008; Svízenská, Dubový, & Sulcová, 2008).

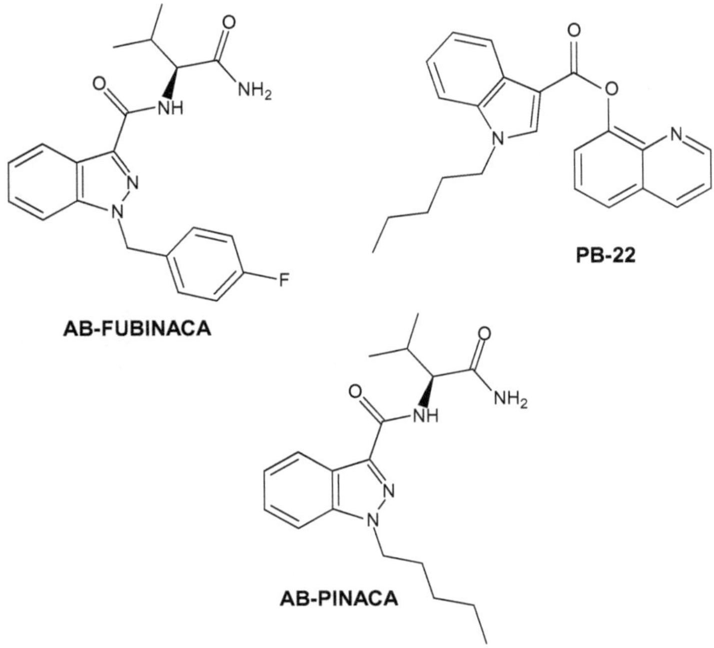

Fig. 6 The structures of two indazole carboxiamides (AB-PINACA and AB-FUBINACA) and one quinolinyl ester (PB22).

Learning and memory regulation involves neuronal networks that operate by means of glutamate (excitatory) and GABA (γ-aminobutyric acid, inhibitory) and that are modulated by endocannabinoids. Endocannabinoids act within both presynaptic and postsynaptic neuronal compartments and exert neuroplastic changes of synaptic function in glutamatergic and GABA-ergic pathways. It has been established that neuronal activity triggers postsynaptic synthesis and release of endocannabinoids that act retrogradely across the synapse and bind to presynaptic CB_1 receptors; it is the nature of the neural network involved that decides about the various neurobiological effects of endocannabinoids mediated by CB_1 receptors. Thus, their actions in the brain regions involved in learning and memory, such as the hippocampus (Davies, Pertwee, & Riedel, 2002), amygdala, and dorsal striatum (Goodman & Packard, 2015) necessarily translate into changes in learning and memory-related functions. Of relevance to memory regulation, endocannabinoid release is affected by glucocorticoids as hormonal mediators of the response to stress, which act at glucocorticoid receptors richly expressed in the hippocampus and amygdala. Glucocorticoids activate postsynaptic glucocorticoid receptors that trigger the postsynaptic synthesis of endocannabinoids, which then act retrogradely via presynaptic CB_1 receptors on glutamatergic terminals and this triggers a signaling cascade which inhibits glutamate transmission, leading to a reduction in the neural activity in the hippocampus and amygdala (Di, Malcher-Lopes, Halmos, & Tasker, 2003). It should be said at this stage that not only can endocannabinoids act at CB_1 receptors but also exogenous cannabinoids, including THC and their synthetic forms.

While it has been accepted that presynaptic hippocampal CB_1 receptors play a role in learning and memory, in line with the fact that the hippocampus has long been implicated in these phenomena, there is a growing interest in the function of mitochondrial cannabinoid receptors as CB_1 receptors are located not only in the presynaptic membrane but also in neuronal mitochondria. Activation of mitochondrial CB_1 receptors can cause an acute change in the energy status, with reductions in the rate of mitochondrial respiration and further long-term consequences of mitochondrial dysfunction, including neuronal aging and degeneration. Thus, the role of mitochondrial CB_1 receptors has emerged as an interesting aspect in the neurobiology of learning and memory (Hebert-Chatelain et al., 2016).

Activation of presynaptic CB_1 receptors affects the release of neurotransmitters such as glutamate or GABA in both short-term and long-term (e.g., review by Puighermanal, Busquets-Garcia, Maldonado, & Ozaita, 2012). Experimental rodent studies in vivo or in vitro, using brain tissue—most often hippocampal sections, are essential in explaining the role of the ECS in memory regulation, and the effects of CB_1 receptor agonists and antagonists, acute or chronic. Experimental in vitro approaches have demonstrated that short-term endocannabinoid actions involve synaptic plasticity responses such as depolarization-induced suppression of inhibition (DSI) or depolarization-induced excitation (DSE) (Heifets & Castillo, 2009; Kano et al., 2009). A long-term inhibition of transmitter release also induces neuroplasticity as it associates with long-term depression (LTD) of synaptic activity; LTD at inhibitory synapses can lead to long-term potentiation (LTP) downstream (Carlson, Wang, & Alger, 2002). The finding that endocannabinoids can facilitate LTP induction in neurons augments our understanding of the behavioral effects of endocannabinoids in health and under the influence of exogenous cannabinoids.

Exogenous cannabinoids such as of THC administered in the course of experimental interventions in animal and human studies, or as recreational drugs in humans, are presumed to interact with the brain ECS at higher concentrations than those of endogenous modulators. Thus exogenous cannabinoids, including new SCB that bind to CB_1 receptors, can affect endocannabinoid-dependent synaptic plasticity including LTP or LTD, and change behavioral learning processes as observed in acute and long-term treatments (Puighermanal et al., 2012).

A single dose of THC has been shown to abolish endocannabinoid-induced LTD in rat hippocampus, while chronic administration of THC abolishes LTP generated by high-frequency stimulation in vitro, with reductions in glutamate release in rat hippocampal slices. In the hippocampus in vivo, THC preferentially decreases GABA release and has less effect on glutamate release, as there are more CB_1 receptors in GABA-ergic neurons and those CB_1 receptors have a higher sensitivity to cannabinoid agonists. Therefore, memory impairment caused by exogenous cannabinoids could be predominantly a consequence of a disruption of hippocampal network function that is mediated by synchronized GABAergic activity (for review, see Puighermanal et al., 2012).

A useful experimental tool in studies on the role of the ECS in learning and memory is a genetic modification whereby the *Cnr1* gene that encodes the CB_1 receptors is deleted in mice. Mice lacking CB_1 receptors have increased hippocampal LTP and improved memory retention when compared with the wild strain (Bohme, Laville, Ledent, Parmentier, & Imperato, 2000; Martin, Ledent, Parmentier, Maldonado, & Valverde, 2002). Interestingly, mature and old Cnr1 knockout mice, unlike young ones, tend to display deficits in procedural learning, spatial memory, and social recognition abilities. These cognitive deficits associate with neuronal losses in the hippocampal areas CA1 and CA3 that are involved in memory consolidation, consistent with the neuroprotective effects mediated via the CB_1 receptor. On the other hand, CB_1-deficient mice show significantly impaired short-term and long-term extinction of memory, as tested in auditory fear-conditioning paradigms, although no effects have been found in their memory acquisition and consolidation (Marsicano et al., 2002). Similar effects have been observed in control (wild strain) mice treated with the CB_1 receptor antagonist SR141716A (rimonabant), which confirms that the CB_1 receptor is paramount in the process of memory extinction (Marsicano et al., 2002). Extinction of traumatic/aversive memories is essential in the recovery from posttraumatic stress disorder (PTSD) and maladaptive rumination in clinical depression, where persistent negative memories can cause retraumatization and relapse of mental illness. There is growing evidence that exogenous cannabinoids could exert normalizing effects on aversive memories in PTSD and phobias.

While there is consensus that CB_1 receptors located in the hippocampus play a necessary role in the memory impairments caused by cannabinoid agonists, including THC (e.g., Wise, Thorpe, & Lichtman, 2009) other brain regions also contribute to memory regulation with their CB_1 receptors. For example, the prefrontal cortex plays a role in CB_1 receptor-mediated memory as demonstrated in a study where THC infusion into the prefrontal cortex disrupted rat memory in a radial arm maze (Silva de Melo et al., 2005). It should be said, however, that in situ infusion of exogenous cannabinoids may bring about different effects to those observed after a systemic administration (for review, see Zanettini et al., 2011).

4.2 Cannabinoids and Dorsal Striatal Memory

CB_1 receptors are also present in the striatum; they are localized on presynaptic terminals of glutamatergic corticostriatal projection neurons and GABA-ergic medium spiny neurons. CB_1 receptors have not been found on cholinergic interneurons in the striatum nor nigrostriatal projections to the striatum. The ECS plays an important role in the types of learning and memory mediated by the dorsal striatum, which includes stimulus–response (S–R) habit memory. Studies of this kind of memory involve maze learning and instrumental learning tasks in mostly rodents although they can be adapted to humans. There is a growing body of evidence that manipulating the ECS by means of either infusion or a chronic exposure to exogenous cannabinoids can alter dorsal striatum-dependent habit memory (for review, see Goodman & Packard, 2015). Exogenous cannabinoid agonist or antagonist administration associates with impairment of dorsal striatum-dependent S–R habit memory, while THC tolerance can associate with enhancement of that type of memory. It is a complex area of research as appetitive paradigms also engage the ventral striatum. As in the case of hippocampal memory, endocannabinoid-dependent striatal memory implicates CB_1 receptors with synaptic plasticity (Goodman & Packard, 2015).

It is appropriate to note that the very wide range of endocannabinoid roles superimposes with the complexity of the neuronal circuits involved with their other neurotransmitter systems that respond to *endo-* and *exo*cannabinoid actions as a matter of secondary effects. This justifies an opinion that the effects of the ECS also depend on environmental conditions when it comes to memory impairment produced by exogenous cannabinoids (Zanettini et al., 2011). On the basis of the limited human studies on the effects of SCB on learning and memory, it would be fair to say that SCB bioactivity is mediated via CB_1 receptor agonism in humans (Gunderson, Haughey, Ait-Daoud, Joshi, & Hart, 2012).

4.3 Cognitive Changes in SCB Users

A recent study by Cohen et al. (2017) has assessed executive functions in a group of participants comprising SCB users, recreational cannabis users and nonusers by means of cognitive function tests, the Stroop word-color task, and the n-back and free-recall memory tasks. SCB users have performed significantly worse than the other participants in all the tests applied. In addition, they have had higher depression and anxiety scores when compared with the two other groups. Thus, executive functions were impaired in SCB users (Cohen et al., 2017). It is consistent with CB_1 receptor involvement.

4.4 Role of CB_1 Receptors in Psychosis

Synaptic activity closely involves membrane potential changes and gives rise to transmembrane currents that can be measured in the extracellular field to which all neuron types contribute; they time their action potentials with millisecond precision depending on their membrane potential fluctuations (Buzsáki & Wang, 2012). The spatial alignment of neurons and the temporal synchrony of neuronal firing determine the strength of the extracellular field. The synchrony, which results from network oscillations, determines the different magnitudes of local field potentials that represent different brain states (Buzsáki, Anastassiou, & Koch, 2012). In the intact brain, endogenous oscillations result in high-frequency patterns, of which most ubiquitous are rhythms in the gamma-frequency range (30–90 Hz) (Buzsáki & Wang, 2012). Another rhythm of relevance to psychosis is theta oscillations (4–7 Hz) that represent the net activity of the hippocampus; they are generated mainly by the entorhinal cortical inputs. Theta rhythm is thought to be critical for temporal coding and decoding of active neuronal ensembles and modifications of synaptic strength (Buzsáki, 2002). It has been known that high level cognitive activities, such as working memory, closely associate with gamma oscillations in the prefrontal cortex (Fries, 2009). Typically, patients with schizophrenia who show working memory impairments have also reduced gamma and theta oscillations; deficits in cortical oscillations and impairments of memory associate in schizophrenia and psychosis (Minzenberg et al., 2010; Skosnik, Cortes-Briones, & Hajós, 2016). There is consensus that abnormal neural synchrony and impaired auditory gating indicate of distorted information processing in patients with psychosis.

Interestingly, exogenous cannabinoids, such as THC can also lead to disruptions in neural oscillations, as shown in human studies (for review, see Skosnik et al., 2016). It is of direct relevance to psychotic-like behavior observed after exogenous cannabinoid exposure in humans and can be explained by the fact that oscillations in the cortical and limbic brain areas, including the hippocampus, are controlled by CB_1 receptors. There are lines of evidence derived from animal experiments that activation of CB_1 receptors interferes with neuronal network oscillations and impairs sensory gating function in the cortical and limbic brain areas, including the hippocampus. For example, a CB_1 receptor agonist, CP-55940, has been found to disrupt auditory gating and interrupt theta field potential oscillations in the hippocampus and entorhinal cortex in anesthetized and awake rats. In addition, novelty-induced theta and gamma activities were also significantly diminished by CP-55940 in the same material (Hajós, Hoffmann, & Kocsis, 2008). Findings of this kind have a translational value and support the idea that activation of CB_1 receptors by exogenous cannabinoids impairs theta and gamma oscillations that are known to be affected in cannabis abuse-related psychosis spectrum disorders in vulnerable subjects (Skosnik et al., 2016). Case studies of psychotic SCB users are described later.

To sum up, there are similarities between disruptions of neuronal network oscillations in psychosis and those in psychosis-like conditions triggered by exogenous cannabinoids (e.g., THC). There is evidence that activation of CB_1 receptors disrupts neuronal network oscillations. Exogenous cannabinoids that act as CB_1 receptor agonists, which includes new synthetic forms, can trigger psychosis-like behavior through this mechanism.

5. CLINICAL ADVERSE EFFECTS OF SCB

The health risks associated with using SCB cannot be assumed to be similar to those from taking cannabis because, as described elsewhere, SCB tend to be much more potent at CB_1 receptors and do not contain cannabidiol or cannabinol (among others), which mitigates against many adverse effects. The adverse clinical effects of SCB have previously been reviewed by Cooper (2016), and case reports are the main source of information. The main findings are that acute SC intoxication is usually characterized by tachycardia, hypertension, visual and auditory hallucinations, mydriasis, agitation and anxiety, tachypnea, nausea, and vomiting (Heath, Burroughs, Thompson, & Tecklenburg, 2012; Schneir, Cullen, & Ly, 2011). However, in some cases SC misuse can precipitate stroke, seizures (Harris & Brown, 2013; Hermanns-Clausen, Kneisel, Szabo, & Auwarter, 2013; Hoyte et al., 2012; McQuade, Hudson, Dargan, et al., 2013; Spaderna, Addy, & D'Souza, 2013; Winstock & Barratt, 2013) and what appears to be serotonin syndrome, possibly mediated through mild MAOI (Rosenbaum, Carreiro, & Babu, 2012).

5.1 Adverse Cardiovascular Effects

Although quite uncommon, the use of cannabis is associated with some serious cardiovascular conditions (Thomas, Kloner, & Rezkalla, 2014) and case studies highlighting coronary artery thrombosis, vasospasm, and myocardial infarction have been reported (Gunawardena, Rajapakse, Herath, & Amarasena, 2014; Mittleman, Lewis, Maclure, Sherwood, & Muller, 2001; Tatli, Yilmaztepe, Altun, & Altun, 2007). It is likely that these effects are mediated through TCH evoked increases in catecholamines, increased cardiac workload (with increased heart rate and blood pressure) with decreased supply of oxygen (Aryana & Williams, 2007). Given that SC have much higher affinity at CB_1 receptors, and potentially have effects at other receptors, we may expect more frequent cardiovascular problems with SC. SC use is associated with acute myocardial infarction, found in both adults and children (Ibrahim, Al-Saffar, & Wannenburg, 2014; McKeever et al., 2015; Mir, Obafemi, Young, & Kane, 2011; Tse, Kodur, Squires, & Collins, 2014).

The SC "K2" is associated with tachycardia (Chinnadurai, Shrestha, & Ayinla, 2016). McKeever et al. (2015) reported a 16-year-old male who had taken the SC "K2" 60–120 min prior to complaining of sustained substernal pressure, dyspnea, nausea, and vomiting; ECG revealed ST elevations and increased troponin and creatinine kinase MB. The SC "Black Mamba," smoked 3 h prior to symptoms onset, led to myocardial infarction with ST elevation and high Troponin-T levels. Analysis revealed that the substance ingested was an adamantyl SC (McIlroy et al., 2016).

5.2 Adverse Pulmonary Effects of SCB

Long-term SCB users have reported chronic coughs with pneumothorax and diffuse pulmonary infiltrates were also reported (Froberg & Bauer, 2012). Alhadi et al. (2013) reported on a 21-year-old male with a cannabis habit who had been using SC for 4 months prior to presenting with a 2 month history of chronic cough. Laboratory workup suggested that the diffuse pulmonary infiltrates were probably inflammatory-mediated, possibly through macrophage activation. The authors confirmed SC presence through blood, urine, and saliva testing with AM-2201, JWH-122, JWH-210, and JWH-018 all present, but could not rule out allergic alveolitis caused simply by heat or smoke particulate inhalation. Similarly, Bajantri et al. reported the case of a 21-year-old woman, also a long-term cannabis user, who had started smoking SC (K2) in the last 2 months and who presented with nausea, vomiting, and upper abdominal pain. Chest CT revealed pneumomediastinum, hypothesized to be secondary to SC use and increased alveolar pressure leading to barotrauma. Another case report described a 29-year-old man presenting with severe agitation after smoking "K2." Tests revealed fever and tachycardia, but also leukocytosis and interstitial infiltrates on chest radiography (Chinnadurai et al., 2016). Taken together, these studies suggest that SC can cause adverse pulmonary events not seen with cannabis use.

5.3 Acute Kidney Injury From SCB

In a case series, Bhanushali, Jain, Fatima, Leisch, and Thornley-Brow (2013) described four males, aged 20–30 who had been using "spice" for weeks up to 2 years, two of whom recently changed supplier, all presenting with nausea and vomiting for more than 2 days. Renal biopsy in three of the patients revealed acute tubular necrosis. The Centre for Disease Control and Prevention (USA; 2013) also describe a case series of 16 SC users from a variety of US states presenting with nausea and vomiting and either flank or abdominal pain and were found to have high creatinine levels. Patients were aged between 15 and 33 years and toxicological analysis (urine, blood, or serum) from seven patients revealed XLR-11 *N*-pentanoic acid metabolites in four of these seven patients, who had taken the SC products Phantom Wicked Dreams, Mr. Happy, Clown Loyal, Lava, or Flame 2.0. In another case series, Buser et al. (2014) identified nine persons (all males, 15–27 years) who presented to Oregon and Southwest Washington hospitals (USA) during May–October 2012 with acute kidney injury after smoking SCB products. The first patient presented to the emergency department after 4 days of flank pain, emesis, and oliguria examinations revealed hypertension and bilaterally enlarged hyperechoic kidneys. Symptoms began after smoking an SC product called "Clown Loyal." The second patient presented to an emergency department complaining of abdominal pain, nausea, and lower back discomfort lasting 3 days. He was euvolemic, but hypertensive. A renal ultrasound revealed bilateral hyperechoic kidneys with poor corticomedullary differentiation. In cases who recalled their last exposure, they reported symptom onset between approximately 30 min and 24 h (median: 8–12 h) after smoking a SC product. The SCs were marketed as Spice, Mad Monkey, Clown Loyal, Jonny Clearwater, Feel Good, Lava, and Orgazmo. At least two of these products contained XLR-11. The authors suggest that this drug is a potent and long-acting agonist at CB_2 receptor and that this effect may underlie its kidney toxicity.

5.4 Adverse Neurological Effects of SCB: Psychosis and Catatonia

An increase in susceptibility to schizophrenia has long been hypothesized with cannabis use, with clear data finally confirmed in Swedish conscripts in 1987 (Andréasson, Engström, Allebeck, & Rydberg, 1987). It is then no surprise that SCB have been associated with psychotic events in users and there are numerous case studies in this area (e.g., Glue, Al-Shaqsi, Hancock, et al., 2013). Papanti et al. (2013) have reviewed these cases and coined the term "spiceophrenia" to describe the psychotic symptoms associated with SCB or "Spice" use. In addition to hallucinations, SCB users can exhibit violent and self-injuring behavior (Thomas, Bliss, & Malik, 2012). More recent studies in Europe suggest that 15% of SCB users who report to emergency departments exhibit psychotic symptoms (Vallersnes et al., 2016), interestingly this was a lower percentage of patients compared those taking tryptamines, methylenedioxypyrovalerone, methylphenidate, LSD, or mushrooms.

Catatonia has been seen with SCB use in two patients (Khan, Pace, Truong, Gordon, & Moukaddam, 2016). One patient (21-year-old male) used SC (Kush) almost daily for 18 months, while the other (17-year-old male) used a large quantity of SCB (Spice) over a 2-week period. Both were admitted with catatonia but no mood disturbance or psychosis. To our knowledge, there have been no studies linking cannabis use to catatonia.

5.5 Adverse Neurological Effects of SCB: Seizures, Epilepsy, and Tremor

Rosenberg, Tsien, Whalley, and Devinsky (2015) have recently reviewed the role of cannabinoids in epilepsy; highlighting proconvulsive effects (e.g., THC) and anticonvulsive effects (e.g., cannabidiol). The mechanisms of action of cannabidiol in epilepsy have also been recently reviewed (Reddy & Golub, 2016). Much work with SCB in epilepsy has focused on WIN55,212-2. WIN55,212-22 potentiated the effects of four antiepileptic drugs (carbamazepine, phenytoin, phenobarbital, and valproate) in mice (Luszczki et al., 2011). However, the authors also caution that impairment of motor coordination, long-term memory, and a reduction of skeletal muscular strength was also seen with these combination treatments. The same group found WIN 55,212-2 in combination with lamotrigine, pregabalin, and topiramate and second- and third-generation anticonvulsants gabapentin, levetiracetam but not lacosamide, oxcarbazepine, pregabalin, and tiagabine to potentiate anticonvulsant effects in mice (Florek-Luszczki et al., 2015; Luszczki, Wlaz, Karwan, Florek-Luszczki, & Czuczwar, 2013).

Clinical cases are now being described where SC users are presenting with seizures or convulsions. In the United States, there have been reports of seizure activity after smoking various SCB and these were likely JWH-018, JWH-081, JWH-250, and AM-2201 (Lapoint et al., 2011; Schneir & Baumbacher, 2012; Simmons, Cookman, Kang, & Skinner, 2011). In Europe, McQuade et al. (2013) reported a 20-year-old male who had smoked "Black Mamba" and quickly went into tonic–clonic convulsions. Urine analysis revealed metabolites of AM-2201.

More recently, seizure-like activity has been seen following SCB use. Schep, Slaughter, Hudson, Place, and Watts (2015) described a 23-year-old male, with a history of daily SCB misuse, who had smoked a SCB (K2) and 6 h later appeared to exhibit generalized tonic–clonic seizures. Blood analysis revealed that the patient had ingested SCB BB-22, AM2233, PB-22, 5F-PB-22, and JWH-122.

Cannabinoids have long been considered as potential treatments for tremors associated with various CNS disorders, e.g., multiple sclerosis, Parkinson's and Huntington's disease (Arjmand et al., 2015) and this is described later. However, some studies suggest caution in the use of SCB in these diseases and in mice the synthetic CB receptor agonists CP55,940 and HU-210 evoked motor impairment (DeSanty & Dar, 2001). The phytocannabinoid nabilone increases choreatic movements in

Huntington's disease (Müller-Vahl, Schneider, & Emrich, 1999). The motor centers of the brain including the basal ganglia and the cerebellum contain very high CB_1 receptor levels and thus one might expect SCB to have a significant effect on such symptoms as tremor.

5.6 SCB Withdrawal Effects

In addition to acute toxic effects of SCB, described earlier, there are serious withdrawal effects, recently reviewed by Macfarlane and Christie (2015) in a sample of 47 New Zealanders presenting at detoxification centers. The most common withdrawal symptoms described were agitation (89% of inpatients), irritability (83%), anxiety (55%), and mood swings (55%) and these typically appeared within 1–2 h of last use but peaked on day 2 of withdrawal and remain high for at least 5 days. Other common withdrawal symptoms include nausea and vomiting (44%) and loss of appetite (17%). Elsewhere, a chronic SCB use withdrawal syndrome has also been described where symptoms include drug craving, sweating, insomnia, headache, depression, and anxiety (Nacca et al., 2013; Rominger et al., 2013; Seely et al., 2012; Vandrey, Dunn, Fry, & Girling, 2012; Zimmermann et al., 2009). There have been no longitudinal studies so long-term health risks can only be suggested.

5.7 SCB-Associated Deaths

A small number of drug-related deaths have been reported after SCB ingestion; sometimes with SCB ingested alone, or more often in combination with other drugs. There are some analytically confirmed reports. The National Program for Substance Abuse Deaths (np-SAD) reports on such deaths annually. Their most recent report (2014) reveals only about 5–6 SC-related deaths in the United Kingdom with STS-135 present in three cases (Corkery, Claridge, Loi, Goodair, & Schifano, 2014). In a US case series in 2012, three males (29, 52, and 57 years old) were found to have JWH-018 or JWH-073 postmortem (Shanks, Dahn, & Terrell, 2012). In Japan, a 59-year-old man was found to have MAM-2201 postmortem (Saito et al., 2013). In Germany, a 36-year-old male was taken to hospital suffering from seizures, but died shortly after admission. He had been smoking an SC (Mary Joy Annihilation) which was found to contain JWH-018 and JWH-210. However, blood analysis revealed JWH-018,

JWH-122, AM-2201, MAM-2201, UR-144, and amphetamine (Schaefer et al., 2013). These case studies hint at a possible susceptibility to SC-related deaths in older users.

5.8 Potential Therapeutic Use of SCB

It may not all be bad news. Cannabis preparations are reported to be analgesic, antiemetic, antiinflammatory, antineoplastic (Patil, Goyal, Sharma, Patil, & Ojha, 2015), and sedative and more recently have been associated with lower body mass index and lower incidence of diabetes (Penner, Buettner, & Mittleman, 2013). As mentioned earlier, SCB were originally developed for medicinal reasons; to increase analgesic effects seen with THC. Hill, Williams, Whalley, and Stephens (2012) have reviewed the use of THC in preclinical animal models and suggest potential use in epilepsy, neurodegenerative diseases, and affective disorders. The role of CB receptor ligands in disease and their potential therapeutic effects have recently been reviewed (Alexander, 2016; Arevalo-Martin, Molina-Holgado, & Garcia-Ovejero, 2016; Gómez-Gálvez, Palomo-Garo, Fernández-Ruiz, & García, 2016; Mursaleen & Stamford, 2016; Velasco, Hernández-Tiedra, Dávila, & Lorente, 2016) with therapeutic potential found in numerous diseases including cancer, spinal cord injury, and Parkinson's disease.

Admittedly, most of the therapeutic effects are mediated via CB_2 receptors but one should never discount the possibility of new therapeutic agents from unlikely places (Davidson & Molina-Holgado, 2016). For example, Nutt and colleagues (Danforth, Struble, Yazar-Klosinski, & Grob, 2016) are advocating MDMA for the treatment of anxiety-related disorders, while ketamine may be a fast acting antidepressant (Rasmussen, 2016). More research is needed on these SC, not only to better understand their adverse effects, but also to assess therapeutic potential, particularly in those drugs with a better activity profile at CB_2 receptors compared to CB_1 receptors. We recently wrote a speculative review where we considered which NPS might have potential therapeutic value (Davidson & Schifano, 2016). With respect to SCB such as WIN-55,212-2 and HU-210, they have been found to be neuroprotective in animal models of Parkinson's disease (More & Choi, 2015) and may be useful in Alzheimer's disease through blocking microglia activation (Ramírez, Blázquez, Gómez del Pulgar, Guzmán, & de Ceballos, 2005).

6. CONCLUSION

In this overview, we have reviewed the structure and pharmacology of SCB and highlighted the detrimental psychological effects of SCB, particularly on learning and memory and psychosis, and adverse clinical effects including on the cardiovascular system, brain, and kidneys. However, further work is required to identify the downstream targets, which may include different cellular targets, cell cycle regulatory transcription factors, or interaction with other signaling pathways. Taken together, it is clear that many SCB are extremely dangerous and a major public health problem, especially in Western societies.

Our present knowledge of SCB highlights important differences between the detrimental effects of SCB and the physiological relevance of the ECS as a neuromodulatory network with several protective actions in the human body. This is not simply related to differential activities at CB_1 and CB_2 receptors. We would advocate a ban on the recreational use of SCB but suggest that much has yet to be learned from the study of cannabinoids (including SCB), which will undoubtedly be of clinical use.

CONFLICT OF INTEREST

The authors have no conflicts of interest to declare.

REFERENCES

Adamowicz, P., & Tokarczyk, B. (2016). Simple and rapid screening procedure for 143 new psychoactive substances by liquid chromatography-tandem mass spectrometry. *Drug Testing and Analysis*, *8*(7), 652–667.

Alexander, S. P. H. (2016). Therapeutic potential of cannabis-related drugs. *Progress in Neuro-Psychopharmacology & Biological Psychiatry*, *64*, 157–166.

Alhadi, S., Tiwari, A., Vohra, R., Gerona, R., Acharya, J., & Bilello, K. (2013). High times, low SATS: Diffuse pulmonary infiltrates associated with chronic synthetic cannabinoid use. *Journal of Medical Toxicology*, *9*(2), 199–206.

Andre, C. M., Hausman, J. F., & Guerriero, G. (2016). *Cannabis sativa*: The plant of the thousand and one molecules. *Frontiers in Plant Science*, 7, 19.

Andréasson, S., Engström, A., Allebeck, P., & Rydberg, U. (1987). Cannabis and schizophrenia: A longitudinal study of Swedish conscripts. *Lancet*, *330*, 1483–1486.

Arevalo-Martin, A., Molina-Holgado, E., & Garcia-Ovejero, D. (2016). Cannabinoids to treat spinal cord injury. *Progress in Neuro-Psychopharmacology & Biological Psychiatry*, *64*, 190–199.

Arjmand, S., Vaziri, Z., Behzadi, M., Abbassian, H., Stephens, G. J., & Shabani, M. (2015). Cannabinoids and tremor induced by motor-related disorders: Friend or foe? *Neurotherapeutics*, *12*(4), 778–787.

Aryana, A., & Williams, M. A. (2007). Marijuana as a trigger of cardiovascular events: Speculation or scientific certainty? *International Journal of Cardiology*, *118*(2), 141–144.

Asimaki, O., & Mangoura, D. (2011). Cannabinoid receptor 1 induces a biphasic ERK activation via multiprotein signaling complex formation of proximal kinases PKCε, Src, and Fyn in primary neurons. *Neurochemistry International*, *58*, 135–144.

Bhanushali, G. K., Jain, G., Fatima, H., Leisch, L. J., & Thornley-Brow, D. (2013). AKI associated with synthetic cannabinoids: A case series. *Clinical Journal of the American Society of Nephrology*, *8*, 523–526.

Bohme, G. A., Laville, M., Ledent, C., Parmentier, M., & Imperato, A. (2000). Enhanced long-term potentiation in mice lacking cannabinoid CB1 receptors. *Neuroscience*, *95*, 5–7.

Buser, G., Gerona, R., Horowitz, B., Vian, K., Troxell, M., Hendrickson, R., et al. (2014). Acute kidney injury associated with smoking synthetic cannabinoid. *Clinical Toxicology (Philadelphia, Pa.)*, *52*(7), 664–673.

Buzsáki, G. (2002). Theta oscillations in the hippocampus. *Neuron*, *33*, 325–340.

Buzsáki, G., Anastassiou, C. A., & Koch, C. (2012). The origin of extracellular fields and currents EEG, ECoG, LFP and spikes. *Nature Reviews. Neuroscience*, *13*, 407–420.

Buzsáki, G., & Wang, X.-J. (2012). Mechanisms of gamma oscillations. *Annual Review of Neuroscience*, *35*, 203–225.

Calles, J. L. (2013). New drugs of abuse in the 21st century (2013). In D. E. Greydanus, G. Kaplan, D. R. Patel, & J. Merrick (Eds.), *Substance abuse in adolescents and young adults*: Berlin, Germany: De Gruyter.

Carlson, G., Wang, Y., & Alger, B. E. (2002). Endocannabinoids facilitate the induction of LTP in the hippocampus. *Nature Neuroscience*, *5*, 723–724.

Castaneto, M. S., Gorelick, D. A., Desrosiers, N. A., Hartman, R. L., Pirard, S., & Huestis, M. A. (2014). Synthetic cannabinoids: Epidemiology, pharmacodynamics, and clinical implications. *Drug and Alcohol Dependence*, *144*, 12–14.

Centers for Disease Control and Prevention. (2013). Acute kidney injury associated with synthetic cannabinoid use—Multiple states (2012). *MMWR. Morbidity and Mortality Weekly Report*, *62*, 93–98.

Chinnadurai, T., Shrestha, S., & Ayinla, R. (2016). A curious case of inhalation fever caused by synthetic cannabinoid. *The American Journal of Case Reports*, *17*, 379–383.

Cohen, K., Kapitány-Fövény, M., Mama, Y., Arieli, M., Rosca, P., Demetrovics, Z., et al. (2017). The effects of synthetic cannabinoids on executive function. *Psychopharmacology*, *234*, 1121–1134. http://dx.doi.org/10.1007/s00213-017-4546-4 [Epub ahead of print].

Cooper, Z. D. (2016). Adverse effects of synthetic cannabinoids: Management of acute toxicity and withdrawal. *Current Psychiatry Reports*, *18*(5), 52.

Corkery, J., Claridge, H., Loi, B., Goodair, C., & Schifano, F. (2014). *NPSAD annual report 2013—Drug-related deaths in the UK: January–December 2012*. Cranmer Terrace, London SW17 0RE: International Centre for Drug Policy (ICDP), St George's, University of London. ISBN: 978-1-897778-9-2.

Danforth, A. L., Struble, C. M., Yazar-Klosinski, B., & Grob, C. S. (2016). MDMA-assisted therapy: A new treatment model for social anxiety in autistic adults. *Progress in Neuro-Psychopharmacology & Biological Psychiatry*, *64*, 237–249.

Davidson, C., & Molina-Holgado, F. (2016). Drugs of abuse-its not all bad news. *Progress in Neuro-Psychopharmacology & Biological Psychiatry*, *64*, 155–156.

Davidson, C., & Schifano, F. (2016). The potential utility of some legal highs in CNS disorders. *Progress in Neuro-Psychopharmacology & Biological Psychiatry*, *64*, 267–274.

Davies, S. N., Pertwee, R. G., & Riedel, G. (2002). Functions of cannabinoid receptors in the hippocampus. *Neuropharmacology*, *42*, 993–1007.

Davis, M. I., Ronesi, J., & Lovinger, D. M. (2003). A predominant role for inhibition of the adenylate cyclase/protein kinase a pathway in ERK activation by cannabinoid receptor 1 in N1E-115 neuroblastoma cells. *The Journal of Biological Chemistry*, *278*, 48973–48980.

DeSanty, K. P., & Dar, M. S. (2001). Cannabinoid-induced motor incoordination through the cerebellar CB(1) receptor in mice. *Pharmacology, Biochemistry, and Behavior, 69*, 251–259.

Devane, W. A., Dysarz, F. A., 3rd, Johnson, M. R., Melvin, L. S., & Howlett, A. C. (1988). Determination and characterization of a cannabinoid receptor in rat brain. *Molecular Pharmacology, 34*(5), 605–613.

Di, S., Malcher-Lopes, R., Halmos, K. C., & Tasker, J. G. (2003). Nongenomic glucocorticoid inhibition via endocannabinoid release in the hypothalamus: A fast feedback mechanism. *The Journal of Neuroscience, 23*, 4850–4857.

Di Marzo, V., & Piscitelli, F. (2015). The endocannabinoid system and its modulation by Phytocannabinoids. *Neurotherapeutics, 12*(4), 692–698.

Drug Enforcement Administration. (2010). Schedules of controlled substances: Temporary placement of five synthetic cannabinoids into schedule I. *Federal Register, 75*, 71635–71638.

Dunne, S. J., & Rosengren-Holmberg, J. P. (2016). Quantification of synthetic cannabinoids in herbal smoking blends using NMR. *Drug Testing and Analysis, 9*(5), 734–743. http://dx.doi.org/10.1002/dta.2032[Epub ahead of print].

EMCDDA. (2009). *Addiction; 2009. Addiction. Understanding the 'Spice' phenomenon*. Lisbon: European Monitoring Centre for Drugs and Drug Addiction (EMCDDA).

EMCDDA. (2014). *European Drug Report 2014: Trends and developments*. Lisbon: European Monitoring Centre for Drugs and Drug Addiction (EMCDDA).

EMCDDA. (2015). *European Drug Report 2014: Trends and developments*. Lisbon: European Monitoring Centre for Drugs and Drug Addiction (EMCDDA).

Florek-Luszczki, M., Wlaz, A., Zagaja, M., Andres-Mach, M., Kondrat-Wrobel, M. W., & Luszczki, J. J. (2015). Effects of WIN 55,212-2 (a synthetic cannabinoid CB1 and CB2 receptor agonist) on the anticonvulsant activity of various novel antiepileptic drugs against 6Hz-induced psychomotor seizures in mice. *Pharmacology, Biochemistry, and Behavior, 130*, 53–58.

Ford, L. T., & Berg, J. D. (2016). 1-Adamantylamine a simple urine marker for screening for third generation adamantyl-type synthetic cannabinoids by ultra-performance liquid chromatography tandem mass spectrometry. *Annals of Clinical Biochemistry, 53*(6), 640–646.

Ford, B. M., Tai, S., Fantegrossi, W. E., & Prather, P. L. (2017). Synthetic pot: Not your Grandfather's marijuana. *Trends in Pharmacological Sciences*, 53–78.

Fries, P. (2009). Neuronal gamma-band synchronization as a fundamental process in cortical computation. *Annual Review of Neuroscience, 32*, 209–224.

Froberg, B. A., & Bauer, B. D. (2012). Pneumorachis, pneumomediastinum, and subcutaneous emphysema after synthetic cannabinoid use. *Clinical Toxicology, 50*(7), 705.

Galve-Roperh, I., Rueda, D., Gómez del Pulgar, T., Velasco, G., & Guzmán, M. (2002). Mechanism of extracellular signal-regulated kinase activation by the CB (1) cannabinoid receptor. *Molecular Pharmacology, 62*, 1385–1392.

Glass, M., & Felder, C. C. (1997). Concurrent stimulation of cannabinoid CB1 and dopamine D2 receptors augments cAMP accumulation in striatal neurons: Evidence for a Gs linkage to the CB1 receptor. *Journal of Neuroscience, 17*, 5327–5333.

Glue, P., Al-Shaqsi, S., Hancock, D., et al. (2013). Hospitalisation associated with use of the synthetic cannabinoid K2. *The New Zealand Medical Journal, 126*, 18–23.

Gomez, O., Arevalo-Martin, A., Garcia-Ovejero, D., Ortega-Gutierrez, S., Cisneros, J. A., Almazan, G., et al. (2010). The constitutive production of the endocannabinoid 2-arachidonoylglycerol participates in oligodendrocyte differentiation. *Glia, 58*, 1913–1927.

Gomez del Pulgar, T., de Ceballos, M. L., Guzman, M., & Velasco, G. (2002). Cannabinoids protect astrocytes from ceramide-induced apoptosis through the phosphatidylinositol 3-kinase/protein kinase B pathway. *Journal of Biological Chemistry*, *277*, 36527–36533.

Gomez, O., Sanchez-Rodriguez, A., Le, M. Q. U., Sanchez-Caro, C., Molina-Holgado, F., & Molina-Holgado, E. (2011). Cannabinoid receptor agonists modulate oligodendrocyte differentiation by activating PI3K/Akt and the mammalian target of rapamycin (mTOR) pathways. *British Journal of Pharmacology*, *163*, 1520–1532.

Gómez-Gálvez, Y., Palomo-Garo, C., Fernández-Ruiz, J., & García, C. (2016). Potential of the cannabinoid CB2 receptor as a pharmacological target against inflammation in Parkinson's disease. *Progress in Neuro-Psychopharmacology & Biological Psychiatry*, *64*, 200–208.

Goodman, J., & Packard, M. G. (2015). The influence of cannabinoids on learning and memory processes of the dorsal striatum. *Neurobiology of Learning and Memory*, *125*, 1–14.

Gunawardena, M. D. V. M., Rajapakse, S., Herath, J., & Amarasena, N. (2014). Myocardial infarction following cannabis induced coronary vasospasm. *BMJ Case Reports*, *2014*. pii: bcr2014207020.

Gunderson, E. W., Haughey, H. M., Ait-Daoud, N., Joshi, A. S., & Hart, C. L. (2012). "Spice" and "K2" herbal highs: A case series and systematic review of the clinical effects and biopsychosocial implications of synthetic cannabinoid use in humans. *The American Journal on Addictions*, *21*, 320–326.

Hajós, M., Hoffmann, W. E., & Kocsis, B. (2008). Activation of cannabinoid-1 receptors disrupts sensory gating and neuronal oscillation: Relevance to schizophrenia. *Biological Psychiatry*, *63*, 1075–1083.

Harris, C. R., & Brown, A. (2013). Synthetic cannabinoid intoxication: A case series and review. *The Journal of Emergency Medicine*, *44*(2), 360–366.

Heath, T. S., Burroughs, Z., Thompson, A. J., & Tecklenburg, F. W. (2012). Acute intoxication caused by a synthetic cannabinoid in two adolescents. *Journal of Pediatric Pharmacology and Therapeutics*, *17*(2), 177–181.

Hebert-Chatelain, E., Desprez, T., Serrat, R., Bellocchio, L., Soria-Gomez, E., Busquets-Garcia, A., et al. (2016). A cannabinoid link between mitochondria and memory. *Nature*, *539*(7630), 555–559.

Heifets, B. D., & Castillo, P. E. (2009). Endocannabinoid signaling and long-term synaptic plasticity. *Annual Review of Physiology*, *71*, 283–306.

Herkenham, M., Lynn, A. B., Johnson, M. R., Melvin, L. S., de Costa, B. R., & Rice, K. C. (1991). Characterization and localization of cannabinoid receptors in rat brain: A quantitative in vitro autoradiographic study. *The Journal of Neuroscience*, *11*, 563–583.

Hermanns-Clausen, M., Kneisel, S., Szabo, B., & Auwarter, V. (2013). Acute toxicity due to the confirmed consumption of synthetic cannabinoids: Clinical and laboratory findings. *Addiction*, *108*(3), 534–544.

Hill, A. J., Williams, C. M., Whalley, B. J., & Stephens, G. J. (2012). Phytocannabinoids as novel therapeutic agents in CNS disorders. *Pharmacology & Therapeutics*, *133*, 79–97.

Howlett, A. C., Johnson, M. R., Melvin, L. S., & Milne, G. M. (1988). Nonclassical cannabinoid analgetics inhibit adenylate cyclase: Development of a cannabinoid receptor model. *Molecular Pharmacology*, *33*, 297–302.

Hoyte, C. O., Jacob, J., Monte, A. A., Al-Jumaan, M., Bronstein, A. C., & Heard, K. J. (2012). A Characterization of synthetic cannabinoid exposures reported to the national poison data system in 2010. *Annals of Emergency Medicine*, *60*(4), 435–438.

Hudson, S., & Ramsey, J. (2011). The emergence and analysis of synthetic cannabinoids. *Drug Testing and Analysis*, *3*(7–8), 466–478. http://dx.doi.org/10.1002/dta.268.

Huffman, J. W., Dai, D., Martin, B. R., & Compton, D. R. (1994). Design, synthesis and pharmacology of cannabimimetic indoles. *Bioorganic & Medicinal Chemistry Letters*, *4*, 563–566.

Huffman, J. W., & Padgett, L. W. (2005). Recent developments in the medicinal chemistry of cannabimimetic indoles, pyrroles and indenes. *Current Medicinal Chemistry*, *12*(12), 1395–1411.

Ibrahim, S., Al-Saffar, F., & Wannenburg, T. (2014). A unique case of cardiac arrest following K2 abuse. *Case Reports in Cardiology*, *2014*, 120607.

Izzo, A. A., Borrelli, F., Capasso, R., Di Marzo, V., & Mechoulam, R. (2009). Non-psychotropic plant cannabinoids: New therapeutic opportunities from an ancient herb. *Trends in Pharmacological Sciences*, *30*(10), 515–527.

Kano, M., Ohno-Shosaku, T., Hashimotodani, Y., Uchigashima, M., & Watanabe, M. (2009). Endocannabinoid-mediated control of synaptic transmission. *Physiological Reviews*, *89*, 309–380.

Katona, I., & Freund, T. F. (2012). Multiple functions of endocannabinoid signaling in the brain. *Annual Review of Neuroscience*, *35*, 529–558.

Khan, M., Pace, L., Truong, A., Gordon, M., & Moukaddam, N. (2016). Catatonia secondary to synthetic cannabinoid use in two patients with no previous psychosis. *The American Journal on Addictions/American Academy of Psychiatrists in Alcoholism and Addictions*, *25*(1), 25–27.

Lapoint, J., James, L. P., Moran, C. L., Nelson, L. S., Hoffman, R. S., & Moran, J. H. (2011). Severe toxicity following synthetic cannabinoid ingestion. *Clinical Toxicology (Philadelphia, Pa.)*, *49*, 760–764.

Lauckner, J. E., Hille, B., & Mackie, K. (2005). The cannabinoid agonist WIN55,212-2 increases intracellular calcium via CB1 receptor coupling to Gq/11 G proteins. *Proceedings of the National Academy of Sciences of the United States of America*, *102*, 19144–19149.

Ligresti, A., De Petrocellis, L., & Di Marzo, V. (2016). From Phytocannabinoids to cannabinoid receptors and endocannabinoids: Pleiotropic physiological and pathological roles through complex pharmacology. *Physiological Reviews*, *96*(4), 1593–1659.

Lobo Vicente, J., Chassaigne, H., Holland, M. V., Reniero, F., Kolář, K., Tirendi, S., et al. (2016). Systematic analytical characterization of new psychoactive substances: A case study. *Forensic Science International*, *265*, 107–115.

Luszczki, J. J., Wlaz, A., Karwan, S., Florek-Luszczki, M., & Czuczwar, S. J. (2013). Effects of WIN 55,212-2 mesylate on the anticonvulsant action of lamotrigine, oxcarbazepine, pregabalin and topiramate against maximal electroshock-induced seizures in mice. *European Journal of Pharmacology*, *720*(1–3), 247–254.

Luszczki, J. J., et al. (2011). Synthetic cannabinoid WIN 55,212-2 mesylate enhances the protective action of four classical antiepileptic drugs against maximal electroshock-induced seizures in mice. *Pharmacology, Biochemistry, and Behavior*, *98*, 261–267.

Macfarlane, V., & Christie, G. (2015). Synthetic cannabinoid withdrawal: A new demand on detoxification services. *Drug and Alcohol Review*, *34*(2), 147–153.

Mackie, K. (2008). Cannabinoid receptors: Where they are and what they do. *Journal of Neuroendocrinology*, *20*(Suppl. 1), 10–14.

Marsicano, G., Wotjak, C. T., Azad, S. C., Bisogno, T., Rammes, G., Cascio, M. G., et al. (2002). The endogenous cannabinoid system controls extinction of aversive memories. *Nature*, *418*, 530–534.

Martin, M., Ledent, C., Parmentier, M., Maldonado, R., & Valverde, O. (2002). Involvement of CB1 cannabinoid receptors in emotional behaviour. *Psychopharmacology*, *159*, 379–387.

Matsuda, L. A., Lolait, S. J., Brownstein, M. J., Young, A. C., & Bonner, T. I. (1990). Structure of a cannabinoid receptor and functional expression of the cloned cDNA. *Nature*, *346*(6284), 561–564.

McIlroy, G., Ford, L., & Khan, J. M. (2016). Acute myocardial infarction, associated with the use of a synthetic adamantyl-cannabinoid: A case report. *BMC Pharmacology & Toxicology*, *17*, 2.

McKeever, R. G., Vearrier, D., Jacobs, D., LaSala, G., Okaneku, J., & Greenberg, M. I. (2015). K2—Not the spice of life; Synthetic cannabinoids and ST elevation myocardial infarction: A case report. *Journal of Medical Toxicology*, *11*(1), 129–131.

McQuade, D., Hudson, S., Dargan, P. I., et al. (2013). First European case of convulsions related to analytically confirmed use of the synthetic cannabinoid receptor agonist AM-2201. *European Journal of Clinical Pharmacology*, *69*, 373–376.

Mechoulam, R., & Hanus, L. (2000). A historical overview of chemical research on cannabinoids. *Chemistry and Physics of Lipids*, *108*(1–2), 1–13.

Minzenberg, M. J., Firl, A. J., Yoon, J. H., Gomes, G. C., Reinking, C., & Carter, C. S. (2010). Gamma oscillatory power is impaired during cognitive control independent of medication status in first-episode schizophrenia. *Neuropsychopharmacology*, *35*, 2590–2599.

Mir, A., Obafemi, A., Young, A., & Kane, C. (2011). Myocardial infarction associated with use of the synthetic cannabinoid K2. *Pediatrics*, *128*(6), e1622–e1627.

Mittleman, M. A., Lewis, R. A., Maclure, M., Sherwood, J. B., & Muller, J. E. (2001). Triggering myocardial infarction by marijuana. *Circulation*, *103*(23), 2805–2809.

More, S. V., & Choi, D.-K. (2015). Promising cannabinoid-based therapies for Parkinson's disease: Motor symptoms to neuroprotection. *Molecular Neurodegeneration*, *10*, 17.

Müller-Vahl, K. R., Schneider, U., & Emrich, H. M. (1999). Nabilone increases choreatic movements in Huntington's disease. *Movement Disorders*, *14*(6), 1038–1040.

Munro, S., Thomas, K. L., & Abu-Shaar, M. (1993). Molecular characterization of a peripheral receptor for cannabinoids. *Nature*, *365*(6441), 61–65.

Mursaleen, L. R., & Stamford, J. A. (2016). Drugs of abuse and Parkinson's disease. *Progress in Neuro-Psychopharmacology & Biological Psychiatry*, *64*, 209–217.

Nacca, N., Vatti, D., Sullivan, R., Sud, P., Su, M., & Marraffa, J. (2013). The synthetic cannabinoid withdrawal syndrome. *Journal of Addiction Medicine*, 7, 296–298.

Navarrete, M., & Araque, A. (2008). Endocannabinoids mediate neuron–astrocyte communication. *Neuron*, *57*, 883–893.

Navarrete, M., Díez, A., & Araque, A. (2014). Astrocytes in endocannabinoid signalling. *Philosophical Transactions of the Royal Society of London. Series B, Biological Sciences*, *369*, 20130599.

Nogueras-Ortiz, C., & Yudowski, G. A. (2016). Multiple waves of cannabinoid 1 receptor signaling. *Molecular Pharmaceutics*, *90*, 620–626.

Pacher, P., & Kunos, G. (2013). Modulating the endocannabinoid system in human health and disease—Successes and failures. *The FEBS Journal*, *280*(9), 1918–1943.

Papanti, D., Schifano, F., Botteon, G., Bertossi, F., Mannix, J., Vidoni, D., et al. (2013). Spiceophrenia: A systematic overview of 'Spice'-related psychopathological issues and a case report. *Human Psychopharmacology: Clinical and Experimental*, *28*, 379–389.

Patil, K. R., Goyal, S. N., Sharma, C., Patil, C. R., & Ojha, S. (2015). Phytocannabinoids for cancer therapeutics: Recent updates and future prospects. *Current Medicinal Chemistry*, *22*(30), 3472–3501.

Penner, E. A., Buettner, H., & Mittleman, M. M. (2013). The impact of marijuana use on glucose, insulin, and insulin resistance among US adults. *The American Journal of Medicine*, *126*, 583–589.

Pertwee, R. G., Howlett, A. C., Abood, M. E., Alexander, S. P., Di Marzo, V., Elphick, M. R., et al. (2010). International union of basic and clinical pharmacology. LXXIX. Cannabinoid receptors and their ligands: Beyond CB(1) and CB(2). *Pharmacological Reviews*, *62*(4), 588–631.

Piomelli, D. (2003). The molecular logic of endocannabinoid signalling. *Nature Reviews Neuroscience*, *4*, 873–884.

Presley, B. C., Gurney, S. M., Scott, K. S., Kacinko, S. L., & Logan, B. K. (2016). Metabolism and toxicological analysis of synthetic cannabinoids in biological fluids and tissues. *Forensic Science Review*, *28*(2), 103–169.

Puighermanal, E., Busquets-Garcia, A., Maldonado, R., & Ozaita, A. (2012). Cellular and intracellular mechanisms involved in the cognitive impairment of cannabinoids. *Philosophical Transactions of the Royal Society of London. Series B, Biological Sciences*, *367*, 3254–3263.

Ramírez, B. G., Blázquez, C., Gómez del Pulgar, T., Guzmán, M., & de Ceballos, M. L. (2005). Prevention of Alzheimer's disease pathology by cannabinoids: Neuroprotection mediated by blockade of microglial activation. *The Journal of Neuroscience*, *25*(8), 1904–1913.

Rasmussen, K. G. (2016). Has psychiatry tamed the "ketamine tiger?" Considerations on its use for depression and anxiety. *Progress in Neuro-Psychopharmacology & Biological Psychiatry*, *64*, 218–224.

Reddy, D. S., & Golub, V. M. (2016). The pharmacological basis of cannabis therapy for epilepsy. *The Journal of Pharmacology and Experimental Therapeutics*, *357*(1), 45–55.

Rominger, A., Cumming, P., Xiong, G., Koller, G., Förster, S., Zwergal, A., et al. (2013). Effects of acute detoxification of the herbal blend 'Spice Gold' on dopamine D2/3 receptor availability: A [18F]fallypride PET study. *European Neuropsychopharmacology: The Journal of the European College of Neuropsychopharmacology*, *23*, 1606–1610.

Rosenbaum, C. D., Carreiro, S. P., & Babu, K. M. (2012). Here today, gonetomorrow…and back again? A review of herbal marijuana alternatives (K2, Spice), synthetic cathinones (bath salts), kratom, *Salvia divinorum*, methoxetamine, and piperazines. *Journal of Medical Toxicology: Official Journal of the American College of Medical Toxicology*, *8*(1), 15–32.

Rosenberg, E. C., Tsien, R. W., Whalley, B. J., & Devinsky, O. (2015). Cannabinoids and epilepsy. *Neurotherapeutics*, *12*(4), 747–768.

Rozenfeld, R., & Devi, L. A. (2008). Regulation of CB1 cannabinoid receptor trafficking by the adaptor protein AP-3. *FASEB Journal*, *22*, 2311–2322.

Sahai, M. A., Davidson, C., Khelashvili, G., Barrese, V., Dutta, N., Weinstein, H., et al. (2016). Combined in vitro and in silico approaches to the assessment of stimulant properties of novel psychoactive substances—The case of the benzofuran 5-MAPB. *Progress in Neuro-Psychopharmacology & Biological Psychiatry*, *75*, 1–9.

Saito, T., Namera, A., Miura, N., Ohta, S., Shota Miyazaki, S., Osawa, M., et al. (2013). A fatal case of MAM-2201 poisoning. *Forensic Toxicology*, *31*(2), 333–337.

Schaefer, N., Peters, B., Bregel, D., Kneisel, S., Auwa¨ rter, V., Schmidt, P. H., & Ewald, A. H. (2013). A fatal case involving several synthetic cannabinoids. *Toxichem Krimtech*, *80*(Special Issue), 248–251.

Schep, L., Slaughter, R., Hudson, S., Place, R., & Watts, M. (2015). Delayed seizure-like activity following analytically confirmed use of previously unreported synthetic cannabinoid analogues. *Human & Experimental Toxicology*, *34*(5), 557–560.

Schifano, F., Orsolini, L., Duccio Papanti, G., & Corkery, J. M. (2015). Psychoactive substances of interest for psychiatry. *World Psychiatry*, *14*(1), 15–26.

Schneir, A., & Baumbacher, T. (2012). Convulsions associated with theuse of a synthetic cannabinoid product. *Journal of Medical Toxicology*, *8*, 62–64.

Schneir, A. B., Cullen, J., & Ly, B. T. (2011). Spice girls: Synthetic cannabinoid intoxication. *The Journal of Emergency Medicine*, *40*(3), 296–299.

Scocard, A., Benyamina, A., Coscas, S., & Karila, L. (2017). Synthetic cannabinoids: A new addiction matrix. *Presse Médicale*, *46*(1), 11–22. http://dx.doi.org/10.1016/j.lpm.2016.11.014.

Seely, K. A., Lapoint, J., Moran, J. H., & Fattore, L. (2012). Spice drugs are more than harmless herbal blends: A review of the pharmacology and toxicology of synthetic cannabinoids. *Progress in Neuro-Psychopharmacology & Biological Psychiatry*, *39*(2), 234–243.

Seely, K. A., Prather, P. L., James, L. P., & Moran, J. H. (2011). Marijuan-based drugs: Innovative therapeutics or designer drugs of abuse? Mol. *Intervirology*, *11*(1), 36–51.

Shanks, K. G., Dahn, T., & Terrell, A. R. (2012). Detection of JWH-018 and JWH-073 by UPLC–MS-MS in postmortem whole blood casework. *Journal of Analytical Toxicology*, *36*(3), 145–152.

Silva de Melo, L. C., Cruz, A. P., Rios Valentim, S. J., Jr., Marinho, A. R., Mendonca, J. B., & Nakamura-Palacios, E. M. (2005). Δ9-THC administered into the medial prefrontal cortex disrupts the spatial working memory. *Psychopharmacology*, *183*, 54–64.

Simmons, J., Cookman, L., Kang, C., & Skinner, C. (2011). Three cases of "spice" exposure. *Clinical Toxicology (Philadelphia, Pa.)*, *49*, 431–433.

Skosnik, P. D., Cortes-Briones, J. A., & Hajós, M. (2016). It's all in the rhythm: The role of cannabinoids in neural oscillations and psychosis. *Biological Psychiatry*, *79*, 568–577.

Spaderna, M., Addy, P. H., & D'Souza, D. C. (2013). Spicing things up: Synthetic cannabinoids. *Psychopharmacology*, *228*(4), 525–540.

Strano-Rossi, S., Anzillotti, L., Dragoni, S., Pellegrino, R. M., Goracci, L., Pascali, V. L., et al. (2014). Metabolism of JWH-015, JWH-098, JWH-251, and JWH-307 in silico and in vitro: A pilot study for the detection of unknown synthetic cannabinoids metabolites. *Analytical and Bioanalytical Chemistry*, *406*(15), 3621–3636.

Svízenská, I., Dubový, P., & Sulcová, A. (2008). Cannabinoid receptors 1 and 2 (CB1 and CB2), their distribution, ligands and functional involvement in nervous system structures—A short review. *Pharmacology, Biochemistry, and Behavior*, *90*, 501–511.

Tatli, E., Yilmaztepe, M., Altun, G., & Altun, A. (2007). Cannabis-induced coronary arterythrombosis and acute anterior myocardial infarction in a young man. *International Journal of Cardiology*, *120*(3), 420–422.

Thomas, S., Bliss, S., & Malik, M. (2012). Suicidal ideation and self-harm following K2 use. *The Journal of the Oklahoma State Medical Association*, *105*, 430–433.

Thomas, G., Kloner, R. A., & Rezkalla, S. (2014). Adverse cardiovascular, cerebrovascular, and peripheral vascular effects of marijuana inhalation: What cardiologists need to know. *The American Journal of Cardiology*, *113*(1), 187–190.

Trazzi, S., Steger, M., Mitrugno, V. M., Bartesaghi, R., & Ciani, E. (2010). CB1 cannabinoid receptors increase neuronal precursor proliferation through AKT/glycogen synthase kinase-3beta/beta-catenin signaling. *The Journal of Biological Chemistry*, *285*, 10098–10109.

Tse, R., Kodur, S., Squires, B., & Collins, N. (2014). Sudden cardiac death complicating acute myocardial infarction following synthetic cannabinoid use. *Internal Medicine Journal*, *44*(9), 934–936.

Vallersnes, O. M., Dines, A. M., Wood, D. M., Yates, C., Heyerdahl, F., Hovda, K. E., et al. (2016). Psychosis associated with acute recreational drug toxicity: A European case series. *BMC Psychiatry*, *16*, 293.

Vandrey, R., Dunn, K. E., Fry, J. A., & Girling, E. R. (2012). A survey study to characterize use of spice products (synthetic cannabinoids). *Drug and Alcohol Dependence*, *120*(1–3), 238–241.

Velasco, G., Hernández-Tiedra, S., Dávila, D., & Lorente, M. (2016). The use of cannabinoids as anticancer agents. *Progress in Neuro-Psychopharmacology & Biological Psychiatry*, *64*, 259–266.

Vemuri, V. K., & Makriyannis, A. (2015). Medicinal chemistry of cannabinoids. *Clinical Pharmacology and Therapeutics*, *97*(6), 553–558.

Verrotti, A., Castagnino, M., Maccarrone, M., & Fezza, F. (2016). Plant-derived and endogenous cannabinoids in epilepsy. *Clinical Drug Investigation*, *36*(5), 331–340.

Winstock, A. R., & Barratt, M. J. (2013). The 12-month prevalence and nature of adverse experiences resulting in emergency medical presentations associated with the use of synthetic cannabinoid products. *Human Psychopharmacology: Clinical and Experimental*, *28*, 390–393.

Wise, L. E., Thorpe, A. J., Lichtman, A. H. (2009). Hippocampal CB1 receptors mediate the memory impairing effects of Δ9-tetrahydrocannabinol. Neuropsychopharmacology 34: 2072–2080.

Zanettini, C., Panlilio, L. V., Alicki, M., Goldberg, S. R., Haller, J., & Yasar, S. (2011). Effects of endocannabinoid system modulation on cognitive and emotional behavior. *Frontiers in Behavioral Neuroscience*, *5*, 57. http://dx.doi.org/10.3389/fnbeh.2011.00057.

Zawilska, J. B., & Wojcieszak, J. (2014). Spice/K2 drugs—More than innocent substitutes for marijuana. *International Journal of Neuropsychopharmacology*, *17*(3), 509–525.

Zimmermann, U. S., Winkelmann, P. R., Pilhatsch, M., Nees, J. A., Spanagel, R., & Schulz, K. (2009). Withdrawal phenomena and dependence syndrome after the consumption of 'spice gold. *Deutsches Ärzteblatt International*, *106*, 464–467.

FURTHER READING

Abouchedid, R., Ho, J., Hudson, S., Dines, A., Archer, J., Wood, D., et al. (2016). Acute toxicity associated with use of 5F-derivations of synthetic cannabinoid receptor agonists with analytical confirmation. *Journal of Medical Toxicology: Official Journal of the American College of Medical Toxicology*, *12*, 396–401.

Adamowicz, P., & Gieroń, J. (2016). Acute intoxication of four individuals following use of the synthetic cannabinoid MAB-CHMINACA. *Clinical Toxicology (Philadelphia, Pa.)*, *54*(8), 650–654.

Ai, R., & Chang, C. A. (2012). Ligand-specific homology modeling of human cannabinoid (CB1) receptor. *Journal of Molecular Graphics & Modelling*, *38*, 155–164.

Assi, S., Fergus, S., Stair, J., Corazza, O., & Schifano, F. (2011). Emergence and identification of new designer drug products from the internet. *European Pharmaceutical Review*, *16*(4), 68–72.

Blevins, C., Banes, K., Stephens, R., Walker, D., & Roffman, R. (2016). A preliminary evaluation of synthetic cannabinoid use among adolescent cannabis users: Characteristics and treatment outcomes. *Addictive Behaviors*, *63*, 114–119.

Bramblett, R. D., Panu, A. M., Ballesteros, J. A., & Reggio, P. H. (1995). Construction of a 3D model of the cannabinoid CB1 receptor: Determination of helix ends and helix orientation. *Life Sciences*, *56*, 1971–1982.

De Luca, M. A., Castelli, M. P., Loi, B., Porcu, A., Martorelli, M., Miliano, C., et al. (2016). Native CB1 receptor affinity, intrisic activity and accumbens shell dopamine stimulant properties of third generation SPICE/K2 cannabinoids: BB-22, 5F-PB-22, 5F-AKB-48 and STS-135. *Neuropharmacology*, *105*, 630–638.

Dillon, P., & Copeland, J. (2012). Synthetic cannabinoids: The Australian experience. *NCPIC Bulletin Series*, *13*, 1–10.

Feng, Z., Alqarni, M. H., Yang, P., Tong, Q., Chowdhury, A., Wang, L., et al. (2014). Modeling, molecular dynamics simulation, and mutation validation for structure of cannabinoid receptor 2 based on known crystal structures of GPCRs. *Journal of Chemical Information and Modeling*, *54*, 2483–2499.

Freeman, W. D., Jacksonville, F. L., & Louh, I. K. (2014). Ischemic stroke after use of the synthetic marijuana 'spice'. *Neurology*, *81*, 2090–2093.

Freeman, M. J., Rose, D. Z., Myers, M. A., Gooch, C. L., Bozeman, A. C., & Burgin, W. S. (2013). Ischemic stroke after use of the synthetic marijuana 'spice'. *Neurology*, *81*(24), 2090–2093.

Gugelmann, H., Gerona, R., Li, C., Tsutaoka, B., Olson, K., & Lung, D. (2014). 'Crazy Monkey' poisons man and dog: Human and canine seizures due to PB-22, a novel synthetic cannabinoid. *Clinical Toxicology (Philadelphia, Pa.)*, *52*(6), 635–638.

Heltsley, R., Shelby, M. K., Crouch, D. J., Black, D. L., Robert, T. A., Marshall, L., et al. (2012). Prevalence of synthetic cannabinoids in US athletes: Initial findings. *Journal of Analytical Toxicology*, *36*(8), 588–593.

Hill, S., Najafi, J., Dunn, M., Acheampong, P., Kamour, A., Grundlingh, J., et al. (2016). Clinical toxicity following analytically confirmed use of the synthetic cannabinoid receptor agonist MDMB-CHMICA. A report from the Identification of Novel psychoActive substances (IONA) study. *Clinical Toxicology (Philadelphia, Pa.)*, *54*(8), 638–643.

Hua, T., Vemuri, K., Pu, M., Qu, L., Han, G. W., Wu, Y., et al. (2016). Crystal structure of the human cannabinoid receptor CB1. *Cell*, *167*, 750–762.

Hurst, D. P., Grossfield, A., Lynch, D. L., Feller, S., Romo, T. D., Gawrisch, K., et al. (2010). A lipid pathway for ligand binding is necessary for a cannabinoid G protein-coupled receptor. *The Journal of Biological Chemistry*, *285*, 17954–17964.

Hurst, D. P., Schmeisser, M., & Reggio, P. H. (2013). Endogenous lipid activated G protein-coupled receptors: Emerging structural features from crystallography and molecular dynamics simulations. *Chemistry and Physics of Lipids*, *169*, 46–56.

Keyes, K., Rutherford, C., Hamilton, A., & Palamar, J. (2016). Age, period, and cohort effects in synthetic cannabinoid use among US adolescents, 2011-2015. *Drug and Alcohol Dependence*, *166*, 159–167.

Kronstrand, R., Roman, M., Andersson, M., & Eklund, A. (2013). Toxicological findings of synthetic cannabinoids in recreational users. *Journal of Analytical Toxicology*, *37*(8), 534–541.

Lynch, D. L., & Reggio, P. H. (2005). Molecular dynamics simulations of the endocannabinoid N- arachidonoylethanolamine (anandamide) in a phospholipid bilayer: Probing structure and dynamics. *Journal of Medicinal Chemistry*, *48*, 4824–4833.

Maccarrone, M., Guzman, M., Mackie, K., Doherty, P., & Harkany, T. (2014). Programming of neural cells by (endo)cannabinoids: From physiological rules to emerging therapies. *Nature Reviews. Neuroscience*, *15*(12), 786–801.

McAllister, S. D., Tao, Q., Barnett-Norris, J., Buehner, K., Hurst, D. P., Guarnieri, F., et al. (2002). A critical role for a tyrosine residue in the cannabinoid receptors for ligand recognition. *Biochemical Pharmacology*, *63*, 2121–2136.

Morales, P., Hurst, D. P., & Reggio, P. H. (2017). Molecular targets of the Phytocannabinoids: A complex picture. *Progress in the Chemistry of Organic Natural Products*, *103*, 103–131.

Munk, C., Isberg, V., Mordalski, S., Harpsoe, K., Rataj, K., Hauser, A. S., et al. (2016). GPCRdb: The G protein-coupled receptor database—An introduction. *British Journal of Pharmacology*, *173*, 2195–2207.

Reggio, P. H. (2010). Endocannabinoid binding to the cannabinoid receptors: What is known and what remains unknown. *Current Medicinal Chemistry*, *17*, 1468–1486.

Shanks, K., & Behonick, G. (2016). Death after use of the synthetic cannabinoid 5F-AMB. *Forensic Science International*, *262*, e21–e24.

Shim, J. Y., Khurana, L., & Kendall, D. A. (2016). Computational analysis of the CB1 carboxyl-terminus in the receptor-G protein complex. *Proteins, Structure, Function, and Bioinformatics*, *84*, 532–543.

Shore, D. M., Baillie, G. L., Hurst, D. H., Navas, F., Seltzman, H. H., Marcu, J. P., et al. (2014). Allosteric modulation of a cannabinoid G protein-coupled receptor: Binding site elucidation and relationship to G protein signaling. *The Journal of Biological Chemistry*, *289*, 5828–5845.

Sirikantaramas, S., Taura, F., Morimoto, S., & Shoyama, Y. (2007). Recent advances in *Cannabis sativa* research: Biosynthetic studies and its potential in biotechnology. *Current Pharmaceutical Biotechnology*, *8*(4), 237–243.

Song, Z. H., Slowey, C. A., Hurst, D. P., & Reggio, P. H. (1999). The difference between the CB(1) and CB(2) cannabinoid receptors at position 5.46 is crucial for the selectivity of WIN55212-2 for CB(2). *Molecular Pharmacology*, *56*, 834–840.

Tuccinardi, T., Ferrarini, P. L., Manera, C., Ortore, G., Saccomanni, G., & Martinelli, A. (2006). Cannabinoid CB2/CB1 selectivity. Receptor modeling and automated docking analysis. *Journal of Medicinal Chemistry*, *49*, 984–994.

Ulfers, A. L., McMurry, J. L., Kendall, D. A., & Mierke, D. F. (2002). Structure of the third intracellular loop of the human cannabinoid 1 receptor. *Biochemistry*, *41*, 11344–11350.

Vroling, B., Sanders, M., Baakman, C., Borrmann, A., Verhoeven, S., Klomp, J., et al. (2011). GPCRDB: An information system for G protein-coupled receptors. *Nucleic Acids Research*, *39*, D309–D319.

Walker, D., Neighbors, C., Walton, T., Pierce, A., Mbilinyi, L., Kaysen, D., et al. (2014). Spicing up the military: Use and effects of synthetic cannabis in substance abusing army personnel. *Addictive Behaviors*, *39*(7), 1139–1144.

CHAPTER FIVE

CB_1 and CB_2 Receptor Pharmacology

Allyn C. Howlett*, **Mary E. Abood**[†,1]
*Center for Research on Substance Use and Addiction, Wake Forest University Health Sciences, Winston-Salem, NC, United States
[†]Center for Substance Abuse Research, Lewis Katz School of Medicine at Temple University, Philadelphia, PA, United States
[1]Corresponding author: e-mail address: mabood@temple.edu

Contents

Abstract

The CB_1 and CB_2 cannabinoid receptors (CB_1R, CB_2R) are members of the G protein-coupled receptor (GPCR) family that were identified over 20 years ago. CB_1Rs and CB_2Rs mediate the effects of Δ^9-tetrahydrocannabinol (Δ^9-THC), the principal psychoactive constituent of marijuana, and subsequently identified endogenous cannabinoids (endocannabinoids) anandamide and 2-arachidonoyl glycerol. CB_1Rs and CB_2Rs have both similarities and differences in their pharmacology. Both receptors recognize multiple classes of agonist and antagonist compounds and produce an array of distinct downstream effects. Natural polymorphisms and alternative splice variants may also contribute to their pharmacological diversity. As our knowledge of the distinct

Advances in Pharmacology, Volume 80
ISSN 1054-3589
http://dx.doi.org/10.1016/bs.apha.2017.03.007

differences grows, we may be able to target select receptor conformations and their corresponding pharmacological responses. This chapter will discuss their pharmacological characterization, distribution, phylogeny, and signaling pathways. In addition, the effects of extended agonist exposure and how that affects signaling and expression patterns of the receptors are considered.

ABBREVIATIONS

ACEA arachidonyl-2-chloroethanolamide
AMPK AMP-activated protein kinase
AP-1 activating protein 1
CREBH cAMP-responsive element-binding protein H
ER endoplasmic reticulum
ERK extracellular signal-regulated kinase
FAK focal adhesion kinase
FAS fatty acid synthase
GAP GTPase-activating protein
GPCR G protein-coupled receptor
GRK G protein receptor kinase
IRS1 insulin receptor substrate 1
LXRα liver X receptor-α
MAPK mitogen-activated protein kinase
MTfam mtDNA transcription factor A
NOS nitric oxide synthase
NRF-1 nuclear respiratory factor-1
PGC-1α PPARγ-coactivator-1α
Phlpp1 *PH* domain leucine-rich repeat protein phosphatase-1
PI3K phosphatidylinositol-3-kinase
PPAR peroxisome proliferator-activated receptor
SRE sterol response element
SREBP-1c sterol regulatory element-binding protein 1c
Δ^9-THC delta9-tetrahydrocannabinol

1. INTRODUCTION

The CB_1 cannabinoid receptor was discovered (Devane, Dysarz, Johnson, Melvin, & Howlett, 1988) and subsequently cloned (Matsuda, Lolait, Brownstein, Young, & Bonner, 1990) on the basis of its responsiveness to (−)-Δ^9-tetrahydrocannabinol (Δ^9-THC). Δ^9-THC is the primary psychoactive constituent in *Cannabis* (a.k.a. marijuana), hence the name "cannabinoid" receptor. CB_1 is a member of the G protein-coupled receptor

(GPCR) family. An arachidonic acid metabolite, *N*-arachidonylethanolamide, was shown to activate CB_1, and named "anandamide" from the Sanskrit word for "bliss" (Devane et al., 1992), and this was followed by the identification of a second metabolite 2-arachidonoylglycerol (2-AG) (Mechoulam et al., 1995; Sugiura et al., 1995). The identification of endogenous ligands and the availability of novel ligands with cannabinoid receptor activity led to subsequent breakthroughs, elucidating an "endocannabinoid system" (Di Marzo, Melck, Bisogno, & De Petrocellis, 1998). A second cannabinoid receptor (CB_2) was isolated by a PCR-based strategy designed to isolate GPCRs in differentiated myeloid cells (Munro, Thomas, & Abu-Shaar, 1993). The CB_2 receptor shares 44% amino acid homology with CB_1, and a distinct yet similar binding profile, thus representing a receptor subtype. The most current nomenclature for cannabinoid receptors has been reported by a subcommittee of the International Union of Basic and Clinical Pharmacology (IUPHAR) (Pertwee et al., 2010).

2. PHARMACOLOGICAL CHARACTERIZATION

A range of pharmacological and genetic tools have been developed and used to delineate "cannabinoid receptor"-mediated activity. Five structurally distinct classes of cannabinoid compounds have been identified: the classical cannabinoids (e.g., Δ^9-THC, Δ^8-THC-dimethylheptyl (HU210)); bicyclic cannabinoids (e.g., CP-55,940); indole-derived cannabinoids (e.g., WIN55,212); eicosanoids (e.g., the endogenous ligands, such as anandamide, 2-arachidonylglycerol); and antagonist/inverse agonists (e.g., SR141716A for CB_1, SR145528 for CB_2) (Devane et al., 1992; Eissenstat et al., 1995; Howlett, 1995; Mechoulam & Fride, 1995; Rinaldi-Carmona et al., 1994; Rinaldi-Carmona et al., 1998; Xie, Melvin, & Makriyannis, 1996). While many of the agonists show little selectivity between the CB_1 and CB_2 receptors, the antagonist compounds are highly selective (>1000-fold selective for CB_1 vs CB_2 and vice versa with nanomolar affinity at the relevant receptor). The selectivity of these antagonists allows the discrimination of CB_1- vs CB_2-mediated effects *in vitro* and *in vivo*. There are some very selective CB_1 and CB_2 agonists. One example is arachidonyl-2′-chloroethylamide (ACEA) (Kearn, Greenberg, DiCamelli, Kurzawa, & Hillard, 1999), which is highly selective for CB_1 (nanomolar affinity at CB_1 and >1000-fold selectivity for CB_1 vs CB_2). HU-308, a Δ^9-THC analog, is a highly selective CB_2 agonist with nanomolar affinity at CB_2 and >1000-fold selectivity for CB_2 vs CB_1 (Hanus et al., 1999). Several other compounds show >100-fold selectivity and are generally classified as selective agonists. However, these compounds are used at micromolar concentrations *in vitro*, and therefore may be acting at both receptors (see Pertwee et al., 2010 for more examples). Thus, additional controls should be performed to ensure the site of action of these compounds.

3. NATURAL POLYMORPHISMS AND ALTERNATIVE SPLICE VARIANTS

Natural polymorphisms have been identified in both the CB_1 and CB_2 receptors. In addition, alternative splice variants have been identified for both receptors. This literature is summarized below.

The CB_1 receptor gene (CNR1) is located on human chromosome 6q14-15 (Bonner, 1996). Several human CB_1 receptor polymorphisms have been identified. The initial polymorphism found was a restriction fragment length polymorphism in the intron preceding the coding exon of the receptor (Caenazzo et al., 1991). The CB_1 receptor gene is intronless in its coding region, but possesses an intron 5′ to the coding exon with three putative upstream exons (Bonner, 1996; Zhang et al., 2004). The genomic structure of the human CB_1 receptor has been reported (Zhang et al., 2004). In this study, three exons upstream of the coding exon were identified (a total of four exons), with a variation in the first exon. Five distinct variant exonic structures were demonstrated.

A positive association between a microsatellite polymorphism ($(AAT)_n$) in the CB_1 gene and IV drug abuse has been described (Comings et al., 1997). This polymorphism has subsequently been localized 3′ to the coding exon of the CB_1 receptor (Zhang et al., 2004). Although there are differences between populations, the CB_1 $(AAT)_n$ polymorphism has also been associated with schizophrenia (Ujike et al., 2002) as well as with depression in Parkinson's disease (Barrero et al., 2005), providing genetic evidence for a role of the cannabinoid system in these disorders. A recent systematic review of this and other polymorphisms in addictive disorders showed a significant association with illicit substance dependence but only in the Caucasian population samples and using a risk allele definition of $\geq$16 repeats (Benyamina, Kebir, Blecha, Reynaud, & Krebs, 2011).

Zhang and colleagues studied several polymorphisms in control and drug-abusing individuals from European, African, and Japanese ethnicities and found association with a 5′ "TAG" haplotype that was highly associated with substance abuse in all three populations (Zhang et al., 2004). Analysis of mRNA levels from postmortem brain samples of individuals with the TAG haplotype showed reduced expression for individuals expressing this allele.

The rs806371 polymorphism in the CNR1 promoter is a common functional variant associated with high-density lipoprotein cholesterol levels (Feng et al., 2013). Using 1% of 100,000 BioVU subject records claiming European ancestry for further study (50% female and 50% male subjects), as well as functional assays, this polymorphism was found to alter HDL-C level in humans by generating a novel regulatory DNA-binding site capable of reducing CNR1 expression.

The rs2180619 polymorphism in the CNR1 promoter has recently been found to be associated with working memory in a Mexican-mestizo population (Ruiz-Contreras et al., 2016), where the G allele was associated with a decrement. A previous report found that the G allele was more frequent in subjects with polysubstance abuse (Zhang et al., 2004). The GG genotype of the rs2180619 in combination with the SS genotype of a polymorphism in the promoter of the 5-HTTLPR gene (which encodes a serotonin transporter) was associated with higher anxiety compared with other genotypes (Lazary et al., 2009). This polymorphism is, therefore, associated with a variety of symptoms, but further work is needed to confirm these reports.

The first polymorphism in the coding exon described was a silent mutation in T453 (G to A), a conserved amino acid present in the C terminal region of the CB_1 and CB_2 receptors, that was a common polymorphism in the German population (Gadzicki, Muller-Vahl, & Stuhrmann, 1999). While this mutation is silent, analysis of several human sequences present in the database reveals that CB1K5 (accession #AF107262), a full-length sequence, contains five nucleotide changes, three of which result in amino acid differences. Coincidentally, two amino acid differences are in the third transmembrane domain, F200L and I216V. The third variant is in the fourth transmembrane domain, V246A. A report by the group that submitted the sequence to the database revealed that this was a somatic mutation in an epilepsy patient, i.e., DNA obtained from their blood was unaltered, but DNA from the hippocampus showed the mutation (Kathmann, Haug, Heils, Nothen, & Schlicker, 2000). The presence of a somatic mutation rather than a polymorphism is generally indicative of the disease process in cancers (e.g., mutant p53 or APC expression in tumors, but not normal tissues (Baker et al., 1989; Lamlum et al., 2000)). CB_1 receptor polymorphisms may affect responsiveness to cannabinoids.

Shortly after its molecular cloning, splice variants of the human CB_1 receptor were identified. A PCR amplification product was isolated that lacked 167 bp of the coding region of the human CB_1 receptor (Shire et al., 1995). This alternative splice form (CB_{1a}) is unusual in that it is generated from the mRNA encoding CB_1, and not from a separate exon (Shire et al., 1995). When expressed, the CB_{1a} clone would translate to a receptor truncated by 61 amino acid residues with 28 amino acid residues different at the amino-terminal. A second splice variant of the coding region has been reported in which a 99 base portion of the coding exon is spliced out of the human mRNA, leading to an in-frame deletion of 33 amino acids (Ryberg et al., 2005). This hCB_{1b} cDNA was isolated while cloning the previously reported splice variant. Both the CB_{1a} and CB_{1b} variants showed altered ligand binding and [^{35}S]GTPγS-binding activity compared with CB_1 when the cDNAs were expressed in HEK293 cells (Ryberg et al., 2005). Of the six cannabinoids tested, only 2-AG showed significant affinity for hCB_{1b}; furthermore, 2-AG acted as an inverse agonist at both variants. Anandamide was able to activate the variants at concentrations >10 μM. However, Δ^9-THC, CP55940, WIN55212, HU210, and SR141716 exhibited good affinity and [^{35}S]GTPγS-binding activity with the variants. hCB_{1a} and hCB_{1b} expression has been detected at very low levels in many human tissues by RT-PCR, less than 5% of hCB_1 (Ryberg et al., 2005; Shire et al., 1995; Xiao et al., 2008). However, a subsequent study found no differences in the pharmacology of the variants with respect to the wild-type receptor when each was expressed in CHO cells (Xiao et al., 2008). Also, when the splice variants were expressed in mouse hippocampal neurons cultured from CB_1 null mice, a different profile arose (Straiker, Wager-Miller, Hutchens, & Mackie, 2012). In this expression system, the splice variants were less efficacious than the full-length version in producing the measured response, which was depolarization-induced suppression of excitation. Neither splice variant is present in rat or mouse, because the splice consensus sequence is absent in these genes (Bonner, 1996). The presence of the splice variants was reported in human and macaque brains using a commercially available antibody (Bagher, Laprairie, Kelly, & Denovan-Wright, 2013). These authors found that each splice variant could form heterodimers with hCB_1 and increase its cell surface expression, when the constructs were coexpressed in HEK293 cells. These data suggest that the splice variants may play an important physiological role as regulators of the endocannabinoid system. In sum, the genomic studies implicate the CB_1 receptor in drug addiction and disease.

Polymorphisms in the CB_2 receptor have also been associated with disease phenotypes (Karsak et al., 2005; Sipe, Arbour, Gerber, & Beutler, 2005). The human CB_2 gene (CNR2) is located at chromosome 1p36. Polymorphisms of the human CB_2 gene are linked to osteoporosis in several studies (Karsak et al., 2005; Karsak et al., 2009; Yamada, Ando, & Shimokata, 2007). Karsak et al. examined CB_1 and CB_2 receptor DNA in a sample of French postmenopausal patients and female controls. The authors report that certain changes in CB_2 receptor, but not the CB_1 receptor, were strongly associated with osteoporosis (Karsak et al., 2005). A second study replicated these findings in a group of pre- and postmenopausal Japanese women (Yamada et al., 2007). In contrast, a recent study has found only nominally significant correlations with CB_2 polymorphisms and osteoporosis in a Chinese population; the role of the CNR2 gene in the etiology of Chinese osteoporosis thus requires further study in larger samples (Huang, Li, & Kung, 2009).

A related study examined the role of CB_2 DNA or genes on hand bone strength (Karsak et al., 2009). The authors analyzed radiographic images and DNA samples from a Chevashian population, an ethnically homogeneous population of people of Bulgaric ancestry that live along the Volga river. Several SNPs (small nucleotide polymorphisms) were significantly associated with certain bone phenotypes as previously reported (Karsak et al., 2005). Two of the associated SNPs were in adjacent nucleotides ("double SNP" rs2502992–rs2501432) within the coding region of CB_2 and result in a nonconservative missense variant (Gln63Arg, also referred to as the Q63 variant and the CB2-63 nonsynonymous polymorphism). This Q63 variant is probably functionally relevant as demonstrated by a differentially endocannabinoid-induced inhibition of T lymphocyte proliferation (Sipe et al., 2005). A less functional form of the CB_2 receptor appears to lead to weak hand bone strength and is associated with osteoporosis.

Because the CB_2 receptor is associated with immunomodulation, many studies have investigated a link between CNR2 polymorphisms and various immune disorders. The most widely studied is the Q63 variant, which has been found to be associated with hepatitis (Coppola et al., 2015), as well as other immune-mediated disorders (Coppola et al., 2016), such as chronic child immune thrombocytopenia (Mahmoud Gouda & Mohamed Kamel, 2013).

Intriguingly, this polymorphism along with two others in the CNR2 gene has been associated with schizophrenia in a Japanese population (Ishiguro, Horiuchi, et al., 2010). These authors also found reduced responsiveness of the R63 variant when it was heterologously expressed, confirming the earlier report (Sipe et al., 2005). These same authors found an association with eating disorders and this CNR2 polymorphism (Ishiguro, Carpio, et al., 2010) as well as with depression in a Japanese population (Onaivi et al., 2008a, 2008b).

Another study has reported an association between bipolar disorder and the 524A/C (Leu133Ile, rs41311993) polymorphism in an Italian population (Minocci et al., 2011). This residue is present in the third transmembrane domain and has been suggested to be important for the stability and/or the functionality of the receptor, but this has not been directly examined (Xie, Chen, & Billings, 2003). Although the presence of CB_2 in the normal brain has been controversial, there is a consensus that CB_2 is expressed in microglia during neuroinflammation, and a neuroimmunological etiology of bipolar disorder has been suggested (Minocci et al., 2011), thereby providing a link between CB_2, neuroinflammation, and psychiatric diseases.

4. PHYLOGENY

Comprehensive reviews of cannabinoid receptor phylogeny have been published (Elphick, 2012; McPartland, 2004); we provide here a brief summary of their pharmacology. The CB_1 receptors are highly conserved among vertebrate species and have also been found in some invertebrates (Elphick & Egertova, 2001; McPartland & Glass, 2003; Murphy et al., 2001). The cannabinoid receptor was originally cloned from rat (Matsuda et al., 1990); shortly thereafter, isolation of a human CB_1 receptor cDNA was reported (Gerard, Mollereau, Vassart, & Parmentier, 1991). The human CB_1 receptor has one less amino acid in the N-terminus as compared to the other mammalian species (472 amino acids vs 473 amino acids). The rat and human receptors are highly conserved, 93% identity at the nucleic acid level and 97% at the amino acid level. Similarly, the mouse and rat clones have 95% nucleic acid identity (100% amino acid identity) and the mouse and human clones have 90% nucleic acid identity (97% amino acid identity) (Abood, Ditto, Noel, Showalter, & Tao, 1997; Chakrabarti, Onaivi, & Chaudhuri, 1995; Ho & Zhao, 1996). A meta-analysis of the literature examining cannabinoid ligand-binding affinity revealed subtle interspecies differences for the binding affinities of some ligands (Δ^9-THC, CP55,940, WIN55,212-2, SR141716A) for rat vs human CB_1 receptors (McPartland, Glass, & Pertwee, 2007).

The sequence diversity of the CB_1 receptor showed a variance from 0.41% to 27% in 62 mammalian species using a molecular phylogenetic analysis (Murphy et al., 2001). In addition to mammals, the CB_1 receptor has been isolated from birds (Soderstrom, Leid, Moore, & Murray, 2000), fish (Yamaguchi, Macrae, & Brenner, 1996), amphibia (Cottone, Salio, Conrath, & Franzoni, 2003; Soderstrom et al., 2000), and an invertebrate, *Ciona intestinalis* (Elphick, Satou, & Satoh, 2003), among others. This deuterostomian invertebrate CB receptor contains 28% amino acid identity with CB_1, and 24% with CB_2 (Elphick et al., 2003). Since a CB receptor ortholog has not been found in *Drosophila melanogaster* or *Caenorhabditis elegans*, it has been suggested that the ancestor of vertebrate CB_1 and CB_2 receptors originated in a deuterostomian invertebrate (Elphick et al., 2003).

The CB_2 receptor was initially isolated from HL60 cells, a human promyelocytic leukemic cell line (Munro et al., 1993). In addition to the human CB_2 receptor, clones have been isolated from mouse (Shire et al., 1996; Valk et al., 1997), rat (Brown, Wager-Miller, & Mackie, 2002; Griffin, Tao, & Abood, 2000; Liu et al., 2009), dog (Ndong, O'Donnell, Ahmad, & Groblewski, 2011), the puffer fish *Fugu rubripes* (Elphick, 2002), as well as zebrafish (McPartland, Glass, Matias, Norris, & Kilpatrick, 2007). There is also information in the GenBank database on additional species. The CB_2 receptor shows less homology between species than does CB_1; for instance the human and mouse CB_2 receptors share 82% amino acid identity (Shire et al., 1996), and the mouse and rat 93% amino acid identity. The human, rat, and mouse sequences diverge at the C-terminus; the mouse sequence is 13 amino acids shorter, whereas the rat clone is 50 amino acids longer than the human CB_2 (Brown et al., 2002).

The first evidence for alternative splice forms of CB_2 was in the C-terminus of the rat CB_2 receptor (Brown et al., 2002; Griffin et al., 2000). That this may give rise to rat-specific pharmacology of the CB_2 receptor was suggested by differences in ligand recognition with a number of compounds at the rat CB_2 receptor compared to the human CB_2 receptor in transfected cells (Griffin et al., 2000). The clone described in these studies was amplified from genomic DNA rat CB_2; however, this isoform has subsequently been shown to be the major splice form of rat CB_2 (Liu et al., 2009). Now, variants of the human and mouse CB_2 receptors have been reported as well (Liu et al., 2009).

In summary, from what we know so far, the diversity in the regulatory regions of the CB_1 and CB_2 genes may provide extensive flexibility in gene regulation of these receptors in health and disease. A "clinical endocannabinoid deficiency syndrome" resulting from defects in the endocannabinoid system (i.e., receptor mutations, alterations in endocannabinoid production) has already been proposed to underlie certain diseases including treatment-resistant conditions (Russo, 2008). To date a mutation is yet to be identified in the human cannabinoid receptor that results in conclusive alteration of ligand–receptor interactions; however, we have discovered amino acids residues important for selective ligand recognition and maintaining receptor–ligand interactions *in vitro* (Kapur, Samaniego, Thakur, Makriyannis, & Abood, 2008; Song & Bonner, 1996). The efficacy of future cannabis-based clinical trials could be enhanced by developing patient screening methods for polymorphisms or mutations in genes associated with the endocannabinoid system.

5. DISTRIBUTION

The CB_1 receptor is one of the most abundant GPCRs in the brain; it is highly expressed in the basal ganglia nuclei, hippocampus, cortex, and cerebellum (Glass, Dragunow, & Faull, 1997; Herkenham et al., 1990; Tsou, Brown, Sanudo-Pena, Mackie, & Walker, 1998) (reviewed in Howlett et al., 2002). The distribution of this receptor within the central nervous system correlates with its role in the control of motor function, cognition and memory, and analgesia. CB_1 receptors are primarily localized to the terminals of central and peripheral neurons, where they mediate inhibition of neurotransmitter release (reviewed in Szabo & Schlicker, 2005). CB_1 receptors are found at significantly higher levels on GABAergic than glutamatergic neurons in various brain regions (Katona et al., 1999; Puighermanal et al., 2009). CB_1 receptors are also present in astrocytes, where they are expressed at much lower levels than in neurons, but where they have been shown to modulate synaptic transmission and plasticity (Han et al., 2012) (reviewed in Oliveira da Cruz, Robin, Drago, Marsicano, & Metna-Laurent, 2016). There has been some controversy regarding CB_1 receptor expression in other glial subtypes in situ (Stella, 2010).

The CB_1 receptor is also expressed throughout the periphery, albeit at much lower levels than in the CNS (reviewed in Howlett et al., 2002). Early after its identification, the CB_1 receptor was detected in a variety of circulating immune cells (Bouaboula, Dussossoy, & Casellas, 1999; Galiegue et al., 1995). Furthermore, the level of CB_1 expression appears to be increased or decreased during immune cell activation (reviewed in Klein, 2005). This is also the case with CB_2 expression as described below. CB_1 is expressed in numerous peripheral tissues, including the adrenal gland, heart, lung, prostate, liver, uterus, ovary, testis, vas deferens, bone marrow, thymus, and tonsils (Galiegue et al., 1995).

The CB_2 receptor is abundantly expressed in peripheral organs with immune function, including macrophages, spleen, tonsils, thymus, and leukocytes, as well as the lung and testes (Brown et al., 2002; Galiegue et al., 1995; Munro et al., 1993). Initial studies suggested that CB_2 receptors were absent from the healthy brain (Brown et al., 2002; Griffin et al., 1999). Subsequently, studies have now shown CB_2 receptor expression in diseased brain cells, including astrocytomas (Ellert-Miklaszewska, Grajkowska, Gabrusiewicz, Kaminska, & Konarska, 2007; Sanchez et al., 2001), microglia and astrocytes in Alzheimer's disease (Benito et al., 2003; Esposito et al., 2007), and T cells, microglia, and astrocytes in multiple sclerosis (Benito et al., 2007). These studies and others indicate that the CB_2 receptor is upregulated in response to immune cell activation and inflammation (Klein, 2005; Stella, 2010). More recently, CB_2 receptor expression has been reported in the healthy CNS (Van Sickle et al., 2005), although its presence in adult native brain tissue remains somewhat controversial (Atwood & Mackie, 2010; Soethoudt et al., 2017).

6. CANNABINOID RECEPTOR SIGNALING PATHWAYS ASSOCIATED WITH DIFFERENTIATED TISSUES

The CB_1 cannabinoid receptor was originally discovered based upon its signaling as a GPCR coupled to the Gi/o α proteins that inhibit adenylyl cyclase, thereby reducing cellular cAMP levels (for overview, see Howlett, 1990, 1995). For an overview, please consult the following excellent reviews that have highlighted CB_1 signal transduction (Console-Bram, Marcu, & Abood, 2012; Howlett, 2005; Howlett et al., 2002; McAllister & Glass, 2002; Turu & Hunyady, 2010). The CB_2 receptor cellular signaling has been characterized as Gi/o-coupled signaling, although Gi/o inhibits cAMP production with varying efficacy depending upon experimental model and agonist used (reviewed in Dhopeshwarkar & Mackie, 2014; Turcotte, Blanchet, Laviolette, & Flamand, 2016). In addition to Gi/o-mediated signaling, CB_1 and CB_2 receptors are phosphorylated by G protein receptor kinases (GRKs) and subsequently associate with β-arrestin1 or β-arrestin2 (Breivogel et al., 2013; Chen et al., 2014), which can serve as a scaffold for interaction with proteins that divert signaling along β-arrestin-mediated pathways. Both CB_1 and CB_2 receptors stimulate extracellular signal-regulated kinase (ERK)1 and 2, involving either Gβγ or β-arrestin interactions. We are just beginning to appreciate the cellular signaling pathways that make up the phenotype for healthy differentiated cell types as well as significant modifications in signaling pathways in states of disease. Some of these pathways are exemplified herein.

6.1 Signaling in Smooth Muscle Cells

The ability of cannabinoid agonists to attenuate contraction of vas deferens smooth muscle was among the first bioassays for this pharmacological class (Howlett et al., 2002) and now extends to clinical relevance for diseases associated with smooth muscle regulation. Several signal transduction pathways have been identified that are regulated by the CB_1 receptor to attenuate smooth muscle cell contraction. Smooth muscle contraction requires a Ca^{2+}-mediated pathway, leading to phosphorylation of myosin light chain. Pathways by which stimulation of CB_1 receptors can signal, culminating in the interference of contraction, have been identified in several model systems.

6.1.1 Vas Deferens

In Syrian hamster vas deferens smooth muscle DDT1MF-2 cells, Δ^9-THC evoked a large capacitative Ca^{2+} influx accompanied by a small release of intracellular Ca^{2+} (Filipeanu, de Zeeuw, & Nelemans, 1997). These responses were demonstrated to be due to CB_1 pathways by sensitivity to SR141716, and the capacitative Ca^{2+} mechanism by sensitivity to the sarcoplasmic/endoplasmic reticulum Ca^{2+} pump inhibitor thapsigargin. The capacitative Ca^{2+} influx was in part responsible for a CP55940-stimulated CB_1 receptor and Gi/o-mediated activation of a large conductance Ca^{2+}-dependent K^+ channel that was dependent upon both an inhibition of cAMP production and the activation of ERK1/2 (Begg, Baydoun, Parsons, & Molleman, 2001). It is likely that the ERK1/2 effects on channel regulation occur via a pathway involving a PLA_2-mediated release of arachidonic acid, which activates a noncapacitative Ca^{2+} entry (Demuth et al., 2005).

6.1.2 *Vascular Arterioles*

Studies of isolated vascular components have identified a cellular mechanism that occurs in vascular smooth muscle cells isolated from cat cerebral microvessels which express the CB_1 receptor (Gebremedhin, Lange, Campbell, Hillard, & Harder, 1999). A nifedipine-sensitive L-type Ca^{2+} current was attenuated by either anandamide or WIN55212-2. The CB_1 and Gi/o dependence of the response was demonstrated by evidence that it was antagonized by SR141716 and precluded by pertussis toxin. These results correlate with the vasorelaxation of serotonin-constricted cat cerebral arterioles by anandamide or WIN55212-2, suggesting that the reduction in Ca^{2+} influx via the L-type channels can account for the vasorelaxation in vascular smooth muscle cells.

6.1.3 *Gastric Smooth Muscle*

The signaling pathway utilized by CB_1 receptors in gastric smooth muscle cells to attenuate acetylcholine (M3 muscarinic)- and Gq-mediated contraction was comprehensively described by Mahavadi, Sriwai, Huang, Grider, and Murthy (2014). In dispersed or cultured rabbit gastric smooth muscle cells, anandamide stimulation of the CB_1 receptor activated predominantly Gi2 and inhibited cAMP accumulation. However, unlike for other Gi-coupled receptors in these cells, the $G\beta\gamma$ released by CB_1 receptor stimulation failed to initiate PLC-mediated phosphatidylinositol hydrolysis required for contraction of the cells. Rather, anandamide attenuated the acetylcholine-mediated contraction by a signaling pathway occurring via GRK5 phosphorylation of the CB_1 receptor and recruitment of β-arrestins, leading to activation of ERK1/2 and Src kinases for a two-pronged attenuation process. The ERK1/2 phosphorylated the regulator of G protein signaling 4 (RGS4) to promote inactivation of $G\alpha q$ and subsequent reduction in acetylcholine-mediated phosphatidylinositol hydrolysis that initiates contraction. The Src kinase promoted interaction of Rho1 with RhoA–myosin phosphatase1-interacting protein, thereby inhibiting Rho kinase as well as activating myosin light chain phosphatase, leading to net dephosphorylation of myosin light chain and inhibition of the sustained contraction.

6.1.4 *Myometrium*

Human myometrial strips, obtained as biopsies during C-section deliveries, express CB_1 receptors and respond to anandamide or Δ^9-THC with an SR141716-sensitive relaxation of oxytocin-induced contractions (Dennedy et al., 2004). Cellular signaling characterized in human myometrial smooth muscle ULTR cells (Brighton et al., 2009) and non-pregnant human myometrial cells in primary culture (Brighton, Marczylo, Rana, Konje, & Willets, 2011) indicated that stimulation of the CB_1 receptor by anandamide or methanandamide could promote an early-phase ERK1/2 phosphorylation in response to the sequential activation of Gi/o, phosphatidylinositol-3-kinase (PI3K), and a Src kinase. In ULTR cells, the role of CB_1 receptors (but not CB_2 receptor or TRP channels) was established (Brighton et al., 2009). Interestingly, the desensitization of the cAMP inhibition response in primary myometrial cells was entirely abolished by transfection with siRNA to negate translation of β-arrestin2. However, after that same β-arrestin2 knockdown, the ERK1/2 phosphorylation was augmented and sustained (Brighton et al., 2011). These findings suggest that β-arrestin2 mediates desensitization of Gi/o-driven responses, but that β-arrestin1 mediates processes associated with a prolonged ERK1/2 activation in myometrial smooth muscle.

6.2 Signaling in Metabolic Regulation and Disease

6.2.1 Liver Development and Function

Studies of zebra fish (*Danio rerio*) embryonic development demonstrated that liver differentiation (but not heart, pancreas, or kidney differentiation) requires functional CB_1 and CB_2 receptor signaling (Liu et al., 2016). Receptor knockout or antagonism resulted in defective biliary morphogenesis, developmental reduction of hepatocyte proliferation and liver mass, as well as a functional reduction in gene expression of liver-specific enzymes, a protective metabolic response in $CB_1{}^{-/-}$ embryos to the physiological insults of either ethanol or "high-fat" egg yolk, and an increased appearance of steatosis in $CB_2{}^{-/-}$ adults (Liu et al., 2016). The deficits induced by cannabinoid receptor deficiency were the result of reduced sterol regulatory element-binding transcription factor(s) (Srebf) expression that persists into adulthood (Jeong et al., 2008; Pai et al., 2013). The decreased Srebf led to reduced methionine pathway intermediates, findings that were also observed in livers from $CB_1{}^{-/-}$ mice (Liu et al., 2016). This resulted in a generalized pattern of reduced methylation of proteins (Liu et al., 2016), implicating a reduction in *S*-adenosylmethionine as a methyl donor for nucleic acid, phospholipid, and protein methylation critical for epigenetic regulation. The aberrant hepatogenesis could be overcome by over-expression of Srebf1 during development, but not entirely overcome by methionine replacement, suggesting that cannabinoid receptors and Srebf exert additional developmental regulatory functions not involving methylation.

The endocannabinoid system plays an integral role in mediating homeostasis in metabolic regulation, as has become evident in pathological states that require adjustment such as high-fat or chronic alcohol diets (as described in Tam et al., 2011). In such perturbations, CB_1 receptors are increased in hepatocytes and contribute to the ensuing insulin resistance and dyslipidemia. CB_1 receptors in stellate cells are engaged in fibrogenic activity in diseased states, and CB_2 receptors are induced in response to pathological states including fatty liver disease and liver fibrosis. Both Δ^9-THC and the CB_2-selective agonist JWH-133 reduced the proliferation rate and promoted apoptosis of stellate cells and myofibroblasts, thereby serving a hepatoprotective function (Tam et al., 2011). Thus, cannabinoid receptor signaling in liver may be uniquely targeted toward attempts to regain metabolic homeostasis.

6.2.2 Liver Hepatocytes

Human hepatocytes express predominantly isoform CB_{1b}, which differs from the CB_1 isoform expressed in the brain and exhibits an efficacious inhibition of adenylyl cyclase in response to CB_1-selective agonist ACEA (Gonzalez-Mariscal et al., 2016). Note that we refer to the more generic term CB_1 for the remainder of this discussion because these isoforms do not appear in rodents. CB_1 receptors are induced in human or mouse hepatocytes under conditions of high-fat or alcohol diets, and this may involve a 2-AG-stimulated, CB_1 receptor-mediated "autoinduction" via the retinoid A receptor γ (Mukhopadhyay et al., 2010; Osei-Hyiaman et al., 2005). The 2-AG required to stimulate hepatocyte CB_1 receptors is generated by neighboring stellate cells in ethanol-induced fatty liver, and this paracrine regulation is required for the ensuing lipogenesis and suppression of fatty acid oxidation by the hepatocytes (Jeong et al., 2008; Osei-Hyiaman et al., 2008).

Increased anandamide or 2-AG levels in response to high-fat diet in obese mice stimulated CB_1 receptor signaling that directs lipogenic gene expression, as CB_1 antagonists could block this pathway (Jourdan et al., 2010; Mukhopadhyay et al., 2010; Osei-Hyiaman et al., 2005). CB_1 receptor activation by 2-AG initiated signaling to induce mRNA for sterol regulatory element-binding protein 1c (SREBP-1c) and thereby induce fatty acid synthase (FAS), leading to increased plasma triglyceride-rich apolipoproteins (Ruby et al., 2008). Similarly, a chronic ethanol diet led to increased expression of lipogenic FAS, an effect that was precluded in hepatic $CB_1^{-/-}$ mice (You, Fischer, Deeg, & Crabb, 2002). *In vitro* experiments in hepatoma cells indicated that this was due to the metabolite acetaldehyde initiating signaling to increase levels of SREBP1 which activated an SRE promoter (You et al., 2002).

Lipogenesis in hepatocytes is stimulated for liver's production of fatty acids for storage in an anabolic state, or inhibited when lipids are needed for energy in a catabolic state. This process is regulated by cAMP activation of PKA, which phosphorylates and inhibits the transcription factor liver X receptor-α (LXRα). When dimerized with retinoic X receptor, LXRα is responsible for inducing SREBP-1c expression. SREBP-1c is the master regulatory transcription factor that promotes expression of lipogenic genes coding for FAS as well as for acetyl CoA carboxylase and stearoyl-CoA desaturase-1. Under conditions in which fatty acids are needed for energy rather than storage, a physiological response to adrenergic stimulation would activate the PKA, which would directly phosphorylate a serine on LXRα, which inhibits the SREBP-1c transcription. Conversely, the CB_1 receptor–Gi/o complex can promote the activation of SREBP-1c in a pertussis toxin-sensitive manner (Wu, Yang, & Kim, 2011). As described in the report by Wu et al. (2011), the CB_1 receptor-stimulated, Gi/o-mediated inhibition of cAMP and subsequent reduction in PKA could be correlated with two separate mechanisms that attenuated SREBP-1c expression. By one mechanism, under conditions of CB_1-mediated reduction in cAMP, the PKA would no longer be activated, such that LXRα serine would be unphosphorylated and would be able to induce SREBP-1c expression. Wu and colleagues showed that when the CB_1 receptor was antagonized by SR141716, PKA could phosphorylate the LXRα-serine and inhibit transcription of SREBP-1c (in much the same way as initiating an adrenergic response). By a second (delayed) mechanism demonstrated by Wu et al. (2011), PKA can initiate a sequential phosphorylation of liver kinase B1, which phosphorylates AMP kinase (AMPK), which phosphorylates a threonine on LXRα to attenuate the induction of SREBP-1c. This delayed pathway would also be attenuated by a CB_1-mediated reduction in cAMP and PKA activity, and was shown to be augmented by the antagonism of the CB_1 receptor by SR141716. In summary, the SREBP-1c transcriptional program leading to lipogenesis can be promoted in pathological states under conditions of increased endocannabinoid-stimulated CB_1 receptor signaling via Gi/o and cAMP inhibition. The competitive antagonism of the CB_1 receptor by SR141716 can intervene to curtail that lipogenic program.

High-fat or ethanol diets also reduced mitochondrial respiration and decreased mitochondrial fatty acid β-oxidation due to reduced entry of fatty acids into the mitochondria via the rate-limiting enzyme carnitine palmitoyltransferase 1 (CPT1) (Flamment et al., 2009; Osei-Hyiaman et al., 2008; Tam et al., 2010). This signaling pathway is mediated by agonist-stimulated CB_1 receptors, reducing CPT1 activity. Studies by Tedesco and colleagues investigated the effects of stimulating the CB_1 receptors in liver after 6 weeks of high-fat diet. The diet-induced increased body mass and adiposity could be further augmented by chronic (4 weeks) treatment with the CB_1-selective agonist ACEA (Tedesco et al., 2008). The signaling pathway for this augmentation involved an increase in p38 MAPK phosphorylation and a reduction in AMPK phosphorylation in ACEA-treated mice. ACEA treatment exacerbated the reduction in endothelial nitric oxide synthase (eNOS) mRNA in the liver of the obese mice. Similar exacerbation was observed for the high-fat diet-induced decrements in total mitochondrial DNA as well as mRNA for mitochondrial functional proteins PPARγ-coactivator-1α (PGC-1α), nuclear respiratory factor-1 (NRF-1) and mtDNA transcription factor A (MTfam), protein levels of cytochrome *c* oxidase IV and cytochrome *c*, and the activity of citrate synthase. These findings demonstrate that the ACEA treatment downregulates mitochondrial biogenesis in the liver of high-fat diet-induced obese mice. However, one caveat is that these experiments failed to include a group treated with ACEA plus a CB_1 receptor-selective antagonist in order to confirm that these responses were occurring solely as the result of a CB_1 receptor mechanism.

High-fat diet induces insulin resistance at the level of hepatocytes, and this is believed to be initiated by endoplasmic reticulum (ER) stress in mice expressing hepatic CB_1 receptors but not $CB_1^{-/-}$ mice (Liu et al., 2012). The injection of anandamide promoted the same markers of ER stress, confirming a role for the endocannabinoid system. CB_1 receptor involvement in high-fat diet-induced pathology began with pertussis toxin-sensitive Gi/o signaling through a pathway that led to the phosphorylation of insulin receptor substrate 1 (IRS1) at ser307 (Liu et al., 2012). This stimulated induction of the ser/thr phosphatase, *PH* domain leucine-rich repeat protein phosphatase-1 (Phlpp1), thereby reversing insulin-stimulated phosphorylation of protein kinase B (also known as akt-2), which increased glycogen phosphorylase a activity, culminating in insulin-resistant glycogenolysis.

The IRS1 phosphorylation also resulted in suppressed expression of hepatic insulin degradation enzyme, resulting in reduced insulin clearance and a consequent hyperinsulinemia (Liu et al., 2012).

Gluconeogenesis is regulated in the liver by the CB_1 receptor via the induction of the liver-specific, ER-bound transcription factor cAMP-responsive element-binding protein H (CREBH). CREBH is an ER stress-associated liver-specific transcription factor (Chanda et al., 2011). In studies of primary cultures of rat or human hepatocytes, 2-AG stimulation of CB_1 receptors promoted phosphorylation of c-Jun N-terminal kinase (JNK) and ERK1/2. JNK could phosphorylate c-Jun, allowing formation of activating protein 1 (AP-1). An AP-1 activation of its binding site on the CREBH promoter would lead to induction of CREBH (Chanda et al., 2011). CREBH, in turn, promotes the induction of gluconeogenic genes (phosphoenolpyruvate carboxykinase, glucose-6-phosphatase catalytic subunit, and PGC-1), leading to glucose production. The CB_1 antagonist AM251 mimicked the response to insulin to reduce CREBH gene expression and attenuate gluconeogenesis in cultured hepatocytes (Chanda et al., 2011). Interestingly, in these same studies, 2-AG also induced CB_1 receptor gene expression in cultured hepatocytes (Chanda et al., 2011), which has the potential to augment subsequent responses.

6.2.3 Liver Stellate Cells, Myofibroblasts, and Bile Duct Epithelial Cholangiocytes

CB_1 receptors were induced in stellate cells and myofibroblasts in human cirrhosis and mouse models of fibrosis, and antagonism by SR141716 could ultimately decrease fibrogenesis. Stimulation of these augmented CB_1 receptors by anandamide could increase TGFβ1 levels, leading to proliferation and cytoprotection of myofibroblast fibrogenic cells, and increased fibrogenesis (Teixeira-Clerc et al., 2006).

CB_2 receptors were induced in hepatic stellate cells and myofibroblasts in conditions of fatty liver disease and liver fibrosis (Julien et al., 2005; Mendez-Sanchez et al., 2007). Anandamide stimulation of CB_2 receptors in cholangiocytes initiated a signaling pathway via induction of AP-1 and thioredoxin 1 (also known as redox factor 1), leading to production of reactive oxygen species and cell death (DeMorrow et al., 2008).

6.2.4 White Adipocytes

Adipocyte differentiation is accompanied by an increased expression of the CB_1 receptor and by increased mitochondrial biogenesis, as an important means of regulating metabolic function (Bensaid et al., 2003; Engeli et al., 2005). The CB_1 receptor plays a key role in reducing energy utilization and increasing adiposity by suppressing mitochondrial mass and function (Tedesco et al., 2008, 2010). The cellular signaling mechanisms can be inferred from studies of mouse primary white adipocytes in culture, in which the antagonism of the CB_1 receptor by SR141716 led to a persistent increase in AMPK phosphorylation and activity (Tedesco et al., 2008, 2010). AMPK can activate eNOS by phosphorylation at Ser1177, leading to NO production (Morrow et al., 2003). In the process of mitochondrial biogenesis, NO regulation of NO-sensitive guanylyl cyclase stimulates cGMP production, PKG activation, and gene expression of signaling enzymes such as PGC-1α (Nisoli & Carruba, 2006). This process can be inhibited by the proinflammatory cytokine TNFα released from white and brown fat stores in obese rodents, which induced iNOS and inhibited eNOS expression (Merial-Kieny et al., 2003; Valerio et al., 2006). The observations that SR141716 increased mitochondrial DNA, and mRNA for key enzymes that regulate mitochondrial biogenesis (PGC-1α, NRF-1, and MTfam) in cultured adipocytes suggests that the CB_1 receptor must exert an inhibitory role in limiting mitochondrial biogenesis (Tedesco et al., 2008, 2010). SR141716 increased mitochondrial oxidative phosphorylation functions by increasing cyclooxygenase IV and cytochrome *c* protein levels, citrate synthase activity, and oxygen consumption (Tedesco et al., 2008, 2010), as would be expected if the CB_1 receptor precluded mitochondrial expansion. The responses to CB_1 antagonism in cultured adipocytes were recapitulated in $CB_1^{-/-}$ mice placed on standard or high-fat diets, lending credence to a role for the CB_1 receptor in impairment of this metabolic signaling pathway *in vivo* (Tedesco et al., 2008, 2010).

High-fat diet alters adipocyte functions in an effort to adjust to the anabolic state. In this fed state, serum endocannabinoid levels are increased (Engeli et al., 2005; Matias et al., 2006). In high-fat diet, epididymal white adipose tissue levels of phosphorylated AMPK (Thr172) and AMPK activity are reduced in WT mice but not in $CB_1^{-/-}$ mice (Tedesco et al., 2008), implicating the CB_1 receptor in the processes associated with this metabolic adjustment. In cultured adipocytes, SR141716 increased AMPK phosphorylation within 10 min, and this phosphorylation was sustained for at least 2 days under the influence of SR141716 (Tedesco et al., 2008). Outcomes that result from SR141716 treatment of mouse 3T3-F442A adipocytes include an induction of the beneficial cytokine adiponectin (also known as Acrp30) mRNA and protein (Bensaid et al., 2003), whereas CB_1 receptor stimulation decreases adiponectin expression (Matias et al., 2006). CB_1 receptor stimulation increases fat storage determined as lipid droplets in cultured 3T3-F442A adipocytes (Matias et al., 2006).

6.3 Cannabinoid Receptor Signaling in Neuronal Cells

Cellular signaling in neurons has been described as several prototypical signal transduction pathways. Excellent reviews have described the neurophysiology associated with retrograde short-term or long-term regulation of neurotransmitter release by CB_1 receptors (Kano, 2014; Lu & Mackie, 2016), signaling to the nucleus to regulate neuronal differentiation, migration, and neurite extension in neurodevelopment (Diaz-Alonso, Guzman, & Galve-Roperh, 2012; Gaffuri, Ladarre, & Lenkei, 2012; Maccarrone, Guzman, Mackie, Doherty, & Harkany, 2014) and synapse remodeling (Busquets Garcia, Soria-Gomez, Bellocchio, & Marsicano, 2016), and the CB_1 and CB_2 receptor functions associated with neuroprotection (Fernandez-Ruiz, Moro, & Martinez-Orgado, 2015; Navarro et al., 2016). We will briefly describe two examples of cellular signaling that extend from CB_1 receptor–Gi/o stimulation that have been investigated in model neuronal systems and brain.

6.3.1 CB_1 Receptor Regulation of Focal Adhesion Kinase and Integrin Signaling for Actin Cytoskeleton Organization and Cell Adhesion

CB_1 receptor signaling is important for cellular matrix interactions at the focal adhesions, actin cytoskeletal reorganization, and the scaffolding to multiple proteins via the tyrosine phosphorylation of pp125 focal adhesion kinase (FAK). FAK is a nonreceptor tyrosine kinase that acts as a scaffolding protein within focal adhesions to participate in organization of the actin cytoskeleton, migration, and cell adhesion (Franchini, 2012; Schaller, 2010). CB_1 receptor–Gi/o signaling promoted phosphorylation of tyrosines on FAK in hippocampal slices (Derkinderen et al., 1996, 2001). Gi/o-mediated inhibition of cAMP synthesis and decreased PKA activity were required for FAK tyrosine phosphorylation (Derkinderen et al., 1996). The FAK autophosphorylation site (tyrosine 397) initiates FAK activation, followed by Src family kinases binding to phosphotyrosine 397 to phosphorylate additional tyrosine residues. The phosphotyrosines serve as scaffolds for proteins that regulate cell adhesion, migration, and survival. In the N18TG2 neuroblastoma model, CB_1 receptor-stimulated FAK tyrosine397 phosphorylation was low in magnitude and dependent upon Src. Once phosphorylated, FAK tyrosine397 bound Src, which phosphorylated tyrosines576/577 to obtain full FAK catalytic activity. FAK tyrosine576/577 phosphorylation was governed by reduced PKA activation, which leads to protein tyrosine phosphatase (PTP1B, Shp1/Shp2)-mediated Src activation. Src-mediated phosphorylation at tyrosine925 creates an SH2-binding site for the adaptor protein Grb2 to initiate the ERK1/2 signaling cascade Ras-Raf-MEK-ERK1/2 (Dalton, Peterson, & Howlett, 2013).

CB_1 receptor signaling to FAK is also dependent upon extracellular matrix engagement by integrins. In the N18TG2 cell, fibronectin (α5β1) and laminin (α6β1, α7β1) integrin receptors are endogenously expressed (Dalton et al., 2013). Cells attached to fibronectin or laminin surfaces exhibited significantly higher basal FAK tyrosine397 and tyrosine576/577 phosphorylation compared with suspended cells, and this phosphorylation could be augmented by CB_1 agonists. The RGDS peptide integrin antagonist significantly reduced CB_1-mediated FAK phosphorylation in adherent N18TG2 cells, and α5 integrin silencing with siRNA also decreased FAK tyrosine576/577 phosphorylation (Dalton et al., 2013). RGDS peptide disrupted CB_1-mediated hippocampal FAK activation, demonstrating that the results from the neuronal model could also be observed in a brain preparation (Karanian, Brown, Makriyannis, & Bahr, 2005).

6.3.2 CB_1 Receptor Regulation of Gene Expression in Neurite Elongation

Neurite elongation in the N2A neuroblastoma model is regulated by CB_1 receptor signaling via Gαi/o (Bromberg, Iyengar, & He, 2008; He et al., 2005; He, Neves, Jordan, & Iyengar, 2006; Jordan et al., 2005). CB_1 receptor-mediated Gαi/o attenuated the ability of the Rap1-GTPase-activating protein (GAP) to terminate Rap1 activation by facilitating the ubiquitination of Rap1-GAP, thereby promoting its degradation by proteasomes (Jordan et al., 2005). Active Rap1-GTP signals to small G protein Ral, which led to phosphorylation and activation of Src (He et al., 2005; Jordan et al., 2005). HU210-stimulated CB_1 receptor evoked a sustained (hours) phosphorylation of Src kinase and transcription factor signal transducer and activator of transcription3 (Stat3) (He et al., 2005). Activation of Stat3 required both a direct phosphorylation at tyrosine by Src kinase, and an indirect activation of the small G protein Rac-GTP by Src kinase, thereby activating JNK to phosphorylate a serine on Stat3. Both Src and JNK were required for the CB_1 receptor-mediated Stat3 activation. Phosphorylated and dimerized Stat3 could enter the nucleus to promote transcription necessary for neurite elongation. This pathway could be reversed by activation of the phosphotyrosine phosphatase SHP2 which dephosphorylated and thereby inactivated Stat3 (Zorina, Iyengar, & Bromberg, 2010).

7. EXTENDED AGONIST EXPOSURE

Cannabinoid tolerance develops in the absence of pharmacokinetic changes (Martin, Dewey, Harris, & Beckner, 1976); therefore, biochemical and/or cellular changes are responsible for this adaptation. One hypothesis for tolerance development is that receptors lose function during chronic agonist treatment leading to diminished biological responses. The phenomenon of receptor downregulation has been observed in many brain receptor systems. While an early study failed to detect changes in either receptor number or mRNA levels in whole brains from mice tolerant to Δ^9-THC (Abood, Sauss, Fan, Tilton, & Martin, 1993), brain region-specific changes are observed (Breivogel et al., 1999; McKinney et al., 2008; Oviedo, Glowa, & Herkenham, 1993; Rodriguez de Fonseca, Gorriti, Fernandez-Ruiz, Palomo, & Ramos, 1994; Romero et al., 1997). A comprehensive study examining the time course of changes in cannabinoid-stimulated [^{35}S]GTPγS binding and cannabinoid receptor binding in both rat brain sections and membranes following daily Δ^9-THC treatments for 3, 7, 14, and 21 days found time-dependent decreases in both [^{35}S]GTPγS binding and [^{3}H]WIN 55212-2 and [^{3}H]SR141716 binding in cerebellum, hippocampus, caudate–putamen, and globus pallidus, with regional differences in the rate and magnitude of downregulation and desensitization (Breivogel et al., 1999). In a parallel study, the time course and regional specificity of expression of the CB_1 receptor were examined (Zhuang et al., 1998). Interestingly, receptor desensitization was found to be greater in brain sections than in brain membranes (Breivogel et al., 1999). These data suggest that cellular components important for desensitization (e.g., soluble kinases or β-arrestins) may be lost in the process of preparation of membranes. Indeed, in a comparison between β-arrestin2 knockout mice and WT mice, distinct regional differences were observed following chronic Δ^9-THC administration (Nguyen et al., 2012). These studies and others suggest that β-arrestin2 regulates CB_1 receptor signaling and adaptation in a central nervous system region-dependent manner (Kendall & Yudowski, 2016; Nguyen et al., 2012).

CB_1 receptor downregulation following chronic cannabis exposure in humans has also been reported using positron emission tomography (D'Souza et al., 2016; Hirvonen et al., 2012). Interestingly, regional specificity of downregulation was also observed in cannabis-dependent people, with reduction in cortical areas but not in noncortical areas (Hirvonen et al., 2012). The receptor downregulation correlated with years of cannabis smoking and was reversible upon cessation (D'Souza et al., 2016; Hirvonen et al., 2012). The authors concluded that cortical CB_1 cannabinoid receptor downregulation is a neuroadaptation that may promote cannabis dependence in human brain.

The CB_2 receptor is also desensitized and internalized following agonist treatment *in vitro* (Atwood, Wager-Miller, Haskins, Straiker, & Mackie, 2012; Bouaboula et al., 1999; Carrier et al., 2004; Grimsey, Goodfellow, Dragunow, & Glass, 2011). The first studies were conducted in human CB_2-transfected CHO cells and demonstrated that phosphorylation at S352 appears to play a key role in the loss of responsiveness of the CB_2 receptor to CP-55,940 (Bouaboula et al., 1999). Furthermore, SR144528 could regenerate the desensitized CB_2 receptors by activating a phosphatase that dephosphorylated the receptor (Bouaboula et al., 1999). A subsequent study demonstrated that this process was dependent on Rab-5 (Grimsey et al., 2011). Interestingly, in another study, marked functional selectivity of cannabinoid receptor internalization was observed, where WIN55,212-2 did not produce internalization, nor did most of the aminoalkylindoles tested (Atwood et al., 2012). They reported that Δ^9-THC did not produce any internalization of HEK-293 cells expressing rat CB_2, but compounds that are structurally similar to Δ^9-THC notably JWH133, THCV, and HU210 did (Atwood et al., 2012). One study utilized cultured rat microglia cells, where chronic exposure to 2-AG increased CB_2 receptor internalization (Carrier et al., 2004). Hence, the pharmacological properties and phosphorylation state of the CB_2 receptor can be regulated by both agonists and antagonists, but this appears to be agonist selective. Whether this is also true *in vivo* remains to be determined.

8. AGONIST-BIASED SIGNALING: TARGETING RECEPTOR CONFORMATIONS LEADING TO SELECTIVE PHARMACOLOGICAL RESPONSES

Early pharmacological studies have identified differences between the CB_1 and CB_2 receptors in their signaling via agonists that can bind to both receptors. A very relevant example is the response to Δ^9-THC, which, in COS or CHO cells expressing either receptor exogenously, serves as a partial agonist for CB_1 receptors, but a weak partial agonist or antagonist at CB_2

receptors to inhibit adenylyl cyclase activity (Bayewitch et al., 1996). Drug design in the new millennium has significantly advanced development of novel ligands that can select for either CB_1 or CB_2 receptors. The endocannabinoids anandamide and 2-AG and their structural analogs have the capacity to interact with other receptors, thereby extending the network of cellular signaling pathways beyond the two cannabinoid receptors (see other reviews in this series).

Beyond selectivity based upon receptor type, the next level of selectivity is based upon the receptor's ability to couple to various signaling pathways. The protein(s) with which the receptor interacts can provide the initial platform directing signaling along a pathway that can lead to preferred outcomes. For 7-transmembrane receptors, the primary divergence in signaling occurs at the selection between pathways generated via G proteins vs pathways generated by β-arrestins (see Fig. 1). In response to the endogenous

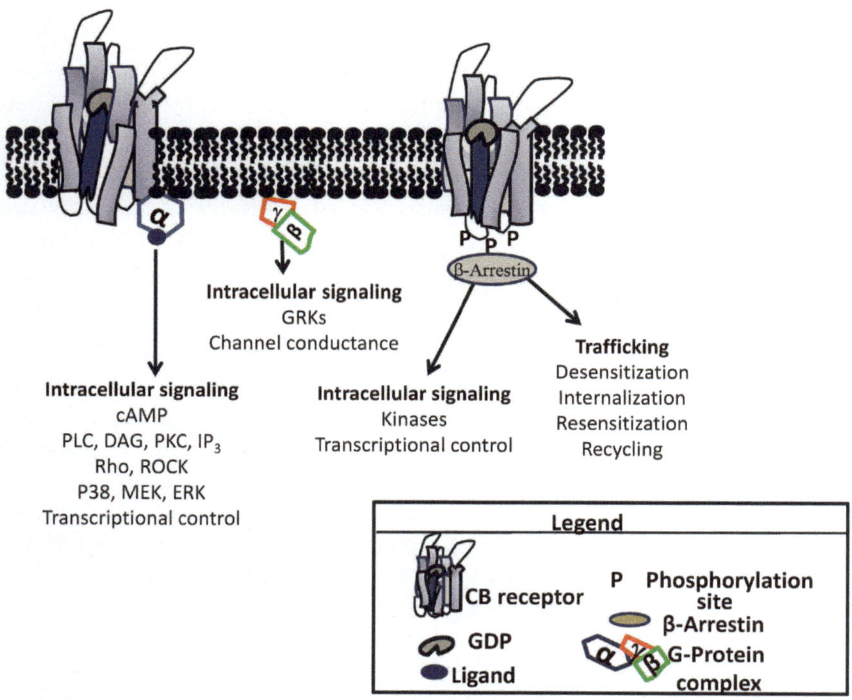

Fig. 1 Biased agonism. Upon agonist binding, G proteins dissociate into α and βγ subunits, and intracellular signaling pathways commence. Phosphorylation of the receptor (by one or more GRKs, not shown) recruits β-arrestin, which, in addition to directing internalization, can also initiate intracellular signaling.

agonists, the determinants between these two signaling outcomes are very likely dependent upon the time course and the strength of the stimulus. Prototypically, the receptor will initiate a pathway determined by the G protein-effector-second messenger-kinase(s) interactome, which can be unique to the differentiated functions of the cell. As the stimulus progresses or strengthens, the phosphorylation by one or several GRKs can direct the interaction with a β-arrestin, which can serve as a scaffold to couple to other signaling proteins, creating one or more signalosomes associated with differentiated functions of the cell. The next level of selectivity is which G protein or which β-arrestin (1 or 2) can be favored, which may depend upon the availability of these proteins due to cotranslational synthesis and trafficking of signaling proteins, intracellular compartmentalization of the receptors and signaling complexes, or the membrane organization (e.g., partitioning to lipid rafts, or scaffolding by protein–protein interactions).

8.1 Functional Selectivity in CB_1 or CB_2 Receptor Signaling

Advances in cannabinoid receptor-based pharmacotherapies are being sought based upon cannabinoid receptor interactions favoring either Gi/o (or other G protein) vs β-arrestin (1 or 2), referred to as "functional selectivity" or "biased agonism." The notion that drugs can be designed to initiate signaling via one of these primary pathways is based upon our understanding that the CB_1 receptor can adopt multiple unique conformations depending upon agonist occupancy (Bosier, Muccioli, Hermans, & Lambert, 2010; Georgieva et al., 2008; Khajehali et al., 2015; Laprairie, Bagher, Kelly, & Denovan-Wright, 2016).

One of the first series of studies to investigate functional ligand selectivity identified a differential regulation by HU210 vs CP55940 in tyrosine hydroxylase gene expression in N1E115 neuroblastoma cells and rat striatum (Bosier et al., 2012; Bosier, Tilleux, Najimi, Lambert, & Hermans, 2007). Further investigations in the N1E115 cells identified cellular signaling pathway divergence by which HU210 stimulated ERK1/2 phosphorylation, whereas CP55940 stimulated JNK phosphorylation preferentially (Bosier, Lambert, & Hermans, 2008).

Investigations have identified agonist biased signaling in a non-Huntington's disease phenotype generated by expressing STHdh(Q7/Q7) in mouse striatal medium spiny neurons. 2-AG, Δ^9-THC, and CP55940 were more potent mediators of β-arrestin2 recruitment than other agonists, whereas 2-AG, anandamide, and WIN55212-2 preferred Gi/o signaling

(Laprairie, Bagher, Kelly, Dupre, & Denovan-Wright, 2014). In the Huntington's disease phenotype of STHdh cells that have been genetically engineered to express the (Q111/Q111 Huntington) (Laprairie, Bagher, Kelly, et al., 2016), WIN55212-2, 2-AG, and anandamide stimulated Gi/o pathways, whereas 2-AG, Δ^9-THC, and CP55940 stimulated β-arrestin pathways concurrently with a reduction in CB_1 and reduced cell viability (Laprairie, Bagher, & Denovan-Wright, 2016; Laprairie, Bagher, Kelly, et al., 2016).

Other recent studies have used model systems that express cannabinoid receptors exogenously in model systems that have been developed to recognize either G protein signaling or β-arrestin mobilization. Example studies have provided predictive clues regarding pathway-preferring ligands for both CB_1 receptors (Baillie et al., 2013; Delgado-Peraza et al., 2016) and CB_2 receptors (Dhopeshwarkar & Mackie, 2016).

9. CONCLUSION

The cannabinoid receptors are expressed throughout the human body and have been shown to play critical roles in nearly all tissues examined. The diversity of signaling pathways, the modulation by chronic exposure, and the presence of splice variants contribute to their unique pharmacology and physiology. While selective agonists and antagonists have been discovered, it can be predicted that more extensive investigations will be appearing in the future that can guide drug design and development based upon conformational selection by agonists and perhaps also antagonist ligands that promote cellular signaling pathways.

CONFLICT OF INTEREST

The authors have no conflicts of interest to declare.

ACKNOWLEDGMENTS

The National Institutes of Health, National Institute on Drug Abuse Grants R01DA03690, R01DA023204, R01DA035926, P30DA013429, and P50DA006634 supported this work. We wish to thank Dr. Linda Console-Bram for her assistance with the figure.

REFERENCES

Abood, M. E., Ditto, K. A., Noel, M. A., Showalter, V. M., & Tao, Q. (1997). Isolation and expression of mouse CB1 cannabinoid receptor gene: Comparison of binding properties with those of native CB1 receptors in mouse brain and N18TG2 neuroblastoma cells. *Biochemical Pharmacology*, *53*, 207–214.

Abood, M. E., Sauss, C., Fan, F., Tilton, C. L., & Martin, B. R. (1993). Development of behavioral tolerance to delta 9-THC without alteration of cannabinoid receptor binding or mRNA levels in whole brain. *Pharmacology, Biochemistry, and Behavior, 46*(3), 575–579.

Atwood, B. K., & Mackie, K. (2010). CB2: A cannabinoid receptor with an identity crisis. *British Journal of Pharmacology, 160*(3), 467–479.

Atwood, B. K., Wager-Miller, J., Haskins, C., Straiker, A., & Mackie, K. (2012). Functional selectivity in CB(2) cannabinoid receptor signaling and regulation: Implications for the therapeutic potential of CB(2) ligands. *Molecular Pharmacology, 81*(2), 250–263.

Bagher, A. M., Laprairie, R. B., Kelly, M. E., & Denovan-Wright, E. M. (2013). Co-expression of the human cannabinoid receptor coding region splice variants (hCB (1)) affects the function of hCB(1) receptor complexes. *European Journal of Pharmacology, 721*(1–3), 341–354.

Baillie, G. L., Horswill, J. G., Anavi-Goffer, S., Reggio, P. H., Bolognini, D., Abood, M. E., et al. (2013). CB(1) receptor allosteric modulators display both agonist and signaling pathway specificity. *Molecular Pharmacology, 83*(2), 322–338.

Baker, S. J., Fearon, E. R., Nigro, J. M., Hamilton, S. R., Preisinger, A. C., Jessup, J. M., et al. (1989). Chromosome 17 deletions and p53 gene mutations in colorectal carcinomas. *Science, 244*(4901), 217–221.

Barrero, F. J., Ampuero, I., Morales, B., Vives, F., de Dios Luna Del Castillo, J., Hoenicka, J., et al. (2005). Depression in Parkinson's disease is related to a genetic polymorphism of the cannabinoid receptor gene (CNR1). *The Pharmacogenomics Journal, 5*(2), 135–141.

Bayewitch, M., Rhee, M. H., Avidor-Reiss, T., Breuer, A., Mechoulam, R., & Vogel, Z. (1996). (-)-Delta9-tetrahydrocannabinol antagonizes the peripheral cannabinoid receptor-mediated inhibition of adenylyl cyclase. *The Journal of Biological Chemistry, 271*(17), 9902–9905.

Begg, M., Baydoun, A., Parsons, M. E., & Molleman, A. (2001). Signal transduction of cannabinoid CB1 receptors in a smooth muscle cell line. *The Journal of Physiology, 531*(Pt. 1), 95–104.

Benito, C., Nunez, E., Tolon, R. M., Carrier, E. J., Rabano, A., Hillard, C. J., et al. (2003). Cannabinoid CB2 receptors and fatty acid amide hydrolase are selectively overexpressed in neuritic plaque-associated glia in Alzheimer's disease brains. *The Journal of Neuroscience, 23*(35), 11136–11141.

Benito, C., Romero, J. P., Tolon, R. M., Clemente, D., Docagne, F., Hillard, C. J., et al. (2007). Cannabinoid CB1 and CB2 receptors and fatty acid amide hydrolase are specific markers of plaque cell subtypes in human multiple sclerosis. *The Journal of Neuroscience, 27*(9), 2396–2402.

Bensaid, M., Gary-Bobo, M., Esclangon, A., Maffrand, J. P., Le Fur, G., Oury-Donat, F., et al. (2003). The cannabinoid CB1 receptor antagonist SR141716 increases Acrp30 mRNA expression in adipose tissue of obese fa/fa rats and in cultured adipocyte cells. *Molecular Pharmacology, 63*(4), 908–914.

Benyamina, A., Kebir, O., Blecha, L., Reynaud, M., & Krebs, M. O. (2011). CNR1 gene polymorphisms in addictive disorders: A systematic review and a meta-analysis. *Addiction Biology, 16*(1), 1–6.

Bonner, T. I. (1996). Molecular biology of cannabinoid receptors. *Journal of Neuroimmunology, 69*(1–2), 15–17.

Bosier, B., Lambert, D. M., & Hermans, E. (2008). Reciprocal influences of CB1 cannabinoid receptor agonists on ERK and JNK signalling in N1E-115 cells. *FEBS Letters, 582*(28), 3861–3867.

Bosier, B., Muccioli, G. G., Hermans, E., & Lambert, D. M. (2010). Functionally selective cannabinoid receptor signalling: Therapeutic implications and opportunities. *Biochemical Pharmacology, 80*(1), 1–12.

Bosier, B., Muccioli, G. G., Mertens, B., Sarre, S., Michotte, Y., Lambert, D. M., et al. (2012). Differential modulations of striatal tyrosine hydroxylase and dopamine metabolism by cannabinoid agonists as evidence for functional selectivity in vivo. *Neuropharmacology, 62*(7), 2328–2336.

Bosier, B., Tilleux, S., Najimi, M., Lambert, D. M., & Hermans, E. (2007). Agonist selective modulation of tyrosine hydroxylase expression by cannabinoid ligands in a murine neuroblastoma cell line. *Journal of Neurochemistry, 102*(6), 1996–2007.

Bouaboula, M., Dussossoy, D., & Casellas, P. (1999). Regulation of peripheral cannabinoid receptor CB2 phosphorylation by the inverse agonist SR 144528. Implications for receptor biological responses. *The Journal of Biological Chemistry, 274*(29), 20397–20405.

Breivogel, C. S., Childers, S. R., Deadwyler, S. A., Hampson, R. E., Vogt, L. J., & Sim-Selley, L. J. (1999). Chronic delta9-tetrahydrocannabinol treatment produces a time-dependent loss of cannabinoid receptors and cannabinoid receptor-activated G proteins in rat brain. *Journal of Neurochemistry, 73*(6), 2447–2459.

Breivogel, C. S., Puri, V., Lambert, J. M., Hill, D. K., Huffman, J. W., & Razdan, R. K. (2013). The influence of beta-arrestin2 on cannabinoid CB1 receptor coupling to G-proteins and subcellular localization and relative levels of beta-arrestin1 and 2 in mouse brain. *Journal of Receptor and Signal Transduction Research, 33*(6), 367–379.

Brighton, P. J., Marczylo, T. H., Rana, S., Konje, J. C., & Willets, J. M. (2011). Characterization of the endocannabinoid system, CB(1) receptor signalling and desensitization in human myometrium. *British Journal of Pharmacology, 164*(5), 1479–1494.

Brighton, P. J., McDonald, J., Taylor, A. H., Challiss, R. A., Lambert, D. G., Konje, J. C., et al. (2009). Characterization of anandamide-stimulated cannabinoid receptor signaling in human ULTR myometrial smooth muscle cells. *Molecular Endocrinology, 23*(9), 1415–1427.

Bromberg, K. D., Iyengar, R., & He, J. C. (2008). Regulation of neurite outgrowth by G(i/o) signaling pathways. *Frontiers in Bioscience, 13*, 4544–4557.

Brown, S. M., Wager-Miller, J., & Mackie, K. (2002). Cloning and molecular characterization of the rat CB2 cannabinoid receptor. *Biochimica et Biophysica Acta, 1576*(3), 255–264.

Busquets Garcia, A., Soria-Gomez, E., Bellocchio, L., & Marsicano, G. (2016). Cannabinoid receptor type-1: Breaking the dogmas. *F1000Research, 5*, 990.

Caenazzo, L., Hoehe, M., Hsieh, W., Berrettini, W., Bonner, T., & Gershon, E. (1991). HindIII identifies a two allele DNA polymorphism of the human cannabinoid receptor gene (CNR). *Nucleic Acids Research, 19*(17), 4798.

Carrier, E. J., Kearn, C. S., Barkmeier, A. J., Breese, N. M., Yang, W., Nithipatikom, K., et al. (2004). Cultured rat microglial cells synthesize the endocannabinoid 2-arachidonylglycerol, which increases proliferation via a CB2 receptor-dependent mechanism. *Molecular Pharmacology, 65*(4), 999–1007.

Chakrabarti, A., Onaivi, E. S., & Chaudhuri, G. (1995). Cloning and sequencing of a cDNA encoding the mouse brain-type cannabinoid receptor protein. *DNA Sequence, 5*, 385–388.

Chanda, D., Kim, D. K., Li, T., Kim, Y. H., Koo, S. H., Lee, C. H., et al. (2011). Cannabinoid receptor type 1 (CB1R) signaling regulates hepatic gluconeogenesis via induction of endoplasmic reticulum-bound transcription factor cAMP-responsive element-binding protein H (CREBH) in primary hepatocytes. *The Journal of Biological Chemistry, 286*(32), 27971–27979.

Chen, X., Zheng, C., Qian, J., Sutton, S. W., Wang, Z., Lv, J., et al. (2014). Involvement of beta-arrestin-2 and clathrin in agonist-mediated internalization of the human cannabinoid CB2 receptor. *Current Molecular Pharmacology*, 7(1), 67–80.

Comings, D. E., Muhleman, D., Gade, R., Johnson, P., Verde, R., Saucier, G., et al. (1997). Cannabinoid receptor gene (CNR1): Association with i.v. drug use. *Molecular Psychiatry, 2*(2), 161–168.

Console-Bram, L., Marcu, J., & Abood, M. E. (2012). Cannabinoid receptors: Nomenclature and pharmacological principles. *Progress in Neuro-Psychopharmacology & Biological Psychiatry, 38*(1), 4–15.

Coppola, N., Zampino, R., Bellini, G., Stanzione, M., Capoluongo, N., Marrone, A., et al. (2015). The impact of the CB2-63 polymorphism on the histological presentation of chronic hepatitis B. *Clinical Microbiology and Infection, 21*(6), 609.e1–609.e4.

Coppola, N., Zampino, R., Bellini, G., Stanzione, M., Capoluongo, N., Marrone, A., et al. (2016). CB2-63 polymorphism and immune-mediated diseases associated with HCV chronic infection. *Digestive and Liver Disease, 48*(11), 1364–1369.

Cottone, E., Salio, C., Conrath, M., & Franzoni, M. F. (2003). *Xenopus laevis* CB1 cannabinoid receptor: Molecular cloning and mRNA distribution in the central nervous system. *The Journal of Comparative Neurology, 464*(4), 487–496.

Dalton, G. D., Peterson, L. J., & Howlett, A. C. (2013). CB(1) cannabinoid receptors promote maximal FAK catalytic activity by stimulating cooperative signaling between receptor tyrosine kinases and integrins in neuronal cells. *Cellular Signalling, 25*(8), 1665–1677.

Delgado-Peraza, F., Ahn, K. H., Nogueras-Ortiz, C., Mungrue, I. N., Mackie, K., Kendall, D. A., et al. (2016). Mechanisms of biased beta-arrestin-mediated signaling downstream from the cannabinoid 1 receptor. *Molecular Pharmacology, 89*(6), 618–629.

DeMorrow, S., Francis, H., Gaudio, E., Ueno, Y., Venter, J., Onori, P., et al. (2008). Anandamide inhibits cholangiocyte hyperplastic proliferation via activation of thioredoxin 1/redox factor 1 and AP-1 activation. *American Journal of Physiology. Gastrointestinal and Liver Physiology, 294*(2), G506–G519.

Demuth, D. G., Gkoumassi, E., Droge, M. J., Dekkers, B. G., Esselink, H. J., van Ree, R. M., et al. (2005). Arachidonic acid mediates non-capacitative calcium entry evoked by CB1-cannabinoid receptor activation in DDT1 MF-2 smooth muscle cells. *Journal of Cellular Physiology, 205*(1), 58–67.

Dennedy, M. C., Friel, A. M., Houlihan, D. D., Broderick, V. M., Smith, T., & Morrison, J. J. (2004). Cannabinoids and the human uterus during pregnancy. *American Journal of Obstetrics and Gynecology, 190*(1), 2–9. discussion 3A.

Derkinderen, P., Toutant, M., Burgaya, F., Le Bert, M., Siciliano, J. C., de Franciscis, V., et al. (1996). Regulation of a neuronal form of focal adhesion kinase by anandamide. *Science, 273*(5282), 1719–1722.

Derkinderen, P., Toutant, M., Kadare, G., Ledent, C., Parmentier, M., & Girault, J. A. (2001). Dual role of Fyn in the regulation of FAK + 6,7 by cannabinoids in hippocampus. *The Journal of Biological Chemistry, 276*(41), 38289–38296.

Devane, W. A., Dysarz, F. A., 3rd, Johnson, M. R., Melvin, L. S., & Howlett, A. C. (1988). Determination and characterization of a cannabinoid receptor in rat brain. *Molecular Pharmacology, 34*(5), 605–613.

Devane, W. A., Hanus, L., Breuer, A., Pertwee, R. G., Stevenson, L. A., Griffin, G., et al. (1992). Isolation and structure of a brain constituent that binds to the cannabinoid receptor. *Science, 258*(5090), 1946–1949.

Dhopeshwarkar, A., & Mackie, K. (2014). CB2 cannabinoid receptors as a therapeutic target-what does the future hold? *Molecular Pharmacology, 86*(4), 430–437.

Dhopeshwarkar, A., & Mackie, K. (2016). Functional selectivity of CB2 cannabinoid receptor ligands at a canonical and noncanonical pathway. *The Journal of Pharmacology and Experimental Therapeutics, 358*(2), 342–351.

Diaz-Alonso, J., Guzman, M., & Galve-Roperh, I. (2012). Endocannabinoids via CB(1) receptors act as neurogenic niche cues during cortical development. *Philosophical Transactions of the Royal Society of London. Series B, Biological Sciences, 367*(1607), 3229–3241.

Di Marzo, V., Melck, D., Bisogno, T., & De Petrocellis, L. (1998). Endocannabinoids: Endogenous cannabinoid receptor ligands with neuromodulatory action. *Trends in Neurosciences*, *21*(12), 521–528.

D'Souza, D. C., Cortes-Briones, J. A., Ranganathan, M., Thurnauer, H., Creatura, G., Surti, T., et al. (2016). Rapid changes in CB1 receptor availability in cannabis dependent males after abstinence from cannabis. *Biological psychiatry: Cognitive Neuroscience and Neuroimaging*, *1*(1), 60–67.

Eissenstat, M. A., Bell, M. R., D'Ambra, T. E., Alexander, E. J., Daum, S. J., Ackerman, J. H., et al. (1995). Aminoalkylindoles: Structure-activity relationships of novel cannabinoid mimetics. *Journal of Medicinal Chemistry*, *38*(16), 3094–3105.

Ellert-Miklaszewska, A., Grajkowska, W., Gabrusiewicz, K., Kaminska, B., & Konarska, L. (2007). Distinctive pattern of cannabinoid receptor type II (CB2) expression in adult and pediatric brain tumors. *Brain Research*, *1137*(1), 161–169.

Elphick, M. R. (2002). Evolution of cannabinoid receptors in vertebrates: Identification of a CB(2) gene in the puffer fish Fugu rubripes. *The Biological Bulletin*, *202*(2), 104–107.

Elphick, M. R. (2012). The evolution and comparative neurobiology of endocannabinoid signalling. *Philosophical Transactions of the Royal Society of London. Series B, Biological Sciences*, *367*(1607), 3201–3215.

Elphick, M. R., & Egertova, M. (2001). The neurobiology and evolution of cannabinoid signalling. *Philosophical Transactions of the Royal Society of London. Series B, Biological Sciences*, *356*(1407), 381–408.

Elphick, M. R., Satou, Y., & Satoh, N. (2003). The invertebrate ancestry of endocannabinoid signalling: An orthologue of vertebrate cannabinoid receptors in the urochordate *Ciona intestinalis*. *Gene*, *302*(1–2), 95–101.

Engeli, S., Bohnke, J., Feldpausch, M., Gorzelniak, K., Janke, J., Batkai, S., et al. (2005). Activation of the peripheral endocannabinoid system in human obesity. *Diabetes*, *54*(10), 2838–2843.

Esposito, G., Scuderi, C., Savani, C., Steardo, L., Jr., De Filippis, D., Cottone, P., et al. (2007). Cannabidiol in vivo blunts beta-amyloid induced neuroinflammation by suppressing IL-1beta and iNOS expression. *British Journal of Pharmacology*, *151*(8), 1272–1279.

Feng, Q., Vickers, K. C., Anderson, M. P., Levin, M. G., Chen, W., Harrison, D. G., et al. (2013). A common functional promoter variant links CNR1 gene expression to HDL cholesterol level. *Nature Communications*, *4*, 1973.

Fernandez-Ruiz, J., Moro, M. A., & Martinez-Orgado, J. (2015). Cannabinoids in neurodegenerative disorders and stroke/brain trauma: From preclinical models to clinical applications. *Neurotherapeutics*, *12*(4), 793–806.

Filipeanu, C. M., de Zeeuw, D., & Nelemans, S. A. (1997). Delta9-tetrahydrocannabinol activates [Ca2+]i increases partly sensitive to capacitative store refilling. *European Journal of Pharmacology*, *336*(1), R1–R3.

Flamment, M., Gueguen, N., Wetterwald, C., Simard, G., Malthiery, Y., & Ducluzeau, P. H. (2009). Effects of the cannabinoid CB1 antagonist rimonabant on hepatic mitochondrial function in rats fed a high-fat diet. *American Journal of Physiology. Endocrinology and Metabolism*, *297*(5), E1162–E1170.

Franchini, K. G. (2012). Focal adhesion kinase—The basis of local hypertrophic signaling domains. *Journal of Molecular and Cellular Cardiology*, *52*(2), 485–492.

Gadzicki, D., Muller-Vahl, K., & Stuhrmann, M. (1999). A frequent polymorphism in the coding exon of the human cannabinoid receptor (CNR1) gene. *Molecular and Cellular Probes*, *13*(4), 321–323.

Gaffuri, A. L., Ladarre, D., & Lenkei, Z. (2012). Type-1 cannabinoid receptor signaling in neuronal development. *Pharmacology*, *90*(1–2), 19–39.

Galiegue, S., Mary, S., Marchand, J., Dussossoy, D., Carriere, D., Carayon, P., et al. (1995). Expression of central and peripheral cannabinoid receptors in human immune tissues and leukocyte subpopulations. *European Journal of Biochemistry, 232*(1), 54–61.

Gebremedhin, D., Lange, A. R., Campbell, W. B., Hillard, C. J., & Harder, D. R. (1999). Cannabinoid CB1 receptor of cat cerebral arterial muscle functions to inhibit L-type Ca2+ channel current. *The American Journal of Physiology, 276*(6 Pt. 2), H2085–H2093.

Georgieva, T., Devanathan, S., Stropova, D., Park, C. K., Salamon, Z., Tollin, G., et al. (2008). Unique agonist-bound cannabinoid CB1 receptor conformations indicate agonist specificity in signaling. *European Journal of Pharmacology, 581*(1–2), 19–29.

Gerard, C. M., Mollereau, C., Vassart, G., & Parmentier, M. (1991). Molecular cloning of a human cannabinoid receptor which is also expressed in testis. *Biochemical Journal, 279*, 129–134.

Glass, M., Dragunow, M., & Faull, R. L. (1997). Cannabinoid receptors in the human brain: A detailed anatomical and quantitative autoradiographic study in the fetal, neonatal and adult human brain. *Neuroscience, 77*(2), 299–318.

Gonzalez-Mariscal, I., Krzysik-Walker, S. M., Doyle, M. E., Liu, Q. R., Cimbro, R., Santa-Cruz Calvo, S., et al. (2016). Human CB1 receptor isoforms, present in hepatocytes and beta-cells, are involved in regulating metabolism. *Scientific Reports, 6*, 33302.

Griffin, G., Tao, Q., & Abood, M. E. (2000). Cloning and pharmacological characterization of the rat CB2 cannabinoid receptor. *Journal of Pharmacology and Experimental Therapeutics, 292*(3), 886–894.

Griffin, G., Wray, E. J., Tao, Q., McAllister, S. D., Rorrer, W. K., Aung, M. M., et al. (1999). Evaluation of the cannabinoid CB2 receptor-selective antagonist, SR144528: Further evidence for cannabinoid CB2 receptor absence in the rat central nervous system. *European Journal of Pharmacology, 377*(1), 117–125.

Grimsey, N. L., Goodfellow, C. E., Dragunow, M., & Glass, M. (2011). Cannabinoid receptor 2 undergoes Rab5-mediated internalization and recycles via a Rab11-dependent pathway. *Biochimica et Biophysica Acta, 1813*(8), 1554–1560.

Han, J., Kesner, P., Metna-Laurent, M., Duan, T., Xu, L., Georges, F., et al. (2012). Acute cannabinoids impair working memory through astroglial CB1 receptor modulation of hippocampal LTD. *Cell, 148*(5), 1039–1050.

Hanus, L., Breuer, A., Tchilibon, S., Shiloah, S., Goldenberg, D., Horowitz, M., et al. (1999). HU-308: A specific agonist for CB(2), a peripheral cannabinoid receptor. *Proceedings of the National Academy of Sciences of the United States of America, 96*(25), 14228–14233.

He, J. C., Gomes, I., Nguyen, T., Jayaram, G., Ram, P. T., Devi, L. A., et al. (2005). The G alpha(o/i)-coupled cannabinoid receptor-mediated neurite outgrowth involves Rap regulation of Src and Stat3. *The Journal of Biological Chemistry, 280*(39), 33426–33434.

He, J. C., Neves, S. R., Jordan, J. D., & Iyengar, R. (2006). Role of the Go/i signaling network in the regulation of neurite outgrowth. *Canadian Journal of Physiology and Pharmacology, 84*(7), 687–694.

Herkenham, M., Lynn, A. B., Little, M. D., Johnson, M. R., Melvin, L. S., de Costa, B. R., et al. (1990). Cannabinoid receptor localization in brain. *Proceedings of the National Academy of Sciences of the United States of America, 87*(5), 1932–1936.

Hirvonen, J., Goodwin, R. S., Li, C. T., Terry, G. E., Zoghbi, S. S., Morse, C., et al. (2012). Reversible and regionally selective downregulation of brain cannabinoid CB1 receptors in chronic daily cannabis smokers. *Molecular Psychiatry, 17*(6), 642–649.

Ho, B. Y., & Zhao, J. (1996). Determination of the cannabinoid receptors in mouse x rat hybridoma NG108-15 cells and rat GH4C1 cells. *Neuroscience Letters, 212*(2), 123–126.

Howlett, A. C. (1990). Reverse pharmacology applied to the cannabinoid receptor. *Trends in Pharmacological Sciences, 11*(10), 395–397.

Howlett, A. C. (1995). Pharmacology of cannabinoid receptors. *Annual Review of Pharmacology and Toxicology*, *35*, 607–634.
Howlett, A. C. (2005). Cannabinoid receptor signaling. *Handbook of Experimental Pharmacology*, (168), 53–79.
Howlett, A. C., Barth, F., Bonner, T. I., Cabral, G., Casellas, P., Devane, W. A., et al. (2002). International Union of Pharmacology. XXVII. Classification of cannabinoid receptors. *Pharmacological Reviews*, *54*(2), 161–202.
Huang, Q. Y., Li, G. H., & Kung, A. W. (2009). Multiple osteoporosis susceptibility genes on chromosome 1p36 in Chinese. *Bone*, *44*(5), 984–988.
Ishiguro, H., Carpio, O., Horiuchi, Y., Shu, A., Higuchi, S., Schanz, N., et al. (2010a). A nonsynonymous polymorphism in cannabinoid CB2 receptor gene is associated with eating disorders in humans and food intake is modified in mice by its ligands. *Synapse*, *64*(1), 92–96.
Ishiguro, H., Horiuchi, Y., Ishikawa, M., Koga, M., Imai, K., Suzuki, Y., et al. (2010b). Brain cannabinoid CB2 receptor in schizophrenia. *Biological Psychiatry*, *67*(10), 974–982.
Jeong, W. I., Osei-Hyiaman, D., Park, O., Liu, J., Batkai, S., & Mukhopadhyay, P. (2008). Paracrine activation of hepatic CB1 receptors by stellate cell-derived endocannabinoids mediates alcoholic fatty liver. *Cell Metabolism*, 7, 227–235.
Jordan, J. D., He, J. C., Eungdamrong, N. J., Gomes, I., Ali, W., Nguyen, T., et al. (2005). Cannabinoid receptor-induced neurite outgrowth is mediated by Rap1 activation through G(alpha)o/i-triggered proteasomal degradation of Rap1GAPII. *The Journal of Biological Chemistry*, *280*(12), 11413–11421.
Jourdan, T., Djaouti, L., Demizieux, L., Gresti, J., Verges, B., & Degrace, P. (2010). CB1 antagonism exerts specific molecular effects on visceral and subcutaneous fat and reverses liver steatosis in diet-induced obese mice. *Diabetes*, *59*(4), 926–934.
Julien, B., Grenard, P., Teixeira-Clerc, F., Van Nhieu, J. T., Li, L., Karsak, M., et al. (2005). Antifibrogenic role of the cannabinoid receptor CB2 in the liver. *Gastroenterology*, *128*(3), 742–755.
Kano, M. (2014). Control of synaptic function by endocannabinoid-mediated retrograde signaling. *Proceedings of the Japan Academy. Series B, Physical and Biological Sciences*, *90*(7), 235–250.
Kapur, A., Samaniego, P., Thakur, G. A., Makriyannis, A., & Abood, M. E. (2008). Mapping the structural requirements in the CB1 cannabinoid receptor transmembrane helix II for signal transduction. *The Journal of Pharmacology and Experimental Therapeutics*, *325*(1), 341–348.
Karanian, D. A., Brown, Q. B., Makriyannis, A., & Bahr, B. A. (2005). Blocking cannabinoid activation of FAK and ERK1/2 compromises synaptic integrity in hippocampus. *European Journal of Pharmacology*, *508*(1–3), 47–56.
Karsak, M., Cohen-Solal, M., Freudenberg, J., Ostertag, A., Morieux, C., Kornak, U., et al. (2005). Cannabinoid receptor type 2 gene is associated with human osteoporosis. *Human Molecular Genetics*, *14*(22), 3389–3396. Epub 2005 Oct 4.
Karsak, M., Malkin, I., Toliat, M. R., Kubisch, C., Nurnberg, P., Zimmer, A., et al. (2009). The cannabinoid receptor type 2 (CNR2) gene is associated with hand bone strength phenotypes in an ethnically homogeneous family sample. *Human Genetics*, *126*(5), 629–636.
Kathmann, M., Haug, K., Heils, A., Nothen, M., & Schlicker, E. (2000). In *Exchange of three amino acids in the cannabinoid CB1 receptor (CNR1) of an epilepsy patient. Paper presented at the 2000 symposium on the cannabinoids, Burlington, VT.*
Katona, I., Sperlagh, B., Sik, A., Kafalvi, A., Vizi, E. S., Mackie, K., et al. (1999). Presynaptically located CB1 cannabinoid receptors regulate GABA release from axon terminals of specific hippocampal interneurons. *The Journal of Neuroscience*, *19*(11), 4544–4558.

Kearn, C., Greenberg, M., DiCamelli, R., Kurzawa, K., & Hillard, C. (1999). Relationships between ligand affinities for the cerebellar cannabinoid receptor CB1 and the induction of GDP/GTP exchange. *Journal of Neurochemistry*, *72*, 2379–2387.

Kendall, D. A., & Yudowski, G. A. (2016). Cannabinoid receptors in the central nervous system: Their signaling and roles in disease. *Frontiers in Cellular Neuroscience*, *10*, 294.

Khajehali, E., Malone, D. T., Glass, M., Sexton, P. M., Christopoulos, A., & Leach, K. (2015). Biased agonism and biased allosteric modulation at the CB1 cannabinoid receptor. *Molecular Pharmacology*, *88*(2), 368–379.

Klein, T. W. (2005). Cannabinoid-based drugs as anti-inflammatory therapeutics. *Nature Reviews. Immunology*, *5*(5), 400–411.

Lamlum, H., Papadopoulou, A., Ilyas, M., Rowan, A., Gillet, C., Hanby, A., et al. (2000). APC mutations are sufficient for the growth of early colorectal adenomas. *Proceedings of the National Academy of Sciences of the United States of America*, *97*(5), 2225–2228.

Laprairie, R. B., Bagher, A. M., & Denovan-Wright, E. M. (2016a). Cannabinoid receptor ligand bias: Implications in the central nervous system. *Current Opinion in Pharmacology*, *32*, 32–43.

Laprairie, R. B., Bagher, A. M., Kelly, M. E., & Denovan-Wright, E. M. (2016b). Biased type 1 cannabinoid receptor signaling influences neuronal viability in a cell culture model of Huntington disease. *Molecular Pharmacology*, *89*(3), 364–375.

Laprairie, R. B., Bagher, A. M., Kelly, M. E., Dupre, D. J., & Denovan-Wright, E. M. (2014). Type 1 cannabinoid receptor ligands display functional selectivity in a cell culture model of striatal medium spiny projection neurons. *The Journal of Biological Chemistry*, *289*(36), 24845–24862.

Lazary, J., Lazary, A., Gonda, X., Benko, A., Molnar, E., Hunyady, L., et al. (2009). Promoter variants of the cannabinoid receptor 1 gene (CNR1) in interaction with 5-HTTLPR affect the anxious phenotype. *American Journal of Medical Genetics. Part B, Neuropsychiatric Genetics*, *150B*(8), 1118–1127.

Liu, L. Y., Alexa, K., Cortes, M., Schatzman-Bone, S., Kim, A. J., Mukhopadhyay, B., et al. (2016). Cannabinoid receptor signaling regulates liver development and metabolism. *Development*, *143*(4), 609–622.

Liu, Q. R., Pan, C. H., Hishimoto, A., Li, C. Y., Xi, Z. X., Llorente-Berzal, A., et al. (2009). Species differences in cannabinoid receptor 2 (CNR2 gene): Identification of novel human and rodent CB2 isoforms, differential tissue expression and regulation by cannabinoid receptor ligands. *Genes, Brain, and Behavior*, *8*(5), 519–530.

Liu, J., Zhou, L., Xiong, K., Godlewski, G., Mukhopadhyay, B., & Tam, J. (2012). Hepatic cannabinoid receptor-1 mediates diet-induced insulin resistance via inhibition of insulin signaling and clearance in mice. *Gastroenterology*, *142*, 1218–1228.

Lu, H. C., & Mackie, K. (2016). An introduction to the endogenous cannabinoid system. *Biological Psychiatry*, *79*(7), 516–525.

Maccarrone, M., Guzman, M., Mackie, K., Doherty, P., & Harkany, T. (2014). Programming of neural cells by (endo)cannabinoids: From physiological rules to emerging therapies. *Nature Reviews. Neuroscience*, *15*(12), 786–801.

Mahavadi, S., Sriwai, W., Huang, J., Grider, J. R., & Murthy, K. S. (2014). Inhibitory signaling by CB1 receptors in smooth muscle mediated by GRK5/beta-arrestin activation of ERK1/2 and Src kinase. *American Journal of Physiology. Gastrointestinal and Liver Physiology*, *306*(6), G535–G545.

Mahmoud Gouda, H., & Mohamed Kamel, N. R. (2013). Cannabinoid CB2 receptor gene (CNR2) polymorphism is associated with chronic childhood immune thrombocytopenia in Egypt. *Blood Coagulation & Fibrinolysis*, *24*(3), 247–251.

Martin, B. R., Dewey, W. L., Harris, L. S., & Beckner, J. S. (1976). 3H-delta9-tetrahydrocannabinol tissue and subcellular distribution in the central nervous system and tissue distribution in peripheral organs of tolerant and nontolerant dogs. *The Journal of Pharmacology and Experimental Therapeutics*, *196*(1), 128–144.

Matias, I., Gonthier, M. P., Orlando, P., Martiadis, V., De Petrocellis, L., Cervino, C., et al. (2006). Regulation, function, and dysregulation of endocannabinoids in models of adipose and beta-pancreatic cells and in obesity and hyperglycemia. *The Journal of Clinical Endocrinology and Metabolism*, *91*(8), 3171–3180.

Matsuda, L. A., Lolait, S. J., Brownstein, M. J., Young, A. C., & Bonner, T. I. (1990). Structure of a cannabinoid receptor and functional expression of the cloned cDNA. *Nature*, *346*(6284), 561–564.

McAllister, S. D., & Glass, M. (2002). CB(1) and CB(2) receptor-mediated signalling: A focus on endocannabinoids. *Prostaglandins, Leukotrienes, and Essential Fatty Acids*, *66*(2–3), 161–171.

McKinney, D. L., Cassidy, M. P., Collier, L. M., Martin, B. R., Wiley, J. L., Selley, D. E., et al. (2008). Dose-related differences in the regional pattern of cannabinoid receptor adaptation and in vivo tolerance development to delta9-tetrahydrocannabinol. *The Journal of Pharmacology and Experimental Therapeutics*, *324*(2), 664–673.

McPartland, J. M. (2004). Phylogenomic and chemotaxonomic analysis of the endocannabinoid system. *Brain Research. Brain Research Reviews*, *45*(1), 18–29.

McPartland, J. M., & Glass, M. (2003). Functional mapping of cannabinoid receptor homologs in mammals, other vertebrates, and invertebrates. *Gene*, *312*, 297–303.

McPartland, J. M., Glass, M., Matias, I., Norris, R. W., & Kilpatrick, C. W. (2007a). A shifted repertoire of endocannabinoid genes in the zebrafish (*Danio rerio*). *Molecular Genetics and Genomics*, *277*(5), 555–570.

McPartland, J. M., Glass, M., & Pertwee, R. G. (2007b). Meta-analysis of cannabinoid ligand binding affinity and receptor distribution: Interspecies differences. *British Journal of Pharmacology*, *152*(5), 583–593.

Mechoulam, R., Ben-Shabat, S., Hanus, L., Ligumsky, M., Kaminski, N. E., Schatz, A. R., et al. (1995). Identification of an endogenous 2-monoglyceride, present in canine gut, that binds to cannabinoid receptors. *Biochemical Pharmacology*, *50*(1), 83–90.

Mechoulam, R., & Fride, E. (1995). The unpaved road to the endogenous cannabinoid ligand anandamide. *Cannabinoids*, 233–258.

Mendez-Sanchez, N., Zamora-Valdes, D., Pichardo-Bahena, R., Barredo-Prieto, B., Ponciano-Rodriguez, G., Bermejo-Martinez, L., et al. (2007). Endocannabinoid receptor CB2 in nonalcoholic fatty liver disease. *Liver International*, *27*(2), 215–219.

Merial-Kieny, C., Lonchampt, M., Coge, F., Verwaerde, P., Galizzi, J. P., Boutin, J. A., et al. (2003). Endothelin-1 inhibits TNF alpha-induced iNOS expression in 3T3-F442A adipocytes. *British Journal of Pharmacology*, *139*(5), 935–944.

Minocci, D., Massei, J., Martino, A., Milianti, M., Piz, L., Di Bello, D., et al. (2011). Genetic association between bipolar disorder and 524A>C (Leu133Ile) polymorphism of CNR2 gene, encoding for CB2 cannabinoid receptor. *Journal of Affective Disorders*, *134*(1–3), 427–430.

Morrow, V. A., Foufelle, F., Connell, J. M., Petrie, J. R., Gould, G. W., & Salt, I. P. (2003). Direct activation of AMP-activated protein kinase stimulates nitric-oxide synthesis in human aortic endothelial cells. *The Journal of Biological Chemistry*, *278*(34), 31629–31639.

Mukhopadhyay, B., Liu, J., Osei-Hyiaman, D., Godlewski, G., Mukhopadhyay, P., Wang, L., et al. (2010). Transcriptional regulation of cannabinoid receptor-1 expression in the liver by retinoic acid acting via retinoic acid receptor-gamma. *The Journal of Biological Chemistry*, *285*(25), 19002–19011.

Munro, S., Thomas, K. L., & Abu-Shaar, M. (1993). Molecular characterization of a peripheral receptor for cannabinoids. *Nature*, *365*(6441), 61–65.

Murphy, W. J., Eizirik, E., Johnson, W. E., Zhang, Y. P., Ryder, O. A., & O'Brien, S. J. (2001). Molecular phylogenetics and the origins of placental mammals. *Nature*, *409*(6820), 614–618.

Navarro, G., Morales, P., Rodriguez-Cueto, C., Fernandez-Ruiz, J., Jagerovic, N., & Franco, R. (2016). Targeting cannabinoid CB2 receptors in the central nervous system. Medicinal chemistry approaches with focus on neurodegenerative disorders. *Frontiers in Neuroscience*, *10*, 406.

Ndong, C., O'Donnell, D., Ahmad, S., & Groblewski, T. (2011). Cloning and pharmacological characterization of the dog cannabinoid CB(2)receptor. *European Journal of Pharmacology*, *669*(1–3), 24–31.

Nguyen, P. T., Schmid, C. L., Raehal, K. M., Selley, D. E., Bohn, L. M., & Sim-Selley, L. J. (2012). Beta-arrestin2 regulates cannabinoid CB1 receptor signaling and adaptation in a central nervous system region-dependent manner. *Biological Psychiatry*, *71*(8), 714–724.

Nisoli, E., & Carruba, M. O. (2006). Nitric oxide and mitochondrial biogenesis. *Journal of Cell Science*, *119*(Pt. 14), 2855–2862.

Oliveira da Cruz, J. F., Robin, L. M., Drago, F., Marsicano, G., & Metna-Laurent, M. (2016). Astroglial type-1 cannabinoid receptor (CB1): A new player in the tripartite synapse. *Neuroscience*, *323*, 35–42.

Onaivi, E. S., Ishiguro, H., Gong, J. P., Patel, S., Meozzi, P. A., Myers, L., et al. (2008a). Functional expression of brain neuronal CB2 cannabinoid receptors are involved in the effects of drugs of abuse and in depression. *Annals of the New York Academy of Sciences*, *1139*, 434–449.

Onaivi, E. S., Ishiguro, H., Gong, J. P., Patel, S., Meozzi, P. A., Myers, L., et al. (2008b). Brain neuronal CB2 cannabinoid receptors in drug abuse and depression: From mice to human subjects. *PLoS One*, *3*(2), e1640.

Osei-Hyiaman, D., DePetrillo, M., Pacher, P., Liu, J., Radaeva, S., Batkai, S., et al. (2005). Endocannabinoid activation at hepatic CB1 receptors stimulates fatty acid synthesis and contributes to diet-induced obesity. *Journal of Clinical Investigation*, *115*(5), 1298–1305.

Osei-Hyiaman, D., Liu, J., Zhou, L., Godlewski, G., Harvey-White, J., Jeong, W. I., et al. (2008). Hepatic CB1 receptor is required for development of diet-induced steatosis, dyslipidemia, and insulin and leptin resistance in mice. *Journal of Clinical Investigation*, *118*(9), 3160–3169.

Oviedo, A., Glowa, J., & Herkenham, M. (1993). Chronic cannabinoid administration alters cannabinoid receptor binding in rat brain: A quantitative autoradiographic study. *Brain Research*, *616*, 293–302.

Pai, W. Y., Hsu, C. C., Lai, C. Y., Chang, T. Z., Tsai, Y. L., & Her, G. M. (2013). Cannabinoid receptor 1 promotes hepatic lipid accumulation and lipotoxicity through the induction of SREBP-1c expression in zebrafish. *Transgenic Research*, *22*, 823–838.

Pertwee, R. G., Howlett, A. C., Abood, M. E., Alexander, S. P., Di Marzo, V., Elphick, M. R., et al. (2010). International Union of Basic and Clinical Pharmacology. LXXIX. Cannabinoid receptors and their ligands: Beyond CB and CB. *Pharmacological Reviews*, *62*(4), 588–631.

Puighermanal, E., Marsicano, G., Busquets-Garcia, A., Lutz, B., Maldonado, R., & Ozaita, A. (2009). Cannabinoid modulation of hippocampal long-term memory is mediated by mTOR signaling. *Nature Neuroscience*, *12*(9), 1152–1158.

Rinaldi-Carmona, M., Barth, F., Heaulme, M., Shire, D., Calandra, B., Congy, C., et al. (1994). SR141716A, a potent and selective antagonist of the brain cannabinoid receptor. *FEBS Letters*, *350*(2–3), 240–244.

Rinaldi-Carmona, M., Barth, F., Millan, J., Derocq, J. M., Casellas, P., Congy, C., et al. (1998). SR 144528, the first potent and selective antagonist of the CB2 cannabinoid receptor. *The Journal of Pharmacology and Experimental Therapeutics*, *284*(2), 644–650.

Rodriguez de Fonseca, F., Gorriti, M. A., Fernandez-Ruiz, J. J., Palomo, T., & Ramos, J. A. (1994). Downregulation of rat brain cannabinoid binding sites after chronic delta 9-tetrahydrocannabinol treatment. *Pharmacology, Biochemistry, and Behavior, 47*(1), 33–40.

Romero, J., Garcia-Palomero, E., Castro, J. G., Garcia-Gil, L., Ramos, J. A., & Fernandez-Ruiz, J. J. (1997). Effects of chronic exposure to delta9-tetrahydrocannabinol on cannabinoid receptor binding and mRNA levels in several rat brain regions. *Brain Research Molecular Brain Research, 46*(1–2), 100–108.

Ruby, M. A., Nomura, D. K., Hudak, C. S., Mangravite, L. M., Chiu, S., Casida, J. E., et al. (2008). Overactive endocannabinoid signaling impairs apolipoprotein E-mediated clearance of triglyceride-rich lipoproteins. *Proceedings of the National Academy of Sciences of the United States of America, 105*(38), 14561–14566.

Ruiz-Contreras, A. E., Roman-Lopez, T. V., Caballero-Sanchez, U., Rosas-Escobar, C. B., Ortega-Mora, E. I., Barrera-Tlapa, M. A., et al. (2016). Because difficulty is not the same for everyone: The impact of complexity in working memory is associated with cannabinoid 1 receptor genetic variation in young adults. *Memory, 25*, 335–343. 1–9.

Russo, E. B. (2008). Clinical endocannabinoid deficiency (CECD): Can this concept explain therapeutic benefits of cannabis in migraine, fibromyalgia, irritable bowel syndrome and other treatment-resistant conditions? *Neuro Endocrinology Letters, 29*(2), 192–200.

Ryberg, E., Vu, H. K., Larsson, N., Groblewski, T., Hjorth, S., Elebring, T., et al. (2005). Identification and characterisation of a novel splice variant of the human CB1 receptor. *FEBS Letters, 579*(1), 259–264.

Sanchez, C., de Ceballos, M. L., Gomez del Pulgar, T., Rueda, D., Corbacho, C., Velasco, G., et al. (2001). Inhibition of glioma growth in vivo by selective activation of the CB(2) cannabinoid receptor. *Cancer Research, 61*(15), 5784–5789.

Schaller, M. D. (2010). Cellular functions of FAK kinases: Insight into molecular mechanisms and novel functions. *Journal of Cell Science, 123*(Pt. 7), 1007–1013.

Shire, D., Calandra, B., Rinaldi-Carmona, M., Oustric, D., Pessegue, B., Bonnin-Cabanne, O., et al. (1996). Molecular cloning, expression and function of the murine CB2 peripheral cannabinoid receptor. *Biochimica et Biophysica Acta, 1307*(2), 132–136.

Shire, D., Carillon, C., Kaghad, M., Calandra, B., Rinaldi-Carmona, M., Le Fur, G., et al. (1995). An amino-terminal variant of the central cannabinoid receptor resulting from alternative splicing. *The Journal of Biological Chemistry, 270*(8), 3726–3731.

Sipe, J. C., Arbour, N., Gerber, A., & Beutler, E. (2005). Reduced endocannabinoid immune modulation by a common cannabinoid 2 (CB2) receptor gene polymorphism: Possible risk for autoimmune disorders. *Journal of Leukocyte Biology, 78*(1), 231–238. Epub 2005 Apr 21.

Soderstrom, K., Leid, M., Moore, F. L., & Murray, T. F. (2000). Behavioral, pharmacological, and molecular characterization of an amphibian cannabinoid receptor. *Journal of Neurochemistry, 75*(1), 413–423.

Soethoudt, M., Grether, U., Fingerle, J., Grim, T. W., Fezza, F., de Petrocellis, L., et al. (2017). Cannabinoid CB2 receptor ligand profiling reveals biased signalling and off-target activity. *Nature Communications, 8*, 13958.

Song, Z. H., & Bonner, T. I. (1996). A lysine residue of the cannabinoid receptor is critical for receptor recognition by several agonists but not WIN55212-2. *Molecular Pharmacology, 49*(5), 891–896.

Stella, N. (2010). Cannabinoid and cannabinoid-like receptors in microglia, astrocytes, and astrocytomas. *Glia, 58*(9), 1017–1030.

Straiker, A., Wager-Miller, J., Hutchens, J., & Mackie, K. (2012). Differential signalling in human cannabinoid CB1 receptors and their splice variants in autaptic hippocampal neurones. *British Journal of Pharmacology, 165*(8), 2660–2671.

Sugiura, T., Kondo, S., Sukagawa, A., Nakane, S., Shinoda, A., Itoh, K., et al. (1995). 2-Arachidonoylglycerol: A possible endogenous cannabinoid receptor ligand in brain. *Biochemical and Biophysical Research Communications*, *215*(1), 89–97.

Szabo, B., & Schlicker, E. (2005). Effects of cannabinoids on neurotransmission. *Handbook of Experimental Pharmacology*, *168*, 327–365.

Tam, J., Liu, J., Mukhopadhyay, B., Cinar, R., Godlewski, G., & Kunos, G. (2011). Endocannabinoids in liver disease. *Hepatology*, *53*(1), 346–355.

Tam, J., Vemuri, V. K., Liu, J., Batkai, S., Mukhopadhyay, B., Godlewski, G., et al. (2010). Peripheral CB1 cannabinoid receptor blockade improves cardiometabolic risk in mouse models of obesity. *Journal of Clinical Investigation*, *120*(8), 2953–2966.

Tedesco, L., Valerio, A., Cervino, C., Cardile, A., Pagano, C., Vettor, R., et al. (2008). Cannabinoid type 1 receptor blockade promotes mitochondrial biogenesis through endothelial nitric oxide synthase expression in white adipocytes. *Diabetes*, *57*(8), 2028–2036.

Tedesco, L., Valerio, A., Dossena, M., Cardile, A., Ragni, M., Pagano, C., et al. (2010). Cannabinoid receptor stimulation impairs mitochondrial biogenesis in mouse white adipose tissue, muscle, and liver: The role of eNOS, p38 MAPK, and AMPK pathways. *Diabetes*, *59*(11), 2826–2836.

Teixeira-Clerc, F., Julien, B., Grenard, P., Tran Van Nhieu, J., Deveaux, V., Li, L., et al. (2006). CB1 cannabinoid receptor antagonism: A new strategy for the treatment of liver fibrosis. *Nature Medicine*, *12*(6), 671–676.

Tsou, K., Brown, S., Sanudo-Pena, M. C., Mackie, K., & Walker, J. M. (1998). Immunohistochemical distribution of cannabinoid CB1 receptors in the rat central nervous system. *Neuroscience*, *83*(2), 393–411.

Turcotte, C., Blanchet, M. R., Laviolette, M., & Flamand, N. (2016). The CB2 receptor and its role as a regulator of inflammation. *Cellular and Molecular Life Sciences*, *73*(23), 4449–4470.

Turu, G., & Hunyady, L. (2010). Signal transduction of the CB1 cannabinoid receptor. *Journal of Molecular Endocrinology*, *44*(2), 75–85.

Ujike, H., Takaki, M., Nakata, K., Tanaka, Y., Takeda, T., Kodama, M., et al. (2002). CNR1, central cannabinoid receptor gene, associated with susceptibility to hebephrenic schizophrenia. *Molecular Psychiatry*, *7*(5), 515–518.

Valerio, A., Cardile, A., Cozzi, V., Bracale, R., Tedesco, L., Pisconti, A., et al. (2006). TNF-alpha downregulates eNOS expression and mitochondrial biogenesis in fat and muscle of obese rodents. *Journal of Clinical Investigation*, *116*(10), 2791–2798.

Valk, P. J., Hol, S., Vankan, Y., Ihle, J. N., Askew, D., Jenkins, N. A., et al. (1997). The genes encoding the peripheral cannabinoid receptor and alpha-L-fucosidase are located near a newly identified common virus integration site, Evi11. *Journal of Virology*, *71*(9), 6796–6804.

Van Sickle, M. D., Duncan, M., Kingsley, P. J., Mouihate, A., Urbani, P., Mackie, K., et al. (2005). Identification and functional characterization of brainstem cannabinoid CB2 receptors. *Science*, *310*(5746), 329–332.

Wu, H. M., Yang, Y. M., & Kim, S. G. (2011). Rimonabant, a cannabinoid receptor type 1 inverse agonist, inhibits hepatocyte lipogenesis by activating liver kinase B1 and AMP-activated protein kinase axis downstream of Galpha i/o inhibition. *Molecular Pharmacology*, *80*(5), 859–869.

Xiao, J. C., Jewell, J. P., Lin, L. S., Hagmann, W. K., Fong, T. M., & Shen, C. P. (2008). Similar in vitro pharmacology of human cannabinoid CB1 receptor variants expressed in CHO cells. *Brain Research*, *1238*, 36–43.

Xie, X. Q., Chen, J. Z., & Billings, E. M. (2003). 3D structural model of the G-protein-coupled cannabinoid CB2 receptor. *Proteins*, *53*(2), 307–319.

Xie, X. Q., Melvin, L. S., & Makriyannis, A. (1996). The conformational properties of the highly selective cannabinoid receptor ligand CP-55,940. *The Journal of Biological Chemistry*, *271*(18), 10640–10647.

Yamada, Y., Ando, F., & Shimokata, H. (2007). Association of candidate gene polymorphisms with bone mineral density in community-dwelling Japanese women and men. *International Journal of Molecular Medicine*, *19*(5), 791–801.

Yamaguchi, F., Macrae, A. D., & Brenner, S. (1996). Molecular cloning of two cannabinoid type 1-like receptor genes from the puffer fish Fugu rubripes. *Genomics*, *35*(3), 603–605.

You, M., Fischer, M., Deeg, M. A., & Crabb, D. W. (2002). Ethanol induces fatty acid synthesis pathways by activation of sterol regulatory element-binding protein (SREBP). *The Journal of Biological Chemistry*, *277*(32), 29342–29347.

Zhang, P. W., Ishiguro, H., Ohtsuki, T., Hess, J., Carillo, F., Walther, D., et al. (2004). Human cannabinoid receptor 1: 5′ exons, candidate regulatory regions, polymorphisms, haplotypes and association with polysubstance abuse. *Molecular Psychiatry*, *9*(10), 916–931.

Zhuang, S., Kittler, J., Grigorenko, E. V., Kirby, M. T., Sim, L. J., Hampson, R. E., et al. (1998). Effects of long-term exposure to delta9-THC on expression of cannabinoid receptor (CB1) mRNA in different rat brain regions. *Brain Research. Molecular Brain Research*, *62*(2), 141–149.

Zorina, Y., Iyengar, R., & Bromberg, K. D. (2010). Cannabinoid 1 receptor and interleukin-6 receptor together induce integration of protein kinase and transcription factor signaling to trigger neurite outgrowth. *The Journal of Biological Chemistry*, *285*(2), 1358–1370.

CHAPTER SIX

Functional Selectivity at Cannabinoid Receptors

Richard Priestley*, Michelle Glass†, David Kendall‡,1

*Alzheimer's Research UK Drug Discovery Institute, University of Oxford, Oxford, United Kingdom
†Faculty of Medical and Health Sciences, University of Auckland, Auckland, New Zealand
‡PharmNovo UK Ltd. and School of Pharmacy and Biomolecular Sciences, Liverpool John Moores University, Liverpool, United Kingdom
[1]Corresponding author. e-mail address: david.kendall@pharmnovo.com

Contents

Abstract

It is now clear that, in contrast to traditional descriptions of G protein-coupled receptor signaling, agonists can activate or inhibit characteristic patterns of downstream effector pathways depending on their structures and the conformational changes induced in the receptor. This is referred to as functional selectivity (also known as agonist-directed trafficking, ligand-induced differential signaling, or biased agonism). It is important because even small structural differences can result in significant variations in overall agonist effects (wanted and unwanted) depending on which postreceptor signaling systems are engaged by each agonist/receptor pairing.

In addition to the canonical signaling pathways mediated by $G_{i/o}$ proteins, CB_1 and CB_2 receptor agonists can have effects via differential activation not only of G_i subtypes but also of G_s and $G_{q/11}$ proteins. For example, the classical cannabinoid HU-210 produces maximal activation of both G_i and G_o proteins, while the endocannabinoid anandamide and aminoalkylindole WIN 55,212 both produce maximal activation of G_i, but submaximal activation of G_o. Cannabinoid agonists can also signal differentially via β-arrestins coupled to mitogen-activated protein kinases, subsequently promoting varying degrees of receptor internalization and agonist desensitization.

Advances in Pharmacology, Volume 80
ISSN 1054-3589
http://dx.doi.org/10.1016/bs.apha.2017.03.005

A recent extensive characterization of the molecular pharmacology of CB_2 agonists (Soethoudt et al., 2017) identified marked differences (bias) in the ability of certain agonists to activate distinct signaling pathways (cAMP accumulation, ERK phosphorylation, GIRK activation, GTPγS binding, and β-arrestin recruitment) and to cause off-target effects, exemplifying the need to evaluate functional selectivity in agonist drug development.

ABBREVIATIONS

cAMP cyclic adenosine monophosphate
ERK extracellular signal-regulated kinase
GIRK G protein-coupled inwardly rectifying potassium channels
MAP mitogen-activated protein kinase
PI3K phosphatidylinositol 3-kinase

1. INTRODUCTION

A basic tenet of pharmacological theory is the distinction between antagonist drugs that occupy but cannot activate receptors and agonists that both occupy and activate receptors, in essence acting, metaphorically, as the classical key in the lock. Thus, it has been held for decades that G protein-coupled receptors (GPCRs) exist in one of two distinct structural conformations—an active conformational state (R*) which couples to and activates downstream effectors, and an inactive state (R) which does not. It is assumed that, in the basal condition, both states exist in some sort of balance, making a variable degree of constitutive activity possible. Occupation by an agonist is then proposed to shift the balance in one direction or another with classical agonists (R* preferring) promoting a spectrum of activation, reflecting partial or full agonist efficacy. On the other hand, drugs which preferentially bind to the (R) state shift the balance toward inactivity and they are referred to as inverse agonists (Kenakin, 2007). Neutral antagonists, by definition, cannot distinguish one state from another and, therefore, produce no change in basal receptor activity.

This concept of *intrinsic efficacy* can be interpreted as receptors acting as simple on/off switches, an idea that has clearly become unfit for purpose given abundant evidence that different agonists, with equivalent selectivity for a given receptor, can have quite different pharmacological properties (Kenakin & Christopoulos, 2013). Over the years, a variety of pharmacological texts and reviews have attempted to characterize GPCRs on the basis of their coupling to particular postreceptor signaling systems. For example, in relation to the adrenoceptor family, the dogma was that β-receptors activate G_s proteins, α_2-receptors $G_{i/o}$, and α_1-receptors G_q. These relationships with particular G protein families are certainly the most common and can be considered to be the canonical (i.e., established) signaling mechanisms for these receptors. However, under certain circumstances (e.g., cardiovascular disease) signaling preference can change and, for example, cardiac β-adrenoceptors can then activate G_i proteins (Melsom et al., 2014). Furthermore, an individual drug can activate different signaling pathways in particular circumstances. For example, morphine acting via μ-opioid receptors is well known to inhibit cyclic AMP formation promoting analgesia, and short-term morphine treatment achieves this by activation of inhibitory $G\alpha_{i/o}$ proteins. However, after long-term morphine treatment in rats, there is a switch from $G\alpha_{i/o}$ to stimulatory $G\alpha_s$ coupling and morphine then stimulates cyclic AMP formation in a variety of brain regions causing hyperalgesia (Wang & Burns, 2006).

These and many other similar examples imply that GPCRs, like other proteins, can adopt *multiple* distinct structural conformations and, importantly, more than one active conformational state (i.e., R^{*1}, R^{*2}, R^{*3}, R^{*n}). Most GPCRs, including the cannabinoid receptors, orthosterically bind a number of structurally distinct endogenous and exogenous ligands and each ligand may then stabilize a subset of active receptor conformations with each active conformation exhibiting differential affinity for downstream effectors, resulting in ligand-dependent receptor signaling. This concept has been termed functional selectivity (also known as agonist-directed trafficking, ligand-induced differential signaling, or biased agonism) and can be defined as the ability of a ligand to differently activate specific signaling pathways. This can be expressed as differences in ligand potency and/or intrinsic activity in relation to a functional effect (e.g., activation of a particular effector/second messenger) compared to one or more others (Hudson, Hebert, & Kelly, 2010; Urban et al., 2007).

2. WHY DOES FUNCTIONAL SELECTIVITY MATTER?

In the absence of functional selectivity, if two structurally distinct agonists had the same receptor selectivity and very similar pharmacokinetic profiles, then their pharmacological effects in vivo would be expected to be very similar. However, the concept of functional selectivity allows that even small structural differences could result in significant variation in overall effect depending on which postreceptor signaling systems were engaged by each agonist/receptor pairing. A recent pertinent example of how functional selectivity can determine therapeutically important pharmacological properties of agonists is reported by Manglik et al. (2016). They have developed a μ-opioid receptor agonist, PZM21, which is a full agonist with regard to $G_{i/o}$ signaling but which has minimal ability to recruit the adaptor protein β-arrestin-2. PZM21 is similar to morphine with regard to its analgesic efficacy but, unlike morphine, PZM21 is devoid of both respiratory depression and reinforcing activity in mice at equianalgesic doses. Thus, understanding the spectrum of agonist signaling can facilitate the optimization of drugs' medicinal properties.

3. DETERMINATION OF FUNCTIONAL SELECTIVITY

Care must be taken to consider the broader effector system when investigating ligands with distinct functional profiles before concluding that true functional selectivity is present. First, ligands may be acting at more than one pharmacological target. This is certainly true of the cannabinoid signaling system, with ligands such as anandamide being able to activate the vanilloid TRPV1 receptor (Smart et al., 2000) and certain peroxisome proliferator-activated receptor subtypes (O'Sullivan, 2007), and non-CB_1/CB_2 cannabinoid-like receptors such as GPR55 and GPR119 which are yet to be fully characterized (Pertwee et al., 2010). The synthetic cannabinoid ligands, likewise, have been demonstrated to have many off-target effects (e.g., Taylor et al., 2015), and particular care must be taken, particularly with novel, largely uncharacterized compounds in complex systems, to ensure that effects are CB receptor-mediated. Next, partial agonists may be able to maximally activate a particular signaling pathway more strongly than other pathways. When compared to a full agonist maximally activating all coupled signaling pathways, the ligands would appear to have functionally distinct profiles. This phenomenon is known as a *strength-of-signal* effect and differs from true functional selectivity, whereby any receptor-coupled signaling pathway may be selectivity activated, not just the most strongly coupled one(s) (Kenakin, 2007).

Although functional selectivity is an inherent attribute of the receptor–ligand interaction, the receptor is part of a larger signaling complex which includes in addition to direct signaling effectors, mediators of desensitization and internalization, other receptors (with the possibility of forming both homo- and heteromers), and other modulatory proteins. All of these may have a direct and/or indirect effect on receptor function and pharmacology, including the apparent functional selectivity of agonists (Kenakin, 2007). The presence of such modulators is highly tissue/cell type dependent which means that ligand-selective differential signaling observed in one tissue type may be different or absent in another. Experimental conditions are vitally important to control and the extracellular environment, particularly the concentration of Na^+ and Mg^{2+} ions, can alter the receptor's conformational state which may directly affect the binding and functional profile of certain ligands.

It is clearly essential to be able to distinguish "true" functional selectivity from apparent bias introduced by inappropriate data analysis and interpretation. For example, "observational bias" can occur when the relative sensitivity of different assay methods determines the relative potency of agonists in those assays. Traditional quantification of agonist effects is unable to make valid comparisons of agonist signaling; using potency (pEC_{50} values) is inadequate for agonists that produce different maximal responses and using only maximal responses to quantify agonist activity cannot distinguish between full agonists which produce a stimulus that exceeds the signaling capabilities of the system (which would then all appear to be uniformly 100% effective). Thus, comparisons should be based on the calculation of a single parameter that allows statistical methods to be properly employed. It is becoming widely accepted that the theoretically most sound method of quantifying ligand bias in vitro is through ratios of transduction coefficients ($\Delta\Delta\log(\tau/KA)$) or ratios of changes in relative activity ($\Delta\Delta\log(RA)$), and readers are referred to the excellent review by Kenakin and Christopoulos (2013) for a full account of analytical methods and pitfalls.

4. FUNCTIONAL SELECTIVITY AT CANNABINOID RECEPTORS

Cannabinoid receptors provide a particularly appealing model to investigate functional selectivity for a number of reasons: first, members of the receptor family, particularly CB_1, are endogenously expressed in a wide array of mammalian cell and tissue types, as well as being widely expressed in neuronal tissue (Herkenham, 1991; Matsuda, Bonner, & Lolait, 1992). Next, as described below and in other chapters in this volume, cannabinoid receptors couple to multiple intracellular signaling pathways, which increase their potential for ligand-selective specific activation. The various structural groups of cannabinoid ligands may each bind to and activate different active receptor conformations and, with at least five putative endogenous endocannabinoid ligands each with the potential to produce differential signaling via cannabinoid receptors, this system provides a good model for investigating the role of functional selectivity in an endogenous system (Alexander & Kendall, 2007). Finally, the cannabinoid signaling system has huge potential as a target for therapeutic treatment of a number of disorders including pain, inflammation and a variety of psychiatric disorders (Scotter, Abood, & Glass, 2010). It may be possible, in the future, to develop functionally selective compounds which maximize positive effects, while minimizing activation of pathways associated with negative side effects. This is particularly true of compounds targeting CB_1 receptors which often produce unwanted (but on-target) psychotropic side effects.

4.1 Downstream Signaling via Cannabinoid Receptors

A large body of research has shown that both cannabinoid receptor subtypes (CB_1 and CB_2) couple predominantly to $G_{i/o}$ proteins (Howlett et al., 2002), whose activation inhibits adenylyl cyclase (AC) and thus production of cyclic AMP. This is considered to be the canonical signaling pathway. However, CB_1 receptors have been shown to activate other G proteins. Coupling to G_s has been shown in CB_1 receptor-transfected cells and cultured rat striatal neurons (Glass & Felder, 1997), in which cyclic AMP *accumulation* was observed upon stimulation with the CB_1/CB_2 receptor agonist HU-210 and blocked by the selective CB_1 receptor antagonist rimonabant. The structural basis for coupling of CB_1 receptors to both G_i and G_s has been described by Chen et al. (2010). CB_1 receptor-mediated activation of the G_q signaling pathway has also been shown (Lauckner, Hille, & Mackie, 2005), and suggested to be highly ligand dependent, with stimulation of CB_1 receptor-transfected HEK 293 cells and cultured mouse hippocampal neurons with the CB_1/CB_2 receptor agonist WIN 55,212-2 (but not other synthetic cannabinoids) increasing intracellular calcium levels blocked by the transfection of dominant-negative $G\alpha_q$ protein.

Both CB receptor subtypes have also been shown to couple positively to members of the mitogen-activated protein (MAP) kinase family of serine/threonine protein kinases which regulate a variety of cellular responses, including gene expression, growth, cellular transformation, and apoptosis (Pearson et al., 2001). CB_1 receptor-mediated activation of extracellular signal-regulated kinase (ERK) has been shown in U373MG human astrocytoma (Bouaboula et al., 1995), transfected CHO cells (Galve-Roperh, Rueda, Del Pulgar, Velasco, & Guzman, 2002), and Neuro 2a and N1E-115 (both murine neuroblastoma cell lines) (Bosier, Lambert, & Hermans, 2008; Graham et al., 2006), and via CB_2 receptors in HL-60 cells (Kobayashi, Arai, Waku, & Sugiura, 2001) with responses which were pertussis toxin-sensitive, suggesting the involvement of $G_{i/o}$ proteins. The mechanisms by which cannabinoid receptors activate MAP kinases have not been fully elucidated, but a number of pathways have been suggested, including direct actions via activation of phosphatidylinositol 3-kinase (PI3K) (Galve-Roperh et al., 2002). In addition, ERK activation can be mediated via β-arrestin-1 (Ahn, Mahmoud, Shim, & Kendall, 2013), which brings various components of the ERK signaling pathway into close proximity by acting as a protein scaffold (DeWire, Ahn, Lefkowitz, & Shenoy, 2007). β-Arrestin-2 does not appear to have a primary role in CB_1 receptor-mediated ERK signaling, but it is critical for CB_1 receptor internalization (Ahn et al., 2013; Delgado-Peraza et al., 2016). Some studies have shown that mutation of the putative CB_1 receptor G protein receptor kinase phosphorylation sites S426A/S430A to alanine resulted in lower levels of receptor internalization, reduced desensitization, and persistent activation of ERK independently from $G_{i/o}$, suggestive of a β-arrestin-mediated pathway (Daigle, Kearn, & Mackie, 2008), and the facility to bias CB_1 receptor signaling in this direction is a valuable experimental strategy (Delgado-Peraza et al., 2016; Morgan et al., 2014).

Stimulation of CB_1 receptors by different agonists leads to activation of G protein-coupled inwardly rectifying potassium channels (GIRKs) through pertussis toxin-sensitive $G_{i/o}$ proteins, and CB_1 receptor agonists can also inhibit the function of voltage-gated calcium channels (L, N, and P/Q types; see Turu & Hunyady, 2010). Caution in interpretation of agonist-biased signaling through ion channels is, however, necessary as some agents appear to interact with channel elements directly rather than via CB receptors (Pertwee, 2010).

5. CANNABINOID RECEPTOR AGONIST-SELECTIVE SIGNALING

As previously described, cannabinoid receptors predominantly couple to $G_{i/o}$ proteins. However, there are several subtypes of $G_{i/o}$ protein, with certain cannabinoid ligands having distinct selectivity for particular ones. Stimulation of CB_1 receptors exogenously expressed in Sf9 (*Spodoptera frugiperda*) cells with different cannabinoid ligands led to different levels of $G_{i/o}$ protein activation (Glass & Northup, 1999). The classical cannabinoid HU-210 produced maximal activation of both G_i and G_o proteins, while the endocannabinoid anandamide and aminoalkylindole WIN 55,212 both produced maximal activation of G_i, but submaximal activation of G_o. The phytocannabinoid THC produced submaximal activation of both G protein subtypes and the rank order of ligand potency was consistent for both G protein subtypes. Further study of ligand specificity for $G\alpha_i$ subtypes $G\alpha_i1$, $G\alpha_i2$, and $G\alpha_i3$, using a coimmunoprecipitation technique in N18TG2 neuroblastoma cells showed differential effects of chemically distinct ligands (Mukhopadhyay & Howlett, 2005). WIN 55,212-2 exhibited potency for all three subtypes investigated, while the tricyclic cannabinoid desacetyllevonantradol had potency for $G\alpha_i1$ and $G\alpha_i2$, but not $G\alpha_i3$, and the synthetic eicosanoid methanandamide only had an effect on $G\alpha_i3$. This ligand specificity appears to extend to G proteins of other families. In CHO cells exogenously expressing human CB_1 receptors, WIN 55,212-2 was a full agonist for G_i and G_s signaling pathways, measured by the inhibition and accumulation of cyclic AMP, respectively, in forskolin-stimulated cells (Bonhaus, Chang, Kwan, & Martin, 1998), whereas THC was a partial agonist for both signaling pathways. Interestingly, from a functional selectivity perspective, both the nonclassical cannabinoid CP 55,940 and anandamide exhibited significantly higher intrinsic activity at the G_i signaling pathway, acting as full agonists when measuring inhibition of cyclic AMP formation, but acting as partial agonists when measuring cyclic AMP accumulation. CB_1 receptor-mediated activation of $G_{q/11}$ protein also appears to be ligand selective. WIN 55,212-2 was able to stimulate G_q-dependent intracellular Ca^{2+} release in HEK cells via transfected CB_1 receptor activation (Lauckner et al., 2005). A series of other cannabinoid receptor ligands, including THC, HU-210, CP 55,940, and 2-AG, were unable to produce any response in the same assay.

The putative cannabinoid peptide ligands RVD- and VD-hemopressin (Hp) also appear to exhibit functional selectivity at the CB_1 receptor. The peptides produced quantitatively similar responses compared with HU-210 in a series of assays measuring functional consequences of receptor activation, including neuronal outgrowth in neuro 2A cells and internalization of myc-tagged CB_1 receptors expressed in CHO cells (Gomes et al., 2009). The profile of ERK phosphorylation differed between HU-210 and RVD-Hp, with the level and rate of increase in phospho-ERK being lower for RVD-Hp. The study also reported CB_1 receptor-mediated, ligand-selective release of Ca^{2+} from intracellular stores in neuro-2A cells. Treatment with RVD-Hp, HU-210, and the endocannabinoid 2-AG led to a sustained increase in Ca^{2+} levels; however, the RVD-Hp-mediated release was much faster and significantly larger. Interestingly, the effects of RVD-Hp on both pERK levels and intracellular Ca^{2+} levels were only partially blocked by pertussis toxin, whereas the response due to HU-210 was almost abolished, indicating differential G_i protein mediation. A further study showed that both RVD-Hp and VD-Hp were unable to promote G protein activation as measured by accumulation of [^{35}S]GTPγS in mice striatal and cerebellar membranes (Gomes et al., 2010). These results suggest that the peptide ligands activate a G_i-independent signaling pathway distinct from HU-210. One of the family of N-terminally extended peptides (designated Pepcan-12) exhibited potent negative allosteric modulation of orthosteric agonist-induced cAMP accumulation, [^{35}S]GTPγS binding, and CB_1 receptor internalization; therefore, caution is required in interpreting the effects of the RVD-Hp peptides.

Allosteric ligands which bind to sites distinct from the orthosteric site could theoretically generate quite markedly different receptor conformations, and there is a suggestion of highly biased signaling of the allosteric modulator ORG27569. This compound has been suggested to exhibit biased signaling toward ERK pathways via β-arrestin-1 (Ahn et al., 2013). However, this requires further investigation, as two more recent studies (Gamage, Anderson, & Abood, 2016; Khajehali et al., 2015) did not observe that ORG27569 alone induced ERK phosphorylation.

Although most of the work on cannabinoid agonist functional selectivity has been done in relation to the CB_1 receptor, CB_2 receptor signaling has been shown to exhibit bias. Shoemaker, Ruckle, Mayeux, and Prather (2005) reported that endocannabinoids seem to be more "efficient" agonists at CB_2 receptors relative to synthetic agonists such as CP-55,940. Atwood, Wager-Miller, Haskins, Straiker, and Mackie (2012) reported that WIN55,212-2 (and other aminoalkylindoles) failed to promote CB_2 receptor internalization, whereas CP55,940 robustly internalized the receptors. More recently, Dhopeshwarkar and Mackie (2016) investigated mouse CB_2 receptor-transfected HEK cells, signaling via G_i (inhibition of forskolin-stimulated cyclic AMP formation) compared with agonists' ability to recruit β-arrestin-2 and bias factors, were calculated. CP 55,940, AM1710, and A836339 were efficacious and unbiased agonists. On the other hand, 4-*O*-methylhonokiol, STS135, UR144 and GW833972A were more arrestin-biased with the remainder of the compounds tested being either cyclase-biased (particularly so in the cases of THC, 2-AG, HU-308, and MAM2201) and weakly efficacious, or ineffective at either pathway. It is interesting that the classic cannabinoids (L759633 and L759656), the aminoalkylindoles (AM2233 and GW405833) and the carboxamide derivative 4Q3C were inactive in both assays, suggesting that their cannabinoid activity is mediated by other signaling pathways (e.g., MAP kinase, ceramide, PI3K/Akt kinase). It was also notable that there was a good correlation between the agonists' ability to recruit arrestin and their efficacy in internalizing the CB_2 receptor, although whether the differences in internalization have functional consequences, such as variations in their capacity for agonist desensitization, is not known.

Soethoudt et al. (2017) have recently characterized a set of 18 commonly utilized cannabinoid ligands in a wide range of signaling assays (cyclic AMP, pERK, GIRK, GTPγS, and arrestin recruitment) in multiple species of CB_2 receptors. They demonstrated that THC, 2-AG, and (rac)-AM1241 behaved as the most biased agonists on human CB_2 receptors, with each stimulating their most preferred pathway >100-fold stronger than their least preferred pathway. Operational analysis on data from hCB_2 receptors revealed that THC showed statistically significant bias toward pERK signaling compared to β-arrestin and GTPγS. THC did not activate GIRK at any concentration tested, indicative of complete bias against this pathway. (rac)-AM1241 was biased toward β-arrestin coupling and pERK signaling compared to GIRK channel activation. JWH133 was moderately biased toward β-arrestin compared to GIRK, whereas both WIN 55,212-2 and JWH015 showed preference for GIRK compared to cyclic AMP signaling. Intriguingly, 2-AG and AEA had distinct profiles in signaling pathway activation, AEA showed preference for pERK and GIRK signaling compared to cyclic AMP, whereas 2-AG was significantly biased toward GIRK compared to G protein signaling. HU-910 and HU-308 were well-balanced ligands without significant bias toward any signal transduction pathway on the hCB_2 receptor. Importantly, however, this study highlighted species differences with HU-910, HU-308, and JWH133, demonstrating significant biased toward G protein signaling over β-arrestin coupling and cyclic AMP signaling regarding the mouse CB_2 receptor. This study also, intriguingly, provided a potential example of inverse agonist bias, with SR144528 demonstrating less potent antagonism of GIRK and pERK signaling than of cyclic AMP at the human receptor.

6. FUNCTIONAL SELECTIVITY IN COMPLEX SYSTEMS

A cautionary note that should be applied to many studies in this area is that model cells overexpressing CB receptors were used, and it is highly probable that the cellular context of where, how, and in what density the receptors are expressed will have an effect on the agonists' signaling profiles. Encouragingly, however, functional selectivity of CB receptor agonists has been demonstrated in more complex "natural" systems. For example, Diez-Alarcia et al. (2016) studied the pattern of G protein subunit stimulation triggered by three different cannabinoid ligands, THC, WIN 55,212-2, and ACEA in mouse brain cortex. The agonists were able to significantly stimulate, via CB_1 and/or CB_2, not only the classical inhibitory $G\alpha_{i/o}$ but also other G protein subunits such as $G\alpha_s$, $G\alpha_{q/11}$, and $G\alpha_{12/13}$; moreover, the specific pattern of G protein subunit activation was different depending on the ligand.

There is also evidence of cannabinoid functional selectivity in vivo. A structure/activity study of aminoalkylindole derivatives using the behavioral tetrad test demonstrated that while WIN 55,212-2 was more potent in inducing hypolocomotion than hypothermia and catalepsy, several WIN 55,212-2 derivatives were more potent in inducing catalepsy and hypothermia (Wiley et al., 1998). However, differences in the metabolism of ligands in vivo, the possible presence of multiple pharmacological targets and the complex patterns of receptor distribution in various tissues all act to complicate the mechanisms by which ligand-selective responses could occur in vivo. A more recent study (Bosier et al., 2012) has provided a clearer example of a true functionally selective response in vivo. In this study, although both HU-210 and CP 55,940 induced hypolocomotion and catalepsy in male Wistar rats, only HU-210 was able to upregulate tyrosine hydroylase expression in the striatum, in a rimonabant-sensitive manner, despite both agonists exhibiting equivalent levels of brain penetration and receptor occupancy, as determined by ex vivo binding assays.

7. MECHANISMS OF FUNCTIONAL SELECTIVITY

A number of structural studies point to potential mechanisms by which cannabinoid functional selectivity might be mediated. CP 55,940 and WIN 55,212-2 have been shown to induce distinct conformational changes in CB_1 receptors upon binding (Georgieva et al., 2008). Use of the highly sensitive plasmon-wavelength resonance (PWR) spectroscopic technique showed that the two ligands produced changes in the PWR spectra of myc-His6-tagged receptors which were of similar magnitude, but in opposite directions. This study also showed that the abilities of these distinct receptor conformations to activate the G_i1 protein subtype were significantly different, with the WIN 55,212-2-induced receptor conformation being a much more potent signal transducer. Mutant CB_1 receptors with single residue substitutions at position L7.60 in the intracellular C-terminal helix 8 produced ligand-selective receptor activation profiles (Anavi-Goffer et al., 2007). Wild-type receptors containing a leucine residue at position L7.60 gave a maximal response upon stimulation with HU-210, CP 55,940, and WIN 55,212-2, but L7.60I mutation caused a significant decrease in the maximal response produced by all three ligands and a L7.60F mutation only caused a significant decrease in the maximal response produced by CP 55,940 and WIN 55,212-2. Further investigation showed that the H8 domain of the receptor is important in CB_1-$G\alpha_i3$ and $G\alpha_o$ coupling but not $G\alpha_i1$ and $G\alpha_i2$ (Anavi-Goffer et al., 2007). This research supports the contention that different ligands may preferentially activate signaling pathways through distinct receptor domains.

8. CONCLUSION

The lack of success to date of novel cannabinoids in the clinic is disappointing, but the complexity and specificity of cannabinoid receptor signaling networks provides the opportunity to develop new therapeutic compounds with programmed degrees of bias, possibly leading to optimal medicinal effects. For example, it appears that the avoidance of β-arrestin 2 coupling in the design of novel cannabinoid agonists might be advantageous. However, there is still much work to be done in understanding cell-specific CB signaling networks. Most studies have employed comparatively facile assay systems such as inhibition of cyclic AMP formation, arrestin recruitment, and MAP kinase activation, often using commercial kits and model cell lines. The challenge for the future is essentially to produce functional agonist bar codes, better describing the plethora of downstream signals that cascade following receptor activation in complex systems. An attractive possibility is the use of phosphoproteomic analysis as has begun to be applied in studies of the μ-opioid receptor (Moulédous, Froment, Burlet-Schiltz, Schulz, & Mollereau, 2015). The analysis and interpretation of the hugely complex data sets generated will then need to be correlated with relevant functional measures before proceeding to rational chemical design; no easy task but, perhaps, a tantalizing glimpse of the future of cannabinoid pharmacology and therapeutics.

CONFLICT OF INTEREST

The authors have no conflicts of interest to declare.

REFERENCES

Ahn, K. H., Mahmoud, M. M., Shim, J. Y., & Kendall, D. A. (2013). Distinct roles of beta-arrestin 1 and beta-arrestin 2 in ORG27569-induced biased signaling and internalization of the cannabinoid receptor 1 (CB1). *Journal of Biological Chemistry*, *288*, 9790–9800.

Alexander, S. P., & Kendall, D. A. (2007). The complications of promiscuity: Endocannabinoid action and metabolism. *British Journal of Pharmacology*, *152*, 602–623.

Anavi-Goffer, S., Fleischer, D., Hurst, D. P., Lynch, D. L., Barnett-Norris, J., Shi, S. P., et al. (2007). Helix 8 Leu in the CB1 cannabinoid receptor contributes to selective signal transduction mechanisms. *Journal of Biological Chemistry*, *282*, 25100–25113.

Atwood, B. K., Wager-Miller, J., Haskins, C., Straiker, A., & Mackie, K. (2012). Functional selectivity in CB(2) cannabinoid receptor signaling and regulation: Implications for the therapeutic potential of CB(2) ligands. *Molecular Pharmacology*, *81*, 250–263.

Bonhaus, D. W., Chang, L. K., Kwan, J., & Martin, G. R. (1998). Dual activation and inhibition of adenylyl cyclase by cannabinoid receptor agonists: Evidence for agonist-specific trafficking of intracellular responses. *Journal of Pharmacology and Experimental Therapeutics*, *287*, 884–888.

Bosier, B., Lambert, D. M., & Hermans, E. (2008). Reciprocal influences of CB1 cannabinoid receptor agonists on ERK and JNK signalling in N1E-115 cells. *FEBS Letters*, *582*, 3861–3867.

Bosier, B., Muccioli, G. G., Mertens, B., Sarre, S., Michotte, Y., Lambert, D. M., et al. (2012). Differential modulations of striatal tyrosine hydroxylase and dopamine metabolism by cannabinoid agonists as evidence for functional selectivity *in vivo*. *Neuropharmacology*, *62*, 2328–2336.

Bouaboula, M., Poinotchazel, C., Bourrie, B., Canat, X., Calandra, B., Rinaldicarmona, M., et al. (1995). Activation of mitogen-activated protein kinases by stimulation of the central cannabinoid receptor CB1. *The Biochemical Journal*, *312*, 637–641.

Chen, X. P., Yang, W., Fan, Y., Luo, J. S., Hong, K., Wang, Z., et al. (2010). Structural determinants in the second intracellular loop of the human cannabinoid CB1 receptor mediate selective coupling to G(s) and G(i). *British Journal of Pharmacology*, *16*, 1817–1834.

Daigle, T. L., Kearn, C. S., & Mackie, K. (2008). Rapid CB_1 cannabinoid receptor desensitization defines the time course of ERK1/2 MAP kinase signaling. *Neuropharmacology*, *54*, 6–44.

Delgado-Peraza, F., Ahn, K. H., Nogueras-Ortiz, C., Mungrue, I. N., Mackie, K., Kendall, D. A., et al. (2016). Mechanisms of biased β-arrestin-mediated signaling downstream from the cannabinoid 1 receptor. *Molecular Pharmacology*, *89*, 618–629.

DeWire, S. M., Ahn, S., Lefkowitz, R. J., & Shenoy, S. K. (2007). Beta-arrestins and cell signaling. *Annual Review of Physiology*, *69*, 483–510.

Dhopeshwarkar, A., & Mackie, K. (2016). Functional selectivity of CB2 cannabinoid receptor ligands at a canonical and noncanonical pathway. *The Journal of Pharmacology and Experimental Therapeutics*, *358*, 342–351.

Diez-Alarcia, R., Ibarra-Lecue, I., Lopez-Cardona, Á. P., Meana, J., Gutierrez-Adán, A., Callado, L. F., et al. (2016). Biased agonism of three different cannabinoid receptor agonists in mouse brain cortex. *Frontiers in Pharmacology*, 7, 415.

Galve-Roperh, I., Rueda, D., Del Pulgar, T. G., Velasco, G., & Guzman, M. (2002). Mechanism of extracellular signal-regulated kinase activation by the CB1 cannabinoid receptor. *Molecular Pharmacology*, *62*, 1385–1392.

Gamage, T. F., Anderson, J. C., & Abood, M. E. (2016). CB1 Allosteric modulator ORG27569 is an antagonist/inverse agonist of ERK1/2 signalling. *Cannabis and Cannabinoid Research*, *1*(1), 272–280.

Georgieva, T., Devanathan, S., Stropova, D., Park, C. K., Salamon, Z., Tollin, G., et al. (2008). Unique agonist-bound cannabinoid CB1 receptor conformations indicate agonist specificity in signaling. *European Journal of Pharmacology*, *581*, 19–29.

Glass, M., & Felder, C. C. (1997). Concurrent stimulation of cannabinoid CB1 and dopamine D2 receptors augments cAMP accumulation in striatal neurons: Evidence for a G(s) linkage to the CB1 receptor. *Journal of Neuroscience*, *17*, 5327–5333.

Glass, M., & Northup, J. K. (1999). Agonist selective regulation of G proteins by cannabinoid CB1 and CB2 receptors. *Molecular Pharmacology*, *56*, 1362–1369.

Gomes, I., Dale, C. S., Casten, K., Geigner, M. A., Gozzo, F. C., Ferro, E. S., et al. (2010). Hemoglobin-derived peptides as novel type of bioactive signaling molecules. *The AAPS Journal*, *12*, 658–669.

Gomes, I., Grushko, J. S., Golebiewska, U., Hoogendoorn, S., Gupta, A., Heimann, A. S., et al. (2009). Novel endogenous peptide agonists of cannabinoid receptors. *FASEB Journal*, *23*, 3020–3029.

Graham, E. S., Ball, N., Scotter, E. L., Narayan, P., Dragunow, M., & Glass, M. (2006). Induction of Krox-24 by endogenous cannabinoid type 1 receptors in Neuro2a cells is mediated by the MEK-ERK MAPK pathway and is suppressed by the phosphatidylinositol 3-kinase pathway. *Journal of Biological Chemistry*, *281*, 29085–29095.

Herkenham, M. (1991). Characterization and localization of cannabinoid receptors in brain: An in vitro technique using slide-mounted tissue sections. *NIDA Research Monograph*, *112*, 129–145.

Howlett, A. C., Barth, F., Bonner, T. I., Cabral, G., Casellas, P., Devane, W. A., et al. (2002). International Union of Pharmacology. XXVII. Classification of cannabinoid receptors. *Pharmacological Reviews*, *54*, 161–202.

Hudson, B. D., Hebert, T. E., & Kelly, M. E. M. (2010). Ligand- and heterodimer-directed signaling of the CB_1 cannabinoid receptor. *Molecular Pharmacology*, *77*, 1–9.

Kenakin, T. (2007). Functional selectivity through protean and biased agonism: Who steers the ship? *Molecular Pharmacology*, *72*, 1393–1401.

Kenakin, T., & Christopoulos, A. (2013). Signalling bias in new drug discovery: Detection, quantification and therapeutic impact. *Nature Reviews. Drug Discovery*, *12*, 205–216.

Khajehali, E., Malone, D. T., Glass, M., Sexton, P. M., Christopoulos, A., & Leach, K. (2015). Biased agonism and biased allosteric modulation at the CB1 cannabinoid receptor. *Molecular Pharmacology*, *88*, 68–79.

Kobayashi, Y., Arai, S., Waku, K., & Sugiura, T. (2001). Activation by 2-arachidonoylglycerol, an endogenous cannabinoid receptor ligand, of p42/44 mitogen-activated protein kinase in HL-60 cells. *Journal of Biochemistry*, *129*, 665–669.

Lauckner, J. E., Hille, B., & Mackie, K. (2005). The cannabinoid agonist WIN55,212-2 increases intracellular calcium via CB1 receptor coupling to G(q/11) G proteins. *Proceedings of the National Academy of Sciences of the United States of America*, *102*, 19144–19149.

Manglik, A., Lin, H., Aryal, D. K., McCorvy, J. D., Dengler, D., Corder, G., et al. (2016). Structure-based discovery of opioid analgesics with reduced side effects. *Nature*, *2537*, 185–190.

Matsuda, L. A., Bonner, T. I., & Lolait, S. J. (1992). Cannabinoid receptors: Which cells, where, how, and why? *NIDA Research Monograph*, *126*, 48–56.

Melsom, C. B., Hussain, R. I., Ørstavik, Ø., Aronsen, J. M., Sjaastad, I., Skomedal, T., et al. (2014). Non-classical regulation of β1- and β 2-adrenoceptor-mediated inotropic responses in rat heart ventricle by the G protein Gi. *Naunyn-Schmiedeberg's Archives of Pharmacology*, *387*, 1177–1186.

Morgan, D. J., Davis, B. J., Kearn, C. S., Marcus, D., Cook, A. J., Wager-Miller, J., et al. (2014). Mutation of putative GRK phosphorylation sites in the cannabinoid. Receptor 1 (CB1R) confers resistance to cannabinoid tolerance and hypersensitivity to cannabinoids in mice. *The Journal of Neuroscience*, *34*, 5152–5163.

Moulédous, L., Froment, C., Burlet-Schiltz, O., Schulz, S., & Mollereau, C. (2015). Phosphoproteomic analysis of the mouse brain mu-opioid (MOP) receptor. *FEBS Letters*, *589*, 2401–2408.

Mukhopadhyay, S., & Howlett, A. C. (2005). Chemically distinct ligands promote differential CB1 cannabinoid receptor-Gi protein interactions. *Molecular Pharmacology*, *67*, 2016–2024.
O'Sullivan, S. E. (2007). Cannabinoids go nuclear: Evidence for activation of peroxisome proliferator-activated receptors. *British Journal of Pharmacology*, *152*, 576–582.
Pearson, G., Robinson, F., Gibson, T. B., Xu, B. E., Karandikar, M., Berman, K., et al. (2001). Mitogen-activated protein (MAP) kinase pathways: Regulation and physiological functions. *Endocrine Reviews*, *22*, 153–183.
Pertwee, R. G. (2010). Receptors and channels targeted by synthetic cannabinoid receptor agonists and antagonists. *Current Medicinal Chemistry*, *17*, 1360–1381.
Pertwee, R. G., Howlett, A. C., Abood, M. E., Alexander, S. P. H., Di Marzo, V., Elphick, M. R., et al. (2010). International Union of Basic and Clinical Pharmacology. LXXIX. Cannabinoid receptors and their ligands: Beyond CB_1 and CB_2. *Pharmacological Reviews*, *62*, 588–631.
Scotter, E. L., Abood, M. E., & Glass, M. (2010). The endocannabinoid system as a target for the treatment of neurodegenerative disease. *British Journal of Pharmacology*, *160*, 480–498.
Shoemaker, J. L., Ruckle, M. B., Mayeux, P. R., & Prather, P. L. (2005). Agonist-directed trafficking of response by endocannabinoids acting at CB2 receptors. *The Journal of Pharmacology and Experimental Therapeutics*, *315*, 828–838.
Smart, D., Gunthorpe, M. J., Jerman, J. C., Nasir, S., Gray, J., Muir, A. I., et al. (2000). The endogenous lipid anandamide is a full agonist at the human vanilloid receptor (hVR1). *British Journal of Pharmacology*, *129*, 227–230.
Soethoudt, M., Grether, U., Fingerle, J., Grim, T. W., Fezza, F., de Petrocellis, L., et al. (2017). Cannabinoid CB(2) receptor ligand profiling reveals biased signalling and off-target activity. *Nature Communications*, *8*, 13958.
Taylor, L., Christou, I., Kapellos, T. S., Buchan, A., Brodermann, M. H., Gianella-Borradori, M., et al. (2015). Primary macrophage chemotaxis induced by cannabinoid receptor 2 agonists occurs independently of the CB2 receptor. *Scientific Reports*, *5*, 10682.
Turu, G., & Hunyady, L. (2010). Signal transduction of the CB1 cannabinoid receptor. *Journal of Molecular Endocrinology*, *44*, 75–85.
Urban, J. D., Clarke, W. P., von Zastrow, M., Nichols, D. E., Kobilka, B., Weinstein, H., et al. (2007). Functional selectivity and classical concepts of quantitative pharmacology. *Journal of Pharmacology and Experimental Therapeutics*, *320*, 1–13.
Wang, H. Y., & Burns, L. H. (2006). G beta gamma that interacts with adenylyl cyclase in opioid tolerance originates from a Gs protein. *Journal of Neurobiology*, *66*, 1302–1310.
Wiley, J. L., Compton, D. R., Dai, D., Lainton, J. A. H., Phillips, M., Huffman, J. W., et al. (1998). Structure-activity relationships of indole- and pyrrole-derived cannabinoids. *Journal of Pharmacology and Experimental Therapeutics*, *285*, 995–1004.

CHAPTER SEVEN

Cannabinoid Receptor-Related Orphan G Protein-Coupled Receptors

Andrew Irving*[,1], Ghayth Abdulrazzaq[†], Sue L.F. Chan[†], June Penman[‡], Jenni Harvey[‡], Stephen P.H. Alexander[†]

*The Conway Institute, School of Biomolecular and Biomedical Science, University College Dublin, Dublin, Ireland
[†]Life Sciences, University of Nottingham Medical School, Nottingham, United Kingdom
[‡]Division of Neuroscience, Ninewells Hospital and Medical School, University of Dundee, Dundee, Scotland, United Kingdom
[1]Corresponding author: e-mail address: andrew.irving@ucd.ie

Contents

Abstract

Of the druggable group of G protein-coupled receptors in the human genome, a number remain which have yet to be paired with an endogenous ligand—orphan GPCRs.

Advances in Pharmacology, Volume 80
ISSN 1054-3589
http://dx.doi.org/10.1016/bs.apha.2017.04.004

Among these 100 or so entities, 3 have been linked to the cannabinoid system. GPR18, GPR55, and GPR119 exhibit limited sequence homology with the established CB_1 and CB_2 cannabinoid receptors. However, the pharmacology of these orphan receptors displays overlap with CB_1 and CB_2 receptors, particularly for GPR18 and GPR55. The linking of GPR119 to the cannabinoid receptors is less convincing and emanates from structural similarities of endogenous ligands active at these GPCRs, but which do not cross-react. This review describes the evidence for describing these orphan GPCRs as cannabinoid receptor-like receptors.

ABBREVIATIONS

Δ^9-THC Δ^9-tetrahydrocannabinol
2AG 2-arachidonoylglycerol
2OG 2-oleoylglycerol
abn-CBD abnormal cannabidiol, 4-[(1*R*,6*R*)-3-methyl-6-prop-1-en-2-yl-1-cyclohex-2-enyl]-5-pentylbenzene-1,3-diol
CID16020046 4-[4,6-dihydro-4-(3-hydroxyphenyl)-3-(4-methylphenyl)-6-oxopyrrolo [3,4-*c*]pyrazol-5(1*H*)-yl]benzoic acid
CREB cyclic AMP response element binding protein
FAAH fatty acid amide hydrolase
LPA lysophosphatidic acid
LPI *L*-α-lysophosphatidylinositol
NAGly *N*-arachidonoylglycine
NFAT nuclear factor of activated T-cells
O1602 5-methyl-4-[(1*R*,6*R*)-3-methyl-6-prop-1-en-2-ylcyclohex-2-en-1-yl] benzene-1,3-diol
O1918 1,3-dimethoxy-5-methyl-2-[(1*R*,6*R*)-3-methyl-6-(1-methylethenyl)-2-cyclohexen-1-yl]benzene
OEA *N*-oleoylethanolamine
PEA *N*-palmitoylethanolamine

1. INTRODUCTION

The aim of NC-IUPHAR is to provide logical, consistent and long-lasting nomenclature to ensure that scientists spend their time on research and not on discussions/contradictions/arguments about how to describe individual proteins or families of proteins.

The NC-IUPHAR subcommittee on cannabinoid receptors (http://www.guidetopharmacology.org/GRAC/FamilyDisplayForward?familyId=13) considered whether further receptors should be considered additional cannabinoid receptors in a publication in 2010 (Pertwee et al., 2010). In particular, GPCRs other than CB_1 and CB_2 receptors, ligand-gated ion channels such as TRPV1 and nuclear hormone receptors such as PPARs were assessed. At that time, although there was useful, peer-reviewed literature identifying that GPR18, GPR55 and GPR119 had associations with the cannabinoid receptor family, it was too premature to consider them as cannabinoid receptors.

A simple comparison of the primary amino acid sequences of the Family A (rhodopsin) orphan GPCR allows generation of a dendrogram (Fig. 1). Indicated by the blue arrows are GPR18, GPR55 and GPR119. Also indicated are the cannabinoid receptors (CB_1 and CB_2) and the first identified lysophosphatidic acid receptors (LPA_1, LPA_2, and LPA_3). Clearly, there are limited structural similarities between conventional cannabinoid receptors and GPR18, GPR55 and GPR119.

An area of intersection between cannabinoid and LPA receptors with the orphan GPCRs GPR18, GPR55 and GPR119 are the similarities between the putative endogenous agonists (see later). Depicted in Fig. 2 are endogenous agonists at cannabinoid and LPA receptors. Anandamide was identified 25 years ago as a component of pig brain that bound and activated cannabinoid receptors (Devane et al., 1992). Within 3 years, 2-arachidonoylglycerol (2AG) was identified in the gut of dogs (Mechoulam et al., 1995). In the investigation of LPA receptors, the most commonly used agonist is 1-oleoyl-2-lysophosphatidic acid (because of its widespread availability and relatively low cost), although it appears that a family of endogenous LPA analogues exist, which differ in the acyl chain. Depicted in Fig. 2 is one possible endogenous version of LPA, 2-arachidonoyl-lysophosphatidic acid, selected to highlight the similarities of the endogenous agonists at these GPCRs.

Pharmacological profiling of orphan GPCRs has multiple functions. Selective ligands allow investigation of the roles of the GPCRs in complex systems ("native" cells and tissues or in vivo). Nonselective ligands can be useful also, but primarily in recombinant systems where the "masking" effects of other mechanisms are reduced.

2. EVIDENCE FOR NOVEL CANNABINOID RECEPTOR-LIKE GPCR TARGETS

Increasing evidence suggests that there are non-CB_1/CB_2 targets for cannabinoids in the brain (Begg et al., 2005; Breivogel, Griffin, Di Marzo, & Martin, 2001; Di Marzo et al., 2000), in the cardiovascular system (Begg et al., 2005; Jarai et al., 1999), and in the immune system (Rao & Kaminski, 2006). Both anandamide and the synthetic cannabinoid agonist, WIN55212-2, applied to CB_1-knockout mouse brain were observed to stimulate [^{35}S]GTPγS binding mediated by an unknown GPCR which did not

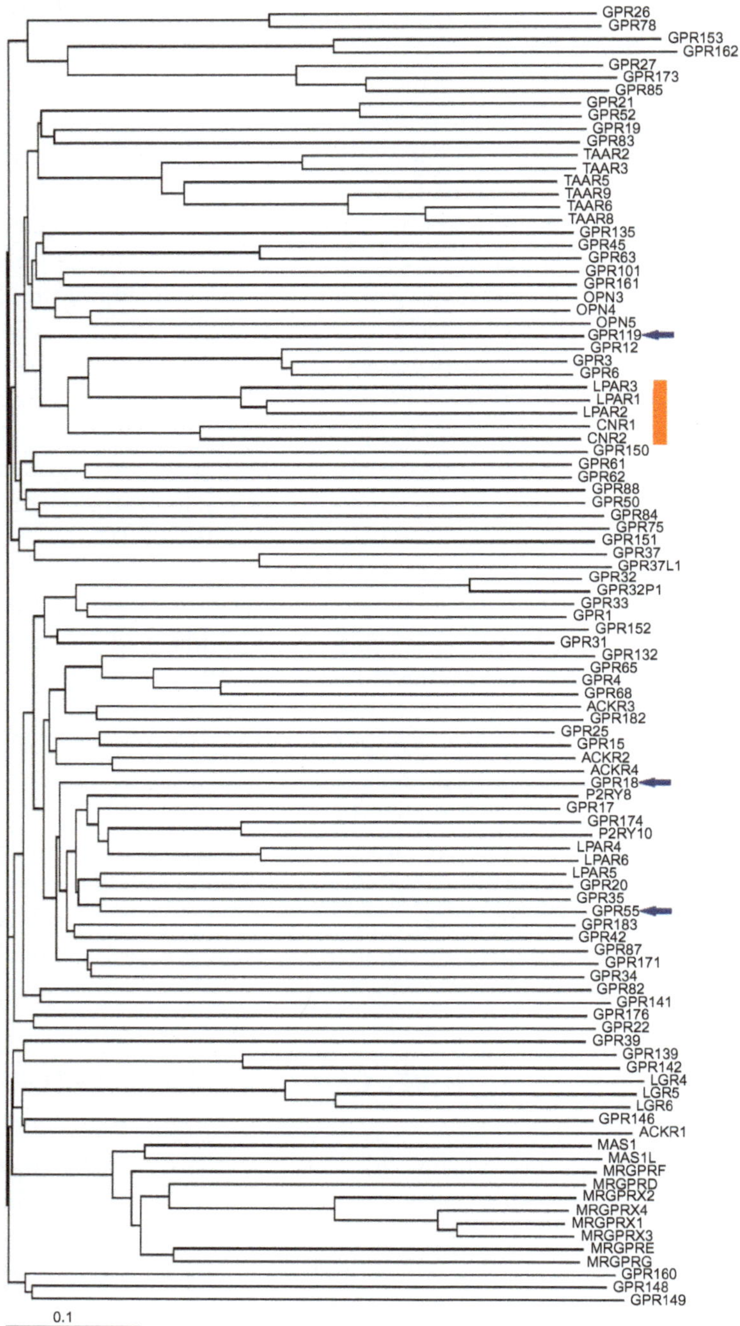

Fig. 1 Dendrogram of orphan GPCRs and selected related receptors.

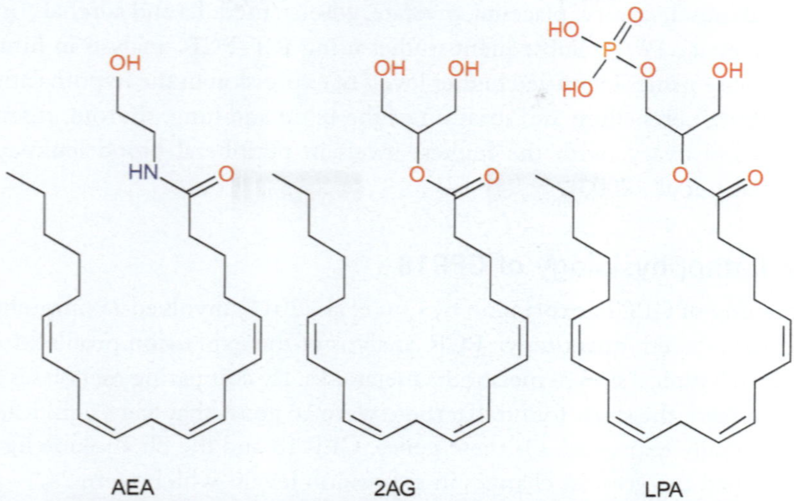

Fig. 2 Endogenous agonists at cannabinoid and lysophosphatidic acid receptors.

bind Δ9-tetrahydrocannabinol (Δ^9-THC) (Breivogel et al., 2001). Moreover, structural analogues of anandamide were ineffective at promoting [^{35}S]GTPγS binding in brain membranes derived from CB_1-knockout mice (Breivogel et al., 2001). The effects of anandamide-induced [^{35}S]GTPγS binding in CB_1-knockout brain membranes were unaffected by CB_1 (rimonabant) or CB_2 (SR144528) receptor antagonists (Di Marzo et al., 2000).

3. GPR18 AS A CANNABINOID RECEPTOR-LIKE GPCR

3.1 Distribution of GPR18

GPR18 was first detected in canine gastric mucosa and the human colonic cancer Colo 320 DM cell line (Gantz et al., 1997). The gene encoding GPR18 was localized to human (13q32), rodent, and canine chromosomes, where it clusters with Epstein–Barr virus-induced receptor 2 (EBI2, GPR183) and the cysteinyl leukotriene receptors $CysLT_1$ and $CysLT_2$ (Gantz et al., 1997; Rosenkilde et al., 2006).

GPR18 is highly expressed in the testis, especially in the most terminally differentiated cells. The density of expression in spleen, thymus, peripheral blood leukocytes, small intestine, appendix and lymph node has prompted the inference of a role in regulation of the immune system (Gantz et al., 1997). By contrast, there appear to be a number of tissues lacking GPR18 mRNA, including brain, heart, lung, liver, kidney, pancreas, colon, skeletal muscle, ovary, placenta, prostate, adrenal medulla and adrenal cortex (Gantz et al., 1997). Subsequent studies using RT-PCR analysis in human and mouse tissues identified higher levels of expression in the hypothalamus, brainstem, cerebellum and striatum of the brain and lung, thyroid, thymes, testes, and ovary, with the highest levels in peripheral blood leukocytes (Vassilatis et al., 2003).

3.2 Pathophysiology of GPR18

Screening of GPCR expression by Qin et al. (2011) involved a comprehensive array-based, quantitative PCR analysis of the expression profile of 130 genes in 3 typical sites of melanoma metastases. By comparing metastases and benign nevi, the study found that there were 16 genes that were significantly differentially expressed. Of these genes, GPR18 and the chemokine ligand CCL4 had the greatest changes in expression levels, which were 24.1- and 27.4-fold higher, respectively, in metastasis (Qin et al., 2011). Subsequently, many experiments in yeast and melanoma were designed to test the ability of GPR18 to mediate proliferative or antiapoptotic signaling. They revealed that the GPR18 sequence deviated from other GPCRs at position 3.35, where an alanine is present in place of a normally highly conserved asparagine. Asparagine to alanine mutations at 3.35 have been previously shown to result in constitutive activity in CXCR3 and CXCR4 chemokine receptors, precluding the requirement of an agonist ligand to activate them (Verzijl et al., 2008; Zhang et al., 2002).

Qin et al. (2011) suggested that mutating alanine back to asparagine at 3.35 resulted in the loss of constitutive activity of GPR18. This result is of interest because malignant cells are dependent on the constitutive or overexpression of driver genes for conservation of cell survival or inhibition of apoptosis. To support this hypothesis, Qin et al. (2011) reported that in vitro siRNA-mediated knockdown of GPR18 in human melanoma cells enhanced death via apoptosis.

3.3 Endogenous Ligand Activity at Recombinant GPR18

Several studies have suggested that *N*-arachidonylglycine (NAGly; Fig. 3) is an endogenous ligand for GPR18. Unlike anandamide, NAGly has no activity on the classical cannabinoid receptors CB_1 and CB_2 (Sheskin, Hanus, Slager, Vogel, & Mechoulam, 1997). The initial description of a deorphanization of GPR18 used a lipid library of almost 200 compounds for screening purposes and identified an elevation of intracellular calcium

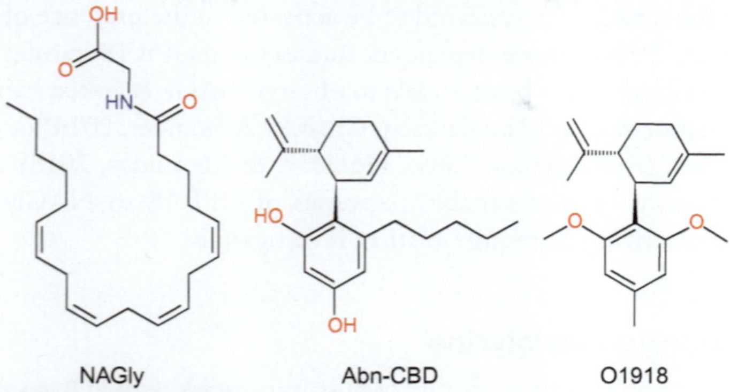

Fig. 3 Ligands active at GPR18.

in response to NAGly when GPR18 was expressed in a variety of host cells (Kohno et al., 2006). The authors also noted that NAGly evoked a concentration-dependent inhibition of forskolin-stimulated cAMP production in GPR18-transfected CHO cells with a pIC_{50} value of 7.7. This NAGly-mediated inhibition was abolished by pertussis toxin, implying a role for $G\alpha_{i/o}$ proteins in this response (Kohno et al., 2006).

Recombinant GPR18 expressed in HEK293 cells was assessed for activation of multiple signaling pathways following NAGly exposure (Console-Bram, Brailoiu, Brailoiu, Sharir, & Abood, 2014). Interpolation of the data presented in this report suggests that NAGly increased intracellular calcium ions with a pEC_{50} value of ~6.2 (Console-Bram et al., 2014). NAGly was also observed to elicit a rapid, long-lasting phosphorylation of ERK1/2, but failed to alter β-arrestin recruitment. This observation was a recapitulation, of sorts, of a previous report examining 16 putative lipid-activated GPCRs, including GPR18, expressed in HEK293 cells, screening a library of about 400 lipid ligands (Yin et al., 2009). Although the authors failed to indicate the concentrations of NAGly employed, they reported a failure of GPR18-expressing cells to couple to β-arrestin.

Lu et al. (2013) expressed epitope-tagged GPR18 in rat sympathetic cervical ganglia and confirmed cell surface expression. Assessing the coupling of the receptor to calcium ion elevations, potassium channels, or cAMP levels, NAGly failed to alter any of these responses in a manner dependent on GPR18 expression (Lu et al., 2013). More recently, tagged GPR18 transfected into HEL cells was assessed for responses to NAGly by monitoring the levels of cAMP and intracellular calcium, as well as ERK phosphorylation and receptor internalization (Finlay, Joseph, Grimsey, & Glass, 2016).

None of these pathways appeared to be activated in the presence of NAGly (Finlay et al., 2016). Our independent studies using GPR18 transfected into HEK293 cells have also been unable to observe NAGly-evoked increases in ERK phosphorylation (Abdulrazzaq, Chan, & Alexander, 2014) or calcium ion elevation (Abdulrazzaq, Chan, Holliday, & Alexander, 2015).

The reasons for the variable responses of GPR18 to NAGly remain unclear, but obviously require further investigation.

3.4 *N*-Arachidonoylglycine

NAGly is a member of a subfamily of lipoamino acids, which have also been termed elmiric acids (Burstein, 2008; Burstein et al., 2007) or *N*-acylamino acids; there is currently a lack of consensus on the most appropriate nomenclature for these compounds. It is present abundantly in mammalian nervous tissues, particularly in brain and spinal cord (Huang et al., 2001). It has two distinct identified biosynthetic pathways (Bradshaw et al., 2009). One involves enzymatically regulated conjugation of arachidonic acid, presumably as a CoA ester, and glycine. The other pathway suggests that NAGly is an enzymatically oxygenated metabolite of anandamide. NAGly has been reported to be hydrolyzed by FAAH (Cascio et al., 2004), although other mechanisms may exist (Garle, Mehrotra, Sandy-Hindmarch, Alharthi, & Alexander, 2016). NAGly is a substrate for cyclooxygenase-2 (Prusakiewicz, Kingsley, Kozak, & Marnett, 2002) and lipoxygenases (Prusakiewicz et al., 2007), although the activity of the products of oxidative metabolism has not been clarified. Intriguingly, NAGly administration to HEK293 cells expressing GPR18 has been identified to increase prostanoid and lipoxin production (Burstein, McQuain, Ross, Salmonsen, & Zurier, 2011).

The pharmacology of NAGly beyond GPR18 is still not well understood, although there is evidence for multiple effects. For example, NAGly acts as a selective inhibitor of the GlyT2 transporter (Wiles, Pearlman, Rosvall, Aubrey, & Vandenberg, 2006). NAGly administration in spinal cord slices selectively enhanced glycine-induced currents, apparently through GlyT2 transporter inhibition (Jeong, Vandenberg, & Vaughan, 2010). NAGly has also been reported to act directly at particular α subunits of the ligand-gated ion channel glycine receptor (Yang et al., 2008).

Using isolated mesenteric arteries from the rat, NAGly was observed to cause a concentration-dependent relaxation primarily through the activation of BK_{Ca} calcium-activated potassium channels in the smooth muscle following nitric oxide release from the endothelium (Parmar & Ho, 2010). In rat pancreatic beta cells, NAGly caused an increase in intracellular calcium levels and enhanced glucose-induced insulin release (Ikeda et al., 2005).

3.5 Pharmacology of Synthetic Ligands at GPR18

Using recombinant GPR18, a number of synthetic ligands have been described to be active as agonists or antagonists (Fig. 3). Thus, abn-CBD (abnormal cannabidiol, 4-[(1*R*,6*R*)-3-methyl-6-prop-1-en-2-yl-1-cyclohex-2-enyl]-5-pentylbenzene-1,3-diol), O1602 (5-methyl-4-[(1*R*,6*R*)-3-methyl-6-prop-1-en-2-ylcyclohex-2-en-1-yl]benzene-1,3-diol), Δ^9-THC and *N*-arachidonoylcyclopropylamide have all been described as full agonists in GPR18-transfected HEK cells (McHugh, Page, Dunn, & Bradshaw, 2012). The endocannabinoid anandamide appears to be a full agonist also (McHugh, Page, et al., 2012), which, together with the activity of Δ^9-THC, leads to some deep thought as to the nomenclature of this receptor (Alexander, 2012). The same study, however, indicated that cells were able to convert anandamide to NAGly with a minute timescale, through both enzymatic pathways indicated earlier.

Cannabidiol and AM251 act as weak partial agonists (McHugh, Page, et al., 2012), while a number of other agonists of CB_1 and CB_2 cannabinoid receptors were inactive (WIN55212-2, CP55940, JWH015, and JWH133).

Examining native GPR18 expression in cultured cells has allowed investigation of receptor function in BV-2 mouse microglial (McHugh et al., 2010; McHugh, Roskowski, Xie, & Bradshaw, 2014; McHugh, Wager-Miller, Page, & Bradshaw, 2012) and HEC-1B human endometrial cells (McHugh, Page, et al., 2012). In these cells, GPR18 mediates a promigratory response and stimulates ERK1/2 phosphorylation. In GPR18-transfected HEK293 cells, NAGly and abn-CBD also promoted migration, which was lost when GPR18 was absent (McHugh et al., 2010). In these cells, CBD and *N*-arachidonoylserine blocked the migratory response, as did the synthetic compound O1918 (1,3-dimethoxy-5-methyl-2-[(1*R*,6*R*)-3-methyl-6-(1-methylethenyl)-2-cyclohexen-1-yl]benzene). The agonist and antagonist actions of abn-CBD and O1918, respectively, were previously noted for an endothelial "anandamide receptor" coupled to $G_{i/o}$ proteins to evoke vasodilatation in vitro and in vivo (Offertaler et al., 2003). Whether the endothelial "anandamide receptor" is GPR18 is clearly the focus of some current research activities.

4. GPR55 AS A CANNABINOID RECEPTOR-LIKE GPCR

Of all the putative cannabinoid receptors, GPR55 has attracted the most attention—based on its intriguing cannabinoid and endogenous lipid sensitivity. In 1999 the orphan G protein-coupled receptor 55 (GPR55) was identified from in silico studies and subsequently cloned. It contains 319 amino acids and the gene is mapped to chromosome 2q37 (Sawzdargo et al., 1999). However, as already mentioned it has only limited homology to the classical cannabinoid receptors—14% and 15% with CB_1 and CB_2, respectively (Oka, Nakajima, Yamashita, Kishimoto, & Sugiura, 2007). Indeed, phylogenetically CB_1 and CB_2 are members of the Rhodopsin class A α-group, whereas GPR55 is a member of the class A δ-group (Civelli et al., 2013). GPR55 shares a higher level of homology with lysophosphatidic acid and other orphan receptors within this group: GPR35 (37%), LPA_5 (GPR92, 30%), LPA_6 (P2Y5, 30%), and LPA_4 (GPR23, 29%) (Baker, Pryce, Davies, & Hiley, 2006). GPR55 does not possess a classical cannabinoid binding pocket (Petitet, Donlan, & Michel, 2006), suggesting that the binding sites for ligands with mixed cannabinoid/GPR55 activity are likely to be different (Garland, 2013).

4.1 GPR55 Pharmacology

Cannabinoid activation of GPR55 was initially described in two industrial patents from GSK and Astra Zeneca (Drmota, Greasley, & Groblewski, 2004; Wise & Brown, 2001), with follow-up data published in peer-reviewed journals in 2007 (Johns et al., 2007; Ryberg et al., 2007). Despite much subsequent research activity in this area, the cannabinoid pharmacology of GPR55 remains disputed, with the most potent endogenous ligand identified to date being a lysophospholipid.

4.1.1 Endogenous Lipids and GPR55

Controversy remains as to whether endocannabinoids, such as anandamide, 2-AG and virodhamine, can activate GPR55. Some groups find that endocannabinoids are active, for example, with a [^{35}S]GTPγS assay in HEK293 cells expressing human GPR55 (Ryberg et al., 2007) and in native cells (Lauckner et al., 2008; Waldeck-Weiermair et al., 2008). However, other groups have not confirmed these findings in recombinant systems (Henstridge et al., 2009; Oka et al., 2009) or that endocannabinoids are only weakly active (Kapur et al., 2009; Yin et al., 2009). Using a β-arrestin assay, it was suggested that anandamide and virodhamine act as partial agonists, enhancing agonist effects at low concentrations and inhibiting them at high concentrations (Sharir et al., 2012). There is also controversy as to whether *N*-palmitoylethanolamine (PEA), a structural analogue of anandamide, activates GPR55. Some groups find that low nanomolar concentrations of PEA activate GPR55 (Ryberg et al., 2007), whereas others found no difference in signaling when PEA was applied to hGPR55-HEK293 cells compared to control HEK293 cells (Lauckner et al., 2008; Oka et al., 2007).

Despite the issues regarding endocannabinoid activity at GPR55, compelling data now suggest that the endogenous lipid, *L*-α-lysophosphatidylinositol (LPI, Fig. 4), is a natural ligand for this receptor. This was first identified by Oka et al. (2007), with a subsequent publication demonstrating that LPI with an arachidonic fatty acid chain (2-arachidonoyl-*sn*-glycero-3-phosphoinositol) is the most biologically active LPI species (Oka et al., 2009). The activity of LPI at GPR55 has now been confirmed by a number of groups (Henstridge et al., 2009; Kapur et al., 2009; Yin et al., 2009). Interestingly, the related endogenous lipid, LPA, does not activate GPR55 (Henstridge et al., 2009; Oka et al., 2007). Furthermore, other lysophospholipids including lysophosphatidylserine, lysophosphatidylcholine and lysophosphatidylethanolamine did not induce GPR55-mediated

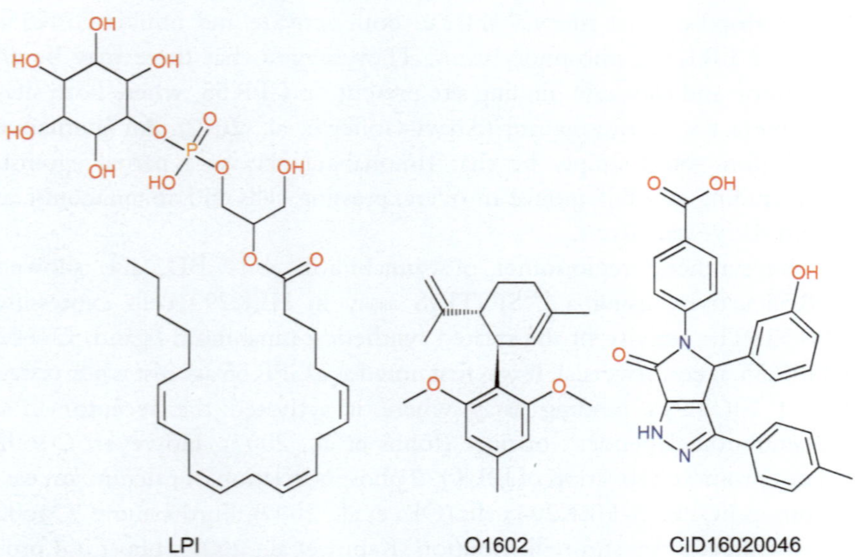

Fig. 4 Ligands active at GPR55.

ERK1/2 phosphorylation (Oka et al., 2007). It should be emphasized that LPI is not selective for GPR55 and clearly has additional biological activities (Bondarenko et al., 2010). Whether additional endogenous lipid species can bind GPR55 remains to be established, but is likely, given that it is often a feature of lipid-sensing GPCRs. Indeed, the *N*-acylamino acid, *N*-arachidonoylserine, promotes phosphorylation of ERK1/2 and Akt and endothelial functions in human dermal microvascular endothelial cells through an effect that is partially sensitive to GPR55 siRNA (Zhang, Maor, Wang, Kunos, & Groopman, 2010).

4.1.2 Synthetic GPR55 Ligands

Increasing experimental data suggest that some synthetic cannabinoid ligands can activate GPR55 (Anavi-Goffer et al., 2012; Henstridge et al., 2010), although the pharmacology can be somewhat inverted, with cannabinoid receptor antagonists acting as GPR55 agonists and some cannabinoid agonists acting as GPR55 antagonists. There is also pharmacological crossover, with some CB_2 agonists, including HU210, also exhibiting GPR55 agonist activity (Anavi-Goffer et al., 2012). The CB_1 antagonists, AM251 and rimonabant, are reported as agonists of GPR55 (Henstridge et al., 2010; Kapur et al., 2009; Yin et al., 2009). However, in some studies, rimonabant also acted as a GPR55 antagonist (Lauckner et al., 2008; Pineiro, Maffucci, & Falasca, 2011). Interestingly, Anavi-Goffer et al. (2012) proposed that rimonabant can both activate and inhibit GPR55-mediated ERK1/2 phosphorylation. They suggest that there may be an orthosteric and allosteric binding site present on GPR55, where both sites may interact with rimonabant (Anavi-Goffer et al., 2012). An alternative explanation could simply be that rimonabant acts as a partial agonist, masquerading as a full agonist in overexpressing cells and an antagonist in certain native cell assays.

The synthetic regioisomer of cannabidiol, abn-CBD, also showed GPR55 activity using a $[^{35}S]GTP\gamma S$ assay in HEK293 cells expressing GPR55. The activity of the related synthetic cannabinoid ligand, O1602 at GPR55, is controversial. It was first noted as a GPR55 agonist when tested in a $[^{35}S]GTP\gamma S$ binding assay where it activated the receptor in a concentration-dependent manner (Johns et al., 2007). However, O1602 did not promote activation of ERK1/2 phosphorylation or calcium ion elevations in hGPR55-HEK293 cells (Oka et al., 2009). Furthermore, O1602 did not affect β-arrestin redistribution (Kapur et al., 2009), but it did promote GPR55-mediated inhibition of osteoclastogenesis, an effect that was not observed in GPR55-knockout mice (Whyte et al., 2009). Also,

O1602 decreased the contractility of colonic strips, which was blocked in GPR55-knockout mice. These data suggest that O1602 may exhibit some activity at GPR55, but this depends on the host cell type being studied. It should be noted that the most prominent actions of O1602 and abn-CBD in native systems are thought to be via GPR18 (see earlier).

The further development of antagonists selective for GPR55 is required to help clarify the role of GPR55 in normal and pathological states. CID16020046 (4-[4,6-dihydro-4-(3-hydroxyphenyl)-3-(4-methylphenyl)-6-oxopyrrolo[3,4-*c*]pyrazol-5(1*H*)-yl]benzoic acid) was identified in a high-throughput screen (Heynen-Genel et al., 2010b) and shown to be a selective GPR55 antagonist against LPI-induced ERK1/2 phosphorylation, PKC βII translocation, calcium mobilization and transcription factor activation in HEK293 cells stably transfected with GPR55 (Kargl et al., 2013). These effects were not observed in CB_1- and CB_2-transfected HEK293 cells. CID16020046 was also effective in endogenous GPR55-expressing cells with similar potencies to those noted in recombinant expression (Kargl et al., 2013). A new generation of synthetic GPR55 agonists has also been recently identified (Heynen-Genel et al., 2010a), with potent activity demonstrated for *N*-aryl substituted sulfonamides (Yrjölä et al., 2016). The use of these new pharmacological compounds will help clarify the physiological and pathological roles of GPR55.

4.1.3 Phytocannabinoids as GPR55 Ligands?

Cannabidiol is suggested to be an antagonist for GPR55 and many studies show that cannabidiol can antagonize GPR55 responses to LPI (Ryberg et al., 2007; Whyte et al., 2009), although no antagonist activity of cannabidiol was observed during a GPR55 antagonist screen. Cannabidiol is known to act at various targets; for example, it has affinity for the abn-CBD receptor in the vasculature (Jarai et al., 1999) and as described earlier it may also be a weak, partial agonist for GPR18 (McHugh, Page, et al., 2012). Cannabidiol is also reported to be a CB_1 and CB_2 antagonist in $[^{35}S]GTP\gamma S$ binding assays in vitro (Thomas et al., 2007). Cannabidiol also acts at $TRPV_1$ to promote antihyperalgesic effects (Costa, Giagnoni, Franke, Trovato, & Colleoni, 2004) and activates PPARγ, promoting 3T3-L1 differentiation into adipocytes (O'Sullivan, Sun, Bennett, Randall, & Kendall, 2009). The prototypic phytocannabinoid Δ^9-THC, on the other hand, exhibits weak activity at GPR55 expressed in HEK293 cells using calcium signaling as the assay (μM range; Lauckner et al., 2008). However, no effect of Δ^9-THC on GPR55-mediated ERK activation was observed in the study carried out by Oka et al. (2007).

4.2 Downstream Signaling in Heterologous Expression Systems and Native Cells

Many groups have evaluated GPR55 pharmacology and downstream signaling in heterologous expression systems, with HEK293 cells being a popular host. Activation of ERK1/2 signaling (Oka et al., 2007), Rho activation, calcium ion elevations and the activation of transcription factors, including nuclear factor of activated T-cells (NFAT) and cAMP response element binding protein (CREB), have been identified (Henstridge et al., 2009). The heterotrimeric G-proteins $G\alpha_{13}$ and $G\alpha_q$ have been implicated in GPR55-mediated signaling (Henstridge et al., 2009; Lauckner et al., 2008; Obara, Ueno, Yanagihata, & Nakahata, 2011). The canonical signaling downstream of GPR55 is via $G\alpha_{13}$, and some of the putative $G\alpha_q$ signaling could reflect off-target actions of the ligands. GPR55-mediated β-arrestin recruitment has also been demonstrated and is an effective screening assay for GPR55 ligands (Kotsikorou et al., 2013). The potential for GPR55 to heterodimerize may further confound the observed pharmacology. Notably GPR55 and CB_2 receptors can associate, which impacts on cell signaling (Moreno et al., 2014), possibly leading to enhanced MAP kinase activation and reduced transcription factor generation (Balenga et al., 2014). Identification and characterization of additional heterodimer partners are an important avenue for future research. Additional complications may arise from agonist bias, for example, with suggestions that certain GPR55 ligands may be more effective at promoting CREB activation in comparison with calcium mobilization (Henstridge et al., 2010).

In the context of native GPR55 expression, there is consensus with the data from recombinant systems, while there are also some notable differences. In endothelial cells, anandamide-promoted GPR55-mediated calcium mobilization is distinct requiring the activation of PI3K–Bmx–PLCγ signaling. Moreover, integrin clustering is necessary to release the inhibition of GPR55 calcium signaling, mediated by CB_1 activation (Waldeck-Weiermair et al., 2008). It remains to be determined if $G\alpha_{13}$ or $G\alpha_q$ is required for calcium mobilization in endothelial cells. LPI-mediated calcium signaling has also been observed in some cancer cells (Pineiro et al., 2011) and at presynaptic nerve terminals in the hippocampus (Sylantyev, Jensen, Ross, & Rusakov, 2013). These effects have been attributed to GPR55, but off-target activity of LPI may complicate the overall picture.

Effects on ERK1/2 phosphorylation have been observed in native cells, for example, in murine BV2 microglia cells treated with interferon γ, LPI-induced ERK1/2 phosphorylation in a concentration-dependent manner (Pietr et al., 2009). ERK phosphorylation is also reported in some cancer cells treated with LPI (Andradas et al., 2011; Pineiro et al., 2011). A kinase thought to be downstream of GPR55 in native cells is AKT. Treatment of prostate cancer cells with LPI results in GPR55-mediated AKT phosphorylation (Pineiro et al., 2011).

4.3 Native Expression of GPR55

GPR55 has a widespread distribution and is implicated in modulating multiple physiological processes, both in the CNS and in the periphery. GPR55 mRNA is expressed in various brain regions, including caudate, putamen, hippocampus, frontal cortex, cerebellum, striatum, hypothalamus, and brainstem (Ryberg et al., 2007; Sawzdargo et al., 1999). Notably, there is evidence of GPR55 mRNA in the immune system (spleen; Ryberg et al., 2007), and it is expressed in microglia (Pietr et al., 2009), large diameter dorsal root ganglion (Lauckner et al., 2008), bone (Whyte et al., 2009), pancreas (Romero-Zerbo et al., 2011), and metastatic cancer cells (Andradas et al., 2011; Ford et al., 2010) including the prostate cancer cell line DU145 (Pineiro et al., 2011). GPR55 mRNA was also detected in the adrenal glands, jejunum and ileum (Ryberg et al., 2007). Although a number of studies have published data using GPR55 antibodies (commercial and generated in-house) or fluorescent probes (Daly et al., 2010) to evaluate the cellular expression of GPR55 protein, these tools remain to be thoroughly validated and may require the use of very specific conditions to work effectively.

4.4 Exploring the (Patho)physiology of GPR55

The diverse physiological and pathophysiological roles of GPR55 are now being established, with much new and exciting data emerging. A detailed evaluation of the specific areas of interest is beyond the scope of this review. However, it is clear that GPR55 plays an important role in cancer (Andradas et al., 2011; Ford et al., 2010; Pineiro et al., 2011), immune regulation (Balenga et al., 2011; Pietr et al., 2009), pain modulation (Schuelert & McDougall, 2011; Staton et al., 2008), diabetes, obesity (Moreno-Navarrete et al., 2012), and osteoarthritis (Whyte et al., 2009). Recent developments in GPR55 pharmacology, in particular, GPR55-selective antagonists, will help clarify its role (Kargl et al., 2013) and help validate data from gene silencing studies. Here the use of siRNA and GPR55-knockout animals has helped to evaluate GPR55 in native systems. This has been used successfully with prostate cancer cells where increases in AKT and ERK1/2 phosphorylation and calcium mobilization are all reduced by GPR55 silencing (Pineiro et al., 2011). However, this approach is not always effective; for example, siRNA applied to breast cancer cells did not lower the endogenous level of GPR55 in the cells (Ford et al., 2010). Many other studies have employed GPR55 siRNA to gain an understanding of the effect GPR55 has in areas as diverse as neuroprotection (Kallendrusch et al., 2013), breast and brain cancer proliferation (Andradas et al., 2011), and calcium mobilization in endothelial cells (Waldeck-Weiermair et al., 2008). Another method for deciphering GPR55-mediated effects is to use GPR55-knockout mice, where they have allowed an assessment of GPR55 in inflammatory pain (Staton et al., 2008). Knockout mice have also highlighted that GPR55 is necessary for regulating increases in bone mass (Whyte et al., 2009).

5. GPR119 AS A CANNABINOID RECEPTOR-LIKE GPCR

GPR119 was initially identified in rodent pancreatic islets, with an enhancing role on glucose-dependent insulin secretion (Soga et al., 2005), with immunoreactivity detected in β and PP (pancreatic polypeptide) cells (Sakamoto et al., 2006). Subsequently, GPR119 was also located in the gut, in L cells responsible for the secretion of glucagon-like peptide 1 (Chu et al., 2008; Lauffer, Iakoubov, & Brubaker, 2009). These two locations appear to be the primary loci for GPR119 expression, although GPR119 appears to be functional in skeletal muscle (Cornall et al., 2013) and liver (Yang et al., 2016).

5.1 Pathophysiology of GPR119

GPR119 expression is increased rapidly in human gut following acute fat exposure in otherwise healthy lean individuals (Cvijanovic et al., 2016), indicating potential involvement in type 2 diabetes, metabolic disorder, and obesity. Indeed, synthetic GPR119 agonists have shown promising results in Phase II clinical trials in type 2 diabetes (Nunez et al., 2014). An alternative therapeutic option, which is currently poorly treated, is the treatment of nonalcoholic fatty liver disease (Yang et al., 2016).

5.2 Endogenous Ligand Activity at Recombinant GPR119

GPR119 has a potential association with cannabinoid receptor-like receptors because of the similar structures of the proposed endogenous ligands (Fig. 5). Thus, *N*-oleoylethanolamine (OEA) is a monounsaturated analogue of the first identified endocannabinoid, AEA, and was shown to

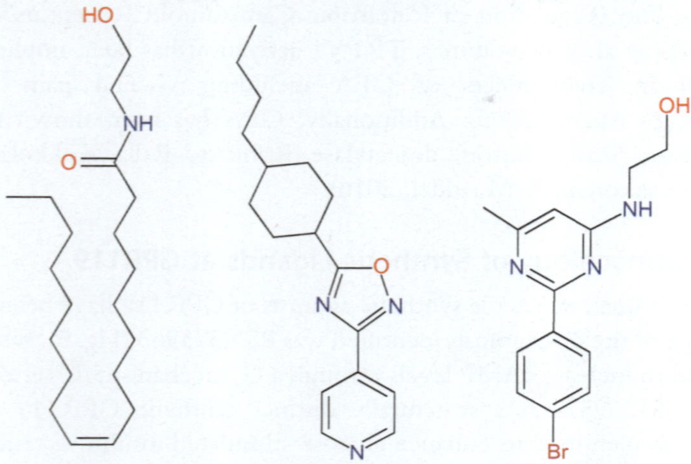

Fig. 5 Ligands active at GPR119.

activate GPR119 in the initial attempt to deorphanize the receptor (Overton et al., 2006), as well as several subsequent independent studies (Chu et al., 2010; Lauffer et al., 2009; Syed et al., 2012). Intriguingly, 2-oleoylglycerol, a monounsaturated analogue of the second identified endocannabinoid, 2AG, has also been identified as a GPR119 agonist (Hansen et al., 2011). A third endogenous GPR119 activator has also been identified with some structural commonality with the endogenous ligand of GPR55, oleoyllysophosphatidylcholine (Soga et al., 2005). However, none of the "classical" cannabinoid ligands, such as THC, have been shown to act through GPR119 in contrast to GPR18 and GPR55.

5.3 *N*-Oleoylethanolamine

OEA was identified as a PPARα ligand (Fu et al., 2003), before the association of OEA with GPR119. For a review of the extended pattern of cannabinoids and related molecules as ligands at PPARs, see chapter "The Role of Nuclear Hormone Receptors in Cannabinoid Function" by Pistis and O′Sullivan (this volume). PPARα activation has been implicated in multiple in vivo effects of OEA including feeding (Fu et al., 2003), neuroprotection (Sun et al., 2007), sleep–wake cycling (Soria-Gomez et al., 2010), cocaine-induced behaviors (Bilbao et al., 2013), and atherosclerosis (Fan et al., 2014).

OEA was also identified as a TRPV1 agonist (Ahern, 2003), also before the association of OEA with GPR119. For a review of the extended pattern of cannabinoids and related molecules as ligands at TRPV1, see chapter

"Actions and Regulation of Ionotropic Cannabinoid Receptors" by De Petrocellis et al. (this volume). TRPV1 activation has been implicated in multiple in vivo effects of OEA including visceral pain (Wang, Miyares, & Ahern, 2005). Additionally, OEA has been shown to bind and activate Sirt6, a histone deacetylase (Rahnasto-Rilla, Kokkola, Jarho, Lahtela-Kakkonen, & Moaddel, 2016).

5.4 Pharmacology of Synthetic Ligands at GPR119

Numerous small-molecule synthetic agonists of GPR119 have been identified. One of the first agonists identified was PSN375963 (Fig. 5), which was observed to increase cAMP levels through a G_s mechanism (Overton et al., 2006). AS1269574 is a structurally distinct synthetic GPR119 agonist, which was identified to enhance glucose-stimulated insulin secretion both in vitro and in vivo (Yoshida, Ohishi, Matsui, & Shibasaki, 2010). This compound, but not OEA, however, has also been shown to activate TRPA1 (Chepurny, Holz, Roe, & Leech, 2016). In an intestinal neuroendocrine cell, AS1269574 evoked GLP-1 secretion through the activation of TRPA1 channels (Chepurny et al., 2016). What contribution TRPA1 channels make to in vivo responses to this and other GPR119 agonists is unclear. To date, no antagonists of GPR119 have been described, presumably because there appears to be little therapeutic potential for them. Of course, a clear therapeutic potential may only become evident when a selective antagonist is identified.

6. CONCLUSION

Since the last publication from NC-IUPHAR considering the status of cannabinoid receptors beyond CB_1 and CB_2 receptors, there has been a major increase in information about the three orphan GPCRs with the closest associations to the classical cannabinoid receptors. However, despite the interest, these receptors are probably best considered less as orphans but rather as "foster children" of the cannabinoid receptors. Given our current understanding of the pharmacology of these three receptors, it appears that GPR18 and GPR55 are the closest relatives to the classical cannabinoid receptors, more cousins than siblings, while GPR119 may represent a more distant relative, a second cousin, perhaps.

CONFLICT OF INTEREST

The authors have no conflict of interest to disclose.

ACKNOWLEDGMENT

G.A. is supported by the Higher Committee for Education Development of Iraq.

REFERENCES

Abdulrazzaq, G. M., Chan, S., & Alexander, S. P. H. (2014). In *Effect of N-arachidonoyl glycine (NAGly) and D⁹tetrahydrocannabinol (D⁹THC) on ERK1/2 phosphorylation in native HEK293 cells* (pp. 1–46). *24th annual symposium on the cannabinoids.*

Abdulrazzaq, G. M., Chan, S. L. F., Holliday, N. D., & Alexander, S. P. H. (2015). Assessment of calcium mobilization induced by the cannabinoid ligands N-arachidonoyl glycine (NAGly) and delta 9Tetrahydrocannabinol (Δ9THC) in GPR18-transfected HEK293TR cells. *pA2 Online, 13,* 230.

Ahern, G. P. (2003). Activation of TRPV1 by the satiety factor oleoylethanolamide. *The Journal of Biological Chemistry, 278,* 30429–30434.

Alexander, S. P. H. (2012). So what do we call GPR18 now? *British Journal of Pharmacology, 165,* 2411–2413.

Anavi-Goffer, S., Baillie, G., Irving, A. J., Gertsch, J., Greig, I. R., Pertwee, R. G., et al. (2012). Modulation of L-α-lysophosphatidylinositol/GPR55 mitogen-activated protein kinase (MAPK) signaling by cannabinoids. *The Journal of Biological Chemistry, 287,* 91–104.

Andradas, C., Caffarel, M. M., Perez-Gomez, E., Salazar, M., Lorente, M., Velasco, G., et al. (2011). The orphan G protein-coupled receptor GPR55 promotes cancer cell proliferation via ERK. *Oncogene, 30,* 245–252.

Baker, D., Pryce, G., Davies, W. L., & Hiley, C. R. (2006). In silico patent searching reveals a new cannabinoid receptor. *Trends in Pharmacological Sciences, 27,* 1–4.

Balenga, N. A., Aflaki, E., Kargl, J., Platzer, W., Schroder, R., Blattermann, S., et al. (2011). GPR55 regulates cannabinoid 2 receptor-mediated responses in human neutrophils. *Cell Research, 21,* 1452–1469.

Balenga, N. A., Martinez-Pinilla, E., Kargl, J., Schroder, R., Peinhaupt, M., Platzer, W., et al. (2014). Heteromerization of GPR55 and cannabinoid CB2 receptors modulates signaling. *British Journal of Pharmacology, 171,* 5387–5406.

Begg, M., Pacher, P., Batkai, S., Osei-Hyiaman, D., Offertaler, L., Mo, F. M., et al. (2005). Evidence for novel cannabinoid receptors. *Pharmacology & Therapeutics, 106,* 133–145.

Bilbao, A., Blanco, E., Luque-Rojas, M. J., Suarez, J., Palomino, A., Vida, M., et al. (2013). Oleoylethanolamide dose-dependently attenuates cocaine-induced behaviours through a PPARα receptor-independent mechanism. *Addiction Biology, 18,* 78–87.

Bondarenko, A., Waldeck-Weiermair, M., Naghdi, S., Poteser, M., Malli, R., & Graier, W. F. (2010). GPR55-dependent and -independent ion signalling in response to lysophosphatidylinositol in endothelial cells. *British Journal of Pharmacology, 161,* 308–320.

Bradshaw, H. B., Rimmerman, N., Hu, S. S., Benton, V. M., Stuart, J. M., Masuda, K., et al. (2009). The endocannabinoid anandamide is a precursor for the signaling lipid *N*-arachidonyl glycine through two distinct pathways. *BMC Biochemistry, 10,* 14.

Breivogel, C. S., Griffin, G., Di Marzo, V., & Martin, B. R. (2001). Evidence for a new G protein-coupled cannabinoid receptor in mouse brain. *Molecular Pharmacology, 60,* 155–163.

Burstein, S. (2008). The elmiric acids: Biologically active anandamide analogs. *Neuropharmacology, 55,* 1259–1264.

Burstein, S. H., Adams, J. K., Bradshaw, H. B., Fraioli, C., Rossetti, R. G., Salmonsen, R. A., et al. (2007). Potential anti-inflammatory actions of the elmiric (lipoamino) acids. *Bioorganic & Medicinal Chemistry, 15,* 3345–3355.

Burstein, S. H., McQuain, C. A., Ross, A. H., Salmonsen, R. A., & Zurier, R. E. (2011). Resolution of inflammation by N-arachidonoylglycine. *Journal of Cellular Biochemistry*, *112*, 3227–3233.

Cascio, M. G., Minassi, A., Ligresti, A., Appendino, G., Burstein, S., & Di Marzo, V. (2004). A structure-activity relationship study on *N*-arachidonoyl-amino acids as possible endogenous inhibitors of fatty acid amide hydrolase. *Biochemical and Biophysical Research Communications*, *314*, 192–196.

Chepurny, O. G., Holz, G. G., Roe, M. W., & Leech, C. A. (2016). GPR119 agonist AS1269574 activates TRPA1 cation channels to stimulate GLP-1 secretion. *Molecular Endocrinology*, *30*, 614–629.

Chu, Z. L., Carroll, C., Alfonso, J., Gutierrez, V., He, H., Lucman, A., et al. (2008). A role for intestinal endocrine cell-expressed G protein-coupled receptor 119 in glycemic control by enhancing glucagon-like peptide-1 and glucose-dependent insulinotropic peptide release. *Endocrinology*, *149*, 2038–2047.

Chu, Z. L., Carroll, C., Chen, R., Alfonso, J., Gutierrez, V., He, H., et al. (2010). N-Oleoyldopamine enhances glucose homeostasis through the activation of GPR119. *Molecular Endocrinology*, *24*, 161–170.

Civelli, O., Reinscheid, R. K., Zhang, Y., Wang, Z., Fredriksson, R., & Schioth, H. B. (2013). G protein-coupled receptor deorphanizations. *Annual Review of Pharmacology and Toxicology*, *53*, 127–146.

Console-Bram, L., Brailoiu, E., Brailoiu, G. C., Sharir, H., & Abood, M. E. (2014). Activation of GPR18 by cannabinoid compounds: A tale of biased agonism. *British Journal of Pharmacology*, *171*, 3908–3917.

Cornall, L. M., Mathai, M. L., Hryciw, D. H., Simcocks, A. C., O'Brien, P. E., Wentworth, J. M., et al. (2013). GPR119 regulates genetic markers of fatty acid oxidation in cultured skeletal muscle myotubes. *Molecular and Cellular Endocrinology*, *365*, 108–118.

Costa, B., Giagnoni, G., Franke, C., Trovato, A. E., & Colleoni, M. (2004). Vanilloid TRPV1 receptor mediates the antihyperalgesic effect of the nonpsychoactive cannabinoid, cannabidiol, in a rat model of acute inflammation. *British Journal of Pharmacology*, *143*, 247–250.

Cvijanovic, N., Isaacs, N. J., Rayner, C. K., Feinle-Bisset, C., Young, R. L., & Little, T. J. (2016). Duodenal fatty acid sensor and transporter expression following acute fat exposure in healthy lean humans. *Clinical Nutrition (Edinburgh, Scotland)*, *36*, 564–569.

Daly, C. J., Ross, R. A., Whyte, J., Henstridge, C. M., Irving, A. J., & McGrath, J. C. (2010). Fluorescent ligand binding reveals heterogeneous distribution of adrenoceptors and 'cannabinoid-like' receptors in small arteries. *British Journal of Pharmacology*, *159*, 787–796.

Devane, W. A., Hanus, L., Breuer, A., Pertwee, R. G., Stevenson, L. A., Griffin, G., et al. (1992). Isolation and structure of a brain constituent that binds to the cannabinoid receptor. *Science*, *258*, 1946–1949.

Di Marzo, V., Breivogel, C. S., Tao, Q., Bridgen, D. T., Razdan, R. K., Zimmer, A. M., et al. (2000). Levels, metabolism, and pharmacological activity of anandamide in CB_1 cannabinoid receptor knockout mice: Evidence for non-CB_1, non-CB_2 receptor-mediated actions of anandamide in mouse brain. *Journal of Neurochemistry*, *75*, 2434–2444.

Drmota, T., Greasley, P., & Groblewski, T. (2004). *Screening assays for cannabinoid-ligand-type modulators of GPR55*. WO2004GB00571 20040213.

Fan, A., Wu, X., Wu, H., Li, L., Huang, R., Zhu, Y., et al. (2014). Atheroprotective effect of oleoylethanolamide (OEA) targeting oxidized LDL. *PLoS One*, *9*. e85337.

Finlay, D. B., Joseph, W. R., Grimsey, N. L., & Glass, M. (2016). GPR18 undergoes a high degree of constitutive trafficking but is unresponsive to N-arachidonoyl glycine. *PeerJ*, *4*, e1835.

Ford, L. A., Roelofs, A. J., Anavi-Goffer, S., Mowat, L., Simpson, D. G., Irving, A. J., et al. (2010). A role for L-α-lysophosphatidylinositol and GPR55 in the modulation of migration, orientation and polarization of human breast cancer cells. *British Journal of Pharmacology, 160,* 762–771.

Fu, J., Gaetani, S., Oveisi, F., Lo Verme, J., Serrano, A., Rodriguez De Fonseca, F., et al. (2003). Oleylethanolamide regulates feeding and body weight through activation of the nuclear receptor PPAR-α. *Nature, 425,* 90–93.

Gantz, I., Muraoka, A., Yang, Y. K., Samuelson, L. C., Zimmerman, E. M., Cook, H., et al. (1997). Cloning and chromosomal localization of a gene (GPR18) encoding a novel seven transmembrane receptor highly expressed in spleen and testis. *Genomics, 42,* 462–466.

Garland, S. L. (2013). Are GPCRs still a source of new targets? *Journal of Biomolecular Screening, 18,* 947–966.

Garle, M. J., Mehrotra, P., Sandy-Hindmarch, O., Alharthi, N., & Alexander, S. P. H. (2016). In *N-Acylglycine hydrolysis by rat liver microsomes* (p. 77). *26th annual symposium on the cannabinoids.*

Hansen, K. B., Rosenkilde, M. M., Knop, F. K., Wellner, N., Diep, T. A., Rehfeld, J. F., et al. (2011). 2-Oleoyl glycerol is a GPR119 agonist and signals GLP-1 release in humans. *The Journal of Clinical Endocrinology and Metabolism, 96,* E1409–E1417.

Henstridge, C. M., Balenga, N. A. B., Ford, L. A., Ross, R. A., Waldhoer, M., & Irving, A. J. (2009). The GPR55 ligand L-α-lysophosphatidylinositol promotes RhoA-dependent Ca^{2+} signaling and NFAT activation. *The FASEB Journal, 23,* 183–193.

Henstridge, C. M., Balenga, N. A., Schroder, R., Kargl, J. K., Platzer, W., Martini, L., et al. (2010). GPR55 ligands promote receptor coupling to multiple signalling pathways. *British Journal of Pharmacology, 160,* 604–614.

Heynen-Genel, S., Dahl, R., Shi, S., Milan, L., Hariharan, S., Bravo, Y., et al. (2010a). *Screening for selective ligands for GPR55—Agonists.* Probe Reports from the NIH Molecular Libraries Program [Internet].

Heynen-Genel, S., Dahl, R., Shi, S., Milan, L., Hariharan, S., Sergienko, E., et al. (2010b). *Screening for selective ligands for GPR55—Antagonists.* Probe Reports from the NIH Molecular Libraries Program [Internet].

Huang, S. M., Bisogno, T., Petros, T. J., Chang, S. Y., Zavitsanos, P. A., Zipkin, R. E., et al. (2001). Identification of a new class of molecules, the arachidonyl amino acids, and characterization of one member that inhibits pain. *The Journal of Biological Chemistry, 276,* 42639–42644.

Ikeda, Y., Iguchi, H., Nakata, M., Ioka, R. X., Tanaka, T., Iwasaki, S., et al. (2005). Identification of *N*-arachidonylglycine, U18666A, and 4-androstene-3,17-dione as novel insulin secretagogues. *Biochemical and Biophysical Research Communications, 333,* 778–786.

Jarai, Z., Wagner, J. A., Varga, K., Lake, K. D., Compton, D. R., Martin, B. R., et al. (1999). Cannabinoid-induced mesenteric vasodilation through an endothelial site distinct from CB1 or CB2 receptors. *Proceedings of the National Academy of Sciences of the United States of America, 96,* 14136–14141.

Jeong, H. J., Vandenberg, R. J., & Vaughan, C. W. (2010). N-Arachidonyl-glycine modulates synaptic transmission in superficial dorsal horn. *British Journal of Pharmacology, 161,* 925–935.

Johns, D. G., Behm, D. J., Walker, D. J., Ao, Z., Shapland, E. M., Daniels, D. A., et al. (2007). The novel endocannabinoid receptor GPR55 is activated by atypical cannabinoids but does not mediate their vasodilator effects. *British Journal of Pharmacology, 152,* 825–831.

Kallendrusch, S., Kremzow, S., Nowicki, M., Grabiec, U., Winkelmann, R., Benz, A., et al. (2013). The G protein-coupled receptor 55 ligand L-α-lysophosphatidylinositol exerts microglia-dependent neuroprotection after excitotoxic lesion. *Glia, 61,* 1822–1831.

Kapur, A., Zhao, P., Sharir, H., Bai, Y., Caron, M. G., Barak, L. S., et al. (2009). Atypical responsiveness of the orphan receptor GPR55 to cannabinoid ligands. *The Journal of Biological Chemistry*, *284*, 29817–29827.

Kargl, J., Brown, A. J., Andersen, L., Dorn, G., Schicho, R., Waldhoer, M., et al. (2013). A selective antagonist reveals a potential role of G protein-coupled receptor 55 in platelet and endothelial cell function. *The Journal of Pharmacology and Experimental Therapeutics*, *346*, 54–66.

Kohno, M., Hasegawa, H., Inoue, A., Muraoka, M., Miyazaki, T., Oka, K., et al. (2006). Identification of *N*-arachidonylglycine as the endogenous ligand for orphan G-protein-coupled receptor GPR18. *Biochemical and Biophysical Research Communications*, *347*, 827–832.

Kotsikorou, E., Sharir, H., Shore, D. M., Hurst, D. P., Lynch, D. L., Madrigal, K. E., et al. (2013). Identification of the GPR55 antagonist binding site using a novel set of high-potency GPR55 selective ligands. *Biochemistry*, *52*, 9456–9469.

Lauckner, J. E., Jensen, J. B., Chen, H. Y., Lu, H. C., Hille, B., & Mackie, K. (2008). GPR55 is a cannabinoid receptor that increases intracellular calcium and inhibits M current. *Proceedings of the National Academy of Sciences of the United States of America*, *105*, 2699–2704.

Lauffer, L. M., Iakoubov, R., & Brubaker, P. L. (2009). GPR119 is essential for oleoylethanolamide-induced glucagon-like peptide-1 secretion from the intestinal enteroendocrine L-cell. *Diabetes*, *58*, 1058–1066.

Lu, V. B., Puhl, H. L., & Ikeda, S. R. (2013). N-Arachidonyl glycine does not activate G protein-coupled receptor 18 signaling via canonical pathways. *Molecular Pharmacology*, *83*, 267–282.

McHugh, D., Hu, S. S. J., Rimmerman, N., Juknat, A., Vogel, Z., Walker, J. M., et al. (2010). N-arachidonoyl glycine, an abundant endogenous lipid, potently drives directed cellular migration through GPR18, the putative abnormal cannabidiol receptor. *BMC Neuroscience*, *11*, 44.

McHugh, D., Page, J., Dunn, E., & Bradshaw, H. B. (2012). Δ^9-THC and *N*-arachidonyl glycine are full agonists at GPR18 and cause migration in the human endometrial cell line, HEC-1B. *British Journal of Pharmacology*, *165*, 2414–2424.

McHugh, D., Roskowski, D., Xie, S., & Bradshaw, H. B. (2014). Δ^9-THC and N-arachidonoyl glycine regulate BV-2 microglial morphology and cytokine release plasticity: Implications for signaling at GPR18. *Frontiers in Pharmacology*, *4*, 162.

McHugh, D., Wager-Miller, J., Page, J., & Bradshaw, H. B. (2012). siRNA knockdown of GPR18 receptors in BV-2 microglia attenuates N-arachidonoyl glycine-induced cell migration. *Journal of Molecular Signaling*, *7*, 10.

Mechoulam, R., Benshabat, S., Hanus, L., Ligumsky, M., Kaminski, N. E., Schatz, A. R., et al. (1995). Identification of an endogenous 2-monoglyceride, present in canine gut, that binds to cannabinoid receptors. *Biochemical Pharmacology*, *50*, 83–90.

Moreno, E., Andradas, C., Medrano, M., Caffarel, M. M., Perez-Gomez, E., Blasco-Benito, S., et al. (2014). Targeting CB2-GPR55 receptor heteromers modulates cancer cell signaling. *The Journal of Biological Chemistry*, *289*, 21960–21972.

Moreno-Navarrete, J. M., Catalan, V., Whyte, L., Diaz-Arteaga, A., Vazquez-Martinez, R., Rotellar, F., et al. (2012). The L-α-lysophosphatidylinositol/GPR55 system and its potential role in human obesity. *Diabetes*, *61*, 281–291.

Nunez, D. J., Bush, M. A., Collins, D. A., McMullen, S. L., Gillmor, D., Apseloff, G., et al. (2014). Gut hormone pharmacology of a novel GPR119 agonist (GSK1292263), metformin, and sitagliptin in type 2 diabetes mellitus: Results from two randomized studies. *PLoS One*, *9*, e92494.

Obara, Y., Ueno, S., Yanagihata, Y., & Nakahata, N. (2011). Lysophosphatidylinositol causes neurite retraction via GPR55, G13 and RhoA in PC12 cells. *PLoS One*, *6*, e24284.

Offertaler, L., Mo, F. M., Batkai, S., Liu, J., Begg, M., Razdan, R. K., et al. (2003). Selective ligands and cellular effectors of a G protein-coupled endothelial cannabinoid receptor. *Molecular Pharmacology*, *63*, 699–705.

Oka, S., Nakajima, K., Yamashita, A., Kishimoto, S., & Sugiura, T. (2007). Identification of GPR55 as a lysophosphatidylinositol receptor. *Biochemical and Biophysical Research Communications*, *362*, 928–934.

Oka, S., Toshida, T., Maruyama, K., Nakajima, K., Yamashita, A., & Sugiura, T. (2009). 2-Arachidonoyl-*sn*-glycero-3-phosphoinositol: A possible natural ligand for GPR55. *Journal of Biochemistry*, *145*, 13–20.

O'Sullivan, S. E., Sun, Y., Bennett, A. J., Randall, M. D., & Kendall, D. A. (2009). Time-dependent vascular actions of cannabidiol in the rat aorta. *European Journal of Pharmacology*, *612*, 61–68.

Overton, H. A., Babbs, A. J., Doel, S. M., Fyfe, M. C., Gardner, L. S., Griffin, G., et al. (2006). Deorphanization of a G protein-coupled receptor for oleoylethanolamide and its use in the discovery of small-molecule hypophagic agents. *Cell Metabolism*, *3*, 167–175.

Parmar, N., & Ho, W.-S. V. (2010). N-Arachidonoyl glycine, an endogenous lipid that acts as a vasorelaxant via nitric oxide and large conductance calcium-activated potassium channels. *British Journal of Pharmacology*, *160*, 594–603.

Pertwee, R. G., Howlett, A. C., Abood, M. E., Alexander, S. P. H., Di Marzo, V., Elphick, M. R., et al. (2010). International union of basic and clinical pharmacology. LXXIX. Cannabinoid receptors and their ligands: Beyond CB_1 and CB_2. *Pharmacological Reviews*, *62*, 588–631.

Petitet, F., Donlan, M., & Michel, A. (2006). GPR55 as a new cannabinoid receptor: Still a long way to prove it. *Chemical Biology & Drug Design*, *67*, 252–253.

Pietr, M., Kozela, E., Levy, R., Rimmerman, N., Lin, Y. H., Stella, N., et al. (2009). Differential changes in GPR55 during microglial cell activation. *FEBS Letters*, *583*, 2071–2076.

Pineiro, R., Maffucci, T., & Falasca, M. (2011). The putative cannabinoid receptor GPR55 defines a novel autocrine loop in cancer cell proliferation. *Oncogene*, *30*, 142–152.

Prusakiewicz, J. J., Kingsley, P. J., Kozak, K. R., & Marnett, L. J. (2002). Selective oxygenation of *N*-arachidonylglycine by cyclooxygenase-2. *Biochemical and Biophysical Research Communications*, *296*, 612–617.

Prusakiewicz, J. J., Turman, M. V., Vila, A., Ball, H. L., Al-Mestarihi, A. H., Di Marzo, V., et al. (2007). Oxidative metabolism of lipoamino acids and vanilloids by lipoxygenases and cyclooxygenases. *Archives of Biochemistry and Biophysics*, *464*, 260–268.

Qin, Y., Verdegaal, E. M., Siderius, M., Bebelman, J. P., Smit, M. J., Leurs, R., et al. (2011). Quantitative expression profiling of G-protein-coupled receptors (GPCRs) in metastatic melanoma: The constitutively active orphan GPCR GPR18 as novel drug target. *Pigment Cell & Melanoma Research*, *24*, 207–218.

Rahnasto-Rilla, M., Kokkola, T., Jarho, E., Lahtela-Kakkonen, M., & Moaddel, R. (2016). N-Acylethanolamines bind to SIRT6. *Chembiochem*, *17*, 77–81.

Rao, G. K., & Kaminski, N. E. (2006). Induction of intracellular calcium elevation by Δ^9-tetrahydrocannabinol in T cells involves TRPC1 channels. *Journal of Leukocyte Biology*, *79*, 202–213.

Romero-Zerbo, S. Y., Rafacho, A., Diaz-Arteaga, A., Suarez, J., Quesada, I., Imbernon, M., et al. (2011). A role for the putative cannabinoid receptor GPR55 in the islets of Langerhans. *The Journal of Endocrinology*, *211*, 177–185.

Rosenkilde, M. M., Benned-Jensen, T., Andersen, H., Holst, P. J., Kledal, T. N., Luttichau, H. R., et al. (2006). Molecular pharmacological phenotyping of EBI2. An orphan seven-transmembrane receptor with constitutive activity. *The Journal of Biological Chemistry*, *281*, 13199–13208.

Ryberg, E., Larsson, N., Sjogren, S., Hjorth, S., Hermansson, N. O., Leonova, J., et al. (2007). The orphan receptor GPR55 is a novel cannabinoid receptor. *British Journal of Pharmacology*, *152*, 1092–1101.
Sakamoto, Y., Inoue, H., Kawakami, S., Miyawaki, K., Miyamoto, T., Mizuta, K., et al. (2006). Expression and distribution of Gpr119 in the pancreatic islets of mice and rats: Predominant localization in pancreatic polypeptide-secreting PP-cells. *Biochemical and Biophysical Research Communications*, *351*, 474–480.
Sawzdargo, M., Nguyen, T., Lee, D. K., Lynch, K. R., Cheng, R., Heng, H. H. Q., et al. (1999). Identification and cloning of three novel human G protein-coupled receptor genes GPR52, Psi GPR53 and GPR55: GPR55 is extensively expressed in human brain. *Molecular Brain Research*, *64*, 193–198.
Schuelert, N., & McDougall, J. J. (2011). The abnormal cannabidiol analogue O-1602 reduces nociception in a rat model of acute arthritis via the putative cannabinoid receptor GPR55. *Neuroscience Letters*, *500*, 72–76.
Sharir, H., Console-Bram, L., Mundy, C., Popoff, S. N., Kapur, A., & Abood, M. E. (2012). The endocannabinoids anandamide and virodhamine modulate the activity of the candidate cannabinoid receptor GPR55. *Journal of Neuroimmune Pharmacology*, *7*, 856–865.
Sheskin, T., Hanus, L., Slager, J., Vogel, Z., & Mechoulam, R. (1997). Structural requirements for binding of anandamide-type compounds to the brain cannabinoid receptor. *Journal of Medicinal Chemistry*, *40*, 659–667.
Soga, T., Ohishi, T., Matsui, T., Saito, T., Matsumoto, M., Takasaki, J., et al. (2005). Lysophosphatidylcholine enhances glucose-dependent insulin secretion via an orphan G-protein-coupled receptor. *Biochemical and Biophysical Research Communications*, *326*, 744–751.
Soria-Gomez, E., Guzman, K., Pech-Rueda, O., Montes-Rodriguez, C. J., Cisneros, M., & Prospero-Garcia, O. (2010). Oleoylethanolamide affects food intake and sleep-waking cycle through a hypothalamic modulation. *Pharmacological Research*, *61*, 379–384.
Staton, P. C., Hatcher, J. P., Walker, D. J., Morrison, A. D., Shapland, E. M., Hughes, J. P., et al. (2008). The putative cannabinoid receptor GPR55 plays a role in mechanical hyperalgesia associated with inflammatory and neuropathic pain. *Pain*, *139*, 225–236.
Sun, Y., Alexander, S. P. H., Garle, M. J., Gibson, C. L., Hewitt, K., Murphy, S. P., et al. (2007). Cannabinoid activation of PPARα: A novel neuroprotective mechanism. *British Journal of Pharmacology*, *152*, 734–743.
Syed, S. K., Bui, H. H., Beavers, L. S., Farb, T. B., Ficorilli, J., Chesterfield, A. K., et al. (2012). Regulation of GPR119 receptor activity with endocannabinoid-like lipids. *American Journal of Physiology. Endocrinology and Metabolism*, *303*, E1469–E1478.
Sylantyev, S., Jensen, T. P., Ross, R. A., & Rusakov, D. A. (2013). Cannabinoid- and lysophosphatidylinositol-sensitive receptor GPR55 boosts neurotransmitter release at central synapses. *Proceedings of the National Academy of Sciences of the United States of America*, *110*, 5193–5198.
Thomas, A., Baillie, G. L., Phillips, A. M., Razdan, R. K., Ross, R. A., & Pertwee, R. G. (2007). Cannabidiol displays unexpectedly high potency as an antagonist of CB_1 and CB_2 receptor agonists in vitro. *British Journal of Pharmacology*, *150*, 613–623.
Vassilatis, D. K., Hohmann, J. G., Zeng, H., Li, F., Ranchalis, J. E., Mortrud, M. T., et al. (2003). The G protein-coupled receptor repertoires of human and mouse. *Proceedings of the National Academy of Sciences of the United States of America*, *100*, 4903–4908.
Verzijl, D., Storelli, S., Scholten, D. J., Bosch, L., Reinhart, T. A., Streblow, D. N., et al. (2008). Noncompetitive antagonism and inverse agonism as mechanism of action of nonpeptidergic antagonists at primate and rodent CXCR3 chemokine receptors. *The Journal of Pharmacology and Experimental Therapeutics*, *325*, 544–555.
Waldeck-Weiermair, M., Zoratti, C., Osibow, K., Balenga, N., Goessnitzer, E., Waldhoer, M., et al. (2008). Integrin clustering enables anandamide-induced Ca^{2+}

signaling in endothelial cells via GPR55 by protection against CB_1-receptor-triggered repression. *Journal of Cell Science*, *121*, 1704–1717.
Wang, X., Miyares, R. L., & Ahern, G. P. (2005). Oleoylethanolamide excites vagal sensory neurones, induces visceral pain and reduces short-term food intake in mice via capsaicin receptor TRPV1. *The Journal of Physiology*, *564*, 541–547.
Whyte, L. S., Ryberg, E., Sims, N. A., Ridge, S. A., Mackie, K., Greasley, P. J., et al. (2009). The putative cannabinoid receptor GPR55 affects osteoclast function in vitro and bone mass in vivo. *Proceedings of the National Academy of Sciences of the United States of America*, *106*, 16511–16516.
Wiles, A. L., Pearlman, R. J., Rosvall, M., Aubrey, K. R., & Vandenberg, R. J. (2006). N-Arachidonyl-glycine inhibits the glycine transporter, GLYT2a. *Journal of Neurochemistry*, *99*, 781–786.
Wise, A., & Brown, A. J. (2001). *Screening for modulators of G-protein coupled receptor 55*. https://www.google.com/patents/WO2001086305A3?cl=un.
Yang, Z., Aubrey, K. R., Alroy, I., Harvey, R. J., Vandenberg, R. J., & Lynch, J. W. (2008). Subunit-specific modulation of glycine receptors by cannabinoids and N-arachidonyl-glycine. *Biochemical Pharmacology*, *76*, 1014–1023.
Yang, J. W., Kim, H. S., Im, J. H., Kim, J. W., Jun, D. W., Lim, S. C., et al. (2016). GPR119: A promising target for nonalcoholic fatty liver disease. *The FASEB Journal*, *30*, 324–335.
Yin, H., Chu, A., Li, W., Wang, B., Shelton, F., Otero, F., et al. (2009). Lipid G-protein-coupled receptor ligand identification using β-arrestin pathhunter assay. *The Journal of Biological Chemistry*, *284*, 12328–12338.
Yoshida, S., Ohishi, T., Matsui, T., & Shibasaki, M. (2010). Identification of a novel GPR119 agonist, AS1269574, with in vitro and in vivo glucose-stimulated insulin secretion. *Biochemical and Biophysical Research Communications*, *400*, 437–441.
Yrjölä, S., Parkkari, T., Navia-Paldanius, D., Laitinen, T., Kaczor, A. A., Kokkola, T., et al. (2016). Potent and selective *N*-(4-sulfamoylphenyl)thiourea-based GPR55 agonists. *European Journal of Medicinal Chemistry*, *107*, 119–132.
Zhang, X., Maor, Y., Wang, J. F., Kunos, G., & Groopman, J. E. (2010). Endocannabinoid-like *N*-arachidonoyl serine is a novel pro-angiogenic mediator. *British Journal of Pharmacology*, *160*, 1583–1594.
Zhang, W. B., Navenot, J. M., Haribabu, B., Tamamura, H., Hiramatu, K., Omagari, A., et al. (2002). A point mutation that confers constitutive activity to CXCR4 reveals that T140 is an inverse agonist and that AMD3100 and ALX40-4C are weak partial agonists. *The Journal of Biological Chemistry*, *277*, 24515–24521.

CHAPTER EIGHT

Actions and Regulation of Ionotropic Cannabinoid Receptors

Luciano De Petrocellis*, Massimo Nabissi†, Giorgio Santoni†, Alessia Ligresti*,[1]

*National Research Council of Italy, Institute of Biomolecular Chemistry, Endocannabinoid Research Group, Naples, Italy
†School of Pharmacy, University of Camerino, Camerino, Italy
[1]Corresponding author: e-mail address: aligresti@icb.cnr.it

Contents

Abstract

Almost three decades have passed since the identification of the two specific metabotropic receptors mediating cannabinoid pharmacology. Thereafter, many cannabinoid effects, both at central and peripheral levels, have been well documented and characterized. However, numerous evidences demonstrated that these pharmacological actions could not be attributable solely to the activation of CB1 and CB2 receptors since several important cannabimimetic actions have been found in biological systems lacking CB1 or CB2 gene such as in specific cell lines or transgenic mice. It is now well accepted that, beyond their receptor-mediated effects, these molecules can act also via CB1/CB2-receptor-independent mechanism. Cannabinoids have been demonstrated to modulate several voltage-gated channels (including Ca^{2+}, Na^{+}, and various type of K^{+} channels), ligand-gated ion channels (i.e., GABA, glycine), and ion-transporting membranes proteins such as transient potential receptor class (TRP) channels. The first direct, cannabinoid receptor-independent interaction was reported on the function of serotonin 5-HT_3 receptor-ion channel complex. Similar effects were reported also on the other above mentioned ion channels. In the early ninety, studies searching for endogenous modulators of L-type Ca^{2+} channels identified anandamide as ligand for L-type Ca^{2+} channel. Later investigations indicated that other types of Ca^{2+} currents are also affected by endocannabinoids, and, in the late ninety, it was discovered that endocannabinoids

Advances in Pharmacology, Volume 80
ISSN 1054-3589
http://dx.doi.org/10.1016/bs.apha.2017.04.001

activate the vanilloid receptor subtype 1 (TRPV1), and nowadays, it is known that (endo) cannabinoids gate at least five distinct TRP channels. This chapter focuses on cannabinoid regulation of ion channels and lays special emphasis on their action at transient receptor channels.

ABBREVIATIONS

2-AG 2-arachidonoylglycerol
AEA *N*-arachidonoylethanolamine, anandamide
CB1R cannabinoid receptor type-1
CB2R cannabinoid receptor type-2
CBD cannabidiol
CBDA cannabidiolic acid
CBDV cannabidivarin
CBG cannabigerol
CBGV cannabigevarin
CBN cannabinol
DRG dorsal root ganglia
PIP_2 phosphatidylinositol (4,5) bisphospahate
PKA protein kinase A
PKC protein kinase C
PLC phospholipase C
TG trigeminal ganglia
THC tetrahydrocannabinol
THCA tetrahydrocannabinolic acid
THCV tetrahydrocannabivarin
THCVA tetrahydrocannabivarin carboxylic acid
TRP channels transient receptor potential channels

1. INTRODUCTION

The characterization of tetrahydrocannabinol (THC), the main ingredient of *Cannabis sativa*, represents a milestone in the striking era of cannabinoid research. After that, a significant series of findings led to the discovery of the endocannabinoid system, a physiological signaling system composed of cannabinoid receptor type-1 (CB1R) and cannabinoid receptor type-2 (CB2R) receptors, their endogenous ligands (endocannabinoids), and the biochemical machinery to produce and to degrade these lipids. Such a complex system is involved in most, if not all, aspects of mammalian physiology and pathology (Di Marzo, 2008b).

The two major cannabinoid receptors cloned that have been expressed functionally (Matsuda, 1997) belong to the G-protein-coupled receptor family (GPCR) and couple to inhibition of adenylyl cyclase as well as other second messenger systems such as protein kinase C (PKC) and Ca^{2+} (Howlett & Mukhopadhyay, 2000). However, numerous evidences demonstrated that many of the cannabinoid-receptor-mediated actions both at central and peripheral level could not be attributable solely to the activation of CB1R and CB2R since several important cannabimimetic actions have been found in biological systems lacking CB1R or CB2R gene such as specific cell lines or transgenic mice. It is now well accepted that, beyond their receptor-mediated effects, these molecules can act also via CB1/CB2-receptor-independent mechanism and particularly via ion channels.

Ion channel receptors are usually multimeric proteins located in the plasma membrane. Each protein is arranged in a way that forms a passageway from one side of the membrane to the other. These passageways, or ion channels, have the ability to open and close in response to chemical or mechanical signals. When an ion channel is open, ions move into or out of the cell in single-file fashion. Individual ion channels are specific to particular ions, meaning that they usually allow only a single type of ion to pass through them. The factors that determine how ions wiggle from the cell exterior to its interior (and vice versa) are the type of amino acids that line the channel and the physical width of the channel. The opening of an ion channel is a transitory event. Within a few milliseconds of opening, most ion channels close and enter a resting state, where they are unresponsive to signals for a certain period of time known as desensitization time.

Among the ionotropic cannabinoid receptors a key role is played by the members of the family of transient receptor potential (TRP) channels including TRPV1, TRPV2, TRPV4, TRPM1, TRPM8, and TRPA1. Generally, TRP channels mediate the transmembrane flux of cations down their electrochemical gradients leading to an increase of calcium and sodium intracellular concentration and to cell depolarization (Montell, 2005). Within this context, voltage plays a crucial role by directing the driving force for calcium entry and by controlling the gating of voltage-dependent cation channels (Clapham, Montell, Schultz, & Julius, 2003). Although specific cellular contexts (such as phosphorylation status, ligand concentration, lipid environment, and proteins) differently modulate TRP, three particular ways of activation have been established as fundamental. The first mechanism regards the activation of phospholipase C (PLC) via GPCRs or tyrosine kinase receptors. These specific activations lead to Ca^{2+} release from intracellular stores due to the one of the following cellular events: (a) hydrolysis of phosphatidylinositol (4,5) bisphospahate (PIP_2); (b) production of diacylglycerol (DAG); and (c) production of inositol (1,4,5) trisphosphate (IP_3) (Clapham, 1995). The second mechanism regards the direct activation by ligands, which range from natural products (capsaicin (CPS), menthol) to endogenous lipids, i.e., 2-arachidonoylglycerol (2-AG) and *N*-arachidonoyl ethanolamine (AEA aka anandamide), to inorganic ions (mainly Ca^{2+} and Mg^{2+}) (Ramsey, Delling, & Clapham, 2006). The third mechanism depends on changes in the environment especially pH and ambient temperature (Zheng, 2013). Other mechanisms such as acute posttranslational modifications (phosphorylation), protein kinases (i.e., protein kinase A (PKA), PKC, and PKG), and calcium-calmodulin regulation can also modulate TRP channel activity (Zheng, 2013).

This chapter focuses on cannabinoid-mediated effects on TRP receptors (as summarized in Fig. 1) and provides an overview of the pharmacology of all ion channels that can act as ionotropic cannabinoid receptors.

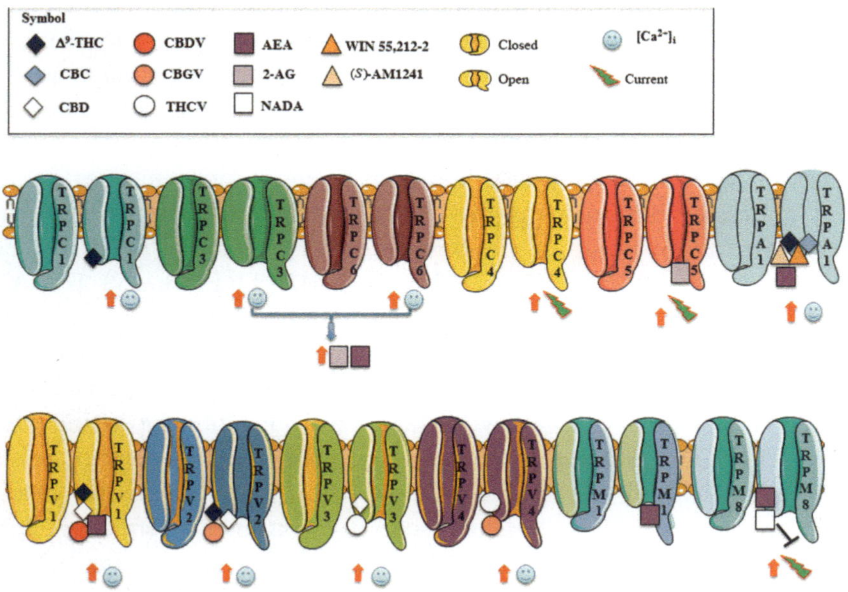

Fig. 1 Actions and regulation of ionotropic cannabinoid receptors. A schematic representation of the TRP channels regulated by cannabinoids is depicted. Cannabinoid molecules are represented bound to the cytoplasmatic domains of open channels. Red arrows, the black bar-headed lines, and green lightning indicate respectively, increase of intracellular calcium, inhibition of intracellular calcium, and inward currents.

2. TRPV CHANNELS AND CANNABINOID-MEDIATED REGULATION

The TRPV channel subfamily consists of six members classifiable in two major groups: the thermosensitive (TRPV1–V4) and the nonthermosensitive (TRPV5 and TRPV6) TRPs. The channels from the former group are moderately permeable to Ca^{2+} and generally activated by extracellular acidification and heat (Nilius, Owsianik, Voets, & Peters, 2007) other than by numerous other stimuli (Benham, Davis, & Randall, 2002). Calcium tightly regulates the channels from the latter group, as these are the only highly Ca^{2+}-selective channels in the TRP family. TRPV5 and TRPV6 conduct calcium under physiological conditions and monovalent cations in absence of extracellular calcium. Moreover, both receptors are voltage dependently blocked by extracellular Mg^{2+} (Pedersen, Owsianik, & Nilius, 2005). All the members of the TRPV subfamily function as tetrameric complexes with each subunit containing six N-terminal ankyrin repeats and they have a TRP box in their C-terminus (Nilius & Szallasi, 2014).

The first mammalian member to be identified and thus one of the most extensively investigated is the TRPV1, a channel widely expressed in spinal and peripheral nerve terminals, as well as in a multiple nonneuronal cell types (Nilius & Szallasi, 2014). The TRPV1 is activated by several molecules including naturally occurring vanilloids such as CPS and resinferatoxin, heat, and endogenous ligands such as protons, *N*-acylamides, arachidonic acid metabolites, as well as *N*-acyl amino acids and *N*-acyl neurotransmitter conjugates (Iannotti, Di Marzo, & Petrosino, 2016). Furthermore, it was shown to be sensitized by PKA, PKC, receptor-activated PLC activity (Mohapatra & Nau, 2003; Premkumar & Ahern, 2000) and by direct binding from PIP_2 originated by PLC-catalyzed PIP_2 hydrolysis (Prescott & Julius, 2003). In the peripheral sensory nerve terminals, it acts as a polymodal receptor, which modulates synaptic transmission at the first sensory synapse (Tominaga et al., 1998). TRPV1 is present in several areas related to pain such as primary afferent neurons, dorsal root ganglia (DRG), the dorsal horn of the spinal cord, and the PAG. However, in term of pain modulation it is worth considering that this channel is not the only major player as numerous evidences indicate intricate interactions with cannabinoid and opioid receptors. These interactions can be bidirectional, inhibitory or excitatory, acute, or chronic, and can arise at molecular level (structurally and functionally) and in physiological processes (Zador & Wollemann, 2015). Although TRPV1 involvement is prevalent in thermal sensory perception, its distribution in regions not subjected to its temperature activation indicates that this receptor plays a role also in other functions. Thus, its expression in the smooth muscle of blood vessels and bronchi is implicated with vasodilatation and bronchoconstriction (Mitchell, Williams, Williams, & Larkin, 1997; Zygmunt et al., 1999), while its presence in the urothelium supports its role in micturition (Birder et al., 2002). Recently, it has been proposed that the temperature-sensitive property of TRPV1 may play an important role in regulating cough reflex (Lee, Ni, Hayes, & Lin, 2011) and airway disease (Wortley, Birrell, & Belvisi, 2016).

Sharing a 50% sequence similarity with TRPV1, the TRPV2 is also expressed in DRG neurons and nonneuronal tissues including gastrointestinal (GI) tract and smooth muscle cells (Beech, Muraki, & Flemming, 2004). TRPV2 is insensitive to CPS or proton but is activated by high temperature and swelling (De Petrocellis & Di Marzo, 2010). A TRPV2-mediated calcium influx has been reported via a stimulation mediated by endogenous lysophospholipids such as lysophosphatidylcoline (LPC) and lysophosphatidylinositol that promote channel translocation to the plasma membrane (Monet et al., 2009). TRPV2 proteins are expressed in CNS, myenteric plexus, nodose ganglion, polymorphonuclear leukocytes, macrophages, and monocytes where they, respectively, mediate cellular effects induced by heat, regulate intestinal movements, and stimulate migration, phagocytosis, and cytokine production (Ramsey et al., 2006).

Showing an important role in thermosensation and several skin functions, TRPV3 channels share only a 43% sequence homology with TRPV1 and are expressed in DRG neurons, trigeminal ganglia (TG) neurons, brain, and various peripheral tissues (hair follicles cells, skin keratinocytes, tongue, and testis). The distribution of this channel resembles its involvement in pain, thermosensation, and itch perception. In particular, genetic deletion of this receptor in mice provoked a reduced scratching behavior compared with wild-type animals (Yamamoto-Kasai et al., 2012). However, it is still controversial whether this phenotype might be directly related to the generation of pruritogenic substances or with the detection of these substances by sensory neurons. TRPV3 is reported to have a role also in maintaining the epidermal homeostasis and dermatitis as well as in promoting the onset of several human skin diseases (Caterina, 2014). TRPV3 is widely present also in the GI tract. Indeed, except for the epithelial cells of stomach, duodenum, and proximal colon, TRPV3 is expressed by epithelial cells of the distal colon, ileum, and jejunum (De Petrocellis, Orlando, et al., 2012). Only recently these receptors have been detected in mouse adipocytes, acinar, and ductal cells, although the physiological relevance of their presence is still debated (Sobhan et al., 2013). TRPV3 receptors are selectively activated by the natural compound camphor and by innocuous warm temperature (Pedersen et al., 2005) and are supposed to form heterooligomers with other TRPVs although the issue is still controversial (Nilius & Szallasi, 2014).

TRPV4 shows some homology with the CPS site of TRPV1 (Nilius & Owsianik, 2011) and can be activated by a plethora of stimuli including moderate heat, cell swelling, shear stress, and several endogenous compounds (Nilius, Vriens, Prenen, Droogmans, & Voets, 2004). This channel exhibits multiple consensus sites for PKC-mediated phosphorylation and its activation is sensitive to PKC analogously to TRPV1 (Nilius et al., 2004). TRPV4 is widely expressed in CNS, but is also easily detectable in non-neuronal tissues such as salivary gland, placenta, chondrocytes, osteoclasts/osteoblasts, lung, keratinocytes, urothelium, vascular endothelial cells, and in a wide range of epithelial cell types in lung, kidney, oviduct, and trachea (Everaerts et al., 2010). Main physiological functions attributable to TRPV4 include central and peripheral thermosensing, mechanosensing, osmosensing, and basal Ca^{2+} homeostasis (O'Neil & Heller, 2005).

Among the others, TRPV5 and TRPV6 constitute a separate group, as they are the only highly Ca^{2+}-selective channels that mutually share almost a 74% amino acid identity with a 23% identity with the other TRPV members. Both channels are voltage dependently blocked by extracellular Mg^{2+} depending on the presence of a ring of negatively charged aspartate residues in the selectivity filter (SF). A voltage-dependent block mediated by intracellular Mg^{2+} has been also reported (Pedersen et al., 2005). TRPV5 and TRPV6 function as homotetramers as well as heterotetramers (TRPV5/6) in expression system via interactions in both the N- and C-termini (Ramsey et al., 2006). Their expression in periphery (small kidney and kidney) is crucial for vitamin D-stimulated calcium uptake across epithelia (Hoenderop, Nilius, & Bindels, 2005).

Cannabinoids target only few members of this subfamily and the first evidence that AEA can activate TRPV1 date back to 1998, when was first noted the chemical similarity between endogenous bioactive lipids and CPS (Di Marzo et al., 1998) that led to the discovery of the endovanilloids. TRPV1 became the first ionotropic cannabinoid receptor identified and the intracellular location of its binding site raised the intriguing hypothesis that AEA, beyond its action as extracellular retrograde messenger, plays a regulatory action on ion channels also as an intracellular messenger (van der Stelt & Di Marzo, 2005). However, the type of cell and the local metabolism of AEA influence the potency and affinity at TRPV1. Moreover, TRPV1 responsiveness and activation is dependent on both AEA metabolism and activation of the "classical" receptors since (1) AEA metabolites affect TRPV1 responses and (2) the convergent physiological actions of AEA and TRPV1 agonists necessarily represent direct effects on TRPV1. In addition, the coactivation of cannabinoid receptors and TRPV1 is a relevant issue that often complicates the distinction between these pathways (van der Stelt & Di Marzo, 2005). Also synthetic analogues of AEA such as *R*-(+)-methanandamide (Met-AEA) and arachidonoyl-2′-chloroethylamide (ACEA) can activate this channel (Ross et al., 2001). Interestingly, although with a low potency, the CB1 blocker SR141617A was reported as a TRPV1 mixed agonist/antagonist in HEK cells (De Petrocellis et al., 2001), isolated blood vessels (Zygmunt et al., 1999), and hippocampal neurons (Gibson, Edwards, Page, Van Hook, & Kauer, 2008). Recently, patch-clamp analysis in transfected HEK-293 cells demonstrated that the nonpsychotropic plant cannabinoids CBD and CBDV dose dependently activate and rapidly desensitize TRPV1 expressed to a varying extent in rat hippocampal slices. Similarly, to CPS, these phytocannabinoids dephosphorylated rat hippocampal TRPV1 in slices kept in an Mg^{2+}-free solution leading to its desensitization, and contrasting TRPV1 participation in neuronal hyperexcitability (Iannotti et al., 2014).

The high-threshold thermosensor TRPV2 is specifically activate by plant cannabinoids. Based on the previously reported agonistic effect of CBD on this channel in cultured rat dorsal root ganglion neurons (Qin et al., 2008), a recent study investigated the effects of 11 pure cannabinoids and botanical extracts in TRPV2-overexpressing HEK-293 cells. Almost all pure compounds increased $[Ca^{2+}]_i$ with a rank of potency as follows: THC > CBD > cannabigevarin (CBGV) > CBG > tetrahydrocannabivarin (THCV) > CBDV > cannabinol (CBN). All the carboxylic acid cannabinoids (i.e., tetrahydrocannabinolic acid (THCA), tetrahydrocannabivarin carboxylic acid (THCVA), cannabidiolic acid (CBDA), and CBGA) as well as CBC were inactive or showed a very weak effect. However, a 5 min preincubation of TRPV2-HEK-293 cells with CBGV, THC, CBG, CBD, and THCV dose dependently abolished the LPC-induced elevation of intracellular calcium $[Ca^{2+}]_i$ suggesting an antagonist/desensitizing behavior. Importantly, the order of potency for desensitization did not merely reflect the rank order of potency for channel activation (De Petrocellis et al., 2011).

Endogenous compounds such as growth factors, hormones, and endocannabinoids are also able to activate TRPV2. In nonmalignant cells, this activation induces a translocation of the receptor from the endosomal compartment to the plasma membrane, which results in abrogation of cell proliferation and induction of cell death. Therefore, the loss of TRPV2 signaling leads to unconstrained proliferation, resistance to apoptotic signals, and increased resistance to CD95-induced apoptotic cell death (Liberati et al., 2014; Nabissi et al., 2010). Other endogenous molecules such as ω-3 polyunsaturated fatty acid docosahexaenoic acid (DHA) have been reported not to have a direct activation of TRPV2, but on the expression of its protein. In fact, DHA in a dose-dependent manner downregulated TRPV2 expression in correlation with DHA's effect on spatial memory (Pan et al., 2011).

Very few evidences have been reported regarding cannabinoid activation of TRPV3 and TRPV4 receptors. A recent paper showed that plant cannabinoids evoke intracellular Ca^{2+} response in both TRPV3- and TRPV4-expressing heterologous cells. In particular, CBD and THCV activated TRPV3 channel with high efficacy and potency, whereas CBGV and CBGA were more prone at desensitizing it upon carvacrol stimulus. Analogously, CBDV and THCV induced TRPV4-mediated calcium influx with moderate efficacy and potency, whereas CBG, CBGV, and CBGA desensitized it efficiently to the response of 4-α-phorbol 12,13-didecanoate (4α-PDD) (De Petrocellis, Orlando, et al., 2012). Moreover, the same study supported the hypothesis of a crucial role for TRPV3 in GI inflammation based on the following evidences: (1) these receptors are widely distributed at GI level and (2) the TRPV3-inactive CBC reduced the mRNA expression in jejunum and ileum of croton oil-treated mice (De Petrocellis, Orlando, et al., 2012).

In addition to plant cannabinoid, TRPV4 is reported to be activated by the endocannabinoid AEA and its metabolite arachidonic acid although in an indirect way involving the cytochrome P450 epoxygenase-dependent formation of epoxyeicosatrienoic acids (Watanabe et al., 2003). The application of a cytochrome P450 metabolite of arachidonic acid (5′,6′-epoxyeicosatrienoic acid; 5,6-EET) activated TRPV4 in a membrane-delimited manner and led to a TRPV4-mediated Ca^{2+} influx in vascular endothelial cells. The idea proposed by the study is that the relaxant effects of endocannabinoids and their P450 epoxygenase-dependent metabolites on vascular tone is supported by TRPV4 activation (Watanabe et al., 2003).

3. TRPA CHANNELS AND CANNABINOID-MEDIATED REGULATION

The TRPA family comprises just one mammalian member, TRPA1, which is primarily expressed in most nociceptors (small neurons of dorsal root, trigeminal, and nodose ganglia) where it contributes to cold, mechanical, and chemical nociception. TRPA1 is also present in nonneuronal tissues such as lung, heart, small intestine, pancreas, as well as in hair cell epithelia where it contributes to nonneurogenic inflammation, basal insulin release, GI, and hearing functions (Cao et al., 2012; Kaji, Yasuoka, Karaki, & Kuwahara, 2012; Nagata, Duggan, Kumar, & Garcia-Anoveros, 2005; Nassini et al., 2012).

Formerly TRPA1 was known as ANKTM1 for its large number of ankyrin repeats at the cytoplasmic N-terminal (the mammalian TRPA1 contains 14–19 ankyrin repeats) in addition to the six-transmembrane domains characteristic of all TRP channels (Story et al., 2003). TRPA1 is activated by many irritants like isothiocyanates, the pungent compound in mustard oil, wasabi, and horse radish (Bandell et al., 2004); allicilin and cinnamaldehyde, the pungent natural compounds present in garlic and cinnamon, respectively (Macpherson et al., 2005); and the plant-derived cannabinoid receptor agonists THC (Jordt et al., 2004).

All these compounds have very different structures, but all are electrophiles that may covalently modify intracellular cysteines and lysines forming Michael adducts that allosterically open the channel (Hinman, Chuang, Bautista, & Julius, 2006; Paulsen, Armache, Gao, Cheng, & Julius, 2015). Structurally, each TRPA1 subunit consists of six-transmembrane α-helices (S1–S6) with a reentrant pore loop between S5 and S6. Apart from this conserved transmembrane core, TRPA1 exhibits numerous distinctive features such as a C-terminal tetrameric parallel coiled-coil domain, which is linked with another extended feature that forms the crescent-shaped element and is surrounded by a five ankyrin repeats (Paulsen et al., 2015). Key cysteine residues that contribute to activation by electrophiles are located within the pre-S1 region at solvent-accessible sites, probably accounting for their relative chemical reactivity. Several studies suggest that TRPA1 functions as an electrophile receptor, with key cysteine and lysine residues that cause channel gating located in ankyrin repeat domains (Kim & Cavanaugh, 2007). However, TRPA1 can be activated by other plant compounds, independently of the reactive cysteines, suggesting the presence of alternative activation mechanisms (Cavanaugh, Simkin, & Kim, 2008).

The idea that the main psychoactive compound from *Cannabis sativa* can stimulate TRPA1 raised up after that THC was shown able to relax hepatic or mesenteric arteries in vitro by activating CPS-sensitive, CGRP-containing perivascular sensory nerve endings that innervate the smooth muscle (Zygmunt, Andersson, & Hogestatt, 2002). This effect was not cannabinoid receptor mediated but similarly to those of CPS and other vanilloid receptor agonists (Zygmunt et al., 1999) it depended on extracellular calcium and was sensitive to ruthenium red, a general inhibitor of TRP channels including TRPA1. Therefore, Jordt and coworkers investigated whether THC and specific TRPA1 ligands excite the same population of CGRP-containing sensory neurons. Indeed, all THC-excitable cells responded to mustard oil in a ruthenium red sensitive way, and a subpopulation of CPS-sensitive cells was dually responsive to mustard oil and THC. All the results obtained suggested that THC and mustard oil excite nociceptors through a similar, if not identical mechanism involving activation of a calcium-permeable, ruthenium-red-blockable channel on CPS-sensitive, CGRP-containing sensory neurons. Finally, they indicated TRPA1 channel as the only molecular target, which met these characteristics (Jordt et al., 2004). Later on, in HEK-293 cells stably expressing the rat TRPA1, the affinity of THC was confirmed with a potency of $EC_{50} = 0.23 \pm 0.03\,\mu M$ (De Petrocellis et al., 2008).

TRPA1 plays a role in thermal, cold, and mechanical nociception in acute pain models and TRPA1 activators induce spontaneous pain and hyperalgesia. Even though its role per se or in respect to other TRP channels (i.e., TRPV1) has been debated (Bautista et al., 2006). Other than in acute nociception TRPA1 is also involved in chronic painful states such as neuropathic pain (Obata et al., 2005) and diabetic neuropathy (Eberhardt et al., 2012; Wei et al., 2010). Cannabinoids produce profound supraspinal, spinal, and peripheral antinociception and antihyperalgesia in several acute and chronic pain states mostly via the $G_{i/o}$-protein-coupled cannabinoid receptors (Croxford, 2003). However, a CB1/CB2-independent peripheral cannabinoid mechanism, including the activation of Ca^{2+} permeable channels, has been also proposed (Duncan, Kendall, & Ralevic, 2004; Ralevic & Kendall, 2001). Indeed, plant, synthetic, and endogenous cannabinoids were reported to elevate $[Ca^{2+}]_i$ in nociceptors by gating TRPV1 or TRPA1 channels (Huang et al., 2002; Jordt et al., 2004; Price, Patwardhan,

Akopian, Hargreaves, & Flores, 2004). Given that, TRPA1 channel can undergo pharmacological desensitization (Ruparel, Patwardhan, Akopian, & Hargreaves, 2008), its activation by cannabinoids could lead ultimately to a channel inhibition. Some aminolakylindole derivatives such as *R*-WIN 55,212-2 and *S*-AM1241 were found to inhibit the responses of trigeminal ganglion neurons to noxious chemical stimuli via a TRPA1 channel-mediated mechanism (Akopian, Ruparel, Patwardhan, & Hargreaves, 2008). Accordingly, these two cannabinoid receptor agonists have been reported to activate rat TRPA1 in HEK-293-overexpressing cells with a potency of $EC_{50} = 2.3 \pm 0.1\,\mu M$ for *R*-WIN 55,212-2 and $19.5 \pm 5.8\,\mu M$ for *S*-AM1241, respectively (Soethoudt et al., 2017).

A different strategy suggested to alleviate pain was the spinal TRPA1 activation by cannabinoids and paracetamol metabolites (Andersson et al., 2011). TRPA1 was reported to be upregulated following inflammatory injury (da Costa et al., 2010) and to mediate carrageenan-induced inflammatory pain response (Bonet, Fischer, Parada, & Tambeli, 2013). Several evidence suggested that endogenous activation of peripheral TRPA1 receptors could play a crucial role in the development of TNFα-induced mechanical hyperalgesia and in sustaining the mechanical hyperalgesia observed after intraarticular injection of Freund's complete adjuvant (CFA). These results indicated the blockade of TRPA1 receptors as a beneficial approach in reducing the chronic pain associated with arthritis (Fernandes et al., 2011). Moreover, some ketones that have been previously shown to inhibit TNFα and IL-6 expression such as the chalcone derivatives were also reported to activate and subsequently desensitize TRPA1 confirming the relevance of antihyperalgesic preparations based on TRPA1 desensitization (Schiano Moriello et al., 2016).

A role in the visceral perception of pain has also been attributed to this channel. In fact, TRPA1 was also reported to be upregulated in colonic afferent DRG of rats exposed to a prolonged water avoidance stress indicating its involvement in the stress-induced visceral hyperalgesia (Yu et al., 2010). The upregulation of TRPA1 was also observed in colitis model induced after intracolonic administration of the TRPA1 activator allyl isothiocyanate (AITC) (Yang et al., 2008). Even though the AITC-induced-colitis has been reported to generate TRPA1-independent effects (Capasso et al., 2012), when the TRPA1 upregulation occurs in humans or mouse colitis models, it leads to protective roles by decreasing the expression of several inflammatory cytokines and chemokines as well as proinflammatory neuropeptides (Kun et al., 2014).

The control of intracellular activities triggering antihyperalgesia and antinociception can occur via two distinct pathways (metabotropic or ionotropic) that can work independently or can functionally cooperate under certain conditions. CB1R agonists, including AEA, are able to directly stimulate the hydrolysis of PIP_2 with release of inositol-1,4,5-phosphate (IP_3) and Ca^{2+} mobilization from the endoplasmic reticulum via either $G_{q/11}$- or $G_{i/o}$-mediated mechanisms (Lauckner, Hille, & Mackie, 2005). In turn, this mechanism may cause the concomitant modulation of several plasma membrane calcium channels, including some TRP channels (Nilius, Owsianik, & Voets, 2008). Likewise, CB1 may also modulate phosphoinositide-3-kinase (PI3K)-mediated signaling cascades via activation of $G_{i/o}$ (Sanchez, Ruiz-Llorente, Sanchez, & Diaz-Laviada, 2003) with consequences on PIP_2 levels, thereby indirectly influencing the activity of Ca^{2+} channels. AEA not only dose dependently stimulates rat recombinant TRPA1 with elevation of cytosolic Ca^{2+}, with a potency of about 10 μM, (De Petrocellis & Di Marzo, 2009) but also was able to desensitize this channel in HEK-293-overexpressing cells (De Petrocellis, Schiano Moriello, et al., 2012). AEA affinity was further confirmed on human TRPA1 (Redmond, Gu, Camo, McIntyre, & Connor, 2014). It is worth noting that also arachidonic acid is reported to activate very strongly mouse, rat, and human TRPA1 (Bandell et al., 2004; Motter & Ahern, 2012; Redmond et al., 2014), and that several arachidonic acid-derived molecules, including highly reactive COX-dependent fatty acid metabolites (Materazzi et al., 2008), prostaglandins (Taylor-Clark et al., 2008), hepoxilins (Gregus et al., 2012), and epoxyeicosatreinoic acids (Sisignano et al., 2012) have been shown to activate TRPA1.

Finally, also several nonpsychoactive phytocannabinoids were shown to potently and efficaciously elevate $[Ca^{2+}]_i$ in rat TRPA1-overexpressing HEK-293 cells and in AITC-responding DRG neurons (De Petrocellis et al., 2011, 2008) being the most potent compound CBC with an $EC_{50} = 34\,\mu M$ in DRG and $EC_{50} = 60\,nM$ in rat TRPA1-HEK-293 cells. The rank of potency observed in TRPA1-HEK-293 cells was the following CBC > CBD > CBN > CBDV > CBG > THCV > CBGV > THCA > CBDA > CBGA > THCVA, indicating that a plenty of plant compounds activated this receptor. Interestingly, all the compounds that activated TRPA1 were also able to desensitize this channel to AITC. In addition, a minor compound such as the cannabinoid sesqui-CBG desensitized TRPA1 ($EC_{50} = 1.7 \pm 0.9\,\mu M$) though more potently ($IC_{50} = 1.2 \pm 0.2\,\mu M$) than its lower prenilogue CBG (Pollastro et al., 2011).

4. TRPM CHANNELS AND CANNABINOID-MEDIATED REGULATION

The TRPM subfamily comprises eight putative members, which are divided in three main groups (TRPM1/3, TRPM4/5, and TRPM6/7) with two separate members (TRPM2 and TRPM8) showing low sequence homology (Fleig & Penner, 2004). Among the TRP channels, these receptors are unique as there are no ankyrin domains in their N-terminus and particularly, TRPM2, TRPM6, and TRPM7 encode enzymatically active protein domains (PKA) fused to their ion channel structures (Ramsey et al., 2006). TRPM channels exhibit highly varying permeability to ions being generally all Ca^{2+} and Mg^{2+} permeable ranging from the Ca^{2+} impermeability of TRPM4 and TRPM5 to the significantly Ca^{2+} permeability of TRPM6 and TRPM7 (Nilius & Owsianik, 2011).

TRPM1 was the first member to be discovered of the melanoma transient receptor potential (TRPM) subfamily. It is an about 180kDa visual transduction channel protein localized in the somas and dendrites of both rod and cone on retinal ON bipolar cells. It is regulated via metabotropic glutamate receptor 6 (mGluR6) by glutamate released from photoreceptors hyperpolarized by an increment of light intensity (Koike et al., 2010; Morgans et al., 2009) and via an heterotrimeric G protein Go (Xu et al., 2016). In the retina, TRPM1 is also primary for night vision, as genetic mutations in the TRPM1 gene are associated with night blindness (Zeitz, Robson, & Audo, 2015). Outside the retina, TRPM1 regulate pigmentation in melanocytes, and its loss is correlated with tumor aggressiveness in human melanoma (Duncan et al., 1998).

TRPM2 is a calcium cation permeable channel first isolated from human brain (Nagamine et al., 1998), but only later assigned to the melastatin subfamily (Montell et al., 2002).

TRPM2 is widely expressed in the CNS as well as in microglia, but also in other tissues such as the bone marrow, spleen, heart, liver, lung, placenta, endometrium, GI tract, as well as in different cell types like pancreatic β-cells, salivary gland, endothelial cells, heart and vasculature, and immune (Faouzi & Penner, 2014). Considering that TRPM2 is highly expressed in brain, its physiological role in the CNS has been suggested to contribute to synaptic transmission as its loss impairs NMDA receptor-dependent LTD (Xie et al., 2011). Furthermore TRPM2 seems to be responsible for microglia activation through ROS- and LPS-mediated signaling

(Faouzi & Penner, 2014). TRPM2-mediated Ca^{2+} influx induced nuclear translocation of nuclear factor-κB, controlling the ROS signaling cascade responsible for chemokine production, which aggravates inflammation and may induce cell death (Haraguchi et al., 2012; Yamamoto et al., 2008).

TRPM3 is highly expressed in nociceptor neurons and in particular in a subset of small diameter sensory neurons from dorsal root (DRG) and trigeminal ganglia (TG) where is activated by heat in general and during the development of inflammatory heat hyperalgesia (Vriens et al., 2011). It has been suggested that channel activation occurs not only via central pore permeation but also via an alternative ion penetration pathway leading to TRPM3-dependent pain (Vriens et al., 2014). An abundant expression of this receptor found in glutamatergic synapses from cerebellar cortex is reported to modulate glutamatergic transmission in developing brain (Zamudio-Bulcock, Everett, Harteneck, & Valenzuela, 2011).

The Ca^{2+}-activated TRPM4, as mentioned earlier, is only permeable to monovalent ions such as K^+ and Na^+ (Launay et al., 2002; Vennekens & Nilius, 2007) and is expressed in a wide range of tissues. In particular, it is present in several areas of the brain, in both vascular and smooth muscle cells, in exocrine cells from the pancreatic tissue, in red blood cells, in adipocytes, in mast cells and in T cells where it is involved in various physiological processes including T cell activation, myogenic vasoconstriction, allergic reactions, and neurotoxicity (Cho, Lee, Kim, Hwang, & Park, 2015; Mathar et al., 2014; Vennekens et al., 2007). TRPM4 is also involved in the nonapoptotic cell death process of oncosis, a physiopathological process characterized by Na^+ influx resulting in cell volume increase, membrane blebbing and membrane rupture, necrotic cell death (Simard, Woo, & Gerzanich, 2012). TRPM4 plays an obligate role in necrotic cell death since the two principal regulators of TRPM4, intracellular ATP and Ca^{2+} are both characteristically altered during necrosis in a way that causes TRPM4 channel opening (Guinamard, Salle, & Simard, 2011). Moreover, TRPM4 levels increase following hypoxia/ischemic stroke, and following spinal cord injury (Loh et al., 2014).

Similarly, the TRPM5 has characteristics of a calcium-activated, nonselective cation channel that carries Na^+ and K^+ equally well, but not Ca^{2+} ions (Prawitt et al., 2003). It is also a highly temperature-sensitive, heat-activated channel showing a steep increase of inward currents at temperatures between 15°C and 35°C (Talavera et al., 2005). This protein plays an important role in taste transduction. Briefly, TRPM5 in a subset of taste bud cells, receptor (type II) taste cells, is coexpressed with taste receptors.

Binding of taste stimuli to G protein-coupled taste receptors leads to dissociation of the heterotrimeric G protein, whose βγ subunits activate PLCβ2 that hydrolyzes PIP_2 into DAG and IP_3, the latter activates IP_3 receptors, which release Ca^{2+} from intracellular stores. Intracellular Ca^{2+} opens TRPM5 with monovalent cation influx and depolarization of the cell (Liman, 2014). Outside the taste buds, TRPM5 is also found in chemical-sensing cells that express "taste" GPCRs located in the GI tract, the respiratory system, and the pancreas. Within these organs, TRPM5 is functional implicated with the regulation of sensation of taste compounds, olfaction of odorants and pheromones (Kaske et al., 2007; Lin, Ogura, Margolskee, Finger, & Restrepo, 2008), and the regulation of normal glucose-stimulated insulin secretion (Brixel et al., 2010). TRPM5 expression in the CNS (particularly in hypothalamus and brainstem) seems involved in energy homeostasis as obesity decreases its expression in these regions (Herrera Moro Chao et al., 2016).

TRPM6 channel, also known as channel kinase 2 (Chak2), for its α-type kinase domain fused to the C-terminal end (Ryazanov, 2002), is detected in a limited number of tissues and mostly in epithelial cells. In particular, TRPM6 transcript is well represented in testis, has limited expression in lung and leukocytes, and is abundant in the intestine and in the kidney where, along to TRPM7, it has a key role in regulating Mg^{2+} homeostasis (Chubanov & Gudermann, 2014). Indeed, the TRPM6-mediated action on Mg^{2+} absorption requires the formation of heteromultimeric channels with TRPM7 and very recently TRPM7 kinase has been proposed to function as part of a Mg^{2+} sensor and transducer of signaling pathways during stressful environmental conditions (Cabezas-Bratesco et al., 2015). Evidences indicating that alterations in TRPM6 function contributed to neural tube defects in humans confirmed the primary role of TRPM6 in Mg^{2+} homeostasis. Mice defective in TRPM6 showed embryonic mortality and neural tube defects suggesting that, in embryonic stem cells and during early embryonic development, TRPM6 expression is required for rapidly dividing cells of the embryo for high amounts of Mg^{2+} (Walder et al., 2009). Accordingly, several hereditary forms of hypomagnesemia have been deciphered with mutations in TRPM6 (de Baaij, Hoenderop, & Bindels, 2015).

Similarly to TRPM6, also TRPM7 belongs to the family of atypical protein kinases known as alpha kinases showing a kinase catalytic domain at C-terminus, but differently to its homologous TRPM7 is ubiquitously expressed in human tissues (Ryazanov, 2002). The kinase domain of TRPM7 directly associates with the C2 domain of PLC. Receptor-mediated activation of PLC results in the hydrolysis of PIP_2, the substrate of PLC, and inhibition of TRPM7 (Runnels, Yue, & Clapham, 2002). The TRPM7 kinase specifically phosphorylates Ser and Thr residues in an Mg^{2+}-dependent manner (Ryazanova, Dorovkov, Ansari, & Ryazanov, 2004) while cations entering through TRPM7 channel may play a crucial role in regulation of the kinase function. As mentioned, TRPM7 plays a crucial role in epithelial Mg^{2+} transport and in its active absorption. It controls cellular Mg^{2+} levels and has an essential role in the control of cellular and whole body Mg^{2+} homeostasis since embryonic stem cells lacking TRPM7 kinase domain displayed a proliferation arrest phenotype that can be rescued by Mg^{2+} supplementation (Ryazanova et al., 2010). This ion channel is also essential for the physiology of proliferating cells regulating cell growth and proliferation and its ablation in proliferating tissue arrests the cell cycle at G_0/G_1 transition. It is involved in apoptosis-induced process in differentiated mast cells (Ng, Jiang, & Lv, 2012) and in hepatic stellate cells (Liu, Li, Huang, & Huang, 2012), while a TRPM7 downregulation has been linked to the differentiation process (Lam, Grant, & Hill, 2012). TRPM7 is involved also in cell adhesion and migration and seems to regulate migration of activated human T cells (Kuras, Yun, Chimote, Neumeier, & Conforti, 2012). Being involved in cell growth, proliferation, differentiation, and migration TRPM7 is a possible target in cancer (Sahni, Tamura, Sweet, & Scharenberg, 2010). Reducing TRPM7 expression inhibits proliferation in human head and neck carcinoma, human gastric adenocarcinoma cells; affects cell migration and invasiveness; and is generally upregulated in human pancreatic adenocarcinoma, human breast cancer, rat hepatoma (Fleig & Chubanov, 2014; Gautier et al., 2016). Interestingly, human pancreatic ductal adenocarcinoma patient survival is inversely related to TRPM7 expression levels (Rybarczyk et al., 2012).

The last member of this family is the TRPM8, also known as the cold- and menthol-activated nonselective channel CMR-1, with prominent voltage-dependent gating properties (McKemy, Neuhausser, & Julius, 2002). TRPM8 is required in the detection of environmental cold temperature and is involved in body temperature regulation (Gavva et al., 2012). The activation of TRPM8 by cold and cooling agents requires also the presence of the membrane phospholipid PIP_2 (Zakharian, Cao, & Rohacs, 2010) as well as a negative shift in the voltage-dependent activation to open the channel at negative potentials (Malkia et al., 2007). Menthol derivative WS-12, icilin, and other synthetic compounds are able to elicit a cooling sensation even with a greater fold of potency rather than menthol

(Bodding, Wissenbach, & Flockerzi, 2007; De Petrocellis, Ortar, Schiano Moriello, Serum, & Rusterholz, 2015). TRPM8 monomers are associated in quaternary structure as homotetramer in a transmembrane protein constituted by six helices similarly to all other TRPs (Pedretti, Marconi, Bettinelli, & Vistoli, 2009). Each subunit consists of six-transmembrane regions (S1–S6), a short pore loop between S5 and S6 that allows the permeation of cations across the membrane, and cytoplasmic N- and C-terminal domains. In particular, between S5 and S6 it is possible to identify a short pore helix (P-helix), a loop, which includes the SF and an extracellular linker (Bidaux et al., 2015). P-helix and other transmembrane regions (S1, S2, and S4) are crucial for menthol- and cold-mediated TRPM8 activity (Bandell et al., 2006; Voets, Owsianik, Janssens, Talavera, & Nilius, 2007), while S6 seems responsible for the ion selectivity (Voets et al., 2007). The C-terminus holds structural elements involved in temperature-dependent gating (Brauchi, Orta, Salazar, Rosenmann, & Latorre, 2006) containing sites for the activation of the channel by PIP_2 (Rohacs, Lopes, Michailidis, & Logothetis, 2005). Some residues at cytosolic N-terminus are PKA phosphorylation sites, which if activated by PKA pathway activators, reduce the response to menthol (De Petrocellis et al., 2007).

TRPM8 is mainly expressed in cold-sensitive peripheral sensory neurons of DRG and TG, which are distinct from those expressing TRPA1 (Kobayashi et al., 2005). However, two different classes of TRPM8-expressing somatosensory neurons were reported, one is menthol-sensitive/CPS-insensitive and the other is menthol-sensitive/CPS-sensitive, ATP-sensitive, prolonged acid response (Xing, Ling, Chen, & Gu, 2006). Apart from its role in thermosensation, TRPM8 seems to play other physiological roles and its altered function or expression has been correlated to different disease states. Other than in somatosensory neurons, TRPM8 is highly expressed by other peripheral tissues especially related to the urogenital tract such as bladder, testis, and prostate where it was first identified. In prostate cancer, as well as in other neoplasms, TRPM8 is upregulated in androgen-sensitive cancer cells and positively regulated by androgens (Zhang & Barritt, 2004). Indeed, testosterone is the only endogenous agonist of TRPM8 so far identified, exerting a potent ionotropic effect at picomolar concentrations, suggesting a crucial role in prostate cancer cell survival (Asuthkar et al., 2015). Consequently, many antagonists and modulators of TRPM8 have been shown useful in the treatment of prostate cancer (Bidaux et al., 2016; Liu et al., 2016). Among these molecules, plant-derived cannabinoids as potent inhibitor of TRPM8 activity were reported potent inhibitors of prostate carcinoma viability in vitro (De Petrocellis et al., 2013). TRPM8 expression is markedly increased in bladder biopsies of patients with bladder pain syndrome or idiopathic detrusor overactivity (Mukerji et al., 2006). Furthermore, pharmacological TRPM8 inhibition acting on the bladder afferent pathway was shown to reduce the frequency of rat bladder contractions and nociceptive reflex responses (Lashinger et al., 2008), or cold stress-induced detrusor over activity (Lei et al., 2013). In mouse sperm, this channel detects temperature changes and may influence the acrosome reaction (Martinez-Lopez et al., 2011). TRPM8 is also present in brown adipocytes where the functional implication of its expression is related to the triggering of UCP1-dependent thermogenesis (Rossato et al., 2014). It is also expressed in corneal cool cells where it regulates ocular surface wetness (Parra et al., 2010). Accordingly, this receptor is reported as a pharmacological target of borneol, which can activate the channel by increasing tear production without evoking nociceptive responses (Chen, Lei, Zhou, Zeng, & Zou, 2016). Only recently it has been described a functional presence of TRPM8 at level of salivary glands and dentin–pulp complexes where this receptor is proposed to be involved in cell differentiation in the submandibular gland during early developmental stage (Fujiseki et al., 2017). Furthermore, the presence of TRPM8 in dentin–pulp complexes is thought to play a crucial role in the nociceptive function of odontoblasts (Tazawa, Ikeda, Kawashima, & Okiji, 2017).

In respect to the regulation of these ion channels from cannabinoids, these molecules can target only TRPM1 and TRPM8. In particular, AEA likely activates mouse TRPM1 on retinal ON bipolar cells independently from TRPV1 and mGluR6 by functioning as modulator of synaptic transmission. One corroborated hypothesis is that, in these cells, the transduction channel is composed of TRPM1, either as a homomer, or in association with other TRP channels, as TRPM1 is localized in the somas and dendrites of both rod and cone on retinal ON bipolar cells where it regulates the darkness/light-sensitivity via glutamate release by mGluR6 (Shen et al., 2009). Briefly, in the retina, during darkness the depolarized photoreceptors release glutamate hyperpolarizing the ON bipolar cells, while the light hyperpolarizes the photoreceptors, reducing presynaptic glutamate release causing the ON bipolar cells to depolarize (Euler, Haverkamp, Schubert, & Baden, 2014). The functional role of TRPM1 in mGluR6 signal transduction was further confirmed as mGluR6 deletion makes the TRPM1 channel in retina inactive (Xu et al., 2012).

AEA, as well as the endovanilloid *N*-arachidonoyldopamine (NADA), can target also TRPM8. In particular, these molecules inhibited a TRPM8-mediated intracellular Ca^{2+} elevation induced by either menthol or icilin (De Petrocellis et al., 2007). In HEK-293 TRPM8-expressing cells, other cannabinoids including plant-derived ones, were able to inhibit agonist-evoked Ca^{2+} increases with a rank order of potency against icilin (0.25 μM) as following: CBD > CBG > Δ^9-THCA > CBN > THCV >CBDV > CBGA > THCVA > CBGV > CBDA (IC_{50} = 0.06–4.8 μM) (De Petrocellis et al., 2011). In icilin-sensitive DRG neurons, CBG inhibited Ca^{2+} elevation with greater potency (IC_{50} = 4.5 μM) than AEA (IC_{50} = 10 μM) (De Petrocellis et al., 2008).

Interestingly, the farnesyl prenylogue of cannabigerol extracted from the variety Carma of fiber hemp (*Cannabis sativa*) showed a decreased inhibitory activity for TRPM8 vs pure cannabigerol (IC_{50} = 0.95 μM vs 0.16 μM; icilin 0.25 μM) (Pollastro et al., 2011).

5. TRPC CHANNELS AND CANNABINOID-MEDIATED REGULATION

Transient receptor potential canonical (TRPC) channels are mammalian homologs of the TRP that in Drosophila function as a Ca^{2+}-permeable channel involved in the light-activated conductance in photoreceptors (Hardie & Minke, 1992). Based on their structural and functional similarities, the TRPC family can be subdivided into four different subfamilies: TRPC1; TRPC2; TRPC3, 6, and 7; and TRPC4 and 5. All channels of this big family can be activated in any of the following three distinct ways: (1) as a consequence of the activation of different isoforms of PLC (by increases in DAGs or by loss of PIP_2), (2) by stimulation of trafficking to the plasma membrane, and (3) by depletion of intracellular Ca^{2+} stores (Putney, 2007). Structurally, all members of the TRPC family are believed to share a common topology where six predicted transmembrane domains (TM1–TM6) with a putative pore region between TM5 and TM6 maintain separated the cytoplasmic N- and C-terminus (Vannier, Zhu, Brown, & Birnbaumer, 1998). Several ankyrin repeats (ranging from three to four) with a predicted coiled-coil region and a putative caveolin binding region compose the N-terminus, while a TRP box (EWKFAR), a highly conserved proline-rich motif, the CIRB (calmodulin/IP_3 receptor binding) region and a predicted coiled-coil region comprise the cytoplasmic

C-terminus (Vazquez, Wedel, Aziz, Trebak, & Putney, 2004). TRPC4 and TRPC5 exhibited an extended C-terminus containing a PDZ-binding motif, which link these channels to PLCβ (Shenolikar, Voltz, Cunningham, & Weinman, 2004). TRPC channels are generally broadly expressed although their functional characterization within a given cell type is complicated by the fact that can form heteromers among themselves (Pedersen et al., 2005).

To date, only few scientific study report correlation between TRPC channels and cannabinoids, evidencing as this issue is almost an unexplored field. In 2005, was first investigated the mechanism by which THC increased $[Ca^{2+}]_i$ in blood-acute lymphoid leukemia (HPB-ALL) cell in correlation with the $[Ca^{2+}]_i$ store depletion and store-operated calcium (SOC) and receptor-operated cation (ROC) channels (Rao & Kaminski, 2006). Based on previous evidences that cannabinoids (particularly THC) robustly elevated intracellular calcium levels in resting human and murine splenic T cells (Rao, Zhang, & Kaminski, 2004), the same authors further examined the mechanism by which THC acted in these cells. TRPC channels have been demonstrated to operate as ROC and SOC channels (Beech, Xu, McHugh, & Flemming, 2003; Philipp et al., 2003; Singh, Liu, & Ambudkar, 2000; Trebak, Vazquez, Bird, & Putney, 2003; Vazquez, Wedel, Trebak, Bird, & Putney, 2003) and both store-depletion-dependent and -independent mechanism have been attributable to these receptors (Trebak, Bird, McKay, & Putney, 2002). Based on these evidences, they first demonstrated that THC-mediated elevation in $[Ca^{2+}]_i$ occurs independently of $[Ca^{2+}]_i$ store depletion and later showed that its mechanism was mediated by TRPC1 (the only TRPC channel expressed in HPB-ALL cells) (Rao & Kaminski, 2006). Since TRPC1 can be activated by analogs of DAG product of PIP_2 hydrolysis by PLC (Albert, 2011), the authors investigated if DAG-sensitive TRPC1 was involved in THC-mediated $[Ca^{2+}]_i$ elevation. By treating HPB-ALL cell with 1-oleoyl-2-acetyl-*sn*-glycerol (OAG), an analog of DAG, an increase of $[Ca^{2+}]_i$ was observed, while THC failed in inducing $[Ca^{2+}]_i$ response after OAG-induced $[Ca^{2+}]_i$, indicating that both compounds increased $[Ca^{2+}]_i$ levels by TRPC1. These results were supported by gene silencing data, since TRPC1 knockdown in HPB-ALL cells produced a reduction of THC-induced $[Ca^{2+}]_i$ elevation, suggesting that this mechanism of THC was partially mediated by the ROC activity carried out by TRPC1.

Several years later, the TRPC channels were also investigated in respect to the endocannabinoid system focusing on the biosynthetic pathways. The synthesis of two major endocannabinoids (AEA and 2-AG) occurs in a calcium-dependent manner (Di Marzo, 2008a) and has been linked to lipid raft microdomains (Placzek, Okamoto, Ueda, & Barker, 2008). In particular, 2-AG was reported to be formed via a calcium-dependent action of sn1-specific DAG lipase from its precursor DAG (Bisogno et al., 2003), via PLC-independent mechanisms (Bisogno, Melck, De Petrocellis, & Di Marzo, 1999; Carrier et al., 2004) as well as via a calcium-independent mechanism (Kondo et al., 1998). Similarly, AEA was also reported to be formed via a calcium-dependent enzyme (NAPE phospholipase D, NAPE PLD) from its precursor, *N*-arachidonoyl phosphatidylethanolamine (NAPE) (Di Marzo et al., 1994; Okamoto, Morishita, Tsuboi, Tonai, & Ueda, 2004; Placzek et al., 2008) as well as via calcium-independent pathways (Vellani et al., 2008). Despite plenty of biosynthetic pathways have been reported, calcium entry remains a critical stimulus for endocannabinoid synthesis (Sugiura et al., 1996), but the calcium channels involved have to be identified yet. Based on previous evidences showing that canonical TRP channels, colocalizing with caveolin-1 are present in caveolae, in 2007 Bardell and coworkers explored the potential role of TRPC3 channels in endocannabinoid synthesis. By using lipid extraction and TLC analysis, they demonstrated that both AEA and 2-AG release were robustly increased upon stimulation of TRPC3 (Bardell & Barker, 2007). Accordingly, endocannabinoid synthesis was blocked by either TRPC3 inhibition or caveolae disruption. Later on, the same authors investigated in neuronal cells whether also other TRPC channels promoted endocannabinoid synthesis. In this study, catecholaminergic neuronal tumor (CAD) cells expressing only the TRPC6 member of TRPC channel family were treated with the DAG analogue, OAG, and endocannabinoid synthesis was evaluated in wild type and TRPC6 knockdown (siTRPC-6) cells. The results showed that OAG-treated wild-type cells synthetized and released AEA and 2-AG, while no effect were observed in siTRPC-6, confirming that TRPC6 activation play a role in promoting endocannabinoid formation (Bardell & Barker, 2010).

A further correlation between TRPC activation and endocannabinoid system was investigated only recently in rat thalamic paraventricular nucleus (PVT) neurons, where activation of thyrotropin-releasing hormone (TRH) receptors was found to engage signaling pathways that include CB1R and CB2R in the activation of TRPC4/5 channels (Zhang, Kolaj, &

Renaud, 2015). PVT, a region that among the thalamus uniquely displays TRH-like immunoreactive axons (Merchenthaler, Csernus, Csontos, Petrusz, & Mess, 1988) and high density of TRH receptors (Heuer, Schafer, O'Donnell, Walker, & Bauer, 2000), has been reported to increase neuron excitability by a TRH-induced inward current coupled with a TRPC-like conductance increase (Kolaj, Zhang, Hermes, & Renaud, 2014; Zhang, Kolaj, & Renaud, 2013). Later on, the same group explored the possibility that this particular signaling pathway involved cannabinoid activation of TRPC4/5 channels. Zhang et al. evidenced as the endocannabinoid 2-AG, a DAG metabolites, CB1R and CB2R were involved in TRPC4/5 current, since TRPC4/5 current was reduced by suppressing DAG hydrolysis as well as by inhibitors of CB1R and CB2R, as rimonabant and SR144528 (Zhang et al., 2015). Since 2-AG is generated by the hydrolysis of DAG by DAGL and may be hydrolyzed to produce arachidonic acid by monoglycerol lipase (MAGL) and/or α/β-hydrolase domain 6 (ABHD6) (Dinh et al., 2002; Marrs et al., 2010). Zhang et al. also reduced the TRH-induced activation of TRPC4/5 channels by using MAGL and ABHD6 inhibitors confirming a pivotal role of 2-AG in this response. Moreover, by using rimonabant and SR144528, they evidenced as TRH-induced regulation of TRPC4/5 channels involved an exclusive participation of CB1R and CB2R (Zhang et al., 2015).

6. NON-TRP ION CHANNELS AND CANNABINOID-MEDIATED REGULATION

As introduced elsewhere in this chapter, it is noteworthy that cannabinoids modulate also other ionotropic channels, although they do not belong to the TRP family.

One of these types of receptors is represented by the ionotropic receptors responsive to the neurotransmitter glutamate, which are integral membrane proteins including the *N*-methyl-D-aspartic acid (NMDAR), the alpha-amino-3-hydroxy-5-methyl-4-isoxazolepropionic acid (AMPAR), and the kainate receptor (KAR) (Traynelis et al., 2010). Glutamate receptor subunits contain four discrete semiautonomous domains: the extracellular amino-terminal domain (ATD), the extracellular ligand-binding domain (LBD), the transmembrane domain (TMD), and an intracellular carboxyl-terminal domain (CTD) (Traynelis et al., 2010). The LBD is highly conserved and is formed by two extracellular stretches of amino acids historically referred to as S1 and S2 and the agonist binding pocket is located within the cleft between these two lobes (Traynelis et al., 2010).

Differently from KAR and AMPAR, NMDAR is activated also by glycine in addition to glutamate, and its activation allows positively charged ions to flow through the cell membrane. NMDAR has a pivotal role in the regulation of synaptic plasticity and memory function (Luscher & Malenka, 2012). Endocannabinoids, postsynaptically synthesized in response to increased intracellular Ca^{2+}, have been reported to modulate calcium flux through NMDAR in a CB1R-dependent manner (Liu, Bhat, Bowen, & Cheng, 2009). In primary DRG neurons, the activation of CB1 receptors inhibits NMDA-mediated calcium influx and cell death via the inositol triphosphate (IP_3) signaling pathway. The effect of WIN 55,212 on CB1R and IP_3 stimulates the release of Ca^{2+} from intracellular stores, raises the cytosolic Ca^{2+} levels, and inhibits the NMDA-mediated Ca^{2+} influx and cell death through a mechanism undetermined yet (Liu et al., 2009). However, THC has been reported to have a neuroprotective effect in AF5 cells exposed to toxic levels of NMDA in a CB1R-independent manner (Chen et al., 2005). Moreover, AEA has been described to enhance NMDAR-mediated field excitatory postsynaptic potentials (fEPSPs) independently from CB1R (Hampson et al., 1998). In acutely isolated CA1 neurons and slices from the hippocampus, NMDA-evoked peak currents were enhanced by the two endocannabinoids 2-AG and AEA, in a CB1R-independent manner. Furthermore, since PKC can upregulate NMDAR currents, the study also demonstrated that the effects of 2-AG and AEA on NMDAR precisely was due to the increasing PKC activity exerted by 2-AG and AEA (Yang, Lei, Xie, MacDonald, & Jackson, 2014).

Another example worthy of note of ionotropic receptors modulated by cannabinoid is represented by the ion channels expressed on beta-cells that regulate insulin secretion. The control mechanism of insulin secretion is finely regulated and, recently, endocannabinoids have been shown to actively participate in it. Briefly, under physiological conditions, voltage-gated calcium channels and ATP-sensitive potassium ion channels are normally open, whereas the calcium ion channels are normally closed. When the glucose concentration outside the cell is high, glucose molecules move into the cell to launch glycolysis. Metabolism of the glucose produces ATP increasing the ATP to ADP ratio, and this increase leads to the closure of ATP-sensitive potassium ion channels. Therefore, the change in potential difference produced opens the voltage-gated calcium channels. The calcium entry leads to insulin release from vesicles by an exocytosis process. An elegant work investigated whether endocannabinoids can influence beta-cells ion channels in the absence of glucose stimulation. Mouse insulinoma cells were used to survey the effects of 2-AG on the high-voltage-activated (HVA) calcium, the delayed rectifier (Kv), and the ATP-sensitive K (K_{ATP}) channels by whole cell patch-clamp recording. The study showed how, at low glucose concentrations, 2-AG stimulates insulin secretion by inhibiting the HVA calcium (the majority of which are L-type channels), Kv, and particularly the K_{ATP} channels in a CB1R-independent manner (Spivak, Kim, Liu, Lupica, & Doyle, 2012).

Finally, it has to be reported that cannabinoids can also modulate glycine receptors (GlyR), the transmitter-gated anion channels of the Cys-loop superfamily which mediate synaptic inhibition at spinal and selected supraspinal sites. GlyRs are pentameric complexes composed of α and β subunits, which can form homomeric (α) or heteromeric (αβ) receptors. Each subunit possesses an amino-terminal extracellular domain (ECD), four-transmembrane domains (TM), and a large intracellular loop (IL) between TM3 and TM4 (Yevenes & Zeilhofer, 2011a). The sites localized in the TM and ECD regions of GlyRs are also subject to allosteric modulation (Yevenes & Zeilhofer, 2011a).

Indeed, chemically neutral *N*-acyl amides such as AEA have been reported to act as positive modulators of α1, α2, and α3 GlyRs, whereas acidic *N*-acyl amino acids such as *N*-arachidonoyl-glycine (NA-Gly) potentiate α1 GlyRs but inhibit α2 and α3 (Yevenes & Zeilhofer, 2011b). Moreover, by patch-clamp recording, a direct action of 2-AG on the functional properties of GlyRs and ionic currents in glycinergic synapses has been reported (Lozovaya et al., 2011). The fact that 2-AG significantly decreased the extent of facilitation of synaptic currents in hypoglossal motoneurons during repetitive stimulation in brainstem slices from CB1R knockout mice, suggested a CB1R-independent mechanism (Lozovaya et al., 2011). Lastly, also plant cannabinoids have been reported to enhance GlyR function. In particular, both THC and CBD significantly potentiate glycine currents in dorsal horn neurons in rat spinal cord slices. Mutagenesis and NMR analyses identified Ser296 in the third transmembrane domain as the critical residue for the potentiation induced by cannabinoids (Xiong et al., 2011, 2012), revealing a new mechanism that could contribute to some of the cannabis-induced analgesic and therapeutic effects.

7. CONCLUSION

The endocannabinoid system is involved in most, if not all, aspects of mammalian physiology and pathology. Since the discovery of the major players involved has been evident that the signal transduction of such a complex system could not be attributable solely to the activation of the "classical" metabotropic cannabinoid CB1R and CB2R. Indeed, it is now well accepted that, beyond their receptor-mediate effects, these molecules can act also via CB1R/CB2R-independent mechanism and particularly via ion channels. As widely discussed within this chapter, TRP channels are multifunctional sensors of environmental signals in the form of physical and chemical stimuli. These channels are widely expressed in multiple cell types both in CNS and in periphery, and are involved in various fundamental cell functions. Accordingly, TRP dysfunctions have now been linked to an increasing number of important pathological conditions. However, especially for some of the latest members of TRP family, many aspects of their physiology and regulation are still elusive. As final point, we believe that a further evaluation of the cellular functions, regulation, and binding partners of TRPs, and their genetic and molecular properties are highly desirable. These findings may have an enormous impact in human pathophysiology and disease and will become an urgent priority in biomedical sciences.

CONFLICT OF INTEREST

The authors declare no conflict of interest.

REFERENCES

Akopian, A. N., Ruparel, N. B., Patwardhan, A., & Hargreaves, K. M. (2008). Cannabinoids desensitize capsaicin and mustard oil responses in sensory neurons via TRPA1 activation. *Journal of Neuroscience*, *28*(5), 1064–1075. http://dx.doi.org/10.1523/Jneurosci.1565-06.2008.

Albert, A. P. (2011). Gating mechanisms of canonical transient receptor potential channel proteins: Role of phosphoinositols and diacylglycerol. *Advances in Experimental Medicine and Biology*, *704*, 391–411. http://dx.doi.org/10.1007/978-94-007-0265-3_22.

Andersson, D. A., Gentry, C., Alenmyr, L., Killander, D., Lewis, S. E., Andersson, A., et al. (2011). TRPA1 mediates spinal antinociception induced by acetaminophen and the cannabinoid Δ^9-tetrahydrocannabiorcol. *Nature Communications*, *2*, 551. http://dx.doi.org/10.1038/Ncomms1559.

Asuthkar, S., Demirkhanyan, L., Sun, X. H., Elustondo, P. A., Krishnan, V., Baskaran, P., et al. (2015). The TRPM8 protein is a testosterone receptor: II. Functional evidence for an ionotropic effect of testosterone on TRPM8. *Journal of Biological Chemistry*, *290*(5), 2670–2688. http://dx.doi.org/10.1074/jbc.M114.610873.

Bandell, M., Dubin, A. E., Petrus, M. J., Orth, A., Mathur, J., Hwang, S. W., et al. (2006). High-throughput random mutagenesis screen reveals TRPM8 residues specifically required for activation by menthol. *Nature Neuroscience*, *9*(4), 493–500. http://dx.doi.org/10.1038/nn1665.

Bandell, M., Story, G. M., Hwang, S. W., Viswanath, V., Eid, S. R., Petrus, M. J., et al. (2004). Noxious cold ion channel TRPA1 is activated by pungent compounds and bradykinin. *Neuron*, *41*(6), 849–857. http://dx.doi.org/10.1016/S0896-6273(04)00150-3.

Bardell, T. K., & Barker, E. L. (2007). Activation of TRPC3 promotes endocannabinoid synthesis. *FASEB Journal*, *21*(6), A1177.

Bardell, T. K., & Barker, E. L. (2010). Activation of TRPC6 channels promotes endocannabinoid biosynthesis in neuronal CAD cells. *Neurochemistry International*, *57*(1), 76–83. http://dx.doi.org/10.1016/j.neuint.2010.05.002. S0197-0186(10)00157-9 [pii].

Bautista, D. M., Jordt, S. E., Nikai, T., Tsuruda, P. R., Read, A. J., Poblete, J., et al. (2006). TRPA1 mediates the inflammatory actions of environmental irritants and proalgesic agents. *Cell*, *124*(6), 1269–1282. http://dx.doi.org/10.1016/j.cell.2006.02.023.

Beech, D. J., Muraki, K., & Flemming, R. (2004). Non-selective cationic channels of smooth muscle and the mammalian homologues of Drosophila TRP. *The Journal of Physiology*, *559*(Pt. 3), 685–706. http://dx.doi.org/10.1113/jphysiol.2004.068734. jphysiol.2004.068734 [pii].

Beech, D. J., Xu, S. Z., McHugh, D., & Flemming, R. (2003). TRPC1 store-operated cationic channel subunit. *Cell Calcium*, *33*(5–6), 433–440. http://dx.doi.org/10.1016/S0143-4160(03)00054-X.

Benham, C. D., Davis, J. B., & Randall, A. D. (2002). Vanilloid and TRP channels: A family of lipid-gated cation channels. *Neuropharmacology*, *42*(7), 873–888. http://dx.doi.org/10.1016/S0028-3908(02)00047-3.

Bidaux, G., Borowiec, A. S., Dubois, C., Delcourt, P., Schulz, C., Vanden Abeele, F., et al. (2016). Targeting of short TRPM8 isoforms induces 4TM-TRPM8-dependent apoptosis in prostate cancer cells. *Oncotarget*, 7(20), 29063–29080. http://dx.doi.org/10.18632/oncotarget.8666.

Bidaux, G., Sgobba, M., Lemonnier, L., Borowiec, A. S., Noyer, L., Jovanovic, S., et al. (2015). Functional and modeling studies of the transmembrane region of the TRPM8 channel. *Biophysical Journal*, *109*(9), 1840–1851. http://dx.doi.org/10.1016/j.bpj.2015.09.027.

Birder, L. A., Nakamura, Y., Kiss, S., Nealen, M. L., Barrick, S., Kanai, A. J., et al. (2002). Altered urinary bladder function in mice lacking the vanilloid receptor TRPV1. *Nature Neuroscience*, *5*(9), 856–860. http://dx.doi.org/10.1038/nn902. nn902 [pii].

Bisogno, T., Howell, F., Williams, G., Minassi, A., Cascio, M. G., Ligresti, A., et al. (2003). Cloning of the first sn1-DAG lipases points to the spatial and temporal regulation of endocannabinoid signaling in the brain. *Journal of Cell Biology*, *163*(3), 463–468. http://dx.doi.org/10.1083/jcb.200305129.

Bisogno, T., Melck, D., De Petrocellis, L., & Di Marzo, V. (1999). Phosphatidic acid as the biosynthetic precursor of the endocannabinoid 2-arachidonoylglycerol in intact mouse neuroblastoma cells stimulated with ionomycin. *Journal of Neurochemistry*, *72*(5), 2113–2119. http://dx.doi.org/10.1046/j.1471-4159.1999.0722113.x.

Bodding, M., Wissenbach, U., & Flockerzi, V. (2007). Characterisation of TRPM8 as a pharmacophore receptor. *Cell Calcium*, *42*(6), 618–628. http://dx.doi.org/10.1016/j.ceca.2007.03.005.

Bonet, I. J. M., Fischer, L., Parada, C. A., & Tambeli, C. H. (2013). The role of transient receptor potential A 1 (TRPA1) in the development and maintenance of carrageenan-induced hyperalgesia. *Neuropharmacology*, *65*, 206–212. http://dx.doi.org/10.1016/j.neuropharm.2012.09.020.

Brauchi, S., Orta, G., Salazar, M., Rosenmann, E., & Latorre, R. (2006). A hot-sensing cold receptor: C-terminal domain determines thermosensation in transient receptor potential channels. *Journal of Neuroscience*, *26*(18), 4835–4840. http://dx.doi.org/10.1523/Jneurosci.5080-05.2006.

Brixel, L. R., Monteilh-Zoller, M. K., Ingenbrandt, C. S., Fleig, A., Penner, R., Enklaar, T., et al. (2010). TRPM5 regulates glucose-stimulated insulin secretion. *Pflugers Archiv: European Journal of Physiology*, *460*(1), 69–76. http://dx.doi.org/10.1007/s00424-010-0835-z.

Cabezas-Bratesco, D., Brauchi, S., Gonzalez-Teuber, V., Steinberg, X., Valencia, I., & Colenso, C. (2015). The different roles of the channel-kinases TRPM6 and TRPM7. *Current Medicinal Chemistry*, *22*(25), 2943–2953. http://dx.doi.org/10.2174/0929867322666150716115644.

Cao, D. S., Zhong, L. L., Hsieh, T. H., Abooj, M., Bishnoi, M., Hughes, L., et al. (2012). Expression of transient receptor potential ankyrin 1 (TRPA1) and its role in insulin release from rat pancreatic beta cells. *PloS One*, 7(5). e38005. http://dx.doi.org/10.1371/journal.pone.0038005.

Capasso, R., Aviello, G., Romano, B., Borrelli, F., De Petrocellis, L., Di Marzo, V., et al. (2012). Modulation of mouse gastrointestinal motility by allyl isothiocyanate, a constituent of cruciferous vegetables (Brassicaceae): Evidence for TRPA1-independent effects. *British Journal of Pharmacology*, *165*(6), 1966–1977. http://dx.doi.org/10.1111/j.1476-5381.2011.01703.x.

Carrier, E. J., Kearn, C. S., Barkmeier, A. J., Breese, N. M., Yang, W. Q., Nithipatikom, K., et al. (2004). Cultured rat microglial cells synthesize the endocannabinoid 2-arachidonylglycerol, which increases proliferation via a CB2 receptor-dependent mechanism. *Molecular Pharmacology*, *65*(4), 999–1007. http://dx.doi.org/10.1124/Mol.65.4.999.

Caterina, M. J. (2014). TRP channel cannabinoid receptors in skin sensation, homeostasis, and inflammation. *ACS Chemical Neuroscience*, *5*(11), 1107–1116. http://dx.doi.org/10.1021/cn5000919.

Cavanaugh, E. J., Simkin, D., & Kim, D. (2008). Activation of transient receptor potential A1 channels by mustard oil, tetrahydrocannabinol and Ca^{2+} reveals different functional channel states. *Neuroscience*, *154*(4), 1467–1476. http://dx.doi.org/10.1016/j.neuroscience.2008.04.048.

Chen, J., Lee, C. T., Errico, S., Deng, X. L., Cadet, J. L., & Freed, W. J. (2005). Protective effects of Δ^9-tetrahydrocannabinol against N-methyl-D-aspartate-induced AF5 cell death. *Molecular Brain Research*, *134*(2), 215–225. http://dx.doi.org/10.1016/j.molbrainres.2004.10.044.

Chen, G. L., Lei, M., Zhou, L. P., Zeng, B., & Zou, F. D. (2016). Borneol is a TRPM8 agonist that increases ocular surface wetness. *PloS One*, *11*(7). e0158868. http://dx.doi.org/10.1371/journal.pone.0158868.

Cho, C. H., Lee, Y. S., Kim, E., Hwang, E. M., & Park, J. Y. (2015). Physiological functions of the TRPM4 channels via protein interactions. *BMB Reports*, *48*(1), 1–5. http://dx.doi.org/10.5483/BMBRep.2015.48.1.252.

Chubanov, V., & Gudermann, T. (2014). TRPM6. In B. Nilius & V. Flockerzi (Eds.), *Mammalian transient receptor potential (Trp) cation channels*: *Vol. 222. Handbook of experimental pharmacology* (pp. 503–520). Germany: Springer-Verlag Berlin Heidelberg. http://dx.doi.org/10.1007/978-3-642-54215-2_20.

Clapham, D. E. (1995). Calcium signaling. *Cell*, *80*(2), 259–268. http://dx.doi.org/10.1016/0092-8674(95)90408-5.

Clapham, D. E., Montell, C., Schultz, G., & Julius, D. (2003). International Union of Pharmacology. XLIII. Compendium of voltage-gated ion channels: Transient receptor potential channels. *Pharmacological Reviews*, *55*(4), 591–596. http://dx.doi.org/10.1124/pr.55.4.6.

Croxford, J. L. (2003). Therapeutic potential of cannabinoids in CNS disease. *CNS Drugs*, *17*(3), 179–202. http://dx.doi.org/10.2165/00023210-200317030-00004.

da Costa, D. S. M., Meotti, F. C., Andrade, E. L., Leal, P. C., Motta, E. M., & Calixto, J. B. (2010). The involvement of the transient receptor potential A1 (TRPA1) in the maintenance of mechanical and cold hyperalgesia in persistent inflammation. *Pain, 148*(3), 431–437. http://dx.doi.org/10.1016/j.pain.2009.12.002.

de Baaij, J. H. F., Hoenderop, J. G. J., & Bindels, R. J. M. (2015). Magnesium in man: Implications for health and disease. *Physiological Reviews, 95*(1), 1–46. http://dx.doi.org/10.1152/physrev.00012.2014.

De Petrocellis, L., Bisogno, T., Maccarrone, M., Davis, J. B., Finazzi-Agro, A., & Di Marzo, V. (2001). The activity of anandamide at vanilloid VR1 receptors requires facilitated transport across the cell membrane and is limited by intracellular metabolism. *Journal of Biological Chemistry, 276*(16), 12856–12863. http://dx.doi.org/10.1074/jbc.M008555200.

De Petrocellis, L., & Di Marzo, V. (2009). Role of endocannabinoids and endovanilloids in Ca^{2+} signalling. *Cell Calcium, 45*(6), 611–624. http://dx.doi.org/10.1016/j.ceca.2009.03.003.

De Petrocellis, L., & Di Marzo, V. (2010). Non-CB1, non-CB2 receptors for endocannabinoids, plant cannabinoids, and synthetic cannabimimetics: Focus on G-protein-coupled receptors and transient receptor potential channels. *Journal of Neuroimmune Pharmacology, 5*(1), 103–121. http://dx.doi.org/10.1007/s11481-009-9177-z.

De Petrocellis, L., Ligresti, A., Schiano Moriello, A., Allara, M., Bisogno, T., Petrosino, S., et al. (2011). Effects of cannabinoids and cannabinoid-enriched cannabis extracts on TRP channels and endocannabinoid metabolic enzymes. *British Journal of Pharmacology, 163*(7), 1479–1494. http://dx.doi.org/10.1111/j.1476-5381.2010.01166.x.

De Petrocellis, L., Ligresti, A., Schiano Moriello, A., Iappelli, M., Verde, R., Stott, C. G., et al. (2013). Non-THC cannabinoids inhibit prostate carcinoma growth in vitro and in vivo: Pro-apoptotic effects and underlying mechanisms. *British Journal of Pharmacology, 168*(1), 79–102. http://dx.doi.org/10.1111/j.1476-5381.2012.02027.x.

De Petrocellis, L., Schiano Moriello, A., Imperatore, R., Cristino, L., Starowicz, K., & Di Marzo, V. (2012a). A re-evaluation of 9-HODE activity at TRPV1 channels in comparison with anandamide: Enantioselectivity and effects at other TRP channels and in sensory neurons. *British Journal of Pharmacology, 167*(8), 1643–1651. http://dx.doi.org/10.1111/j.1476-5381.2012.02122.x.

De Petrocellis, L., Orlando, P., Schiano Moriello, A., Aviello, G., Stott, C., Izzo, A. A., et al. (2012b). Cannabinoid actions at TRPV channels: Effects on TRPV3 and TRPV4 and their potential relevance to gastrointestinal inflammation. *Acta Physiologica, 204*(2), 255–266. http://dx.doi.org/10.1111/j.1748-1716.2011.02338.x.

De Petrocellis, L., Ortar, G., Schiano Moriello, A., Serum, E. M., & Rusterholz, D. B. (2015). Structure-activity relationships of the prototypical TRPM8 agonist icilin. *Bioorganic & Medicinal Chemistry Letters, 25*(11), 2285–2290. http://dx.doi.org/10.1016/j.bmcl.2015.04.032.

De Petrocellis, L., Starowicz, K., Schiano Moriello, A., Vivese, M., Orlando, P., & Di Marzo, V. (2007). Regulation of transient receptor potential channels of melastatin type 8 (TRPM8): Effect of cAMP, cannabinoid CB, receptors and endovanilloids. *Experimental Cell Research, 313*(9), 1911–1920. http://dx.doi.org/10.1016/j.yexcr.2007.
01.008.

De Petrocellis, L., Vellani, V., Schiano-Moriello, A., Marini, P., Magherini, P. C., Orlando, P., et al. (2008). Plant-derived cannabinoids modulate the activity of transient receptor potential channels of ankyrin type-1 and melastatin type-8. *Journal of Pharmacology and Experimental Therapeutics, 325*(3), 1007–1015. http://dx.doi.org/10.1124/jpet.107.134809.

Di Marzo, V. (2008a). Targeting the endocannabinoid system: To enhance or reduce? *Nature Reviews Drug Discovery*, 7(5), 438–455. http://dx.doi.org/10.1038/nrd2553. nrd2553 [pii].

Di Marzo, V. (2008b). Endocannabinoids: Synthesis and degradation. *Reviews of Physiology, Biochemistry and Pharmacology*, *160*, 1–24. http://dx.doi.org/10.1007/112_0505.

Di Marzo, V., Bisogno, T., Melck, D., Ross, R., Brockie, H., Stevenson, L., et al. (1998). Interactions between synthetic vanilloids and the endogenous cannabinoid system. *FEBS Letters*, *436*(3), 449–454. http://dx.doi.org/10.1016/S0014-5793(98)01175-2.

Di Marzo, V., Fontana, A., Cadas, H., Schinelli, S., Cimino, G., Schwartz, J. C., et al. (1994). Formation and inactivation of endogenous cannabinoid anandamide in central neurons. *Nature*, *372*(6507), 686–691. http://dx.doi.org/10.1038/372686a0.

Dinh, T. P., Carpenter, D., Leslie, F. M., Freund, T. F., Katona, I., Sensi, S. L., et al. (2002). Brain monoglyceride lipase participating in endocannabinoid inactivation. *Proceedings of the National Academy of Sciences of the United States of America*, *99*(16), 10819–10824. http://dx.doi.org/10.1073/pnas.152334899.

Duncan, L. M., Deeds, J., Hunter, J., Shao, J., Holmgren, L. M., Woolf, E. A., et al. (1998). Down-regulation of the novel gene melastatin correlates with potential for melanoma metastasis. *Cancer Research*, *58*(7), 1515–1520.

Duncan, M., Kendall, D. A., & Ralevic, V. (2004). Characterization of cannabinoid modulation of sensory neurotransmission in the rat isolated mesenteric arterial bed. *Journal of Pharmacology and Experimental Therapeutics*, *311*(1), 411–419. http://dx.doi.org/10.1124/jpet.104.067587.

Eberhardt, M. J., Filipovic, M. R., Leffler, A., de la Roche, J., Kistner, K., Fischer, M. J., et al. (2012). Methylglyoxal activates nociceptors through transient receptor potential channel A1 (TRPA1) a possible mechanism of metabolic neuropathies. *Journal of Biological Chemistry*, *287*(34), 28291–28306. http://dx.doi.org/10.1074/jbc.M111.328674.

Euler, T., Haverkamp, S., Schubert, T., & Baden, T. (2014). Retinal bipolar cells: Elementary building blocks of vision. *Nature Reviews Neuroscience*, *15*(8), 507–519. http://dx.doi.org/10.1038/nrn3783.

Everaerts, W., Vriens, J., Owsianik, G., Appendino, G., Voets, T., De Ridder, D., et al. (2010). Functional characterization of transient receptor potential channels in mouse urothelial cells. *American Journal of Physiology Renal Physiology*, *298*(3), F692–F701. http://dx.doi.org/10.1152/ajprenal.00599.2009. 00599.2009 [pii].

Faouzi, M., & Penner, R. (2014). TRPM2. In B. Nilius & V. Flockerzi (Eds.), *Mammalian transient receptor potential (Trp) cation channels*: *Vol. 222. Handbook of experimental pharmacology* (pp. 403–426). Germany: Springer-Verlag Berlin Heidelberg. http://dx.doi.org/10.1007/978-3-642-54215-2_16.

Fernandes, E. S., Russell, F. A., Spina, D., McDougall, J. J., Graepel, R., Gentry, C., et al. (2011). A distinct role for transient receptor potential ankyrin 1, in addition to transient receptor potential vanilloid 1, in tumor necrosis factor alpha-induced inflammatory hyperalgesia and Freund's complete adjuvant-induced monarthritis. *Arthritis and Rheumatism*, *63*(3), 819–829. http://dx.doi.org/10.1002/art.30150.

Fleig, A., & Chubanov, V. (2014). Trpm7. In *Mammalian transient receptor potential (Trp) cation channels. Handbook of experimental pharmacology*: *Vol. 222* (pp. 521–546). http://dx.doi.org/10.1007/978-3-642-54215-2_21.

Fleig, A., & Penner, R. (2004). The TRPM ion channel subfamily: Molecular, biophysical and functional features. *Trends in Pharmacological Sciences*, *25*(12), 633–639. http://dx.doi.org/10.1016/j.tips.2004.10.004.

Fujiseki, M., Yamamoto, M., Ubaidus, S., Shinomiya, T., Abe, S., Tazaki, M., et al. (2017). Localization and expression patterns of TRP channels in submandibular gland development. *Archives of Oral Biology*, *74*, 46–50. http://dx.doi.org/10.1016/j.archoralbio.2016.09.011.

Gautier, M., Perriere, M., Monet, M., Vanlaeys, A., Korichneva, I., Dhennin-Duthille, I., et al. (2016). Recent advances in oncogenic roles of the TRPM7 chanzyme. *Current Medicinal Chemistry, 23*(36), 4092–4107. http://dx.doi.org/10.2174/0929867323666160907162002.

Gavva, N. R., Davis, C., Lehto, S. G., Rao, S., Wang, W. Y., & Zhu, D. X. D. (2012). Transient receptor potential melastatin 8 (TRPM8) channels are involved in body temperature regulation. *Molecular Pain, 8*, 36. http://dx.doi.org/10.1186/1744-8069-8-36.

Gibson, H. E., Edwards, J. G., Page, R. S., Van Hook, M. J., & Kauer, J. A. (2008). TRPV1 channels mediate long-term depression at synapses on hippocampal interneurons. *Neuron, 57*(5), 746–759. http://dx.doi.org/10.1016/j.neuron.2007.12.027.

Gregus, A. M., Doolen, S., Dumlao, D. S., Buczynski, M. W., Takasusuki, T., Fitzsimmons, B. L., et al. (2012). Spinal 12-lipoxygenase-derived hepoxilin $A_{(3)}$ contributes to inflammatory hyperalgesia via activation of TRPV1 and TRPA1 receptors. *Proceedings of the National Academy of Sciences of the United States of America, 109*(17), 6721–6726. http://dx.doi.org/10.1073/pnas.1110460109.

Guinamard, R., Salle, L., & Simard, C. (2011). The non-selective monovalent cationic channels TRPM4 and TRPM5. *Advances in Experimental Medicine and Biology, 704*, 147–171. http://dx.doi.org/10.1007/978-94-007-0265-3_8.

Hampson, A. J., Bornheim, L. M., Scanziani, M., Yost, C. S., Gray, A. T., Hansen, B. M., et al. (1998). Dual effects of anandamide on NMDA receptor-mediated responses and neurotransmission. *Journal of Neurochemistry, 70*(2), 671–676. http://dx.doi.org/10.1046/j.1471-4159.1998.70020671.x.

Haraguchi, K., Kawamoto, A., Isami, K., Maeda, S., Kusano, A., Asakura, K., et al. (2012). TRPM2 contributes to inflammatory and neuropathic pain through the aggravation of pronociceptive inflammatory responses in mice. *Journal of Neuroscience, 32*(11), 3931–3941. http://dx.doi.org/10.1523/Jneurosci.4703-11.2012.

Hardie, R. C., & Minke, B. (1992). The trp gene is essential for a light-activated Ca^{2+} channel in Drosophila photoreceptors. *Neuron, 8*(4), 643–651. http://dx.doi.org/10.1016/0896-6273(92)90086-S.

Herrera Moro Chao, D., Argmann, C., Van Eijk, M., Boot, R. G., Ottenhoff, R., Van Roomen, C., et al. (2016). Impact of obesity on taste receptor expression in extra-oral tissues: Emphasis on hypothalamus and brainstem. *Scientific Reports, 6*, 29094. http://dx.doi.org/10.1038/Srep29094.

Heuer, H., Schafer, M. K. H., O'Donnell, D., Walker, P., & Bauer, K. (2000). Expression of thyrotropin-releasing hormone receptor 2 (TRH-R2) in the central nervous system of rats. *Journal of Comparative Neurology, 428*(2), 319–336.

Hinman, A., Chuang, H. H., Bautista, D. M., & Julius, D. (2006). TRP channel activation by reversible covalent modification. *Proceedings of the National Academy of Sciences of the United States of America, 103*(51), 19564–19568. http://dx.doi.org/10.1073/pnas.0609598103.

Hoenderop, J. G., Nilius, B., & Bindels, R. J. (2005). Calcium absorption across epithelia. *Physiological Reviews, 85*(1), 373–422. http://dx.doi.org/10.1152/physrev.00003.2004.

Howlett, A. C., & Mukhopadhyay, S. (2000). Cellular signal transduction by anandamide and 2-arachidonoylglycerol. *Chemistry and Physics of Lipids, 108*(1–2), 53–70. http://dx.doi.org/10.1016/S0009-3084(00)00187-0.

Huang, S. M., Bisogno, T., Trevisani, M., Al-Hayani, A., De Petrocellis, L., Fezza, F., et al. (2002). An endogenous capsaicin-like substance with high potency at recombinant and native vanilloid VR1 receptors. *Proceedings of the National Academy of Sciences of the United States of America, 99*(12), 8400–8405. http://dx.doi.org/10.1073/pnas.122196999.

Iannotti, F. A., Di Marzo, V., & Petrosino, S. (2016). Endocannabinoids and endocannabinoid-related mediators: Targets, metabolism and role in neurological disorders. *Progress in Lipid Research, 62*, 107–128. http://dx.doi.org/10.1016/j.plipres.2016.02.002.

Iannotti, F. A., Hill, C. L., Leo, A., Alhusaini, A., Soubrane, C., Mazzarella, E., et al. (2014). Nonpsychotropic plant cannabinoids, cannabidivarin (CBDV) and cannabidiol (CBD), activate and desensitize transient receptor potential vanilloid 1 (TRPV1) channels in vitro: Potential for the treatment of neuronal hyperexcitability. *ACS Chemical Neuroscience*, *5*(11), 1131–1141. http://dx.doi.org/10.1021/cn5000524.

Jordt, S. E., Bautista, D. M., Chuang, H. H., McKemy, D. D., Zygmunt, P. M., Hogestatt, E. D., et al. (2004). Mustard oils and cannabinoids excite sensory nerve fibres through the TRP channel ANKTM1. *Nature*, *427*(6971), 260–265. http://dx.doi.org/10.1038/nature02282.

Kaji, I., Yasuoka, Y., Karaki, S., & Kuwahara, A. (2012). Activation of TRPA1 by luminal stimuli induces EP4-mediated anion secretion in human and rat colon. *American Journal of Physiology. Gastrointestinal and Liver Physiology*, *302*(7), G690–G701. http://dx.doi.org/10.1152/ajpgi.00289.2011.

Kaske, S., Krasteva, G., Konig, P., Kummer, W., Hofmann, T., Gudermann, T., et al. (2007). TRPM5, a taste-signaling transient receptor potential ion-channel, is a ubiquitous signaling component in chemosensory cells. *BMC Neuroscience*, *8*, 49. http://dx.doi.org/10.1186/1471-2201-8-49.

Kim, D., & Cavanaugh, E. J. (2007). Requirement of a soluble intracellular factor for activation of transient receptor potential A1 by pungent chemicals: Role of inorganic polyphosphates. *Journal of Neuroscience*, *27*(24), 6500–6509. http://dx.doi.org/10.1523/Jneurosci.0623-07.2007.

Kobayashi, K., Fukuoka, T., Obata, K., Yamanaka, H., Dai, Y., Tokunaga, A., et al. (2005). Distinct expression of TRPM8, TRPA1, and TRPV1 mRNAs in rat primary afferent neurons with aδ/c-fibers and colocalization with trk receptors. *Journal of Comparative Neurology*, *493*(4), 596–606. http://dx.doi.org/10.1002/cne.20794.

Koike, C., Obara, T., Uriu, Y., Numata, T., Sanuki, R., Miyata, K., et al. (2010). TRPM1 is a component of the retinal ON bipolar cell transduction channel in the mGluR6 cascade. *Proceedings of the National Academy of Sciences of the United States of America*, *107*(1), 332–337. http://dx.doi.org/10.1073/pnas.0912730107.

Kolaj, M., Zhang, L., Hermes, M. L., & Renaud, L. P. (2014). Intrinsic properties and neuropharmacology of midline paraventricular thalamic nucleus neurons. *Frontiers in Behavioral Neuroscience*, *8*, 132. http://dx.doi.org/10.3389/Fnbeh.2014.00132.

Kondo, S., Kondo, H., Nakane, S., Kodaka, T., Tokumura, A., Waku, K., et al. (1998). 2-Arachidonoylglycerol, an endogenous cannabinoid receptor agonist: Identification as one of the major species of monoacylglycerols in various rat tissues, and evidence for its generation through Ca^{2+}-dependent and -independent mechanisms. *FEBS Letters*, *429*(2), 152–156. http://dx.doi.org/10.1016/S0014-5793(98)00581-X.

Kun, J., Szitter, I., Kemeny, A., Perkecz, A., Kereskai, L., Pohoczky, K., et al. (2014). Upregulation of the transient receptor potential ankyrin 1 ion channel in the inflamed human and mouse colon and its protective roles. *PloS One*, *9*(9), e108164. http://dx.doi.org/10.1371/journal.pone.0108164.

Kuras, Z., Yun, Y. H., Chimote, A. A., Neumeier, L., & Conforti, L. (2012). KCa3.1 and TRPM7 channels at the uropod regulate migration of activated human T cells. *PloS One*, 7(8), e43859. http://dx.doi.org/10.1371/journal.pone.0043859.

Lam, D. H., Grant, C. E., & Hill, C. E. (2012). Differential expression of TRPM7 in rat hepatoma and embryonic and adult hepatocytes. *Canadian Journal of Physiology and Pharmacology*, *90*(4), 435–444. http://dx.doi.org/10.1139/Y11-136.

Lashinger, E. S. R., Steiginga, M. S., Hieble, J. P., Leon, L. A., Gardner, S. D., Nagilla, R., et al. (2008). AMTB, a TRPM8 channel blocker: Evidence in rats for activity in overactive bladder and painful bladder syndrome. *American Journal of Physiology. Renal Physiology*, *295*(3), F803–F810. http://dx.doi.org/10.1152/ajprenal.90269.2008.

Lauckner, J. E., Hille, B., & Mackie, K. (2005). The cannabinoid agonist WIN55,212-2 increases intracellular calcium via CB1 receptor coupling to $G_{(q/11)}$ G proteins. *Proceedings of the National Academy of Sciences of the United States of America*, *102*(52), 19144–19149. http://dx.doi.org/10.1073/pnas.0509588102.

Launay, P., Fleig, A., Perraud, A. L., Scharenberg, A. M., Penner, R., & Kinet, J. P. (2002). TRPM4 is a Ca^{2+}-activated nonselective cation channel mediating cell membrane depolarization. *Cell*, *109*(3), 397–407. http://dx.doi.org/10.1016/S0092-8674(02)00719-5.

Lee, L. Y., Ni, D., Hayes, D., & Lin, R. L. (2011). TRPV1 as a cough sensor and its temperature-sensitive properties. *Pulmonary Pharmacology & Therapeutics*, *24*(3), 280–285. http://dx.doi.org/10.1016/j.pupt.2010.12.003.

Lei, Z., Ishizuka, O., Imamura, T., Noguchi, W., Yamagishi, T., Yokoyama, H., et al. (2013). Functional roles of transient receptor potential melastatin 8 (TRPM8) channels in the cold stress-induced detrusor overactivity pathways in conscious rats. *Neurourology and Urodynamics*, *32*(5), 500–504. http://dx.doi.org/10.1002/nau.22325.

Liberati, S., Morelli, M. B., Amantini, C., Farfariello, V., Santoni, M., Conti, A., et al. (2014). Loss of TRPV2 homeostatic control of cell proliferation drives tumor progression. *Cell*, *3*(1), 112–128. http://dx.doi.org/10.3390/cells3010112. cells3010112 [pii].

Liman, E. R. (2014). TRPM5. In B. Nilius & V. Flockerzi (Eds.), *Mammalian transient receptor potential (Trp) cation channels*: *Vol. 222. Handbook of experimental pharmacology* (pp. 489–502). Germany: Springer-Verlag Berlin Heidelberg. http://dx.doi.org/10.1007/978-3-642-54215-2_19.

Lin, W. H., Ogura, T., Margolskee, R. F., Finger, T. E., & Restrepo, D. (2008). TRPM5-expressing solitary chemosensory cells respond to odorous irritants. *Journal of Neurophysiology*, *99*(3), 1451–1460. http://dx.doi.org/10.1152/jn.01195.2007.

Liu, Q., Bhat, M., Bowen, W. D., & Cheng, J. G. (2009). Signaling pathways from cannabinoid receptor-1 activation to inhibition of N-methyl-D-aspartic acid mediated calcium influx and neurotoxicity in dorsal root ganglion neurons. *Journal of Pharmacology and Experimental Therapeutics*, *331*(3), 1062–1070. http://dx.doi.org/10.1124/jpet.109.156216.

Liu, T., Fang, Z. H., Wang, G., Shi, M. J., Wang, X., Jiang, K., et al. (2016). Anti-tumor activity of the TRPM8 inhibitor BCTC in prostate cancer DU145 cells. *Oncology Letters*, *11*(1), 182–188. http://dx.doi.org/10.3892/ol.2015.3854.

Liu, H., Li, J., Huang, Y., & Huang, C. (2012). Inhibition of transient receptor potential melastain 7 channel increases HSCs apoptosis induced by TRAIL. *Life Sciences*, *90*(15–16), 612–618. http://dx.doi.org/10.1016/j.lfs.2012.02.012.

Loh, K. P., Ng, G., Yu, C. Y., Fhu, C., Yu, D. J., Vennekens, R., et al. (2014). TRPM4 inhibition promotes angiogenesis after ischemic stroke. *Pflugers Archiv: European Journal of Physiology*, *466*(3), 563–576. http://dx.doi.org/10.1007/s00424-013-1347-4.

Lozovaya, N., Mukhtarov, M., Tsintsadze, T., Ledent, C., Burnashev, N., & Bregestovski, P. (2011). Frequency-dependent cannabinoid receptor-independent modulation of glycine receptors by endocannabinoid 2-AG. *Frontiers in Molecular Neuroscience*, *4*, 13. http://dx.doi.org/10.3389/Fnmol.2011.00013.

Luscher, C., & Malenka, R. C. (2012). NMDA receptor-dependent long-term potentiation and long-term depression (LTP/LTD). *Cold Spring Harbor Perspectives in Biology*, *4*(6). http://dx.doi.org/10.1101/cshperspect.a005710.

Macpherson, L. J., Geierstanger, B. H., Viswanath, V., Bandell, M., Eid, S. R., Hwang, S., et al. (2005). The pungency of garlic: Activation of TRPA1 and TRPV1 in response to allicin. *Current Biology*, *15*(10), 929–934. http://dx.doi.org/10.1016/j/cub.2005.04.018.

Malkia, A., Madrid, R., Meseguer, V., de la Pena, E., Valero, M., Belmonte, C., et al. (2007). Bidirectional shifts of TRPM8 channel gating by temperature and chemical agents modulate the cold sensitivity of mammalian thermoreceptors. *The Journal of Physiology*, *581*(1), 155–174. http://dx.doi.org/10.1113/jphysiol.2006.123059.

Marrs, W. R., Blankman, J. L., Horne, E. A., Thomazeau, A., Lin, Y. H., Coy, J., et al. (2010). The serine hydrolase ABHD6 controls the accumulation and efficacy of 2-AG at cannabinoid receptors. *Nature Neuroscience*, *13*(8), 951–957. http://dx.doi.org/10.1038/nn.2601.

Martinez-Lopez, P., Trevino, C. L., De la Vega-Beltran, J. L., De Blas, G., Monroy, E., Beltran, C., et al. (2011). TRPM8 in mouse sperm detects temperature changes and may influence the acrosome reaction. *Journal of Cellular Physiology*, *226*(6), 1620–1631. http://dx.doi.org/10.1002/jcp.22493.

Materazzi, S., Nassini, R., Andre, E., Campi, B., Amadesi, S., Trevisani, M., et al. (2008). Cox-dependent fatty acid metabolites cause pain through activation of the irritant receptor TRPA1. *Proceedings of the National Academy of Sciences of the United States of America*, *105*(33), 12045–12050. http://dx.doi.org/10.1073/pnas.0802354105.

Mathar, I., Jacobs, G., Kecskes, M., Menigoz, A., Philippaert, K., & Vennekens, R. (2014). TRPM4. In B. Nilius & V. Flockerzi (Eds.), *Mammalian transient receptor potential (Trp) cation channels: Vol. 222. Handbook of experimental pharmacology* (pp. 461–487). Germany: Springer-Verlag Berlin Heidelberg. http://dx.doi.org/10.1007/978-3-642-54215-2_18.

Matsuda, L. A. (1997). Molecular aspects of cannabinoid receptors. *Critical Reviews in Neurobiology*, *11*(2–3), 143–166.

McKemy, D. D., Neuhausser, W. M., & Julius, D. (2002). Identification of a cold receptor reveals a general role for TRP channels in thermosensation. *Nature*, *416*(6876), 52–58. http://dx.doi.org/10.1038/Nature719.

Merchenthaler, I., Csernus, V., Csontos, C., Petrusz, P., & Mess, B. (1988). New data on the immunocytochemical localization of thyrotropin-releasing hormone in the rat central nervous system. *The American Journal of Anatomy*, *181*(4), 359–376. http://dx.doi.org/10.1002/aja.1001810404.

Mitchell, J. A., Williams, F. M., Williams, T. J., & Larkin, S. W. (1997). Role of nitric oxide in the dilator actions of capsaicin-sensitive nerves in the rabbit coronary circulation. *Neuropeptides*, *31*(4), 333–338. http://dx.doi.org/10.1016/S0143-4179(97)90068-8.

Mohapatra, D. P., & Nau, C. (2003). Desensitization of capsaicin-activated currents in the vanilloid receptor TRPV1 is decreased by the cyclic AMP-dependent protein kinase pathway. *Journal of Biological Chemistry*, *278*(50), 50080–50090. http://dx.doi.org/10.1074/jbc.M306619200.

Monet, M., Gkika, D., Lehen'kyi, V., Pourtier, A., Vanden Abeele, F., Bidaux, G., et al. (2009). Lysophospholipids stimulate prostate cancer cell migration via TRPV2 channel activation. *Biochimica et Biophysica Acta*, *1793*(3), 528–539. http://dx.doi.org/10.1016/j.bbamcr.2009.01.003. S0167-4889(09)00005-6 [pii].

Montell, C. (2005). The TRP superfamily of cation channels. *Science STKE*, *2005*(272), re3. stke.2722005re3 [pii] http://dx.doi.org/10.1126/stke.2722005re3.

Montell, C., Birnbaumer, L., Flockerzi, V., Bindels, R. J., Brudorf, E. A., Caterina, M. J., et al. (2002). A unified nomenclature for the superfamily of TRP cation channels. *Molecular Cell*, *9*(2), 229–231. http://dx.doi.org/10.1016/S1097-2765(02)00448-3.

Morgans, C. W., Zhang, J. M., Jeffrey, B. G., Nelson, S. M., Burke, N. S., Duvoisin, R. M., et al. (2009). TRPM1 is required for the depolarizing light response in retinal ON-bipolar cells. *Proceedings of the National Academy of Sciences of the United States of America*, *106*(45), 19174–19178. http://dx.doi.org/10.1073/pnas.0908711106.

Motter, A. L., & Ahern, G. P. (2012). TRPA1 is a polyunsaturated fatty acid sensor in mammals. *PloS One*, 7(6), e38439. http://dx.doi.org/10.1371/journal.pone.0038439.

Mukerji, G., Yiangou, Y., Corcoran, S. L., Selmer, I. S., Smith, G. D., Benham, C. D., et al. (2006). Cool and menthol receptor TRPM8 in human urinary bladder disorders and clinical correlations. *BMC Urology*, *6*, 6. http://dx.doi.org/10.1186/1471-2490-6-6.

Nabissi, M., Morelli, M. B., Amantini, C., Farfariello, V., Ricci-Vitiani, L., Caprodossi, S., et al. (2010). TRPV2 channel negatively controls glioma cell proliferation and resistance to Fas-induced apoptosis in ERK-dependent manner. *Carcinogenesis*, *31*(5), 794–803. http://dx.doi.org/10.1093/carcin/bgq019. bgq019 [pii].

Nagamine, K., Kudoh, J., Minoshima, S., Kawasaki, K., Asakawa, S., Ito, F., et al. (1998). Molecular cloning of a novel putative Ca^{2+} channel protein (TRPC7) highly expressed in brain. *Genomics*, *54*(1), 124–131. http://dx.doi.org/10.1006/geno.1998.5551.

Nagata, K., Duggan, A., Kumar, G., & Garcia-Anoveros, J. (2005). Nociceptor and hair cell transducer properties of TRPA1, a channel for pain and hearing. *Journal of Neuroscience*, *25*(16), 4052–4061. http://dx.doi.org/10.1523/Jneurosci.0013-05.2005.

Nassini, R., Pedretti, P., Moretto, N., Fusi, C., Carnini, C., Facchinetti, F., et al. (2012). Transient receptor potential ankyrin 1 channel localized to non-neuronal airway cells promotes non-neurogenic inflammation. *PloS One*, 7(8), e42454. http://dx.doi.org/10.1371/journal.pone.0042454.

Ng, N. M., Jiang, S. P., & Lv, Z. Q. (2012). Retrovirus-mediated siRNA targeting TRPM7 gene induces apoptosis in RBL-2H3 cells. *European Review for Medical and Pharmacological Sciences*, *16*(9), 1172–1178.

Nilius, B., & Owsianik, G. (2011). The transient receptor potential family of ion channels. *Genome Biology*, *12*(3), 218. http://dx.doi.org/10.1186/gb-2011-12-3-218.

Nilius, B., Owsianik, G., & Voets, T. (2008). Transient receptor potential channels meet phosphoinositides. *EMBO Journal*, *27*(21), 2809–2816. http://dx.doi.org/10.1038/emboj.2008.217.

Nilius, B., Owsianik, G., Voets, T., & Peters, J. A. (2007). Transient receptor potential cation channels in disease. *Physiological Reviews*, *87*(1), 165–217. http://dx.doi.org/10.1152/physrev.00021.2006.

Nilius, B., & Szallasi, A. (2014). Transient receptor potential channels as drug targets: From the science of basic research to the art of medicine. *Pharmacological Reviews*, *66*(3), 676–814. http://dx.doi.org/10.1124/pr.113.008268.

Nilius, B., Vriens, J., Prenen, J., Droogmans, G., & Voets, T. (2004). TRPV4 calcium entry channel: A paradigm for gating diversity. *American Journal of Physiology Cell Physiology*, *286*(2), C195–C205. http://dx.doi.org/10.1152/ajpcell.00365.2003. 286/2/C195[pii].

O'Neil, R. G., & Heller, S. (2005). The mechanosensitive nature of TRPV channels. *Pflügers Archiv*, *451*(1), 193–203. http://dx.doi.org/10.1007/s00424-005-1424-4.

Obata, K., Katsura, H., Mizushima, T., Yamanaka, H., Kobayashi, K., Dai, Y., et al. (2005). TRPA1 induced in sensory neurons contributes to cold hyperalgesia after inflammation and nerve injury. *Journal of Clinical Investigation*, *115*(9), 2393–2401. http://dx.doi.org/10.1172/JCI23437.

Okamoto, Y., Morishita, J., Tsuboi, K., Tonai, T., & Ueda, N. (2004). Molecular characterization of a phospholipase D generating anandamide and its congeners. *Journal of Biological Chemistry*, *279*(7), 5298–5305. http://dx.doi.org/10.1074/jbc.M306642200.

Pan, J. P., Zhang, H. Q., Wang, W., Guo, Y. F., Xiao, N., Cao, X. H., et al. (2011). Some subtypes of endocannabinoid/endovanilloid receptors mediate docosahexaenoic acid-induced enhanced spatial memory in rats. *Brain Research*, *1412*, 18–27. http://dx.doi.org/10.1016/j.brainres.2011.07.015.

Parra, A., Madrid, R., Echevarria, D., del Olmo, S., Morenilla-Palao, C., Acosta, M. C., et al. (2010). Ocular surface wetness is regulated by TRPM8-dependent cold thermoreceptors of the cornea. *Nature Medicine*, *16*(12), 1396–1399. http://dx.doi.org/10.1038/nm.2264.

Paulsen, C. E., Armache, J. P., Gao, Y., Cheng, Y. F., & Julius, D. (2015). Structure of the TRPA1 ion channel suggests regulatory mechanisms. *Nature*, *520*(7548), 511–517. http://dx.doi.org/10.1038/nature14367.

Pedersen, S. F., Owsianik, G., & Nilius, B. (2005). TRP channels: An overview. *Cell Calcium*, *38*(3–4), 233–252. http://dx.doi.org/10.1016/j.ceca.2005.06.028.

Pedretti, A., Marconi, C., Bettinelli, I., & Vistoli, G. (2009). Comparative modeling of the quaternary structure for the human TRPM8 channel and analysis of its binding features. *Biochimica et Biophysica Acta-Biomembranes*, *1788*(5), 973–982. http://dx.doi.org/10.1016/j.bbamem.2009.02.007.

Philipp, S., Strauss, B., Hirnet, D., Wissenbach, U., Mery, L., Flockerzi, V., et al. (2003). TRPC3 mediates T-cell receptor-dependent calcium entry in human T-lymphocytes. *Journal of Biological Chemistry*, *278*(29), 26629–26638. http://dx.doi.org/10.1074/jbc.M304044200.

Placzek, E. A., Okamoto, Y., Ueda, N., & Barker, E. L. (2008). Mechanisms for recycling and biosynthesis of endogenous cannabinoids anandamide and 2-arachidonylglycerol. *Journal of Neurochemistry*, *107*(4), 987–1000. http://dx.doi.org/10.1111/j.1471-4159.2008.05659.x.

Pollastro, F., Taglialatela-Scafati, O., Allara, M., Munoz, E., Di Marzo, V., De Petrocellis, L., et al. (2011). Bioactive prenylogous cannabinoid from fiber hemp (*Cannabis sativa*). *Journal of Natural Products*, *74*(9), 2019–2022. http://dx.doi.org/10.1021/np200500p.

Prawitt, D., Monteilh-Zoller, M. K., Brixel, L., Spangenberg, C., Zabel, B., Fleig, A., et al. (2003). TRPM5 is a transient Ca^{2+}-activated cation channel responding to rapid changes in $[Ca^{2+}]_i$. *Proceedings of the National Academy of Sciences of the United States of America*, *100*(25), 15166–15171. http://dx.doi.org/10.1073/pnas.2334624100.

Premkumar, L. S., & Ahern, G. P. (2000). Induction of vanilloid receptor channel activity by protein kinase C. *Nature*, *408*(6815), 985–990. http://dx.doi.org/10.1038/35050121.

Prescott, E. D., & Julius, D. (2003). A modular PIP2 binding site as a determinant of capsaicin receptor sensitivity. *Science*, *300*(5623), 1284–1288. http://dx.doi.org/10.1126/science.1083646.

Price, T. J., Patwardhan, A., Akopian, A. N., Hargreaves, K. M., & Flores, C. M. (2004). Modulation of trigeminal sensory neuron activity by the dual cannabinoid-vanilloid agonists anandamide, N-arachidonoyl-dopamine and arachidonyl-2-chloroethylamide. *British Journal of Pharmacology*, *141*(7), 1118–1130. http://dx.doi.org/10.1038/sj.bjp.0705711.

Putney, J. W. (2007). Multiple mechanisms of TRPC activation. In W. B. Liedtke & S. Heller (Eds.), *TRP ion channel function in sensory transduction and cellular signaling cascades* (pp. 31–44). Boca Raton (FL): CRC Press/Taylor & Francis.

Qin, N., Neeper, M. P., Liu, Y., Hutchinson, T. L., Lubin, M. L., & Flores, C. M. (2008). TRPV2 is activated by cannabidiol and mediates CGRP release in cultured rat dorsal root ganglion neurons. *Journal of Neuroscience*, *28*(24), 6231–6238. http://dx.doi.org/10.1523/Jneurosci.0504-08.2008.

Ralevic, V., & Kendall, D. A. (2001). Cannabinoid inhibition of capsaicin-sensitive sensory neurotransmission in the rat mesenteric arterial bed. *European Journal of Pharmacology*, *418*(1–2), 117–125. http://dx.doi.org/10.1016/S0014-2999(01)00940-2.

Ramsey, I. S., Delling, M., & Clapham, D. E. (2006). An introduction to TRP channels. *Annual Review of Physiology*, *68*, 619–647. http://dx.doi.org/10.1146/annurev.physiol.68.040204.100431.

Rao, G. K., & Kaminski, N. E. (2006). Induction of intracellular calcium elevation by Δ^9-tetrahydrocannabinol in T cells involves TRPC1 channels. *Journal of Leukocyte Biology*, *79*(1), 202–213. http://dx.doi.org/10.1189/jlb.0505274.

Rao, G. K., Zhang, W., & Kaminski, N. E. (2004). Cannabinoid receptor-mediated regulation of intracellular calcium by Δ^9-tetrahydrocannabinol in resting T cells. *Journal of Leukocyte Biology*, *75*(5), 884–892. http://dx.doi.org/10.1189/jlb.1203638.

Redmond, W. J., Gu, L. Q., Camo, M., McIntyre, P., & Connor, M. (2014). Ligand determinants of fatty acid activation of the pronociceptive ion channel TRPA1. *PeerJ*, *2*, e248. http://dx.doi.org/10.7717/peerj.248.

Rohacs, T., Lopes, C. M. B., Michailidis, I., & Logothetis, D. E. (2005). PI(4,5)P-2 regulates the activation and desensitization of TRPM8 channels through the TRP domain. *Nature Neuroscience*, *8*(5), 626–634. http://dx.doi.org/10.1038/nn1451.

Ross, R. A., Gibson, T. M., Brockie, H. C., Leslie, M., Pashmi, G., Craib, S. J., et al. (2001). Structure-activity relationship for the endogenous cannabinoid, anandamide, and certain of its analogues at vanilloid receptors in transfected cells and vas deferens. *British Journal of Pharmacology*, *132*(3), 631–640. http://dx.doi.org/10.1038/sj.bjp.0703850.

Rossato, M., Granzotto, M., Macchi, V., Porzionato, A., Petrelli, L., Calcagno, A., et al. (2014). Human white adipocytes express the cold receptor TRPM8 which activation induces UCP1 expression, mitochondrial activation and heat production. *Molecular and Cellular Endocrinology*, *383*(1–2), 137–146. http://dx.doi.org/10.1016/j.mce.2013.12.005.

Runnels, L. W., Yue, L. X., & Clapham, D. E. (2002). The TRPM7 channel is inactivated by PIP2 hydrolysis. *Nature Cell Biology*, *4*(5), 329–336. http://dx.doi.org/10.1038/ncb781.

Ruparel, N. B., Patwardhan, A. M., Akopian, A. N., & Hargreaves, K. M. (2008). Homologous and heterologous desensitization of capsaicin and mustard oil responses utilize different cellular pathways in nociceptors. *Pain*, *135*(3), 271–279. http://dx.doi.org/10.1016/j.pain.2007.06.005.

Ryazanov, A. G. (2002). Elongation factor-2 kinase and its newly discovered relatives. *FEBS Letters*, *514*(1), 26–29. http://dx.doi.org/10.1016/S0014-5793(02)02299-8.

Ryazanova, L. V., Dorovkov, M. V., Ansari, A., & Ryazanov, A. G. (2004). Characterization of the protein kinase activity of TRPM7/ChaK1, a protein kinase fused to the transient receptor potential ion channel. *The Journal of Biological Chemistry*, *279*(5), 3708–3716. http://dx.doi.org/10.1074/jbc.M308820200.

Ryazanova, L. V., Rondon, L. J., Zierler, S., Hu, Z. X., Galli, J., Yamaguchi, T. P., et al. (2010). TRPM7 is essential for Mg^{2+} homeostasis in mammals. *Nature Communications*, *1*, 109. http://dx.doi.org/10.1038/Ncomms1108.

Rybarczyk, P., Gautier, M., Hague, F., Dhennin-Duthille, I., Chatelain, D., Kerr-Conte, J., et al. (2012). Transient receptor potential melastatin-related 7 channel is overexpressed in human pancreatic ductal adenocarcinomas and regulates human pancreatic cancer cell migration. *International Journal of Cancer*, *131*(6), E851–E861. http://dx.doi.org/10.1002/ijc.27487.

Sahni, J., Tamura, R., Sweet, I. R., & Scharenberg, A. M. (2010). TRPM7 regulates quiescent/proliferative metabolic transitions in lymphocytes. *Cell Cycle*, *9*(17), 3565–3574. http://dx.doi.org/10.4161/cc.9.17.12798.

Sanchez, M. G., Ruiz-Llorente, L., Sanchez, A. M., & Diaz-Laviada, I. (2003). Activation of phosphoinositide 3-kinase/PKB pathway by CB1 and CB2 cannabinoid receptors expressed in prostate PC-3 cells. Involvement in Raf-1 stimulation and NGF induction. *Cellular Signalling*, *15*(9), 851–859. http://dx.doi.org/10.1016/S0898-6568(03)00036-6.

Schiano Moriello, A., Luongo, L., Guida, F., Christodoulou, M. S., Perdicchia, D., Maione, S., et al. (2016). Chalcone derivatives activate and desensitize the transient receptor potential ankyrin 1 cation channel, subfamily A, member 1 TRPA1 ion channel: Structure-activity relationships in vitro and anti-nociceptive and anti-inflammatory activity in vivo. *CNS & Neurological Disorders Drug Targets*, *15*(8), 987–994. http://dx.doi.org/10.1016/j.ienj.2015.05.007.

Shen, Y., Heimel, J. A., Kamermans, M., Peachey, N. S., Gregg, R. G., & Nawy, S. (2009). A transient receptor potential-like channel mediates synaptic transmission in rod bipolar cells. *Journal of Neuroscience*, *29*(19), 6088–6093. http://dx.doi.org/10.1523/Jneurosci.0132-09.2009.

Shenolikar, S., Voltz, J. W., Cunningham, R., & Weinman, E. J. (2004). Regulation of ion transport by the NHERF family of PDZ proteins. *Physiology*, *19*, 362–369. http://dx.doi.org/10.1152/physiol.00020.2004.

Simard, J. M., Woo, S. K., & Gerzanich, V. (2012). Transient receptor potential melastatin 4 and cell death. *Pflugers Archiv: European Journal of Physiology*, *464*(6), 573–582. http://dx.doi.org/10.1007/s00424-012-1166-z.

Singh, B. B., Liu, X. B., & Ambudkar, I. S. (2000). Expression of truncated transient receptor potential protein 1α (Trp1α): Evidence that the Trp1 C terminus modulates store-operated Ca^{2+} entry. *Journal of Biological Chemistry*, *275*(47), 36483–36486. http://dx.doi.org/10.1074/jbc.C000529200.

Sisignano, M., Park, C. K., Angioni, C., Zhang, D. D., von Hehn, C., Cobos, E. J., et al. (2012). 5,6-EET is released upon neuronal activity and induces mechanical pain hypersensitivity via TRPA1 on central afferent terminals. *Journal of Neuroscience*, *32*(18), 6364–6372. http://dx.doi.org/10.1523/Jneurosci.5793-11.2012.

Sobhan, U., Sato, M., Shinomiya, T., Okubo, M., Tsumura, M., Muramatsu, T., et al. (2013). Immunolocalization and distribution of functional temperature-sensitive TRP channels in salivary glands. *Cell and Tissue Research*, *354*(2), 507–519. http://dx.doi.org/10.1007/s00441-013-1691-x.

Soethoudt, M., Grether, U., Fingerle, J., Grim, T. W., Fezza, F., de Petrocellis, L., et al. (2017). Cannabinoid CB2 receptor ligand profiling reveals biased signalling and off-target activity. *Nature Communications*, *8*, 13958. http://dx.doi.org/10.1038/Ncomms13958.

Spivak, C. E., Kim, W., Liu, Q. R., Lupica, C. R., & Doyle, M. E. (2012). Blockade of β-cell K_{ATP} channels by the endocannabinoid, 2-arachidonoylglycerol. *Biochemical and Biophysical Research Communications*, *423*(1), 13–18. http://dx.doi.org/10.1016/j.bbrc.2012.05.042.

Story, G. M., Peier, A. M., Reeve, A. J., Eid, S. R., Mosbacher, J., Hricik, T. R., et al. (2003). ANKTM1, a TRP-like channel expressed in nociceptive neurons, is activated by cold temperatures. *Cell*, *112*(6), 819–829. http://dx.doi.org/10.1016/S0092-8674(03)00158-2.

Sugiura, T., Kondo, S., Sukagawa, A., Tonegawa, T., Nakane, S., Yamashita, A., et al. (1996). Transacylase-mediated and phosphodiesterase-mediated synthesis of N-arachidonoylethanolamine, an endogenous cannabinoid-receptor ligand, in rat brain microsomes. Comparison with synthesis from free arachidonic acid and ethanolamine. *European Journal of Biochemistry*, *240*(1), 53–62. http://dx.doi.org/10.1111/j.1432-1033.1996.0053h.x.

Talavera, K., Yasumatsu, K., Voets, T., Droogmans, G., Shigemura, N., Ninomiya, Y., et al. (2005). Heat activation of TRPM5 underlies thermal sensitivity of sweet taste. *Nature*, *438*(7070), 1022–1025. http://dx.doi.org/10.1038/nature04248.

Taylor-Clark, T. E., Undem, B. J., MacGlashan, D. W., Ghatta, S., Carr, M. J., & McAlexander, M. A. (2008). Prostaglandin-induced activation of nociceptive neurons via direct interaction with transient receptor potential A1 (TRPA1). *Molecular Pharmacology*, *73*(2), 274–281. http://dx.doi.org/10.1124/mol.107.040832.

Tazawa, K., Ikeda, H., Kawashima, N., & Okiji, T. (2017). Transient receptor potential melastatin (TRPM) 8 is expressed in freshly isolated native human odontoblasts. *Archives of Oral Biology*, *75*, 55–61. http://dx.doi.org/10.1016/j.archoralbio.2016.12.007.

Tominaga, M., Caterina, M. J., Malmberg, A. B., Rosen, T. A., Gilbert, H., Skinner, K., et al. (1998). The cloned capsaicin receptor integrates multiple pain-producing stimuli. *Neuron*, *21*(3), 531–543. http://dx.doi.org/10.1016/S0896-6273(00)80564-4.

Traynelis, S. F., Wollmuth, L. P., McBain, C. J., Menniti, F. S., Vance, K. M., Ogden, K. K., et al. (2010). Glutamate receptor ion channels: Structure, regulation, and function. *Pharmacological Reviews*, *62*(3), 405–496. http://dx.doi.org/10.1124/pr.109.002451.

Trebak, M., Bird, G. S. J., McKay, R. R., & Putney, J. W. (2002). Comparison of human TRPC3 channels in receptor-activated and store-operated modes. Differential sensitivity to channel blockers suggests fundamental differences in channel composition. *Journal of Biological Chemistry*, *277*(24), 21617–21623. http://dx.doi.org/10.1074/jbc.M202549200.

Trebak, M., Vazquez, G., Bird, G. S. J., & Putney, J. W. (2003). The TRPC3/6/7 subfamily of cation channels. *Cell Calcium*, *33*(5–6), 451–461. http://dx.doi.org/10.1016/S0143-4160(03)00056-3.

van der Stelt, M., & Di Marzo, V. (2005). Anandamide as an intracellular messenger regulating ion channel activity. *Prostaglandins & Other Lipid Mediators*, 77(1–4), 111–122. http://dx.doi.org/10.1016/j.prostaglandins.2004.09.007.

Vannier, B., Zhu, X., Brown, D., & Birnbaumer, L. (1998). The membrane topology of human transient receptor potential 3 as inferred from glycosylation-scanning mutagenesis and epitope immunocytochemistry. *Journal of Biological Chemistry*, *273*(15), 8675–8679. http://dx.doi.org/10.1074/jbc.273.15.8675.

Vazquez, G., Wedel, B. J., Aziz, O., Trebak, M., & Putney, J. W. (2004). The mammalian TRPC cation channels. *Biochimica et Biophysica Acta*, *1742*(1–3), 21–36. http://dx.doi.org/10.1016/j.bbamer.2004.08.015.

Vazquez, G., Wedel, B. J., Trebak, M., Bird, G. S., & Putney, J. W. (2003). Expression level of the canonical transient receptor potential 3 (TRPC3) channel determines its mechanism of activation. *Journal of Biological Chemistry*, *278*(24), 21649–21654. http://dx.doi.org/10.1074/jbc.M302162200.

Vellani, V., Petrosino, S., De Petrocellis, L., Valenti, M., Prandini, M., Magherini, P. C., et al. (2008). Functional lipidomics. Calcium-independent activation of endocannabinoid/endovanilloid lipid signalling in sensory neurons by protein kinases C and A and thrombin. *Neuropharmacology*, *55*(8), 1274–1279. http://dx.doi.org/10.1016/j.neuropharm.2008.01.010.

Vennekens, R., & Nilius, B. (2007). Insights into TRPM4 function, regulation and physiological role. *Handbook of Experimental Pharmacology*, *179*, 269–285.

Vennekens, R., Olausson, J., Meissner, M., Bloch, W., Mathar, I., Philipp, S. E., et al. (2007). Increased IgE-dependent mast cell activation and anaphylactic responses in mice lacking the calcium-activated nonselective cation channel TRPM4. *Nature Immunology*, *8*(3), 312–320. http://dx.doi.org/10.1038/ni1441.

Voets, T., Owsianik, G., Janssens, A., Talavera, K., & Nilius, B. (2007). TRPM8 voltage sensor mutants reveal a mechanism for integrating thermal and chemical stimuli. *Nature Chemical Biology*, *3*(3), 174–182. http://dx.doi.org/10.1038/nchembio862.

Vriens, J., Held, K., Janssens, A., Toth, B. I., Kerselaers, S., Nilius, B., et al. (2014). Opening of an alternative ion permeation pathway in a nociceptor TRP channel. *Nature Chemical Biology*, *10*(3), 188–195. http://dx.doi.org/10.1038/Nchembio.1428.

Vriens, J., Owsianik, G., Hofmann, T., Philipp, S. E., Stab, J., Chen, X. D., et al. (2011). TRPM3 is a nociceptor channel involved in the detection of noxious heat. *Neuron*, *70*(3), 482–494. http://dx.doi.org/10.1016/j.neuron.2011.02.051.

Walder, R. Y., Yang, B. L., Stokes, J. B., Kirby, P. A., Cao, X., Shi, P. J., et al. (2009). Mice defective in Trpm6 show embryonic mortality and neural tube defects. *Human Molecular Genetics*, *18*(22), 4367–4375. http://dx.doi.org/10.1093/hmg/ddp392.

Watanabe, H., Vriens, J., Prenen, J., Droogmans, G., Voets, T., & Nilius, B. (2003). Anandamide and arachidonic acid use epoxyeicosatrienoic acids to activate TRPV4 channels. *Nature*, *424*(6947), 434–438. http://dx.doi.org/10.1038/nature01807.

Wei, H., Chapman, H., Saarnilehto, M., Kuokkanen, K., Koivisto, A., & Pertovaara, A. (2010). Roles of cutaneous versus spinal TRPA1 channels in mechanical hypersensitivity in the diabetic or mustard oil-treated non-diabetic rat. *Neuropharmacology*, *58*(3), 578–584. http://dx.doi.org/10.1016/j.neuropharm.2009.12.001.

Wortley, M. A., Birrell, M. A., & Belvisi, M. G. (2016). Drugs affecting TRP channels. *Handbook of Experimental Pharmacology*, *237*, 213–241. http://dx.doi.org/10.1007/164_2016_63.

Xie, Y. F., Belrose, J. C., Lei, G., Tymianski, M., Mori, Y., MacDonald, J. F., et al. (2011). Dependence of NMDA/GSK-3 beta mediated metaplasticity on TRPM2 channels at hippocampal CA3-CA1 synapses. *Molecular Brain, 4*, 44. http://dx.doi.org/10.1186/1756-6606-4-44.

Xing, H., Ling, J., Chen, M., & Gu, J. G. (2006). Chemical and cold sensitivity of two distinct populations of TRPM8-expressing somatosensory neurons. *Journal of Neurophysiology, 95*(2), 1221–1230. http://dx.doi.org/10.1152/jn.01035.2005.

Xiong, W., Cheng, K. J., Cui, T. X., Godlewski, G., Rice, K. C., Xu, Y., et al. (2011). Cannabinoid potentiation of glycine receptors contributes to cannabis-induced analgesia. *Nature Chemical Biology*, 7(5), 296–303. http://dx.doi.org/10.1038/nchembio.552.

Xiong, W., Cui, T. X., Cheng, K. J., Yang, F., Chen, S. R., Willenbring, D., et al. (2012). Cannabinoids suppress inflammatory and neuropathic pain by targeting α3 glycine receptors. *Journal of Experimental Medicine, 209*(6), 1121–1134. http://dx.doi.org/10.1084/jem.20120242.

Xu, Y., Dhingra, A., Fina, M. E., Koike, C., Furukawa, T., & Vardi, N. (2012). mGluR6 deletion renders the TRPM1 channel in retina inactive. *Journal of Neurophysiology, 107*(3), 948–957. http://dx.doi.org/10.1152/jn.00933.2011.

Xu, Y., Orlandi, C., Cao, Y., Yang, S. Y., Choi, C. I., Pagadala, V., et al. (2016). The TRPM1 channel in ON-bipolar cells is gated by both the α and the βγ subunits of the G-protein $G_{(o)}$. *Scientific Reports, 6*, 20940. http://dx.doi.org/10.1038/Srep20940.

Yamamoto, S., Shimizu, S., Kiyonaka, S., Takahashi, N., Wajima, T., Hara, Y., et al. (2008). TRPM2-mediated $Ca^{(2+)}$ influx induces chemokine production in monocytes that aggravates inflammatory neutrophil infiltration. *Nature Medicine, 14*(7), 738–747. http://dx.doi.org/10.1038/nm1758.

Yamamoto-Kasai, E., Imura, K., Yasui, K., Shichijou, M., Oshima, I., Hirasawa, T., et al. (2012). TRPV3 as a therapeutic target for itch. *Journal of Investigative Dermatology, 132*(8), 2109–2112. http://dx.doi.org/10.1038/jid.2012.97.

Yang, K., Lei, G., Xie, Y. F., MacDonald, J. F., & Jackson, M. F. (2014). Differential regulation of NMDAR and NMDAR-mediated metaplasticity by anandamide and 2-AG in the hippocampus. *Hippocampus, 24*(12), 1601–1614. http://dx.doi.org/10.1002/hipo.22339.

Yang, J., Li, Y. Q., Zuo, X. L., Zhen, Y. B., Yu, Y. B., & Gao, L. J. (2008). Transient receptor potential ankyrin-1 participates in visceral hyperalgesia following experimental colitis. *Neuroscience Letters, 440*(3), 237–241. http://dx.doi.org/10.1016/j.neulet.2008.05.093.

Yevenes, G. E., & Zeilhofer, H. U. (2011a). Allosteric modulation of glycine receptors. *British Journal of Pharmacology, 164*(2), 224–236. http://dx.doi.org/10.1111/j.1476-5381.2011.01471.x.

Yevenes, G. E., & Zeilhofer, H. U. (2011b). Molecular sites for the positive allosteric modulation of glycine receptors by endocannabinoids. *PloS One, 6*(8), e23886, http://dx.doi.org/10.1371/journal.pone.0023886

Yu, Y. B., Yang, J., Zuo, X. L., Gao, L. J., Wang, P., & Li, Y. Q. (2010). Transient receptor potential vanilloid-1 (TRPV1) and ankyrin-1 (TRPA1) participate in visceral hyperalgesia in chronic water avoidance stress rat model. *Neurochemical Research, 35*(5), 797–803. http://dx.doi.org/10.1007/s11064-010-0137-z.

Zador, F., & Wollemann, M. (2015). Receptome: Interactions between three pain-related receptors or the "triumvirate" of cannabinoid, opioid and TRPV1 receptors. *Pharmacological Research, 102*, 254–263. http://dx.doi.org/10.1016/j.phrs.2015.10.015.

Zakharian, E., Cao, C., & Rohacs, T. (2010). Gating of transient receptor potential melastatin 8 (TRPM8) channels activated by cold and chemical agonists in planar lipid bilayers. *Journal of Neuroscience, 30*(37), 12526–12534. http://dx.doi.org/10.1523/Jneurosci.3189-10.2010.

Zamudio-Bulcock, P. A., Everett, J., Harteneck, C., & Valenzuela, C. F. (2011). Activation of steroid-sensitive TRPM3 channels potentiates glutamatergic transmission at cerebellar Purkinje neurons from developing rats. *Journal of Neurochemistry*, *119*(3), 474–485. http://dx.doi.org/10.1111/j.1471-4159.2011.07441.x.

Zeitz, C., Robson, A. G., & Audo, I. (2015). Congenital stationary night blindness: An analysis and update of genotype-phenotype correlations and pathogenic mechanisms. *Progress in Retinal and Eye Research*, *45*, 58–110. http://dx.doi.org/10.1016/j.preteyeres.2014.09.001.

Zhang, L., & Barritt, G. J. (2004). Evidence that TRPM8 is an androgen-dependent Ca^{2+} channel required for the survival of prostate cancer cells. *Cancer Research*, *64*(22), 8365–8373. http://dx.doi.org/10.1158/0008-5472.Can-04-2146.

Zhang, L., Kolaj, M., & Renaud, L. P. (2013). GIRK-like and TRPC-like conductances mediate thyrotropin-releasing hormone-induced increases in excitability in thalamic paraventricular nucleus neurons. *Neuropharmacology*, *72*, 106–115. http://dx.doi.org/10.1016/j.neuropharm.2013.04.023.

Zhang, L., Kolaj, M., & Renaud, L. P. (2015). Intracellular postsynaptic cannabinoid receptors link thyrotropin-releasing hormone receptors to Trpc-like channels in thalamic paraventricular nucleus neurons. *Neuroscience*, *311*, 81–91. http://dx.doi.org/10.1016/j.neuroscience.2015.10.015.

Zheng, J. (2013). Molecular mechanism of TRP channels. *Comprehensive Physiology*, *3*(1), 221–242. http://dx.doi.org/10.1002/cphy.c120001.

Zygmunt, P. M., Andersson, D. A., & Hogestatt, E. D. (2002). Δ^9-tetrahydrocannabinol and cannabinol activate capsaicin-sensitive sensory nerves via a CB1 and CB2 cannabinoid receptor-independent mechanism. *Journal of Neuroscience*, *22*(11), 4720–4727.

Zygmunt, P. M., Petersson, J., Andersson, D. A., Chuang, H., Sorgard, M., Di Marzo, V., et al. (1999). Vanilloid receptors on sensory nerves mediate the vasodilator action of anandamide. *Nature*, *400*(6743), 452–457. http://dx.doi.org/10.1038/22761.

CHAPTER NINE

The Role of Nuclear Hormone Receptors in Cannabinoid Function

Marco Pistis*, Saoirse E. O'Sullivan†,1
*University of Cagliari, Cittadella Universitaria di Monserrato, Cagliari, Italy
†School of Medicine, Faculty of Medicine & Health Sciences, University of Nottingham, Royal Derby Hospital Centre, Derby, United Kingdom
[1]Corresponding author: e-mail address: s.osullivan@nottingham.ac.uk

Contents

Abstract

Since the early 2000s, evidence has been accumulating that most cannabinoid compounds interact with the nuclear hormone family peroxisome proliferator-activated receptors (PPARs). This can be through direct binding of these compounds to PPARs, metabolism of cannabinoid to other PPAR-activating chemicals, or indirect activation of PPAR through cell signaling pathways. Delivery of cannabinoids to the nucleus may be facilitated by fatty acid-binding proteins and carrier proteins. All PPAR isoforms

Advances in Pharmacology, Volume 80
ISSN 1054-3589
http://dx.doi.org/10.1016/bs.apha.2017.03.008

appear to be activated by cannabinoids, but the majority of evidence is for PPARα and γ. To date, little is known about the potential interaction of cannabinoids with other nuclear hormones. At least some (but not all) of the well-known biological actions of cannabinoids including neuroprotection, antiinflammatory action, and analgesic effects are partly mediated by PPAR-activation, often in combination with activation of the more traditional target sites of action. This has been best investigated for the endocannabinoid-like compounds palmitoylethanolamide and oleoylethanolamine acting at PPARα, and for phytocannabinoids or their derivatives activation acting at PPARγ. However, there are still many aspects of cannabinoid activation of PPAR and the role it plays in the biological and therapeutic effects of cannabinoids that remain to be investigated.

ABBREVIATIONS

CBD cannabidiol
FABPs fatty acid-binding proteins
OEA oleoylethanolamine
PEA palmitoylethanolamide
PPARs peroxisome proliferator-activated receptors
PPRE peroxisome proliferator response elements
RXR 9-cis-retinoic acid receptor
Δ^9-THC Δ^9-tetrahydrocannabinol

1. INTRODUCTION

Peroxisome proliferator-activated receptors (PPARs) are a family of nuclear hormone receptors whose activation leads to changes in the transcription of target genes, which are primarily involved in the regulation of metabolism and energy homeostasis, cell differentiation, and inflammation (Friedland et al., 2012; Menendez-Gutierrez, Roszer, & Ricote, 2012; Neher, Weckbach, Huber-Lang, & Stahel, 2012; Poulsen, Siersbaek, & Mandrup, 2012). PPARs have large ligand-binding domains and can be activated by a number of ligands of different chemical structure, including fatty acids and their derivatives and a number of plant extracts (Wang et al., 2014). Since 2002, evidence has been building that endocannabinoids (such as anandamide and 2-arachidonoylglycerol (2-AG)), endocannabinoid-like compounds (autacoid lipid signaling compounds such as palmitoylethanolamide (PEA) and oleoylethanolamide (OEA)), phytocannabinoids, and synthetic cannabinoid ligands can also activate PPARs (O'Sullivan, 2007, 2016). This has been identified through reporter gene assays, binding studies, the use of selective antagonists in vitro and in vivo, PPARα knockout animals, and small interfering RNA (siRNA) knockdown of PPARs. Although not fully investigated to date, the potential mechanisms of cannabinoid/PPAR interactions include that cannabinoids can either bind directly to PPARs, be converted into PPAR-active metabolites, or that activation of cell surface cannabinoid receptors initiates intracellular signaling cascades that lead to the activation of PPARs indirectly. Another possibility that have recently come to light is that cannabinoids may be actively transported to the nucleus and PPARs by fatty acid-binding proteins (FABPs). FABPs are intracellular lipid-binding proteins that direct fatty acids around a cell. Kaczocha and colleagues first showed that anandamide was transported by FABPs from the plasma membrane to FAAH for hydrolysis (Kaczocha, Glaser, & Deutsch, 2009). They later showed that OEA is transported to the nucleus (and PPARα) by FABP5 and that FABP inhibition reduced the ability of OEA to activate PPARα (Kaczocha, Vivieca, Sun, Glaser, & Deutsch, 2012). Δ^9-tetrahydrocannabinol (Δ^9-THC) and cannabidiol (CBD) were also recently shown to be transported intracellularly by FABPs (Elmes et al., 2015), which may be the mechanism for their delivery to the nucleus for PPAR activation.

In this chapter, we will review the structure and function of each of the PPAR (α, γ, and β/δ) isoforms and examine the evidence that cannabinoids activate this isoform and whether this mediates any of the well-known physiological or therapeutic effects of cannabinoids.

2. PPARα

2.1 PPARα Receptor Structure and Function

PPARα (or NR1C1) was the first member of the PPAR family to be cloned and characterized (Issemann & Green, 1990). Its cloning was the result of several decades of studies on peroxisome proliferators, a group of structurally diverse molecules that lower serum lipids, and induce massive proliferation of peroxisomes in liver cells with transcriptional activation of peroxisomal fatty acid β-oxidation system genes (Hess, Staubli, & Riess, 1965; Thorp & Waring, 1962). This receptor is expressed in several species, including humans, particularly in metabolically active tissues such as liver, kidney, skeletal muscle, heart, brown fat, and in the CNS (Auboeuf et al., 1997; Braissant, Foufelle, Scotto, Dauca, & Wahli, 1996; Galan-Rodriguez et al., 2009; Mandard, Muller, & Kersten, 2004;

Moreno, Farioli-Vecchioli, & Cerù, 2004; Roy et al., 2016; Sher, Yi, McBride, & Gonzalez, 1993). Additionally, PPARα is expressed in the mammalian immune system (monocytes, macrophages, and lymphocytes) (Daynes & Jones, 2002), vascular endothelium (Marx, Duez, Fruchart, & Staels, 2004), and smooth muscle cells (Staels et al., 1998).

Structural studies have confirmed that PPARα, similarly to other PPARs, possesses a C-terminal large (1300 Å) and a complex ligand-binding domain (Bernardes et al., 2013; Desvergne & Wahli, 1999) that interacts with a number of diverse endogenous ligands as well as with synthetic agonists. The ligand-binding domain is also implicated in receptor heterodimerization with the obligatory transcriptional partner, the 9-cis-retinoic acid receptor (RXR). PPARα is activated by both saturated and polyunsaturated fatty acids and fatty acid derivatives (such as resolvins, protectins, maresins, and nitrolipids), with little degree of specificity, and controls important metabolic pathways involved in lipid and energy metabolism. Among fatty acid derivatives, endocannabinoid-like *N*-acylethanolamines (OEA and PEA) display the highest affinity and are considered among endogenous ligands at concentrations normally achieved under physiological conditions (Fu et al., 2003). More recently, other endogenous PPARα agonists have been isolated and characterized in the brain, specifically 3-hydroxy-(2,2)-dimethyl butyrate, hexadecanamide, and 9-octadecenamide (oleamide) (Roy et al., 2016). However, it is unclear if they display higher potency than OEA.

PPARs, in spite of their tissue distributions, ligand specificities and physiological roles, share the same general structure and molecular mechanism of action (Ferre, 2004), and this testifies their importance in the regulation of several physiological functions. In fact, PPARs, together with the other nuclear receptors, are phylogenetically related proteins (Bertrand et al., 2004; Escriva, Bertrand, & Laudet, 2004). Phylogenetic trees showing the evolutionary relationship between the members of the nuclear hormone receptor family suggest that the nuclear hormone receptors appeared early during evolution as they are present in all metazoan phyla (Escriva et al., 2004; Escriva, Delaunay, & Laudet, 2000; Michalik et al., 2002; Zhou et al., 2015). Subsequently, the large number of members in the superfamily is the result of several waves of gene duplication (Michalik et al., 2002). Specifically, the phylogenetic tree of PPARs indicates that a gene duplication event took place, within the PPAR gene family, in bony fish before their separation from birds and mammals. PPARγ is considered the original ancestor gene in the PPAR gene family that, after being firstly duplicated, divided into two subtypes: PPARγ and the common ancestor of PPARα and PPARβ (Zhou et al., 2015).

PPARs can both activate (transactivation) and inhibit (transrepression) gene expression. Their most canonical mechanism of action is regulation of gene transcription via transactivation (Berger & Moller, 2002), to positively regulate gene networks involved in the control of lipid metabolism and glucose homeostasis in several tissues, ultimately influencing circulating lipid and glucose levels. Particularly, ligand binding to PPARs induces recruitment of several coactivator proteins and dissociation of corepressor proteins, heterodimerization with the RXR and then binding to specific regions on DNA, termed peroxisome proliferator response elements (PPRE), localized in the promoter regions of most PPAR-regulated target genes. PPRE contains specific nucleotide repeats (AGGTCA) separated by one or two nucleotides. In the absence of ligands, PPARs bind the promoters of their target genes and repress transcription by recruiting corepressor complexes (ligand-independent repression) (Daynes & Jones, 2002). Besides the canonical genomic mechanisms, PPARα induces several rapid nontranscriptional effects both in the periphery and in the CNS, such as phosphorylation of specific subunits of nicotinic acetylcholine receptors via activation of a tyrosine kinase (Melis et al., 2010, 2013; Pistis & Melis, 2010; Wahli & Michalik, 2012).

2.2 Role in PPARα in Disease

PPARα is considered a lipid sensor that allows adaptation of the rates of fatty acid catabolism, lipogenesis, and ketone body synthesis, in response to feeding and starvation (Desvergne & Wahli, 1999; Hashimoto et al., 2000). Hence, physiological activation of PPARα regulates fatty acid oxidation systems to increase energy combustion. As a consequence, clinically approved PPARα agonists, such as fibrates, induce lowering of serum triglyceride levels, with negligible effects on LDL or HDL cholesterol (Linton & Fazio, 2000). However, as PPARα ligands cause peroxisome proliferation, they induce hepatomegaly and hepatocarcinogenesis in rodents but not in humans (Issemann & Green, 1990).

A great deal of evidence has indicated an important role for PPARα in the control of various types of inflammatory response (Daynes & Jones, 2002). These functions are mediated largely through the abilities of PPARα (but also other PPARs) to transrepress (Ricote & Glass, 2007) functions of many activated transcription factors, such as the transcription factor nuclear factor-κB (NF-κB), signal transducers and activators of transcription (STATs), activator protein 1 (AP1), and nuclear factor of activated T cells (NFAT) (Daynes & Jones, 2002; Wahli & Michalik, 2012). The role of PPARα in inflammation is confirmed by studies in PPARα$^{-/-}$ mice, which display enhanced inflammatory responses, such as increased susceptibility to experimental colitis (Cuzzocrea et al., 2004). Moreover, synthetic PPARα agonists reduce peripheral inflammation in a PPARα-dependent manner (Cuzzocrea et al., 2004; Lo Verme, Fu, et al., 2005; Sheu et al., 2002).

In recent years, there is growing interest in the physiological role of PPARα in the CNS, as well as for the potential implication in the neuropathogenesis and therapy of neurological and psychiatric disorders. PPARα displays a distinct pattern of expression in the CNS, with high levels in the basal ganglia, thalamic, mesencephalic and cranial motor nuclei, the reticular formation and the large motoneurons of the spinal cord (Fidaleo, Fanelli, Ceru, & Moreno, 2014; Moreno et al., 2004). PPARα is also expressed by ependymal and astroglial cells, but not by oligodendrocytes (Moreno et al., 2004). The precise physiological role of PPARα in neurons is still unclear. As in the periphery, these receptors might be involved in lipid metabolism and energy balance in neurons and in protection from neuroinflammation. In the recent years, PPARα has emerged as a key modulator of glial function and of apoptosis and necrosis triggered by inflammation and oxidative stress (Pistis & Melis, 2010). Accordingly, PPARα ligands have been considered as possible protective agents for neurodegenerative neurological diseases. Studies provide evidence for a protective effects in experimental models of Parkinson's disease (Esposito, Impellizzeri, Mazzon, Paterniti, & Cuzzocrea, 2012; Galan-Rodriguez et al., 2009; Gonzalez-Aparicio & Moratalla, 2014; Pistis & Melis, 2010), Alzheimer's disease (D'Agostino et al., 2012; Scuderi et al., 2011a, 2012), multiple sclerosis (Loria et al., 2008), and epilepsy (Auvin, 2012; Lambert, Vandevoorde, Diependaele, Govaerts, & Robert, 2001; Porta et al., 2009; Puligheddu et al., 2013; Sheerin, Zhang, Saucier, & Corcoran, 2004).

2.3 In Vitro Evidence of Cannabinoid Activation of PPARα

2.3.1 Transcriptional, Binding, and Knockdown Studies

One of the earliest studies to demonstrate a nuclear action of a cannabinoid came from Kozak and colleagues who showed in 2002 that a lipoxygenase metabolite of 2-AG activates PPARα (Kozak et al., 2002). In this work, they showed that the 2-AG metabolite 15-hydroxyeicosatetraenoic acid (15-HETE) glyceryl ester was able to increase the transcriptional activity (indicating activation of the receptor and changes in protein transcription and translation) of transiently transfected PPARα (but not γ or β) in NIH3T3 cells. Further studies showed that it was not just the metabolites of endocannabinoids that could activate PPARα, but that the transcriptional activity of PPARα could be activated by most of the extended endocannabinoid family, including OEA (Fu et al., 2003), PEA (Lo Verme, Fu, et al., 2005), anandamide (Sun et al., 2007), noladin ether (Sun et al., 2007), virodhamine (Sun et al., 2007), and oleamide (Dionisi, Alexander, & Bennett, 2012). Specific binding to the PPARα binding domain has been confirmed for OEA (Moreno-Santos et al., 2014), AEA, PEA, noladin ether, virodhamine, and WIN55,212 (all Sun et al., 2007) and for oleamide (Dionisi et al., 2012). Since endocannabinoids are fatty acid derivatives and PPARs are sensors of fatty acids, these results are not surprising, but looking outside of the endocannabinoids, it was also found that the phytocannabinoid Δ^9-THC (Takeda et al., 2014) and the synthetic CB_1/CB_2 agonist WIN55,212 (Sun et al., 2007) can increase the transcriptional activity of PPARα. However, it should be noted that Sun et al. (2007) did not find that Δ^9-THC activated PPARα, so this finding remains to be replicated. Liu and colleagues also found that ajulemic acid (AJA) (a synthetic analogue of a THC metabolite) could neither bind to nor activate the transcriptional activity of PPARα (Liu, Li, Burstein, Zurier, & Chen, 2003).

2.3.2 In Vitro Cannabinoid Responses Mediated by PPARα

With the discovery that many cannabinoids could bind to or activate the transcriptional activity of PPARα, studies began to focus on whether activation of PPARα played a role in modulating some of the cellular or tissue (in vitro) effects of cannabinoids, in addition to the more traditional target sites of action such as CB_1, CB_2, and TRP channels. Probably, the best example of this is the research probing a role for PPARα in mediating the effects of PEA. The neuroprotective effects of PEA in excitotoxic hippocampal slices (Koch et al., 2011) or β-amyloid inflamed astrocytes and astroglial cells (Scuderi et al., 2011b) are inhibited by a PPARα antagonist. In sensory neurons, PEA affects intracellular Ca^{2+} levels that can be inhibited by a PPARα antagonist, and this is thought to mediate the analgesic effects of PEA that have been shown in numerous studies (Ambrosino, Soldovieri, Russo, & Taglialatela, 2013; Khasabova, Xiong, Coicou, Piomelli, & Seybold, 2012). PEA also blocks the nicotine-induced activation of dopamine neurons in vitro that can be inhibited by a PPARα antagonist (Melis et al., 2008). At the blood–brain barrier (BBB), PEA reduces the permeability associated with ischemia/reperfusion damage (a cellular model of stroke), sensitive to PPARα antagonism (Hind et al., 2015). In the periphery, PEA also prevents the permeability changes associated with inflammation or ischemia/reperfusion damage in a cellular model of the intestinal barrier (Karwad et al., 2017) and decreases colon adenocarcinoma cell proliferation and VEGF secretion (Sarnelli et al., 2016) that can be inhibited by a PPARα antagonist. PEA causes time-dependent vasorelaxation of the bovine ophthalmic artery (Romano & Lograno, 2012) and increases aqueous humor outflow ex vivo (Kumar, Qiao, Kumar, & Song, 2012) that can be inhibited by PPARα antagonism. However, not all responses to PEA are mediated by PPARα, as in a cellular model of allergic dermatitis, the antiinflammatory effects of PEA were inhibited by a TRPV1 and not a PPARα antagonist (Petrosino et al., 2010). Together, these studies suggest that PPARα activation is a primary mechanism of action for PEA across a variety of central and peripheral effects of PEA.

Fewer studies have used PPARα antagonists against the actions of OEA in in vitro studies. Like PEA, OEA reduces permeability in a cellular model intestinal inflammation or ischemia/reperfusion (Karwad et al., 2017) and after ischemia/reperfusion in the BBB (Hind et al., 2015) that can be inhibited by PPARα antagonism. Also like PEA, OEA blocks the nicotine-induced activation of dopamine neurons, which is inhibited by a PPARα antagonist (Melis et al., 2008). OEA also has an antiinflammatory effect in human umbilical vein endothelial cells that was inhibited by a CB_2 and a PPARα antagonist (Xu et al., 2016).

AEA causes time-dependent vasorelaxation of the bovine ophthalmic artery that can be inhibited by PPARα (but not PPARγ) antagonism (Romano & Lograno, 2012). No other studies to our knowledge have shown that the in vitro effects of AEA are blocked by a PPARα antagonist, although studies have shown that PPARα is not the mechanism of action for AEA in the modulation of intestinal permeability (Alhamoruni, Lee, Wright, Larvin, & O'Sullivan, 2010; Alhamoruni, Wright, Larvin, & O'Sullivan, 2012) or BBB permeability (Hind et al., 2015). PPARα is also not the mechanism of action for 2-AG, THC, or CBD in the modulation of intestinal permeability (Alhamoruni et al., 2010, 2012). PPARα is also not the mechanism of action for CBD in reduced inflammation in astrocytes treated with β-amyloid (Esposito et al., 2011).

Downer and colleagues showed that the synthetic cannabinoid WIN55,212-2 induces the activation and expression of PPARα mediating its antiinflammatory effects in astrocytes (Downer, Clifford, Amu, Fallon, & Moynagh, 2012).

Although binding to or activation of PPARα has been demonstrated for 2-AG, noladin ether, virodhamine, and oleamide, no studies to our knowledge have investigated PPARα as a potential mechanism of action for these compounds in in vitro studies.

2.4 In Vivo Evidence of Cannabinoid Activation of PPARα

2.4.1 In Vivo Antagonist Studies

As with in vitro studies, the most evidence for a role for PPARα in modulating the physiological or therapeutic effects of a cannabinoid in vivo is for PEA. The antiinflammatory effects of PEA administration in animal models of Alzheimer's (Scuderi, Stecca, et al., 2014), allergic dermatitis (Vaia et al., 2016), colitis (Borrelli et al., 2015; Esposito et al., 2014), and edema (Lo Verme, Gaetani, et al., 2005) can all be reversed by coadministration of a PPARα antagonist. Antiepileptic/anticonvulsant effects of PEA have also been demonstrated in animal models in vivo that were inhibited by a PPARα antagonist (Citraro et al., 2013), and the analgesic effects of brain microinjection of PEA in rats is blocked by coadministration of a PPARα antagonist (de Novellis et al., 2012). However, another study showed that the analgesic effects of PEA in a formalin-evoked pain model were not affected by PPARα antagonism (Okine et al., 2016). The effects of PEA in normalizing intestinal motility in a model of intestinal inflammation were inhibited by CB_1 receptor antagonism, but not by PPARα antagonism (Capasso et al., 2014).

Intracerebral administration of OEA prevented the increase in firing of dopaminergic neurons caused by nicotine that was inhibited by a PPARα antagonist (Melis et al., 2008). Orally administered OEA dose-dependently protects against the neurological damage and edema associated with transient cerebral ischemia and this effect was blocked by a PPARα antagonist (Zhou et al., 2012). Like PEA, OEA also protects against the inflammatory effects of induced edema in animal models that is blocked by PPARα antagonism (Lo Verme, Fu, et al., 2005). However, the effects of OEA on gastrointestinal transit (Cluny, Keenan, Lutz, Piomelli, & Sharkey, 2009) are PPARα independent.

Downer et al. (2012) showed that the synthetic cannabinoid WIN55,212-2 reduces the signs of multiple sclerosis in a mouse model that was inhibited by coadministrating a PPARα antagonist (Downer et al., 2012). Payandemehr et al. (2015) also showed that WIN55,212 has an anticonvulsant effect in a mouse model that was inhibited by a PPARα antagonist.

Few studies have examined the role for PPARα in the responses to AEA, but those that have, have found that the antiepileptic effects of AEA are not via PPARα, but were inhibited by a CB_1 receptor antagonist (Citraro et al., 2013) and behavioral responses to AEA are not via PPARα, but were inhibited by a TRPV1 receptor antagonist (Panlilio et al., 2009).

2.4.2 Knock Out Studies

A number of studies have shown that PPARα activation plays an important role in mediating the effects of OEA and PEA with the use of mice in whom the PPARα protein has been genetically deleted (PPARα null or $^{-/-}$ mice). The first of these was in 2003 when Fu and colleagues demonstrated that OEA administration regulates food intake and body weight that was not observed in PPARα-deficient mice (Fu et al., 2003), and then in 2004, that OEA stimulates lipolysis, but not in PPARα-deficient mice (Guzman et al., 2004). Part of the satiety-inducing effects of OEA are through the central release of oxytocin in the hypothalamus in response to OEA, which is absent in PPARα-deficient mice (Gaetani et al., 2010). The ability of OEA treatment to reduce infarct size in a model of stroke (Sun et al., 2007) is also absent in PPARα-deficient mice, as is the improvement of memory by OEA (Campolongo et al., 2009). The antiinflammatory effects of OEA in a model of liver fibrosis were not observed in PPARα-deficient mice (Chen et al., 2015). However, not all effects of OEA administration in vivo are PPARα mediated; the modulation of cocaine-induced behavior (Bilbao et al., 2013), the inhibition of intestinal motility (Cluny et al., 2009), and the analgesic effects (Suardiaz, Estivill-Torrus, Goicoechea, Bilbao, & Rodriguez de Fonseca, 2007) of OEA are all still observed in PPARα-deficient mice.

Knock out studies have also been used to establish PPARα as a mechanisms of action for PEA. The antiinflammatory effects of PEA in a model of edema-induced inflammation were absent in mice without the PPARα receptor (Lo Verme, Fu, et al., 2005). Similarly in intestinal (Di Paola, Impellizzeri, Torre, et al., 2012), renal (Di Paola, Impellizzeri, Mondello, et al., 2012) or myocardial (Di Paola et al., 2016) injury and inflammation caused by ischemia, the protective effects of PEA are absent in PPARα-deficient mice. PEA reduces pain, edema, and macrophage infiltration in models of neuropathic pain induced chemically (Sasso et al., 2012) or by sciatic nerve damage (Di Cesare Mannelli et al., 2013), and this effect is also absent in PPARα-deficient mice. In a spinal cord injury model (Paterniti et al., 2013) or an experimental model of Alzheimer's disease (D'Agostino et al., 2012), PEA has antiinflammatory and neuroprotective effects (and improvements in memory in the Alzheimer's study) that were less pronounced in a PPARα-deficient mouse.

In summary, many cannabinoids are capable of activating and/or binding to PPARα, although the strongest evidence that this mediates the physiological or therapeutic effects of cannabinoids is for PEA and OEA which have been repeatedly shown to work through PPARα with the use of PPARα antagonists in vitro and in vivo and by the use of PPARα$^{-/-}$ mice.

3. PPARγ

3.1 PPARγ Receptor Structure and Function

PPARγ (NR1C3), cloned and characterized in *Xenopus laevis* in 1992 (Dreyer et al., 1992), is widely expressed in adipose tissue and in immune/inflammatory cells (e.g., monocytes, macrophages), colonic and cecal mucosa, and the placenta (Berger & Moller, 2002; Michalik et al., 2006). Compared with other PPARs, PPARγ expression levels are lower in skeletal muscle and liver, and the most limited in the brain (the basal ganglia, piriform cortex, hippocampus, hypothalamus) (Berger & Moller, 2002; Michalik et al., 2006).

PPARγ plays an important role in differentiation and functioning of brown and white adipocytes and promotes lipid accumulation in adipocytes (Tontonoz & Spiegelman, 2008). PPARγ represents a molecular link between lipid and carbohydrate metabolism, as it is also involved in glucose homeostasis and plays a role in the improvement of insulin sensitivity (Tontonoz & Spiegelman, 2008). For this reason, synthetic PPARγ agonists (thiazolidinediones, i.e., pioglitazone) are in clinical use as insulin sensitizers to treat patients with type 2 diabetes. PPARγ also exerts antiinflammatory actions in a variety of tissues, including the nervous system (Pistis & Melis, 2010).

The PPARγ protein has two N-terminal variants formed by alternative promoters and first exons (Fajas et al., 1997). PPARγ1 contains an additional 30 amino acids at the N-terminal region, involved in ligand-independent activation, but this function is very weak in the whole PPAR family when compared with other nuclear receptors, as activation of gene transcriptions requires ligand binding to PPARs, with little or no constitutive activity in the absence of ligands. Expression of the two PPARγ variants is tissue dependent: PPARγ1 is found in a broad range of tissues; whereas PPARγ2 is more restricted to adipose tissue. The protein also contains a DNA-binding domain and a C-terminal ligand-binding domain (Tontonoz & Spiegelman, 2008).

Similarly to PPARα, agonist binding to PPARγ leads to transactivation, through the formation of heterodimers with RXRs and binding to specific PPRE sequences in the DNA, found on the promoters of PPARγ target genes. Several of these target genes are involved in metabolic homeostasis. In addition, PPARγ induces transrepression of inflammatory-response genes. In contrast to transactivation, transrepression does not involve binding of the nuclear receptor to PPRE, but PPARγ antagonizes signal-dependent activation of its target genes by other classes of transcription factors, including NF-κB, AP-1, STAT, and NFAT proteins, thereby inhibiting inflammatory signaling pathways (Straus & Glass, 2007). PPARγ agonists exert additional beneficial effects on inflammation, such as reduction in the production of proinflammatory molecules in T lymphocytes, promotion of the expression of antiinflammatory mediators in the immune system, and reduction of cytokine levels (TNF-α, IL-1, and IL-6) (Jiang, Ting, & Seed, 1998).

The identity of the endogenous ligands for PPARγ in vivo remains unclear. However, several molecules have been shown to activate PPARγ, such as polyunsaturated fatty acids, prostanoids (i.e., 15-deoxy-D12,14 prostaglandin J2), oxidized fatty acids (i.e., 9-HODE, 13-HODE), nitrated fatty acids, and lysophosphatidic acid, albeit at very high and possibly supraphysiological concentrations.

3.2 Role in PPARγ in Disease

As mentioned, synthetic PPARγ agonists (thiazolidinediones, i.e., pioglitazone) are used in clinical use as insulin sensitizers to treat patients with type 2 diabetes. However, in recent years, the interest in PPARγ therapy was rekindled by the discovery that this receptor is expressed in the CNS and can be exploited as a drug target in neuropsychiatric disorders. In the adult brain, PPARγ shows a relatively low level of expression: granule cells in the dentate gyrus of the hippocampus (Braissant et al., 1996), caudate putamen and globus pallidus in the basal ganglia, thalamus, and the piriform cortex (Moreno et al., 2004). PPARγ expression is also detected in the microglia and astrocytes, which play a significant role in the inflammatory responses in the CNS (Bernardo, Levi, & Minghetti, 2000). Consistently,

PPARγ activation attenuates inflammatory processes associated with chronic and acute neurological disorders as in stroke, spinal cord injury, and traumatic brain injury (Kapadia, Yi, & Vemuganti, 2008). PPARγ ligands have been also reported to be effective in animal models of Parkinson's disease (Carta, 2013; Randy & Guoying, 2007; Schintu et al., 2009), but not in clinical settings (NINDS Exploratory Trials in Parkinson Disease (NET-PD) FS-ZONE Investigators, 2015; see also Brundin & Wyse, 2015).

PPARγ agonists (i.e., pioglitazone, rosiglitazone) have also displayed antidepressant-like properties in preclinical settings (Eissa Ahmed & Al-Rasheed, 2009; Sadaghiani, Javadi-Paydar, Gharedaghi, Fard, & Dehpour, 2011). Consistently, a moderate improvement in depressive symptoms was reported in depressed (and insulin-resistant) patients treated with rosiglitazone (Rasgon et al., 2010) or pioglitazone (Kemp et al., 2014; Sepanjnia, Modabbernia, Ashrafi, Modabbernia, & Akhondzadeh, 2012). Remarkably, in accordance with the antineuroinflammatory actions of PPARγ agonists, a correlation was demonstrated between depressive symptomatology scores and changes in interleukin (IL)-6 levels (Kemp et al., 2014).

3.3 In Vitro Evidence of Cannabinoid Activation of PPARγ

3.3.1 Transcriptional and Binding Studies

The first published evidence that a cannabinoid could activate PPARγ came from Liu et al. (2003) who showed that AJA (a synthetic analogue of a Δ^9-THC metabolite) could bind to and cause the activation of PPARγ (but not α or β) (Liu et al., 2003), later confirmed by Ambrosio and colleagues (Ambrosio et al., 2007). O'Sullivan and colleagues then showed that THC itself was also capable of increasing the transcriptional activity of PPARγ (O'Sullivan, Tarling, Bennett, Kendall, & Randall, 2005), and binding of Δ^9-THC to the PPARγ binding domain was more recently confirmed by Granja and colleagues. Other phytocannabinoids have been investigated and it seems that CBD (Granja et al., 2012; Hegde, Singh, Nagarkatti, & Nagarkatti, 2015; O'Sullivan, Sun, Bennett, Randall, & Kendall, 2009), CBG, CBC, and Cannabigerol quinone (Granja et al., 2012) can all bind to and/or cause the transactivation of PPARγ.

Bouaboula and colleagues showed in 2005 that AEA increases the transcriptional activity of PPARγ in a concentration-dependent manner and binds directly to the PPARγ ligand-binding domain (Bouaboula et al., 2005), more recently confirmed by (Ahn et al., 2015). 2-AG (Rockwell,

Snider, Thompson, Vanden Heuvel, & Kaminski, 2006) or its metabolites (Raman, Kaplan, Thompson, Vanden Heuvel, & Kaminski, 2011) can also activates PPARγ in a reporter gene assay, and NADA and PEA can increase the transcriptional activity of PPARγ (O'Sullivan, Bennett, Kendall, & Randall, 2006; O'Sullivan, Kendall, & Randall, 2006), although this has not been consistently observed for either compound (Ahn et al., 2015; Bouaboula et al., 2005; Lo Verme, Fu, et al., 2005). Oleamide has been shown to both bind to and transactivate PPARγ (Dionisi et al., 2012). Thus, activation of PPARγ appears to be a common trait for endocannabinoids or endocannabinoid-like compounds.

Looking at synthetic cannabinoids, WIN55,212 (O'Sullivan, Kendall, et al., 2006; Fakhfouri et al., 2012) and CP55950 (O'Sullivan, Kendall, et al., 2006) can increase the transcriptional activity of PPARγ, and HU331 has been shown to bind to PPARγ (Granja et al., 2012).

However, the ability of cannabinoids to activate PPARγ is not ubiquitous; O'Sullivan, Kendall, et al. (2006) found that THCV did not increase the transcriptional activity of PPARγ; Kozak et al. (2002) and Ahn et al. (2015) did not find that 2-AG or NADA increased the transcriptional activity of PPARγ; Fu et al. (2003) showed OEA did not to bind to or activate PPARγ; PEA does not increase the transcriptional activity or bind to of PPARγ (Bouaboula et al., 2005; Lo Verme, Fu, et al., 2005); and JWH015 does not bind to PPARγ (Vara, Morell, Rodriguez-Henche, & Diaz-Laviada, 2013).

3.3.2 Cellular/Tissue Responses of Cannabinoids Mediated by PPARγ

The use of PPARγ antagonists in in vitro studies has revealed that some of the cellular and tissue responses to cannabinoids are mediated by PPARγ. In isolated segments of arteries from rats, Δ^9-THC causes a time-dependent vasorelaxation (O'Sullivan et al., 2005) and improves endothelium-dependent vasorelaxation (O'Sullivan, Kendall, et al., 2006) that can be inhibited by a PPARγ antagonist. The neuroprotective effects of THC in neuroblastoma cells exposed to various toxins are inhibited by a PPARγ antagonist but not a CB_1 antagonist (Carroll, Zeissler, Hanemann, & Zajicek, 2012), and the antitumoral effects of Δ^9-THC in hepatocellular carcinoma cells were also blocked by either a PPARγ antagonist or by genetic deletion of PPARγ in the cells with siRNA (Vara et al., 2013). However, the actions of Δ^9-THC on intestinal permeability are not inhibited by a PPARγ antagonist (Alhamoruni et al., 2010, 2012). The antifibrotic effects of AJA (the THC metabolite analogue) in skin fibroblasts from patients with scleroderma were also inhibited by a PPARγ antagonist

(Gonzalez et al., 2012), however, the antiinflammatory effects of AJA in vitro are not mediated by PPARγ (Johnson, Stebulis, Rossetti, Burstein, & Zurier, 2007; Parker et al., 2008). The antiinflammatory and neuroprotective effects of CBD after β-amyloid administration are blocked by a PPARγ antagonist (Esposito et al., 2011). Furthermore, CBD promotes the reduction of β-amyloid expression in a cell model of Alzheimer's and improved cell survival, which could be blocked by a PPARγ antagonist (Scuderi, Steardo, & Esposito, 2014). In a cellular model of the BBB, CBD prevents the increase in permeability caused by 4 h oxygen and glucose deprivation that was inhibited by a PPARγ antagonist and partly reduced by a 5-HT1A receptor antagonist, but was unaffected by CB_1 or CB_2 antagonism (Hind, England, & O'Sullivan, 2016). In isolated rat aortae, CBD causes a time-dependent vasorelaxant effect that was inhibited by a PPARγ antagonist but not CB_1 or CB_2 antagonism (O'Sullivan, Sun, et al., 2009). However, some of the vascular actions of CBD in arteries measured ex vivo are not affected by PPARγ antagonism (Stanley, Hind, Tufarelli, & O'Sullivan, 2015; Wheal, Cipriano, Fowler, Randall, & O'Sullivan, 2014). In biopsies from patients with ulcerative colitis, CBD treatment ex vivo reduces signs of inflammation that can be blocked with a PPARγ antagonist (De Filippis et al., 2011), but PPARγ is not the mechanism of action in CBD's ability to reduce intestinal permeability in vitro (Alhamoruni et al., 2010, 2012) The antiapoptotic effects of CBD in human lung cancer cells were blocked by either a PPARγ antagonist or by genetic deletion of PPARγ with siRNA (Ramer et al., 2013).

The antiinflammatory effects of AEA in mouse splenocytes (white blood cells from the spleen) were not inhibited by CB_1 or CB_2 antagonism but were reduced by COX inhibition and PPARγ antagonism (Rockwell & Kaminski, 2004). Both AEA and NADA also cause a time-dependent vasorelaxant effect that is inhibited by PPARγ antagonism (with a role for CB_1 also mediating the effects of NADA) (O'Sullivan, Kendall, & Randall, 2009). However, modulation of BBB permeability (Hind et al., 2015), time-dependent vasorelaxation of bovine ophthalmic arteries (Romano & Lograno, 2012), and modulation of intestinal permeability (Alhamoruni et al., 2010, 2012) are not mediated by PPARγ for AEA.

Like AEA, the antiinflammatory effects of 2-AG in mouse hippocampal neurons were blocked by PPARγ antagonism (Du, Chen, Zhang, & Chen, 2011) and the ability of 2-AG to suppresses IL-2 secretion in Jurkat T cells is blocked by a PPARγ antagonist (Rockwell et al., 2006). This effect also extends to the metabolites of 2-AG which can decrease IL-2 secretion, partly inhibited by PPARγ antagonism (Raman et al., 2011).

Looking at synthetic cannabinoids, WIN55,212 decreases the expression of adhesion molecules on brain endothelial cell cultures, which was inhibited by a PPARγ antagonist (Mestre et al., 2009). The apoptotic effects of WIN55,212 in two different liver cancer cells were also inhibited by PPARγ antagonists (Giuliano et al., 2009; Hong et al., 2013). Similarly, the antitumoral effects of JWH015 in hepatocellular carcinoma cells were blocked by either a PPARγ antagonist or by genetic deletion of PPARγ in the cells with siRNA (Vara et al., 2013). A role for PPARγ (but not CB_1, CB_2, or TRPV1) in mediating the apoptotic effects of methanandamide was shown in human cervical carcinoma cells by siRNA deletion of PPARγ (Eichele, Ramer, & Hinz, 2009). However, the antiproliferative effects of noladin ether in prostate carcinoma cells are not inhibited by a PPARγ antagonists (Nithipatikom, Isbell, Endsley, Woodliff, & Campbell, 2011). Together, this suggests PPARγ is a key mechanism of action in the antitumoral effects of some, but not all, cannabinoids. Leptin-induced oxidative stress in hypothalamic neuronal cells is also reduced by the synthetic CB_1 agonist ACEA which is blocked by antagonism of both CB_1 and PPARγ (Palomba et al., 2015).

3.4 In Vivo Evidence of Cannabinoid Activation of PPARγ

A more limited number of studies have investigated the role of PPARγ in mediating the response to cannabinoids in in vivo studies. CBD has an immunomodulatory role in vivo by the induction of myeloid-derived suppressor cells that is inhibited by coadministration of a PPARγ antagonist (Hegde et al., 2015). CBD causes tumor regression in a mouse model that was inhibited by a PPARγ antagonist (Ramer et al., 2013). CBD treatment is also neuroprotective in β-amyloid models, and this effect was abolished by coadministration of a PPARγ antagonist (Esposito et al., 2011).

In a spinal cord injury model, the antiinflammatory and neuroprotective effects of PEA administration were reduced by a PPARγ antagonist (Paterniti et al., 2013), and in a sciatic nerve injury model, the analgesic effects of PEA were inhibited by antagonists of CB_1, TRPV1, and PPARγ (Costa, Comelli, Bettoni, Colleoni, & Giagnoni, 2008). However, the analgesic effect of PEA in a formalin-evoked pain model is not affected by PPARγ antagonism (Okine et al., 2016).

WIN55,212 has anticonvulsant effects in a mouse model that were partially inhibited by a PPARγ antagonist (Payandemehr et al., 2015). WIN55,212 treatment also protects against β-amyloid-induced neurodegeneration in rats and improves memory, which is inhibited by CB_1, CB_2, and PPARγ antagonists (Fakhfouri et al., 2012).

Low doses of THC protect the mouse brain from inflammation in a model of lipopolysaccharide (LPS)-induced cognitive damage, which could be blocked by coadministration of a CB_1 or PPARγ antagonist, with no effects of a CB_2 antagonist (Fishbein-Kaminietsky, Gafni, & Sarne, 2014).

In summary, many cannabinoids can bind to or activate PPARγ, although the evidence for this mediating any of the response to cannabinoids is strongest for the phytocannabinoids Δ^9-THC and CBD. PPARγ partially mediates some of the antiinflammatory effects of endocannabinoids and the antitumoral effects of a range of cannabinoids.

4. PPARβ/δ

4.1 PPARβ/δ Receptor Structure and Function

The PPARβ/δ isotype (NR1C2) was first cloned from a *Xenopus* oocyte library and initially termed PPARβ (Dreyer et al., 1992). The mammalian protein, instead, was named PPARδ when identified in the mouse (Kliewer et al., 1994). However, genome sequencing indicated that there were only three PPAR isotypes, and that the mammalian PPARδ was homologous to the amphibian PPARβ. For these reasons, this receptor was denominated as PPARβ/δ (Michalik et al., 2006).

Using quantitative Western blotting experiments, Girroir et al. provided an extensive study on the expression of PPARβ/δ in mouse (Girroir et al., 2008). PPARβ/δ expression is very high in small intestine and keratinocytes; high in liver, colon, kidney, and skin; and relatively low in other tissues including brain, heart, lung, skeletal muscle, testis, spleen, and thymus (Girroir et al., 2008; Neels & Grimaldi, 2014). In the rat brain, PPARβ/δ displays a wide expression both by neurons and glial cells (Moreno et al., 2004), suggesting that it might play a major role in fatty acid metabolism and transport as well as in controlling inflammation (Neels & Grimaldi, 2014), as reported by a number of studies in animal models of multiple sclerosis (experimental autoimmune encephalitis) (Kanakasabai et al., 2010; Polak et al., 2005; Simonini et al., 2009). Expression levels of PPARβ/δ undergo to physiological changes in a tissue-dependent manner: for instance, fasting reduces PPARβ/δ levels in liver and increases in skeletal muscle (Neels & Grimaldi, 2014).

Similar to the other PPARs, PPARβ/δ exerts part of their transcriptional regulation as a heterodimer with RXR and binds to PPRE sequence located in the promoter region or in the transcribed region of the target genes (trans-activation). The PPARβ/δ–RXR heterodimer interacts also with corepressors and other proteins, which results in recruitment of histone deacetylases and subsequent changes toward tight chromatin structure and transcription repression (Neels & Grimaldi, 2014).

Few PPARβ/δ ligands have been reported, when compared with the other PPARs, and they display a certain degree of selectivity for this isoform. The reason might be related by the observation that the ligand-binding pocket is smaller than the corresponding PPARα and PPARγ, which are similar to each other both in shape and in size (Neels & Grimaldi, 2014). Among those ligands, prostacyclin (PGI_2) has been described as a potent PPARβ/δ agonist, with important regulatory roles for the PGI_2/PPARβ/δ interaction axis in embryo hatching and implantation and vascular physiology, but this evidence is still controversial, as other authors have provided contradictory evidence (see Neels & Grimaldi, 2014 and references therein for a comprehensive review). Additionally, the arachidonic acid metabolite 15-hydroxyeicosatetraenoic acid was shown to be a PPARβ/δ agonist, with less affinity for the other PPAR isoforms (Coleman et al., 2007; Naruhn et al., 2010). Lipoperoxidation products, such as 4-hydroxynonenal (4-HNE), 4-hydroperoxynonenal (Coleman et al., 2007), and 4-hydroperoxynonenal hydroxydodeca-(2E,6Z)-dienal (4-HDDE) (Riahi et al., 2010; Rieck, Meissner, Ries, Müller-Brüsselbach, & Müller, 2008) also activate PPARβ/δ. It has been reported that all-*trans*-retinoic acid is also a high-affinity ligand for PPAR-β/δ (Shaw, Elholm, & Noy, 2003), but this finding was not confirmed by other authors (Borland et al., 2008, 2011).

4.2 Role in PPARβ/δ in Disease

PPARβ/δ participates in the control of energy homeostasis by regulating fatty acid catabolism and adaptive thermogenesis, in reproductive physiology in females and in the development of digestive system, muscle physiology, metabolism, and remodeling (Michalik et al., 2006; Neels & Grimaldi, 2014; Wang et al., 2003). Moreover, PPARβ/δ has an important role in the control of cell proliferation, differentiation, and survival and is involved in tissue repair, particularly in keratinocytes (Neels & Grimaldi, 2014). Several phase II clinical trials have been carried out to test the efficacy of two synthetic PPARβ/δ agonists, GW501516, and MBX-8025, providing encouraging findings for the treatment of metabolic disorders in dyslipidemic obese individuals (Bays et al., 2011; Choi et al., 2012; Ooi, Watts, Sprecher, Chan, & Barrett, 2011; Risérus et al., 2008; Sprecher et al., 2007).

Like the other PPAR isoforms, PPARβ/δ activation decreases inflammation in almost all inflammatory disease models (Neels & Grimaldi, 2014). Accordingly, deletion of PPARβ/δ leads to worsening of inflammatory states, i.e., in experimental colitis (Bassaganya-Riera et al., 2011; Neels & Grimaldi, 2014).

4.3 Evidence of Cannabinoid Activation of PPARβ/δ

Very few studies to date have investigated the effects of cannabinoids at PPARβ/δ. Fu et al. (2003) showed that OEA activates the transcriptional activity of PPARβ/δ and Dionisi et al. (2012) showed that oleamide increases the transcriptional activity of and binds to PPARβ/δ, although no further studies have examined this. This effect is not ubiquitous to endocannabinoids, as 2-AG metabolites (Kozak et al., 2002) and PEA (Lo Verme, Fu, et al., 2005) do not activate PPARβ/δ. Despite this, Paterniti et al. (2013) showed that the neuroprotective and antiinflammatory effects of PEA were inhibited by a PPARβ/δ antagonist, and an indirect activation of PPARβ/δ by anandamide (being degraded into arachidonic acid) is speculated to play a role in regulating cognitive function (Yu, Levi, Casadesus, Kunos, & Noy, 2014). Further work is required to explore this research area.

5. MODULATION OF THE ENDOCANNABINOID SYSTEM AND PPAR ACTIVATION

In addition to studying the direct effects of cannabinoids on PPARs, some studies have investigated a potential role for PPAR activation in mediating some of the physiological and therapeutic effects of drugs that upregulate endogenous levels of endocannabinoids by blocking their degradation enzymes, uptake, or intracellular transport.

The analgesic effects of the FAAH inhibitor URB597 (Jhaveri et al., 2008; Sagar, Kendall, & Chapman, 2008) or the COX-inhibitor nimesulide (Jhaveri et al., 2008) can be inhibited by PPARα antagonism. Similarly, FAAH inhibition by URB597 enhances memory acquisition (Mazzola et al., 2009) and blocks the neuronal response to nicotine or cocaine (Luchicchi et al., 2010) in rats that can be blocked by a PPARα antagonist. URB597 also reduces nicotine self-administration in squirrel monkeys that was reversed by a PPARα antagonist (Justinova et al., 2015), although another study in rats found that the effects of URB597 on nicotine seeking were inhibited by CB_1 antagonism and not PPARα antagonism (Forget, Guranda, Gamaleddin, Goldberg, & Le Foll, 2016). Another FAAH inhibitor, PF-3845, supresses nausea in a rat model of conditioned gaping via PPARα (Rock et al., 2015). In the periphery, FAAH inhibition by URB597 increased the migration of human adipose-derived mesenchymal stem cells that is inhibited by PPARα antagonism (Wollank et al., 2015).

The monoacylglycerol lipase inhibitor JZL184 causes antiinflammatory and neuroprotective effects that are inhibited by a PPARγ antagonist (Zhang, Hu, Teng, Tang, & Chen, 2014) and JZL184 (or URB602) increases PPARγ expression (Du et al., 2011).

The *N*-acylethanolamine acid amidase (NAAA, breaks down OEA and PEA) inhibitor ARN077 also causes analgesia in tumor bearing mice (Khasabova et al., 2012) or in inflammatory pain models (Sasso et al., 2013) that can be blocked by a PPARα antagonist. The analgesic effects of another NAAA inhibitor, F96, were absent in mice lacking the PPARα receptor (Yang et al., 2015). A third inhibitor, (S)-OOPP, reduces neutrophil migration and inflammation in mice that was absent in mice lacking PPARα (Solorzano et al., 2009).

The endocannabinoid uptake inhibitor AM404 reduces the inflammatory effects of LPS in rats, which was inhibited by CB_1, CB_2, TRPV1, and PPARγ (Roche, Kelly, O'Driscoll, & Finn, 2008). When AM404 was administered peripherally, it reduced feeding in rats which was inhibited by a PPARα antagonist. Interestingly, the same study showed that AM404 administration directly to the brain stimulated food intake via CB_1 (Reyes-Cabello et al., 2012). Another endocannabinoid uptake inhibitor, UCM707 protects against excitotoxicity in a model of multiple sclerosis which was mediated by CB_1, CB_2, and PPARγ (Loria et al., 2010).

FABPs are suggested to chaperones endocannabinoids intracellularly, for example, to FAAH or NAAA for hydrolysis, or the nucleus for PPAR activation. Kaczocha and colleagues have shown that FABP inhibitors produce analgesia and that this was inhibited by CB_1 or PPARα antagonism, and suggested to be due to reduced hydrolysis of endocannabinoids (Kaczocha et al., 2014).

6. OTHER NUCLEAR HORMONE RECEPTORS

Limited evidence supports the possibility that cannabinoids or endocannabinoids bind to other nuclear hormone receptors. Besides PPARs, this superfamily includes nonsteroid hormone receptors, i.e., those for retinoic acid and thyroid hormones, and steroid hormone receptors, i.e., those for the estrogens and 3-ketosteroids (glucocorticoids, androgens, progestins) (Alexander et al., 2015).

Most studies were focused on potential interaction between cannabinoids and estrogen receptors, as Δ^9-THC has long been known to reduce fertility in males and females (Braude, 1984; Harclerode, 1984). Results were, however, very inconsistent. Early studies indicated that Δ^9-THC displays weak affinity for estrogen receptors in vitro (Rawitch, Schultz, Ebner, & Vardaris, 1977), suggesting that this compound might have a direct estrogenic effect. However, in vivo studies in rats did not agree with these findings (Okey & Truant, 1975). Chakravarty and Naik (Chakravarty, Sheth, & Ghosh, 1975) and Ruh and colleagues (Ruh, Taylor, Howlett, & Welshons, 1997) were also unable to find evidence for Δ^9-THC binding with estrogen receptors in a number of tissues.

Subsequent studies also yielded controversial results. Takeda and colleagues reported that Δ^9-THC induces proliferation in MCF-7 cells via cannabinoid receptor-independent signaling mediated by estrogen receptors (Takeda et al., 2008), while von Bueren, Schlumpf, & Lichtensteiger, (2008) detected inhibition of 17β-estradiol-induced cell division in the same cell line. However, this initial hypothesis was later rejected, as the antiestrogenic effects of Δ^9-THC were attributed to cannabinoid receptor-dependent upregulation of estrogen receptor β (Takeda et al., 2013).

Interestingly, synthetic cannabinoids belonging to the naphthoylindole (JWH-018, JWH-073, JWH-122, and JWH-210) and benzoylindole (AM-694) groups, abused as "spice" drugs, display hormonal actions by binding at estrogen receptors as antagonists with weak antiestrogenic effects at concentrations between 2.1 and 23 μM (Koller, Zlabinger, Auwarter, Fuchs, & Knasmueller, 2013).

Thus, the question whether cannabinoids display affinity for estrogen receptors remains open, even if it is questionable whether this direct interaction displays physiological effects or occurs at concentrations normally achieved in humans.

Some early studies, all from the same group, have investigated whether Δ^9-THC binds to glucocorticoid receptors (Eldridge & Landfield, 1990; Eldridge, Murphy, & Landfield, 1991; Landfield & Eldridge, 1993). They reported that Δ^9-THC displays weak affinity for glucocorticoid receptors in the hippocampus, as binding of [^3H]dexamethasone in vitro was partially inhibited by unlabeled Δ^9-THC and CBD, a nonpsychoactive cannabinoid component of *Cannabis*. Even at large excess, Δ^9-THC could displace only 50% of radiolabeled dexamethasone binding, whereas CBD could inhibit only 22% of tracer binding. Analyses pointed to a possible noncompetitive site for cannabinoid interaction with glucocorticoid receptors (Eldridge & Landfield, 1990). These findings have not been replicated by others, so it is uncertain if this interaction bears pharmacological relevance in vivo.

In conclusion, endocrine effects related to cannabis consumption in humans are not likely to be attributed to direct interactions between these drugs and nuclear hormone receptors. In fact, it is well established that most if not all observed hormonal actions are mediated by cannabinoid receptors that regulate endocrine systems in the hypothalamic–pituitary–gonadal axis, thyroid, and the hypothalamic–pituitary–adrenal axis (see Hillard, 2015 for a recent comprehensive review).

7. CONCLUSION

Most cannabinoids activate or bind to PPARα in cellular assays and PPARα activation modulates some cannabinoid responses, as summarized in Fig. 1 (concentrations and doses used are presented in Table 1). The use of PPARα antagonists in vitro and in vivo has demonstrated that many,

Key points:

- There is much evidence to show that some cannabinoids activate PPARs, although the full picture is still incomplete.
- Intracellularly, cannabinoids are transported by FABPs to enzymes for degradation, or to PPARs for activation. FABP-facilitated metabolism of endocannabinoids can also yield PPAR activators.
- Many cannabinoids have neuroprotective effects in models of stroke, Alzheimer's disease, Parkinson's, multiple sclerosis, and epilepsy that are mediated by both PPARα and γ.
- Modulation of neuronal processes such as nicotine reward and memory by endocannabinoids involves PPARα.
- Endocannabinoids and endocannabinoid-like molecules (especially PEA) have antinociceptive effects through PPARα.
- In many cancer cells lines, PPARγ activation by a range of cannabinoids is involved in their antiproliferative effects.
- In the cardiovascular system, activation of PPARα and γ by a range of cannabinoids causes time-dependent vasorelaxation and reduces endothelial cell activation.
- In the gastrointestinal system, PPARα activation by OEA and PEA reduces intestinal inflammation and permeability.
- OEA regulates body weight through PPARα.
- Inflammation is reduced by cannabinoids via PPARα and γ.

Fig. 1 Summary of the current evidence of the role of PPAR activation by cannabinoids in mediating their responses.

Table 1 In Vivo and In Vitro Concentrations of Cannabinoids Required to Bind to, Activate or Have Responses Mediated by PPAR Nuclear Receptors

	PPARα	PPARγ	PPARβ/δ
Phytocannabinoids and their derivatives			
THC	5–25 μM	EC_{50} 21.2 μM 0.002 mg kg^{-1}	x
CBD	x	1 nM–20 μM, EC_{50} of 20.1 μM 10–20 mg kg^{-1}	x
CBC	x	$EC_{50} > 25$ μM	x
CBG	x	EC_{50} of 12.7 μM	x
AJA	x	1–10 μM	x
Endocannabinoids			
AEA	10 μM	3–30 μM	x
2-AG	x	1–30 μM	x
Endocannabinoid-like compounds			
OEA	5–30 μM 40 mg kg^{-1} 5–10 mg kg^{-1}	x	1–10 μM
PEA	10 nM–10 μM 10–30 mg kg^{-1} 50 μg/paw	1–100 nM, 10 mg kg^{-1}	10 mg kg^{-1}
NADA	x	1–20 μM	x
Noladin ether	10–30 μM	x	x
Virodhamine	10–30 μM	x	x
Oleamide	10–50 μM	10–50 μM	10–50 μM
Synthetic compounds			
WIN55,212	1–30 μM	100 nM–20 μM 10 μg, i.h.p. 0.1 mg kg^{-1}	x
CP55,940	x	1–10 μM	x
ACEA	x	500 nM	x

X denotes no activity or no known activity.

but not all, of the physiological and therapeutic effects of cannabinoids are PPARα dependent, particularly in mediating central effects, although this has only been extensively studied for OEA and PEA. Similarly, most cannabinoids activate or bind to PPARγ in cellular assays (best studied for phytocannabinoids) and PPARγ has been shown to mediate some of the antiinflammatory and antitumoral effects of cannabinoids. For many cannabinoids, the potential role of PPARs (including PPARβ/δ) in mediating their responses has not yet been examined, and there are many gaps in our current knowledge that warrant further investigation. That said, the ability of PPAR activation (either alone or in combination with cannabinoid receptors) to mediate some of the therapeutic effects of cannabinoids adds to the argument that the polypharmacology of cannabinoids is critical to their success.

CONFLICT OF INTEREST

None to report.

REFERENCES

Ahn, S., Yi, S., Seo, W. J., Lee, M. J., Song, Y. K., Baek, S. Y., et al. (2015). A cannabinoid receptor agonist *N*-arachidonoyl dopamine inhibits adipocyte differentiation in human mesenchymal stem cells. *Biomolecules & Therapeutics*, *23*(3), 218–224. http://dx.doi.org/10.4062/biomolther.2014.137.

Alexander, S. P., Cidlowski, J. A., Kelly, E., Marrion, N., Peters, J. A., Benson, H. E., et al. (2015). The concise guide to PHARMACOLOGY 2015/16: Nuclear hormone receptors. *British Journal of Pharmacology*, *172*(24), 5956–5978. http://dx.doi.org/10.1111/bph.13352.

Alhamoruni, A., Lee, A. C., Wright, K. L., Larvin, M., & O'Sullivan, S. E. (2010). Pharmacological effects of cannabinoids on the Caco-2 cell culture model of intestinal permeability. *The Journal of Pharmacology and Experimental Therapeutics*, *335*(1), 92–102. http://dx.doi.org/10.1124/jpet.110.168237.

Alhamoruni, A., Wright, K. L., Larvin, M., & O'Sullivan, S. E. (2012). Cannabinoids mediate opposing effects on inflammation-induced intestinal permeability. *British Journal of Pharmacology*, *165*(8), 2598–2610. http://dx.doi.org/10.1111/j.1476-5381.2011.01589.x.

Ambrosino, P., Soldovieri, M. V., Russo, C., & Taglialatela, M. (2013). Activation and desensitization of TRPV1 channels in sensory neurons by the PPARalpha agonist palmitoylethanolamide. *British Journal of Pharmacology*, *168*(6), 1430–1444. http://dx.doi.org/10.1111/bph.12029.

Ambrosio, A. L., Dias, S. M., Polikarpov, I., Zurier, R. B., Burstein, S. H., & Garratt, R. C. (2007). Ajulemic acid, a synthetic nonpsychoactive cannabinoid acid, bound to the ligand binding domain of the human peroxisome proliferator-activated receptor gamma. *The Journal of Biological Chemistry*, *282*(25), 18625–18633. http://dx.doi.org/10.1074/jbc.M702538200.

Auboeuf, D., Rieusset, J., Fajas, L., Vallier, P., Frering, V., Riou, J. P., et al. (1997). Tissue distribution and quantification of the expression of mRNAs of peroxisome proliferator-activated receptors and liver X receptor-alpha in humans: No alteration in adipose tissue of obese and NIDDM patients. *Diabetes*, *46*(8), 1319–1327.

Auvin, S. (2012). Fatty acid oxidation and epilepsy. *Epilepsy Research*, *100*(3), 224–228. http://dx.doi.org/10.1016/j.eplepsyres.2011.05.022.

Bassaganya-Riera, J., DiGuardo, M., Climent, M., Vives, C., Carbo, A., Jouni, Z. E., et al. (2011). Activation of PPARγ and δ by dietary punicic acid ameliorates intestinal inflammation in mice. *British Journal of Nutrition*, *106*(06), 878–886.

Bays, H. E., Schwartz, S., Littlejohn, T., III, Kerzner, B., Krauss, R. M., Karpf, D. B., et al. (2011). MBX-8025, a novel peroxisome proliferator receptor-δ agonist: Lipid and other metabolic effects in dyslipidemic overweight patients treated with and without atorvastatin. *The Journal of Clinical Endocrinology & Metabolism*, *96*(9), 2889–2897.

Berger, J., & Moller, D. E. (2002). The mechanisms of action of PPARs. *Annual Review of Medicine*, *53*, 409–435.

Bernardes, A., Souza, P. C., Muniz, J. R., Ricci, C. G., Ayers, S. D., Parekh, N. M., et al. (2013). Molecular mechanism of peroxisome proliferator-activated receptor alpha activation by WY14643: A new mode of ligand recognition and receptor stabilization. *Journal of Molecular Biology*, *425*(16), 2878–2893. http://dx.doi.org/10.1016/j.jmb.2013.05.010.

Bernardo, A., Levi, G., & Minghetti, L. (2000). Role of the peroxisome proliferator-activated receptor-gamma (PPAR-gamma) and its natural ligand 15-deoxy-Delta12, 14-prostaglandin J2 in the regulation of microglial functions. *European Journal of Neuroscience*, *12*(7), 2215–2223.

Bertrand, S., Brunet, F. G., Escriva, H., Parmentier, G., Laudet, V., & Robinson-Rechavi, M. (2004). Evolutionary genomics of nuclear receptors: From twenty-five ancestral genes to derived endocrine systems. *Molecular Biology and Evolution*, *21*(10), 1923–1937. http://dx.doi.org/10.1093/molbev/msh200.

Bilbao, A., Blanco, E., Luque-Rojas, M. J., Suarez, J., Palomino, A., Vida, M., et al. (2013). Oleoylethanolamide dose-dependently attenuates cocaine-induced behaviours through a PPARalpha receptor-independent mechanism. *Addiction Biology*, *18*(1), 78–87. http://dx.doi.org/10.1111/adb.12006.

Borland, M. G., Foreman, J. E., Girroir, E. E., Zolfaghari, R., Sharma, A. K., Amin, S., et al. (2008). Ligand activation of peroxisome proliferator-activated receptor-β/δ inhibits cell proliferation in human HaCaT keratinocytes. *Molecular Pharmacology*, *74*(5), 1429–1442.

Borland, M. G., Khozoie, C., Albrecht, P. P., Zhu, B., Lee, C., Lahoti, T. S., et al. (2011). Stable over-expression of PPARβ/δ and PPARγ to examine receptor signaling in human HaCaT keratinocytes. *Cellular Signalling*, *23*(12), 2039–2050.

Borrelli, F., Romano, B., Petrosino, S., Pagano, E., Capasso, R., Coppola, D., et al. (2015). Palmitoylethanolamide, a naturally-occurring lipid, is an orally effective intestinal anti-inflammatory agent. *British Journal of Pharmacology*, *172*, 142–158. http://dx.doi.org/10.1111/bph.12907.

Bouaboula, M., Hilairet, S., Marchand, J., Fajas, L., Le Fur, G., & Casellas, P. (2005). Anandamide induced PPARgamma transcriptional activation and 3T3-L1 preadipocyte differentiation. *European Journal of Pharmacology*, *517*(3), 174–181. http://dx.doi.org/10.1016/j.ejphar.2005.05.032.

Braissant, O., Foufelle, F., Scotto, C., Dauca, M., & Wahli, W. (1996). Differential expression of peroxisome proliferator-activated receptors (PPARs): Tissue distribution of PPAR-alpha, -beta, and -gamma in the adult rat. *Endocrinology*, *137*(1), 354–366.

Braude, M. C. (1984). Marijuana effects on the endocrine and reproductive systems. Discussion and recommendations. *NIDA Research Monograph*, *44*, 124–129.

Brundin, P., & Wyse, R. (2015). Parkinson disease: Laying the foundations for disease-modifying therapies in PD. *Nature Reviews. Neurology*, *11*(10), 553–555. doi: nrneurol.2015.150 [pii]. http://dx.doi.org/10.1038/nrneurol.2015.150.

Campolongo, P., Roozendaal, B., Trezza, V., Cuomo, V., Astarita, G., Fu, J., et al. (2009). Fat-induced satiety factor oleoylethanolamide enhances memory consolidation. *Proceedings of the National Academy of Sciences of the United States of America*, *106*(19), 8027–8031. http://dx.doi.org/10.1073/pnas.0903038106.

Capasso, R., Orlando, P., Pagano, E., Aveta, T., Buono, L., Borrelli, F., et al. (2014). Palmitoylethanolamide normalizes intestinal motility in a model of post-inflammatory accelerated transit: Involvement of CB(1) receptors and TRPV1 channels. *British Journal of Pharmacology*, *171*(17), 4026–4037. http://dx.doi.org/10.1111/bph.12759.

Carroll, C. B., Zeissler, M. L., Hanemann, C. O., & Zajicek, J. P. (2012). Delta(9)-tetrahydrocannabinol (Delta(9)-THC) exerts a direct neuroprotective effect in a human cell culture model of Parkinson's disease. *Neuropathology and Applied Neurobiology*, *38*(6), 535–547. http://dx.doi.org/10.1111/j.1365-2990.2011.01248.x.

Carta, A. R. (2013). PPAR-gamma: Therapeutic prospects in Parkinson's disease. *Current Drug Targets*, *14*(7), 743–751.

Chakravarty, I., Sheth, A. R., & Ghosh, J. J. (1975). Effect of acute delta9-tetrahydrocannabinol treatment on serum luteinizing hormone and prolactin levels in adult female rats. *Fertility and Sterility*, *26*(9), 947–948.

Chen, L., Li, L., Chen, J., Li, L., Zheng, Z., Ren, J., et al. (2015). Oleoylethanolamide, an endogenous PPAR-alpha ligand, attenuates liver fibrosis targeting hepatic stellate cells. *Oncotarget*, *6*(40), 42530–42540. http://dx.doi.org/10.18632/oncotarget.6466.

Choi, Y.-J., Roberts, B. K., Wang, X., Geaney, J. C., Naim, S., Wojnoonski, K., et al. (2012). Effects of the PPAR-δ agonist MBX-8025 on atherogenic dyslipidemia. *Atherosclerosis*, *220*(2), 470–476.

Citraro, R., Russo, E., Scicchitano, F., van Rijn, C. M., Cosco, D., Avagliano, C., et al. (2013). Antiepileptic action of *N*-palmitoylethanolamine through CB1 and PPAR-alpha receptor activation in a genetic model of absence epilepsy. *Neuropharmacology*, *69*, 115–126. http://dx.doi.org/10.1016/j.neuropharm.2012.11.017.

Cluny, N. L., Keenan, C. M., Lutz, B., Piomelli, D., & Sharkey, K. A. (2009). The identification of peroxisome proliferator-activated receptor alpha-independent effects of oleoylethanolamide on intestinal transit in mice. *Neurogastroenterology and Motility*, *21*(4), 420–429. http://dx.doi.org/10.1111/j.1365-2982.2008.01248.x.

Coleman, J. D., Prabhu, K. S., Thompson, J. T., Reddy, P. S., Peters, J. M., Peterson, B. R., et al. (2007). The oxidative stress mediator 4-hydroxynonenal is an intracellular agonist of the nuclear receptor peroxisome proliferator-activated receptor-β/δ (PPARβ/δ). *Free Radical Biology and Medicine*, *42*(8), 1155–1164.

Costa, B., Comelli, F., Bettoni, I., Colleoni, M., & Giagnoni, G. (2008). The endogenous fatty acid amide, palmitoylethanolamide, has anti-allodynic and anti-hyperalgesic effects in a murine model of neuropathic pain: Involvement of CB(1), TRPV1 and PPARgamma receptors and neurotrophic factors. *Pain*, *139*(3), 541–550. http://dx.doi.org/10.1016/j.pain.2008.06.003.

Cuzzocrea, S., Di Paola, R., Mazzon, E., Genovese, T., Muia, C., Centorrino, T., et al. (2004). Role of endogenous and exogenous ligands for the peroxisome proliferators activated receptors alpha (PPAR-[alpha]) in the development of inflammatory bowel disease in mice. *Laboratory Investigation*, *84*(12), 1643–1654.

D'Agostino, G., Russo, R., Avagliano, C., Cristiano, C., Meli, R., & Calignano, A. (2012a). Palmitoylethanolamide protects against the amyloid-beta25-35-induced learning and memory impairment in mice, an experimental model of Alzheimer disease. *Neuropsychopharmacology: Official Publication of the American College of Neuropsychopharmacology*, *37*(7), 1784–1792. http://dx.doi.org/10.1038/npp.2012.25.

Daynes, R. A., & Jones, D. C. (2002). Emerging roles of PPARs in inflammation and immunity. *Nature Reviews. Immunology*, *2*(10), 748–759. http://dx.doi.org/10.1038/nri912.

De Filippis, D., Esposito, G., Cirillo, C., Cipriano, M., De Winter, B. Y., Scuderi, C., et al. (2011). Cannabidiol reduces intestinal inflammation through the control of neuroimmune axis. *PloS One*, *6*(12), e28159. http://dx.doi.org/10.1371/journal.pone.0028159.

de Novellis, V., Luongo, L., Guida, F., Cristino, L., Palazzo, E., Russo, R., et al. (2012). Effects of intra-ventrolateral periaqueductal grey palmitoylethanolamide on thermoceptive threshold and rostral ventromedial medulla cell activity. *European Journal of Pharmacology*, *676*(1–3), 41–50. http://dx.doi.org/10.1016/j.ejphar.2011.11.034.

Desvergne, B., & Wahli, W. (1999). Peroxisome proliferator-activated receptors: Nuclear control of metabolism. *Endocrine Reviews*, *20*(5), 649–688. http://dx.doi.org/10.1210/er.20.5.649.

Di Cesare Mannelli, L., D'Agostino, G., Pacini, A., Russo, R., Zanardelli, M., Ghelardini, C., et al. (2013). Palmitoylethanolamide is a disease-modifying agent in peripheral neuropathy: Pain relief and neuroprotection share a PPAR-alpha-mediated mechanism. *Mediators of Inflammation*, *2013*, 328797. http://dx.doi.org/10.1155/2013/328797.

Di Paola, R., Cordaro, M., Crupi, R., Siracusa, R., Campolo, M., Bruschetta, G., et al. (2016). Protective effects of ultramicronized palmitoylethanolamide (PEA-um) in myocardial ischaemia and reperfusion injury in VIVO. *Shock*, *46*(2), 202–213. http://dx.doi.org/10.1097/shk.0000000000000578.

Di Paola, R., Impellizzeri, D., Mondello, P., Velardi, E., Aloisi, C., Cappellani, A., et al. (2012a). Palmitoylethanolamide reduces early renal dysfunction and injury caused by experimental ischemia and reperfusion in mice. *Shock*, *38*(4), 356–366. http://dx.doi.org/10.1097/SHK.0b013e318267bbb9.

Di Paola, R., Impellizzeri, D., Torre, A., Mazzon, E., Cappellani, A., Faggio, C., et al. (2012b). Effects of palmitoylethanolamide on intestinal injury and inflammation caused by ischemia-reperfusion in mice. *Journal of Leukocyte Biology*, *91*(6), 911–920. http://dx.doi.org/10.1189/jlb.0911485.

Dionisi, M., Alexander, S. P., & Bennett, A. J. (2012). Oleamide activates peroxisome proliferator-activated receptor gamma (PPARgamma) in vitro. *Lipids in Health and Disease*, *11*, 51. http://dx.doi.org/10.1186/1476-511x-11-51.

Downer, E. J., Clifford, E., Amu, S., Fallon, P. G., & Moynagh, P. N. (2012). The synthetic cannabinoid R(+)WIN55,212-2 augments interferon-beta expression via peroxisome proliferator-activated receptor-alpha. *The Journal of Biological Chemistry*, *287*(30), 25440–25453. http://dx.doi.org/10.1074/jbc.M112.371757.

Dreyer, C., Krey, G., Keller, H., Givel, F., Helftenbein, G., & Wahli, W. (1992). Control of the peroxisomal beta-oxidation pathway by a novel family of nuclear hormone receptors. *Cell*, *68*(5), 879–887. http://dx.doi.org/0092-8674(92)90031-7 [pii].

Du, H., Chen, X., Zhang, J., & Chen, C. (2011). Inhibition of COX-2 expression by endocannabinoid 2-arachidonoylglycerol is mediated via PPAR-gamma. *British Journal of Pharmacology*, *163*(7), 1533–1549. http://dx.doi.org/10.1111/j.1476-5381.2011.01444.x.

Eichele, K., Ramer, R., & Hinz, B. (2009). R(+)-methanandamide-induced apoptosis of human cervical carcinoma cells involves a cyclooxygenase-2-dependent pathway. *Pharmaceutical Research*, *26*(2), 346–355. http://dx.doi.org/10.1007/s11095-008-9748-3.

Eissa Ahmed, A. A., & Al-Rasheed, N. M. (2009). Antidepressant-like effects of rosiglitazone, a PPARgamma agonist, in the rat forced swim and mouse tail suspension tests. *Behavioural Pharmacology*, *20*(7), 635–642. http://dx.doi.org/10.1097/FBP.0b013e328331b9bf.

Eldridge, J. C., & Landfield, P. W. (1990). Cannabinoid interactions with glucocorticoid receptors in rat hippocampus. *Brain Research*, *534*(1–2), 135–141.

Eldridge, J. C., Murphy, L. L., & Landfield, P. W. (1991). Cannabinoids and the hippocampal glucocorticoid receptor: Recent findings and possible significance. *Steroids*, *56*(5), 226–231.

Elmes, M. W., Kaczocha, M., Berger, W. T., Leung, K., Ralph, B. P., Wang, L., et al. (2015). Fatty acid-binding proteins (FABPs) are intracellular carriers for Delta9-tetrahydrocannabinol (THC) and cannabidiol (CBD). *The Journal of Biological Chemistry*, *290*(14), 8711–8721. http://dx.doi.org/10.1074/jbc.M114.618447.

Escriva, H., Bertrand, S., & Laudet, V. (2004). The evolution of the nuclear receptor superfamily. *Essays in Biochemistry*, *40*, 11–26.

Escriva, H., Delaunay, F., & Laudet, V. (2000). Ligand binding and nuclear receptor evolution. *BioEssays*, *22*(8), 717–727. http://dx.doi.org/10.1002/1521-1878(200008)22:8<717::AID-BIES5>3.0.CO;2-I.

Esposito, G., Capoccia, E., Turco, F., Palumbo, I., Lu, J., Steardo, A., et al. (2014). Palmitoylethanolamide improves colon inflammation through an enteric glia/toll like receptor 4-dependent PPAR-alpha activation. *Gut*, *63*(8), 1300–1312. http://dx.doi.org/10.1136/gutjnl-2013-305005.

Esposito, E., Impellizzeri, D., Mazzon, E., Paterniti, I., & Cuzzocrea, S. (2012). Neuroprotective activities of palmitoylethanolamide in an animal model of Parkinson's disease. *PloS One*, 7(8), e41880. http://dx.doi.org/10.1371/journal.pone.0041880.

Esposito, G., Scuderi, C., Valenza, M., Togna, G. I., Latina, V., De Filippis, D., et al. (2011). Cannabidiol reduces Abeta-induced neuroinflammation and promotes hippocampal neurogenesis through PPARgamma involvement. *PloS One*, *6*(12), e28668. http://dx.doi.org/10.1371/journal.pone.0028668.

Fajas, L., Auboeuf, D., Raspe, E., Schoonjans, K., Lefebvre, A. M., Saladin, R., et al. (1997). The organization, promoter analysis, and expression of the human PPARgamma gene. *Journal of Biological Chemistry*, *272*(30), 18779–18789.

Fakhfouri, G., Ahmadiani, A., Rahimian, R., Grolla, A. A., Moradi, F., & Haeri, A. (2012). WIN55212-2 attenuates amyloid-beta-induced neuroinflammation in rats through activation of cannabinoid receptors and PPAR-gamma pathway. *Neuropharmacology*, *63*(4), 653–666. http://dx.doi.org/10.1016/j.neuropharm.2012.05.013.

Ferre, P. (2004). The biology of peroxisome proliferator-activated receptors: Relationship with lipid metabolism and insulin sensitivity. *Diabetes*, *53*(Suppl. 1), S43–S50.

Fidaleo, M., Fanelli, F., Ceru, M. P., & Moreno, S. (2014). Neuroprotective properties of peroxisome proliferator-activated receptor alpha (PPARalpha) and its lipid ligands. *Current Medicinal Chemistry*, *21*(24), 2803–2821.

Fishbein-Kaminietsky, M., Gafni, M., & Sarne, Y. (2014). Ultralow doses of cannabinoid drugs protect the mouse brain from inflammation-induced cognitive damage. *Journal of Neuroscience Research*, *92*(12), 1669–1677. http://dx.doi.org/10.1002/jnr.23452.

Forget, B., Guranda, M., Gamaleddin, I., Goldberg, S. R., & Le Foll, B. (2016). Attenuation of cue-induced reinstatement of nicotine seeking by URB597 through cannabinoid CB1 receptor in rats. *Psychopharmacology*, *233*(10), 1823–1828. http://dx.doi.org/10.1007/s00213-016-4232-y.

Friedland, S. N., Leong, A., Filion, K. B., Genest, J., Lega, I. C., Mottillo, S., et al. (2012). The cardiovascular effects of peroxisome proliferator-activated receptor agonists. *The American Journal of Medicine*, *125*(2), 126–133. http://dx.doi.org/10.1016/j.amjmed.2011.08.025.

Fu, J., Gaetani, S., Oveisi, F., Lo Verme, J., Serrano, A., Rodriguez De Fonseca, F., et al. (2003). Oleylethanolamide regulates feeding and body weight through activation of the nuclear receptor PPAR-alpha. *Nature*, *425*(6953), 90–93. http://dx.doi.org/10.1038/nature01921.

Gaetani, S., Fu, J., Cassano, T., Dipasquale, P., Romano, A., Righetti, L., et al. (2010). The fat-induced satiety factor oleoylethanolamide suppresses feeding through central release of oxytocin. *The Journal of Neuroscience*, *30*(24), 8096–8101. http://dx.doi.org/10.1523/jneurosci.0036-10.2010.

Galan-Rodriguez, B., Suarez, J., Gonzalez-Aparicio, R., Bermudez-Silva, F. J., Maldonado, R., Robledo, P., et al. (2009). Oleoylethanolamide exerts partial and dose-dependent neuroprotection of substantia nigra dopamine neurons. *Neuropharmacology*, *56*(3), 653–664.

Girroir, E. E., Hollingshead, H. E., He, P., Zhu, B., Perdew, G. H., & Peters, J. M. (2008). Quantitative expression patterns of peroxisome proliferator-activated receptor-beta/delta (PPARbeta/delta) protein in mice. *Biochemical and Biophysical Research Communications*, *371*(3), 456–461. http://dx.doi.org/10.1016/j.bbrc.2008.04.086.

Giuliano, M., Pellerito, O., Portanova, P., Calvaruso, G., Santulli, A., De Blasio, A., et al. (2009). Apoptosis induced in HepG2 cells by the synthetic cannabinoid WIN: Involvement of the transcription factor PPARgamma. *Biochimie*, *91*(4), 457–465. http://dx.doi.org/10.1016/j.biochi.2008.11.003.

Gonzalez, E. G., Selvi, E., Balistreri, E., Akhmetshina, A., Palumbo, K., Lorenzini, S., et al. (2012). Synthetic cannabinoid ajulemic acid exerts potent antifibrotic effects in experimental models of systemic sclerosis. *Annals of the Rheumatic Diseases*, *71*(9), 1545–1551. http://dx.doi.org/10.1136/annrheumdis-2011-200314.

Gonzalez-Aparicio, R., & Moratalla, R. (2014). Oleoylethanolamide reduces L-DOPA-induced dyskinesia via TRPV1 receptor in a mouse model of Parkinson s disease. *Neurobiology of Disease*, *62*, 416–425. http://dx.doi.org/10.1016/j.nbd.2013.10.008.

Granja, A. G., Carrillo-Salinas, F., Pagani, A., Gomez-Canas, M., Negri, R., Navarrete, C., et al. (2012). A cannabigerol quinone alleviates neuroinflammation in a chronic model of multiple sclerosis. *Journal of Neuroimmune Pharmacology*, 7(4), 1002–1016. http://dx.doi.org/10.1007/s11481-012-9399-3.

Guzman, M., Lo Verme, J., Fu, J., Oveisi, F., Blazquez, C., & Piomelli, D. (2004). Oleoylethanolamide stimulates lipolysis by activating the nuclear receptor peroxisome proliferator-activated receptor alpha (PPAR-alpha). *The Journal of Biological Chemistry*, *279*(27), 27849–27854. http://dx.doi.org/10.1074/jbc.M404087200.

Harclerode, J. (1984). Endocrine effects of marijuana in the male: Preclinical studies. *NIDA Research Monograph*, *44*, 46–64.

Hashimoto, T., Cook, W. S., Qi, C., Yeldandi, A. V., Reddy, J. K., & Rao, M. S. (2000). Defect in peroxisome proliferator-activated receptor alpha-inducible fatty acid oxidation determines the severity of hepatic steatosis in response to fasting. *Journal of Biological Chemistry*, *275*(37), 28918–28928. http://dx.doi.org/10.1074/jbc.M910350199.

Hegde, V. L., Singh, U. P., Nagarkatti, P. S., & Nagarkatti, M. (2015). Critical role of mast cells and peroxisome proliferator-activated receptor gamma in the induction of myeloid-derived suppressor cells by marijuana cannabidiol in vivo. *Journal of Immunology*, *194*(11), 5211–5222. http://dx.doi.org/10.4049/jimmunol.1401844.

Hess, R., Staubli, W., & Riess, W. (1965). Nature of the hepatomegalic effect produced by ethyl-chlorophenoxy-isobutyrate in the rat. *Nature*, *208*(5013), 856–858.

Hillard, C. J. (2015). Endocannabinoids and the endocrine system in health and disease. *Handbook of Experimental Pharmacology*, *231*, 317–339. http://dx.doi.org/10.1007/978-3-319-20825-1_11.

Hind, W. H., England, T. J., & O'Sullivan, S. E. (2016). Cannabidiol protects an in vitro model of the blood-brain barrier from oxygen-glucose deprivation via PPARγ and 5-HT1A receptors. *British Journal of Pharmacology*, *173*(5), 815–825. Epub 2016 Feb 3. http://dx.doi.org/10.1111/bph.13368.

Hind, W. H., Tufarelli, C., Neophytou, M., Anderson, S. I., England, T. J., & O'Sullivan, S. E. (2015). Endocannabinoids modulate human blood-brain barrier permeability in vitro. *British Journal of Pharmacology*, *172*, 3015–3027. http://dx.doi.org/10.1111/bph.13106.

Hong, Y., Zhou, Y., Wang, Y., Xiao, S., Liao, D. J., & Zhao, Q. (2013). PPARgamma mediates the effects of WIN55,212-2, an synthetic cannabinoid, on the proliferation and apoptosis of the BEL-7402 hepatocarcinoma cells. *Molecular Biology Reports*, *40*(11), 6287–6293. http://dx.doi.org/10.1007/s11033-013-2741-x.

Issemann, I., & Green, S. (1990). Activation of a member of the steroid hormone receptor superfamily by peroxisome proliferators. *Nature*, *347*(6294), 645–650. http://dx.doi.org/10.1038/347645a0.

Jhaveri, M. D., Richardson, D., Robinson, I., Garle, M. J., Patel, A., Sun, Y., et al. (2008). Inhibition of fatty acid amide hydrolase and cyclooxygenase-2 increases levels of endocannabinoid related molecules and produces analgesia via peroxisome proliferator-activated receptor-alpha in a model of inflammatory pain. *Neuropharmacology*, *55*(1), 85–93. http://dx.doi.org/10.1016/j.neuropharm.2008.04.018.

Jiang, C., Ting, A. T., & Seed, B. (1998). PPAR-gamma agonists inhibit production of monocyte inflammatory cytokines. *Nature*, *391*(6662), 82–86. http://dx.doi.org/10.1038/34184.

Johnson, D. R., Stebulis, J. A., Rossetti, R. G., Burstein, S. H., & Zurier, R. B. (2007). Suppression of fibroblast metalloproteinases by ajulemic acid, a nonpsychoactive cannabinoid acid. *Journal of Cellular Biochemistry*, *100*(1), 184–190. http://dx.doi.org/10.1002/jcb.21046.

Justinova, Z., Panlilio, L. V., Moreno-Sanz, G., Redhi, G. H., Auber, A., Secci, M. E., et al. (2015). Effects of fatty acid amide hydrolase (FAAH) inhibitors in non-human primate models of nicotine reward and relapse. *Neuropsychopharmacology*, *40*(9), 2185–2197. http://dx.doi.org/10.1038/npp.2015.62.

Kaczocha, M., Glaser, S. T., & Deutsch, D. G. (2009). Identification of intracellular carriers for the endocannabinoid anandamide. *Proceedings of the National Academy of Sciences of the United States of America*, *106*(15), 6375–6380. http://dx.doi.org/10.1073/pnas.0901515106.

Kaczocha, M., Rebecchi, M. J., Ralph, B. P., Teng, Y. H., Berger, W. T., Galbavy, W., et al. (2014). Inhibition of fatty acid binding proteins elevates brain anandamide levels and produces analgesia. *PloS One*, *9*(4), e94200. http://dx.doi.org/10.1371/journal.pone.0094200.

Kaczocha, M., Vivieca, S., Sun, J., Glaser, S. T., & Deutsch, D. G. (2012). Fatty acid-binding proteins transport N-acylethanolamines to nuclear receptors and are targets of endocannabinoid transport inhibitors. *The Journal of Biological Chemistry*, *287*(5), 3415–3424. Epub 2011 Dec 14. http://dx.doi.org/10.1074/jbc.M111.304907.

Kanakasabai, S., Chearwae, W., Walline, C. C., Iams, W., Adams, S. M., & Bright, J. J. (2010). Peroxisome proliferator-activated receptor δ agonists inhibit T helper type 1 (Th1) and Th17 responses in experimental allergic encephalomyelitis. *Immunology*, *130*(4), 572–588.

Kapadia, R., Yi, J. H., & Vemuganti, R. (2008). Mechanisms of anti-inflammatory and neuroprotective actions of PPAR-gamma agonists. *Frontiers in Bioscience*, *13*, 1813–1826.

Karwad, M. A., Macpherson, T., Wang, B., Theophilidou, E., Sarmad, S., Barrett, D. A., et al. (2017). Oleoylethanolamine and palmitoylethanolamine modulate intestinal permeability in vitro via TRPV1 and PPARalpha. *The FASEB Journal*, *31*(2), 469–481. Epub 2016 Sep 13. http://dx.doi.org/10.1096/fj.201500132.

Kemp, D. E., Schinagle, M., Gao, K., Conroy, C., Ganocy, S. J., Ismail-Beigi, F., et al. (2014). PPAR-gamma agonism as a modulator of mood: Proof-of-concept for pioglitazone in bipolar depression. *CNS Drugs*, *28*(6), 571–581. http://dx.doi.org/10.1007/s40263-014-0158-2.

Khasabova, I. A., Xiong, Y., Coicou, L. G., Piomelli, D., & Seybold, V. (2012). Peroxisome proliferator-activated receptor alpha mediates acute effects of palmitoylethanolamide on sensory neurons. *The Journal of Neuroscience*, *32*(37), 12735–12743. http://dx.doi.org/10.1523/jneurosci.0130-12.2012.

Kliewer, S. A., Forman, B. M., Blumberg, B., Ong, E. S., Borgmeyer, U., Mangelsdorf, D. J., et al. (1994). Differential expression and activation of a family of murine peroxisome proliferator-activated receptors. *Proceedings of the National Academy of Sciences of the United States of America*, *91*(15), 7355–7359.

Koch, M., Kreutz, S., Bottger, C., Benz, A., Maronde, E., Ghadban, C., et al. (2011). Palmitoylethanolamide protects dentate gyrus granule cells via peroxisome proliferator-activated receptor-alpha. *Neurotoxicity Research*, *19*(2), 330–340. http://dx.doi.org/10.1007/s12640-010-9166-2.

Koller, V. J., Zlabinger, G. J., Auwarter, V., Fuchs, S., & Knasmueller, S. (2013). Toxicological profiles of selected synthetic cannabinoids showing high binding affinities to the cannabinoid receptor subtype CB(1). *Archives of Toxicology*, *87*(7), 1287–1297. http://dx.doi.org/10.1007/s00204-013-1029-1.

Kozak, K. R., Gupta, R. A., Moody, J. S., Ji, C., Boeglin, W. E., DuBois, R. N., et al. (2002). 15-Lipoxygenase metabolism of 2-arachidonylglycerol. Generation of a peroxisome proliferator-activated receptor alpha agonist. *The Journal of Biological Chemistry*, *277*(26), 23278–23286. http://dx.doi.org/10.1074/jbc.M201084200.

Kumar, A., Qiao, Z., Kumar, P., & Song, Z. H. (2012). Effects of palmitoylethanolamide on aqueous humor outflow. *Investigative Ophthalmology & Visual Science*, *53*(8), 4416–4425. http://dx.doi.org/10.1167/iovs.11-9294.

Lambert, D. M., Vandevoorde, S., Diependaele, G., Govaerts, S. J., & Robert, A. R. (2001). Anticonvulsant activity of *N*-palmitoylethanolamide, a putative endocannabinoid, in mice. *Epilepsia*, *42*(3), 321–327.

Landfield, P. W., & Eldridge, J. C. (1993). Neurotoxicity and drugs of abuse: Cannabinoid interaction with brain glucocorticoid receptors. *NIDA Research Monograph*, *136*, 242–256. discussion 256-247.

Linton, M. F., & Fazio, S. (2000). Re-emergence of fibrates in the management of dyslipidemia and cardiovascular risk. *Current Atherosclerosis Reports*, *2*(1), 29–35.

Liu, J., Li, H., Burstein, S. H., Zurier, R. B., & Chen, J. D. (2003). Activation and binding of peroxisome proliferator-activated receptor gamma by synthetic cannabinoid ajulemic acid. *Molecular Pharmacology*, *63*(5), 983–992.

Lo Verme, J., Fu, J., Astarita, G., La Rana, G., Russo, R., Calignano, A., et al. (2005a). The nuclear receptor peroxisome proliferator-activated receptor-alpha mediates the anti-inflammatory actions of palmitoylethanolamide. *Molecular Pharmacology*, *67*(1), 15–19. http://dx.doi.org/10.1124/mol.104.006353.

Lo Verme, J., Gaetani, S., Fu, J., Oveisi, F., Burton, K., & Piomelli, D. (2005b). Regulation of food intake by oleoylethanolamide. *Cellular and Molecular Life Sciences*, *62*(6), 708–716. http://dx.doi.org/10.1007/s00018-004-4494-0.

Loria, F., Petrosino, S., Hernangomez, M., Mestre, L., Spagnolo, A., Correa, F., et al. (2010). An endocannabinoid tone limits excitotoxicity in vitro and in a model of multiple sclerosis. *Neurobiology of Disease*, *37*(1), 166–176. http://dx.doi.org/10.1016/j.nbd.2009.09.020.

Loria, F., Petrosino, S., Mestre, L., Spagnolo, A., Correa, F., Hernangomez, M., et al. (2008). Study of the regulation of the endocannabinoid system in a virus model of multiple sclerosis reveals a therapeutic effect of palmitoylethanolamide. *The European Journal of Neuroscience*, *28*(4), 633–641. doi:EJN6377 [pii]. http://dx.doi.org/10.1111/j.1460-9568.2008.06377.x.

Luchicchi, A., Lecca, S., Carta, S., Pillolla, G., Muntoni, A. L., Yasar, S., et al. (2010). Effects of fatty acid amide hydrolase inhibition on neuronal responses to nicotine, cocaine and morphine in the nucleus accumbens shell and ventral tegmental area: Involvement of PPAR-alpha nuclear receptors. *Addiction Biology*, *15*(3), 277–288. http://dx.doi.org/10.1111/j.1369-1600.2010.00222.x.

Mandard, S., Muller, M., & Kersten, S. (2004). Peroxisome proliferator-activated receptor alpha target genes. *Cellular and Molecular Life Sciences*, *61*(4), 393–416. http://dx.doi.org/10.1007/s00018-003-3216-3.

Marx, N., Duez, H., Fruchart, J.-C., & Staels, B. (2004). Peroxisome proliferator-activated receptors and atherogenesis. Regulators of gene expression in vascular cells. *Circulation Research*, *94*(9), 1168–1178. http://dx.doi.org/10.1161/01.res.0000127122.22685.0a.

Mazzola, C., Medalie, J., Scherma, M., Panlilio, L. V., Solinas, M., Tanda, G., et al. (2009). Fatty acid amide hydrolase (FAAH) inhibition enhances memory acquisition through activation of PPAR-alpha nuclear receptors. *Learning & Memory*, *16*(5), 332–337. http://dx.doi.org/10.1101/lm.1145209.

Melis, M., Carta, S., Fattore, L., Tolu, S., Yasar, S., Goldberg, S. R., et al. (2010). Peroxisome proliferator-activated receptors-alpha modulate dopamine cell activity through nicotinic receptors. *Biological Psychiatry*, *68*(3), 256–264. http://dx.doi.org/10.1016/j.biopsych.2010.04.016.

Melis, M., Pillolla, G., Luchicchi, A., Muntoni, A. L., Yasar, S., Goldberg, S. R., et al. (2008). Endogenous fatty acid ethanolamides suppress nicotine-induced activation of mesolimbic dopamine neurons through nuclear receptors. *The Journal of Neuroscience*, *28*(51), 13985–13994. http://dx.doi.org/10.1523/jneurosci.3221-08.2008.

Melis, M., Scheggi, S., Carta, G., Madeddu, C., Lecca, S., Luchicchi, A., et al. (2013). PPARalpha regulates cholinergic-driven activity of midbrain dopamine neurons via a novel mechanism involving alpha7 nicotinic acetylcholine receptors. *Journal of Neuroscience*, *33*(14), 6203–6211. http://dx.doi.org/10.1523/JNEUROSCI.4647-12.2013.

Menendez-Gutierrez, M. P., Roszer, T., & Ricote, M. (2012). Biology and therapeutic applications of peroxisome proliferator- activated receptors. *Current Topics in Medicinal Chemistry*, *12*(6), 548–584.

Mestre, L., Docagne, F., Correa, F., Loria, F., Hernangomez, M., Borrell, J., et al. (2009). A cannabinoid agonist interferes with the progression of a chronic model of multiple sclerosis by downregulating adhesion molecules. *Molecular and Cellular Neurosciences*, *40*(2), 258–266. http://dx.doi.org/10.1016/j.mcn.2008.10.015.

Michalik, L., Auwerx, J., Berger, J. P., Chatterjee, V. K., Glass, C. K., Gonzalez, F. J., et al. (2006). International union of pharmacology. LXI. Peroxisome proliferator-activated receptors. *Pharmacological Reviews*, *58*(4), 726–741. http://dx.doi.org/10.1124/pr.58.4.5.

Michalik, L., Desvergne, B., Dreyer, C., Gavillet, M., Laurini, R. N., & Wahli, W. (2002). PPAR expression and function during vertebrate development. *International Journal of Developmental Biology*, *46*(1), 105–114.

Moreno, S., Farioli-Vecchioli, S., & Cerù, M. P. (2004). Immunolocalization of peroxisome proliferator-activated receptors and retinoid X receptors in the adult rat CNS. *Neuroscience*, *123*(1), 131–145.

Moreno-Santos, I., Pavon, F. J., Romero-Cuevas, M., Serrano, A., Cano, C., Suardiaz, M., et al. (2014). Computational and biological evaluation of *N*-octadecyl-*N'*-propylsulfamide, a selective PPARalpha agonist structurally related to *N*-acylethanolamines. *PloS One*, *9*(3), e92195. http://dx.doi.org/10.1371/journal.pone.0092195.

Naruhn, S., Meissner, W., Adhikary, T., Kaddatz, K., Klein, T., Watzer, B., et al. (2010). 15-Hydroxyeicosatetraenoic acid is a preferential peroxisome proliferator-activated receptor β/δ agonist. *Molecular Pharmacology*, 77(2), 171–184.

Neels, J. G., & Grimaldi, P. A. (2014). Physiological functions of peroxisome proliferator-activated receptor beta. *Physiological Reviews*, *94*(3), 795–858. http://dx.doi.org/10.1152/physrev.00027.2013.

Neher, M. D., Weckbach, S., Huber-Lang, M. S., & Stahel, P. F. (2012). New insights into the role of peroxisome proliferator-activated receptors in regulating the inflammatory response after tissue injury. *PPAR Research*, *2012*, 728461. http://dx.doi.org/10.1155/2012/728461.

NINDS Exploratory Trials in Parkinson Disease (NET-PD) FS-ZONE Investigators. (2015). Pioglitazone in early Parkinson's disease: A phase 2, multicentre, double-blind, randomised trial. *The Lancet Neurology*, *14*(8), 795–803. Epub 2015 Jun 23. http://dx.doi.org/10.1016/S1474-4422(15)00144-1.

Nithipatikom, K., Isbell, M. A., Endsley, M. P., Woodliff, J. E., & Campbell, W. B. (2011). Anti-proliferative effect of a putative endocannabinoid, 2-arachidonylglyceryl ether in prostate carcinoma cells. *Prostaglandins & Other Lipid Mediators, 94*(1–2), 34–43. http://dx.doi.org/10.1016/j.prostaglandins.2010.12.002.

Okey, A. B., & Truant, G. S. (1975). Cannabis demasculinizes rats but is not estrogenic. *Life Sciences, 17*(7), 1113–1117.

Okine, B. N., Madasu, M. K., McGowan, F., Prendergast, C., Gaspar, J. C., Harhen, B., et al. (2016). *N*-Palmitoylethanolamide in the anterior cingulate cortex attenuates inflammatory pain behaviour indirectly via a CB1 receptor-mediated mechanism. *Pain, 157*(12), 2687–2696. http://dx.doi.org/10.1097/j.pain.0000000000000687.

Ooi, E. M., Watts, G. F., Sprecher, D. L., Chan, D. C., & Barrett, P. H. R. (2011). Mechanism of action of a peroxisome proliferator-activated receptor (PPAR)-δ agonist on lipoprotein metabolism in dyslipidemic subjects with central obesity. *The Journal of Clinical Endocrinology & Metabolism, 96*(10), E1568–E1576.

O'Sullivan, S. E. (2007). Cannabinoids go nuclear: Evidence for activation of peroxisome proliferator-activated receptors. *British Journal of Pharmacology, 152*(5), 576–582. http://dx.doi.org/10.1038/sj.bjp.0707423.

O'Sullivan, S. E. (2016). An update on PPAR activation by cannabinoids. *British Journal of Pharmacology, 173*(12), 1899–1910. http://dx.doi.org/10.1111/bph.13497.

O'Sullivan, S. E., Bennett, A. J., Kendall, D. A., & Randall, M. D. (2006). Cannabinoids and peroxisome proliferator-activated receptor gamma (PPARg). *Proceedings of the International Cannabinoid Research Society*.

O'Sullivan, S. E., Kendall, D. A., & Randall, M. D. (2006). Further characterization of the time-dependent vascular effects of Δ^{-9}Tetrahydrocannabinol. *Journal of Pharmacology and Experimental Therapeutics, 317*(1), 428–438. http://dx.doi.org/10.1124/jpet.105.095828.

O'Sullivan, S. E., Kendall, D. A., & Randall, M. D. (2009a). Time-dependent vascular effects of endocannabinoids mediated by peroxisome proliferator-activated receptor gamma (PPARgamma). *PPAR Research, 2009*, 425289. http://dx.doi.org/10.1155/2009/425289.

O'Sullivan, S. E., Sun, Y., Bennett, A. J., Randall, M. D., & Kendall, D. A. (2009b). Time-dependent vascular actions of cannabidiol in the rat aorta. *European Journal of Pharmacology, 612*(1–3), 61–68. http://dx.doi.org/10.1016/j.ejphar.2009.03.010.

O'Sullivan, S. E., Tarling, E. J., Bennett, A. J., Kendall, D. A., & Randall, M. D. (2005). Novel time-dependent vascular actions of Delta9-tetrahydrocannabinol mediated by peroxisome proliferator-activated receptor gamma. *Biochemical and Biophysical Research Communications, 337*(3), 824–831. http://dx.doi.org/10.1016/j.bbrc.2005.09.121.

Palomba, L., Silvestri, C., Imperatore, R., Morello, G., Piscitelli, F., Martella, A., et al. (2015). Negative regulation of leptin-induced reactive oxygen species (ROS) formation by cannabinoid CB1 receptor activation in hypothalamic neurons. *The Journal of Biological Chemistry, 290*(22), 13669–13677. http://dx.doi.org/10.1074/jbc.M115.646885.

Panlilio, L. V., Mazzola, C., Medalie, J., Hahn, B., Justinova, Z., Drago, F., et al. (2009). Anandamide-induced behavioral disruption through a vanilloid-dependent mechanism in rats. *Psychopharmacology, 203*(3), 529–538. http://dx.doi.org/10.1007/s00213-008-1399-x.

Parker, J., Atez, F., Rossetti, R. G., Skulas, A., Patel, R., & Zurier, R. B. (2008). Suppression of human macrophage interleukin-6 by a nonpsychoactive cannabinoid acid. *Rheumatology International, 28*(7), 631–635. http://dx.doi.org/10.1007/s00296-007-0489-0.

Paterniti, I., Impellizzeri, D., Crupi, R., Morabito, R., Campolo, M., Esposito, E., et al. (2013). Molecular evidence for the involvement of PPAR-delta and PPAR-gamma in anti-inflammatory and neuroprotective activities of palmitoylethanolamide after spinal cord trauma. *Journal of Neuroinflammation, 10*, 20. http://dx.doi.org/10.1186/1742-2094-10-20.

Payandemehr, B., Ebrahimi, A., Gholizadeh, R., Rahimian, R., Varastehmoradi, B., Gooshe, M., et al. (2015). Involvement of PPAR receptors in the anticonvulsant effects of a cannabinoid agonist, WIN 55,212-2. *Progress in Neuro-Psychopharmacology & Biological Psychiatry*, *57*, 140–145. http://dx.doi.org/10.1016/j.pnpbp.2014.11.005.

Petrosino, S., Cristino, L., Karsak, M., Gaffal, E., Ueda, N., Tuting, T., et al. (2010). Protective role of palmitoylethanolamide in contact allergic dermatitis. *Allergy*, *65*(6), 698–711. http://dx.doi.org/10.1111/j.1398-9995.2009.02254.x.

Pistis, M., & Melis, M. (2010). From surface to nuclear receptors: The endocannabinoid family extends its assets. *Current Medicinal Chemistry*, *17*(14), 1450–1467.

Polak, P. E., Kalinin, S., Russo, C. D., Gavrilyuk, V., Sharp, A., Peters, J. M., et al. (2005). Protective effects of a peroxisome proliferator-activated receptor-β/δ agonist in experimental autoimmune encephalomyelitis. *Journal of Neuroimmunology*, *168*(1), 65–75.

Porta, N., Vallee, L., Lecointe, C., Bouchaert, E., Staels, B., Bordet, R., et al. (2009). Fenofibrate, a peroxisome proliferator-activated receptor-alpha agonist, exerts anticonvulsive properties. *Epilepsia*, *50*(4), 943–948. doi:EPI1901 [pii]. http://dx.doi.org/10.1111/j.1528-1167.2008.01901.x.

Poulsen, L., Siersbaek, M., & Mandrup, S. (2012). PPARs: Fatty acid sensors controlling metabolism. *Seminars in Cell & Developmental Biology*, *23*(6), 631–639. http://dx.doi.org/10.1016/j.semcdb.2012.01.003.

Puligheddu, M., Pillolla, G., Melis, M., Lecca, S., Marrosu, F., De Montis, M. G., et al. (2013). PPAR-alpha agonists as novel antiepileptic drugs: Preclinical findings. *PloS One*, *8*(5), e64541. http://dx.doi.org/10.1371/journal.pone.0064541.

Raman, P., Kaplan, B. L., Thompson, J. T., Vanden Heuvel, J. P., & Kaminski, N. E. (2011). 15-Deoxy-delta12,14-prostaglandin J2-glycerol ester, a putative metabolite of 2-arachidonyl glycerol, activates peroxisome proliferator activated receptor gamma. *Molecular Pharmacology*, *80*(1), 201–209. http://dx.doi.org/10.1124/mol.110.070441.

Ramer, R., Heinemann, K., Merkord, J., Rohde, H., Salamon, A., Linnebacher, M., et al. (2013). COX-2 and PPAR-gamma confer cannabidiol-induced apoptosis of human lung cancer cells. *Molecular Cancer Therapeutics*, *12*(1), 69–82. http://dx.doi.org/10.1158/1535-7163.mct-12-0335.

Randy, L. H., & Guoying, B. (2007). Agonism of peroxisome proliferator receptor-gamma may have therapeutic potential for neuroinflammation and Parkinson's disease. *Current Neuropharmacology*, *5*(1), 35–46.

Rasgon, N. L., Kenna, H. A., Williams, K. E., Powers, B., Wroolie, T., & Schatzberg, A. F. (2010). Rosiglitazone add-on in treatment of depressed patients with insulin resistance: A pilot study. *TheScientificWorldJOURNAL*, *10*, 321–328. http://dx.doi.org/10.1100/tsw.2010.32.

Rawitch, A. B., Schultz, G. S., Ebner, K. E., & Vardaris, R. M. (1977). Competition of delta 9-tetrahydrocannabinol with estrogen in rat uterine estrogen receptor binding. *Science*, *197*(4309), 1189–1191.

Reyes-Cabello, C., Alen, F., Gomez, R., Serrano, A., Rivera, P., Orio, L., et al. (2012). Effects of the anandamide uptake blocker AM404 on food intake depend on feeding status and route of administration. *Pharmacology, Biochemistry, and Behavior*, *101*(1), 1–7. http://dx.doi.org/10.1016/j.pbb.2011.11.011.

Riahi, Y., Sin-Malia, Y., Cohen, G., Alpert, E., Gruzman, A., Eckel, J., et al. (2010). The natural protective mechanism against hyperglycemia in vascular endothelial cells roles of the lipid peroxidation product 4-Hydroxydodecadienal and peroxisome proliferator–activated receptor δ. *Diabetes*, *59*(4), 808–818.

Ricote, M., & Glass, C. K. (2007). PPARs and molecular mechanisms of transrepression. *Biochimica et Biophysica Acta (BBA): Molecular and Cell Biology of Lipids*, *1771*(8), 926–935. http://dx.doi.org/10.1016/j.bbalip.2007.02.013.

Rieck, M., Meissner, W., Ries, S., Müller-Brüsselbach, S., & Müller, R. (2008). Ligand-mediated regulation of peroxisome proliferator-activated receptor (PPAR) β/δ: A comparative analysis of PPAR-selective agonists and all-trans retinoic acid. *Molecular Pharmacology, 74*(5), 1269–1277.

Risérus, U., Sprecher, D., Johnson, T., Olson, E., Hirschberg, S., Liu, A., et al. (2008). Activation of peroxisome proliferator–activated receptor (PPAR) δ promotes reversal of multiple metabolic abnormalities, reduces oxidative stress, and increases fatty acid oxidation in moderately obese men. *Diabetes, 57*(2), 332–339.

Roche, M., Kelly, J. P., O'Driscoll, M., & Finn, D. P. (2008). Augmentation of endogenous cannabinoid tone modulates lipopolysaccharide-induced alterations in circulating cytokine levels in rats. *Immunology, 125*(2), 263–271. http://dx.doi.org/10.1111/j.1365-2567.2008.02838.x.

Rock, E. M., Limebeer, C. L., Ward, J. M., Cohen, A., Grove, K., Niphakis, M. J., et al. (2015). Interference with acute nausea and anticipatory nausea in rats by fatty acid amide hydrolase (FAAH) inhibition through a PPARalpha and CB1 receptor mechanism, respectively: A double dissociation. *Psychopharmacology, 232*(20), 3841–3848. http://dx.doi.org/10.1007/s00213-015-4050-7.

Rockwell, C. E., & Kaminski, N. E. (2004). A cyclooxygenase metabolite of anandamide causes inhibition of interleukin-2 secretion in murine splenocytes. *The Journal of Pharmacology and Experimental Therapeutics, 311*(2), 683–690. http://dx.doi.org/10.1124/jpet.104.065524.

Rockwell, C. E., Snider, N. T., Thompson, J. T., Vanden Heuvel, J. P., & Kaminski, N. E. (2006). Interleukin-2 suppression by 2-arachidonyl glycerol is mediated through peroxisome proliferator-activated receptor gamma independently of cannabinoid receptors 1 and 2. *Molecular Pharmacology, 70*(1), 101–111. http://dx.doi.org/10.1124/mol.105.019117.

Romano, M. R., & Lograno, M. D. (2012). Involvement of the peroxisome proliferator-activated receptor (PPAR) alpha in vascular response of endocannabinoids in the bovine ophthalmic artery. *European Journal of Pharmacology, 683*(1–3), 197–203. http://dx.doi.org/10.1016/j.ejphar.2012.02.049.

Roy, A., Kundu, M., Jana, M., Mishra, R. K., Yung, Y., Luan, C. H., et al. (2016). Identification and characterization of PPARalpha ligands in the hippocampus. *Nature Chemical Biology, 12*(12), 1075–1083. http://dx.doi.org/10.1038/nchembio.2204.

Ruh, M. F., Taylor, J. A., Howlett, A. C., & Welshons, W. V. (1997). Failure of cannabinoid compounds to stimulate estrogen receptors. *Biochemical Pharmacology, 53*(1), 35–41.

Sadaghiani, M. S., Javadi-Paydar, M., Gharedaghi, M. H., Fard, Y. Y., & Dehpour, A. R. (2011). Antidepressant-like effect of pioglitazone in the forced swimming test in mice: The role of PPAR-gamma receptor and nitric oxide pathway. *Behavioural Brain Research, 224*(2), 336–343. http://dx.doi.org/10.1016/j.bbr.2011.06.011.

Sagar, D. R., Kendall, D. A., & Chapman, V. (2008). Inhibition of fatty acid amide hydrolase produces PPAR-alpha-mediated analgesia in a rat model of inflammatory pain. *British Journal of Pharmacology, 155*(8), 1297–1306. http://dx.doi.org/10.1038/bjp.2008.335.

Sarnelli, G., Gigli, S., Capoccia, E., Iuvone, T., Cirillo, C., Seguella, L., et al. (2016). Palmitoylethanolamide exerts antiproliferative effect and downregulates VEGF signaling in Caco-2 human colon carcinoma cell line through a selective PPAR-alpha-dependent inhibition of Akt/mTOR pathway. *Phytotherapy Research, 30*(6), 963–970. http://dx.doi.org/10.1002/ptr.5601.

Sasso, O., Moreno-Sanz, G., Martucci, C., Realini, N., Dionisi, M., Mengatto, L., et al. (2013). Antinociceptive effects of the *N*-acylethanolamine acid amidase inhibitor ARN077 in rodent pain models. *Pain, 154*(3), 350–360. http://dx.doi.org/10.1016/j.pain.2012.10.018.

Sasso, O., Russo, R., Vitiello, S., Raso, G. M., D'Agostino, G., Iacono, A., et al. (2012). Implication of allopregnanolone in the antinociceptive effect of *N*-palmitoylethanolamide in acute or persistent pain. *Pain, 153*(1), 33–41. http://dx.doi.org/10.1016/j.pain.2011.08.010.

Schintu, N., Frau, L., Ibba, M., Caboni, P., Garau, A., Carboni, E., et al. (2009). PPAR-gamma-mediated neuroprotection in a chronic mouse model of Parkinson's disease. *The European Journal of Neuroscience, 29*(5), 954–963.

Scuderi, C., Esposito, G., Blasio, A., Valenza, M., Arietti, P., Steardo, L., Jr., et al. (2011a). Palmitoylethanolamide counteracts reactive astrogliosis induced by beta-amyloid peptide. *Journal of Cellular and Molecular Medicine, 15*(12), 2664–2674. http://dx.doi.org/10.1111/j.1582-4934.2011.01267.x.

Scuderi, C., Steardo, L., & Esposito, G. (2014a). Cannabidiol promotes amyloid precursor protein ubiquitination and reduction of beta amyloid expression in SHSY5YAPP + cells through PPARgamma involvement. *Phytotherapy Research, 28*(7), 1007–1013. http://dx.doi.org/10.1002/ptr.5095.

Scuderi, C., Stecca, C., Valenza, M., Ratano, P., Bronzuoli, M. R., Bartoli, S., et al. (2014b). Palmitoylethanolamide controls reactive gliosis and exerts neuroprotective functions in a rat model of Alzheimer's disease. *Cell Death & Disease, 5*, e1419. http://dx.doi.org/10.1038/cddis.2014.376.

Scuderi, C., Valenza, M., Stecca, C., Esposito, G., Carratu, M. R., & Steardo, L. (2012). Palmitoylethanolamide exerts neuroprotective effects in mixed neuroglial cultures and organotypic hippocampal slices via peroxisome proliferator-activated receptor-alpha. *Journal of Neuroinflammation, 9*, 49. http://dx.doi.org/10.1186/1742-2094-9-21.

Sepanjnia, K., Modabbernia, A., Ashrafi, M., Modabbernia, M. J., & Akhondzadeh, S. (2012). Pioglitazone adjunctive therapy for moderate-to-severe major depressive disorder: Randomized double-blind placebo-controlled trial. *Neuropsychopharmacology, 37*(9), 2093–2100. http://dx.doi.org/10.1038/npp.2012.58.

Shaw, N., Elholm, M., & Noy, N. (2003). Retinoic acid is a high affinity selective ligand for the peroxisome proliferator-activated receptor β/δ. *Journal of Biological Chemistry, 278*(43), 41589–41592.

Sheerin, A. H., Zhang, X., Saucier, D. M., & Corcoran, M. E. (2004). Selective antiepileptic effects of *N*-palmitoylethanolamide, a putative endocannabinoid. *Epilepsia, 45*(10), 1184–1188. doi:EPI16604 [pii]. http://dx.doi.org/10.1111/j.0013-9580.2004.16604.x.

Sher, T., Yi, H. F., McBride, O. W., & Gonzalez, F. J. (1993). cDNA cloning, chromosomal mapping, and functional characterization of the human peroxisome proliferator activated receptor. *Biochemistry, 32*(21), 5598–5604.

Sheu, M. Y., Fowler, A. J., Kao, J., Schmuth, M., Schoonjans, K., Auwerx, J., et al. (2002). Topical peroxisome proliferator activated receptor-alpha activators reduce inflammation in irritant and allergic contact dermatitis models. *The Journal of Investigative Dermatology, 118*(1), 94–101. http://dx.doi.org/10.1046/j.0022-202x.2001.01626.x.

Simonini, M. V., Polak, P. E., Boullerne, A. I., Peters, J. M., Richardson, J. C., & Feinstein, D. L. (2009). Regulation of oligodendrocyte progenitor cell maturation by PPARδ: Effects on bone morphogenetic proteins. *ASN Neuro, 2*(1), AN20090033.

Solorzano, C., Zhu, C., Battista, N., Astarita, G., Lodola, A., Rivara, S., et al. (2009). Selective *N*-acylethanolamine-hydrolyzing acid amidase inhibition reveals a key role for endogenous palmitoylethanolamide in inflammation. *Proceedings of the National Academy of Sciences of the United States of America, 106*(49), 20966–20971. http://dx.doi.org/10.1073/pnas.0907417106.

Sprecher, D. L., Massien, C., Pearce, G., Billin, A. N., Perlstein, I., Willson, T. M., et al. (2007). Triglyceride: High-density lipoprotein cholesterol effects in healthy subjects administered a peroxisome proliferator activated receptor δ agonist. *Arteriosclerosis, Thrombosis, and Vascular Biology, 27*(2), 359–365.

Staels, B., Koenig, W., Habib, A., Merval, R., Lebret, M., Torra, I. P., et al. (1998). Activation of human aortic smooth-muscle cells is inhibited by PPAR[alpha] but not by

PPAR[gamma] activators. *Nature, 393*(6687), 790–793. http://www.nature.com/nature/journal/v393/n6687/suppinfo/393790a0_S1.html.

Stanley, C. P., Hind, W. H., Tufarelli, C., & O'Sullivan, S. E. (2015). Cannabidiol causes endothelium-dependent vasorelaxation of human mesenteric arteries via CB1 activation. *Cardiovascular Research, 107*(4), 568–578. http://dx.doi.org/10.1093/cvr/cvv179.

Straus, D. S., & Glass, C. K. (2007). Anti-inflammatory actions of PPAR ligands: New insights on cellular and molecular mechanisms. *Trends in Immunology, 28*(12), 551–558. http://dx.doi.org/10.1016/j.it.2007.09.003.

Suardiaz, M., Estivill-Torrus, G., Goicoechea, C., Bilbao, A., & Rodriguez de Fonseca, F. (2007). Analgesic properties of oleoylethanolamide (OEA) in visceral and inflammatory pain. *Pain, 133*(1–3), 99–110. http://dx.doi.org/10.1016/j.pain.2007.03.008.

Sun, Y., Alexander, S. P., Garle, M. J., Gibson, C. L., Hewitt, K., Murphy, S. P., et al. (2007). Cannabinoid activation of PPAR alpha; a novel neuroprotective mechanism. *British Journal of Pharmacology, 152*(5), 734–743. http://dx.doi.org/10.1038/sj.bjp.0707478.

Takeda, S., Ikeda, E., Su, S., Harada, M., Okazaki, H., Yoshioka, Y., et al. (2014). Delta(9)-THC modulation of fatty acid 2-hydroxylase (FA2H) gene expression: Possible involvement of induced levels of PPARalpha in MDA-MB-231 breast cancer cells. *Toxicology, 326*, 18–24. http://dx.doi.org/10.1016/j.tox.2014.09.011.

Takeda, S., Yamaori, S., Motoya, E., Matsunaga, T., Kimura, T., Yamamoto, I., et al. (2008). Delta(9)-tetrahydrocannabinol enhances MCF-7 cell proliferation via cannabinoid receptor-independent signaling. *Toxicology, 245*(1–2), 141–146. http://dx.doi.org/10.1016/j.tox.2007.12.019.

Takeda, S., Yoshida, K., Nishimura, H., Harada, M., Okajima, S., Miyoshi, H., et al. (2013). Delta(9)-tetrahydrocannabinol disrupts estrogen-signaling through up-regulation of estrogen receptor beta (ERbeta). *Chemical Research in Toxicology, 26*(7), 1073–1079. http://dx.doi.org/10.1021/tx4000446.

Thorp, J. M., & Waring, W. S. (1962). Modification of metabolism and distribution of lipids by ethyl chlorophenoxyisobutyrate. *Nature, 194*, 948–949.

Tontonoz, P., & Spiegelman, B. M. (2008). Fat and beyond: The diverse biology of PPARgamma. *Annual Review of Biochemistry, 77*, 289–312. http://dx.doi.org/10.1146/annurev.biochem.77.061307.091829.

Vaia, M., Petrosino, S., De Filippis, D., Negro, L., Guarino, A., Carnuccio, R., et al. (2016). Palmitoylethanolamide reduces inflammation and itch in a mouse model of contact allergic dermatitis. *European Journal of Pharmacology, 791*, 669–674. http://dx.doi.org/10.1016/j.ejphar.2016.10.005.

Vara, D., Morell, C., Rodriguez-Henche, N., & Diaz-Laviada, I. (2013). Involvement of PPARgamma in the antitumoral action of cannabinoids on hepatocellular carcinoma. *Cell Death & Disease, 4*, e618. http://dx.doi.org/10.1038/cddis.2013.141.

von Bueren, A. O., Schlumpf, M., & Lichtensteiger, W. (2008). Delta(9)-tetrahydrocannabinol inhibits 17beta-estradiol-induced proliferation and fails to activate androgen and estrogen receptors in MCF7 human breast cancer cells. *Anticancer Research, 28*(1A), 85–89.

Wahli, W., & Michalik, L. (2012). PPARs at the crossroads of lipid signaling and inflammation. *Trends in Endocrinology & Metabolism, 23*(7), 351–363. http://dx.doi.org/10.1016/j.tem.2012.05.001.

Wang, Y. X., Lee, C. H., Tiep, S., Yu, R. T., Ham, J., Kang, H., et al. (2003). Peroxisome-proliferator-activated receptor delta activates fat metabolism to prevent obesity. *Cell, 113*(2), 159–170. http://dx.doi.org/S0092867403002691 [pii].

Wang, L., Waltenberger, B., Pferschy-Wenzig, E. M., Blunder, M., Liu, X., Malainer, C., et al. (2014). Natural product agonists of peroxisome proliferator-activated receptor gamma (PPARgamma): A review. *Biochemical Pharmacology, 92*(1), 73–89. http://dx.doi.org/10.1016/j.bcp.2014.07.018.

Wheal, A. J., Cipriano, M., Fowler, C. J., Randall, M. D., & O'Sullivan, S. E. (2014). Cannabidiol improves vasorelaxation in Zucker diabetic fatty rats through cyclooxygenase activation. *The Journal of Pharmacology and Experimental Therapeutics*, *351*(2), 457–466. http://dx.doi.org/10.1124/jpet.114.217125.

Wollank, Y., Ramer, R., Ivanov, I., Salamon, A., Peters, K., & Hinz, B. (2015). Inhibition of FAAH confers increased stem cell migration via PPARalpha. *Journal of Lipid Research*, *56*(10), 1947–1960. http://dx.doi.org/10.1194/jlr.M061473.

Xu, X., Guo, H., Jing, Z., Yang, L., Chen, C., Peng, L., et al. (2016). *N*-Oleoylethanolamine reduces inflammatory cytokines and adhesion molecules in TNF-alpha-induced human umbilical vein endothelial cells by activating CB2 and PPAR-alpha. *Journal of Cardiovascular Pharmacology*, *68*(4), 280–291. http://dx.doi.org/10.1097/fjc.0000000000000413.

Yang, L., Li, L., Chen, L., Li, Y., Chen, H., Li, Y., et al. (2015). Potential analgesic effects of a novel *N*-acylethanolamine acid amidase inhibitor F96 through PPAR-alpha. *Scientific Reports*, *5*, 13565. http://dx.doi.org/10.1038/srep13565.

Yu, S., Levi, L., Casadesus, G., Kunos, G., & Noy, N. (2014). Fatty acid-binding protein 5 (FABP5) regulates cognitive function both by decreasing anandamide levels and by activating the nuclear receptor peroxisome proliferator-activated receptor beta/delta (PPARbeta/delta) in the brain. *The Journal of Biological Chemistry*, *289*(18), 12748–12758. http://dx.doi.org/10.1074/jbc.M114.559062.

Zhang, J., Hu, M., Teng, Z., Tang, Y. P., & Chen, C. (2014). Synaptic and cognitive improvements by inhibition of 2-AG metabolism are through upregulation of microRNA-188-3p in a mouse model of Alzheimer's disease. *The Journal of Neuroscience*, *34*(45), 14919–14933. http://dx.doi.org/10.1523/jneurosci.1165-14.2014.

Zhou, T., Yan, X., Wang, G., Liu, H., Gan, X., Zhang, T., et al. (2015a). Evolutionary pattern and regulation analysis to support why diversity functions existed within PPAR gene family members. *BioMed Research International*, *2015*, 613910. http://dx.doi.org/10.1155/2015/613910.

Zhou, Y., Yang, L., Ma, A., Zhang, X., Li, W., Yang, W., et al. (2012). Orally administered oleoylethanolamide protects mice from focal cerebral ischemic injury by activating peroxisome proliferator-activated receptor alpha. *Neuropharmacology*, *63*(2), 242–249. http://dx.doi.org/10.1016/j.neuropharm.2012.03.008.

CHAPTER TEN

Cannabinoids in the Cardiovascular System

Wing S.V. Ho*,[1], Melanie E.M. Kelly†
*Vascular Biology Research Centre, St George's University of London, London, United Kingdom
†Dalhousie University, Halifax, NS, Canada
[1]Corresponding author: e-mail address: vho@sgul.ac.uk

Contents

Abstract

Cannabinoids are known to modulate cardiovascular functions including heart rate, vascular tone, and blood pressure in humans and animal models. Essential components of the endocannabinoid system, namely, the production, degradation, and signaling pathways of endocannabinoids have been described not only in the central and peripheral nervous system but also in myocardium, vasculature, platelets, and immune cells. The mechanisms of cardiovascular responses to endocannabinoids are often complex and may involve cannabinoid CB_1 and CB_2 receptors or non-$CB_{1/2}$ receptor targets. Preclinical and some clinical studies have suggested that targeting the endocannabinoid system can improve cardiovascular functions in a number of pathophysiological conditions, including hypertension, metabolic syndrome, sepsis, and atherosclerosis. In this chapter, we summarize the local and systemic cardiovascular effects of cannabinoids and highlight our current knowledge regarding the therapeutic potential of endocannabinoid signaling and modulation.

Advances in Pharmacology, Volume 80
ISSN 1054-3589
http://dx.doi.org/10.1016/bs.apha.2017.05.002

ABBREVIATIONS

2-AG 2-arachidonoyl glycerol
AEA *N*-arachidonoyl ethanolamine
Akt protein kinase B
ApoE apolipoprotein E
CB cannabinoid
CB_1R cannabinoid 1 receptor
CB_2R cannabinoid 2 receptor
CGRP calcitonin gene-related peptide
CIDS CNS injury-induced immunodeficiency syndrome
CNS central nervous system
COX cyclooxygenase
eCB endocannabinoid
ECS endocannabinoid system
FAAH fatty acid amide hydrolase
GPCR G protein-coupled receptor
IL interleukin
I/R ischemia/reperfusion
LDLR low-density lipoprotein receptor
LOX lipoxygenase
MAPK mitogen-activated protein kinase
MGL monoacylglycerol lipase
PEA *N*-palmitoylethanolamine
PPAR peroxisome proliferator-activated receptors
OEA *N*-oleoylethanolamine
THC Δ^9-tetrahydrocannabinol
TLR Toll-like receptors
TRPV1 transient receptor potential vanilloid 1 receptor

1. INTRODUCTION

The plant *Cannabis sativa* has a rich and prolific history of human recreational and medical use spanning several thousand years. Cannabis has been abused for its psychoactive properties. At the same time, Cannabis and its constituents have been used, in various preparations and via different routes of delivery, to treat a plethora of ailments (reviewed in Pisanti & Bifulco, 2017; Russo, 2017). In addition to the psychoactive phytocannabinoid, Δ^9-tetrahydrocannabinol (THC) (first isolated by Gaoni & Mechoulam, 1964), the Cannabis plant contains at least 80 additional phytocannabinoids and other active ingredients (Mechoulam, Hanuš, Pertwee, & Howlett, 2014; Pertwee, 2006; Russo, 2011).

Following identification of THC, several other pivotal events drove the discovery in humans and animals of a ubiquitous endogenous system, coined the endocannabinoid system (ECS), that mediates the effects of Cannabis and cannabinoids. These events included evidence that THC actions are stereospecific (Mechoulam et al., 1988), a tell-tale sign of high-affinity receptor interactions, and the demonstration that cannabinoids signal in cells via a receptor-mediated decrease in adenylyl cyclase (Howlett, 1984). Synthesis of high-affinity synthetic cannabinoids contributed to the cloning of cannabinoid 1 receptor and subsequent analysis of receptor distribution and pharmacology (Gerard, Mollereau, Vassart, & Parmentier, 1991; Matsuda, Lolait, Brownstein, Young, & Bonner, 1990). Both cannabinoid 1 receptor (CB_1R) and cannabinoid 2 receptor (CB_2R) belong to the superfamily of seven-transmembrane, G protein-coupled receptors (GPCRs) and are both coupled to $G_{i/o}$-dependent signaling pathways (Howlett et al., 2002). Activation of CB_1R, but not CB_2R, underlies the behavioral effects of THC and is associated with presynaptic inhibition of neurotransmitter release at central and peripheral sites (Hillard, 2015; Howlett et al., 2002; Ishac et al., 1996). On the other hand, CB_2R is commonly found in immune cells including glial cells and its activation inhibits cytokine production and suppresses immune response (reviewed in Chiurchiu, 2016; Rom & Persidsky, 2013), although CB_2R might also be localized to some neuronal populations (Van Sickle et al., 2005).

A growing number of endogenous lipid ligands (endocannabinoids, eCBs) have been identified that bind to and activate cannabinoid receptors (reviewed in Pertwee, 2015). The first two eCBs to be identified were *N*-arachidonoyl ethanolamine (AEA; Devane et al., 1992) and 2-arachidonoyl glycerol (2-AG; Mechoulam et al., 1995; Sugiura et al., 1995). AEA and 2-AG both activate CB_1R and CB_2R, with 2-AG being a full agonist at both cannabinoid receptors (recently reviewed in Maccarrone et al., 2015; Pertwee, 2015). Endocannabinoids are generated in a Ca^{2+}-dependent manner "on-demand" from cells, including immune cells, via enzymatic production from membrane lipids. The lifetime of these endogenous cannabinoid ligands is transient and limited by degradative enzymes including fatty acid amide hydrolase (FAAH; Cravatt et al., 1996) and monoacylglycerol lipase (MGL; Dinh et al., 2002) that break down AEA and 2-AG, respectively. In addition to CB_1R and CB_2R, eCBs and some cannabinoids may also interact with noncannabinoid receptors (Pertwee et al., 2010). These include the nuclear peroxisome proliferator-activated receptors (PPAR; O'Sullivan, 2016), the GPCRs, GPR55 and

GPR18 (Ross, 2009; Ryberg et al., 2007), as well as ion channels such as the ligand-gated transient receptor potential vanilloid 1 receptor, TRPV1 (Zygmunt et al., 1999) and 5-HT3 receptors (Xiong et al., 2012).

Elements of ECS, including eCBs, receptors, and enzymes, are present ubiquitously in both peripheral tissues and the central nervous system (CNS), and contribute to key homeostatic functions including metabolic, cardiovascular, and immune regulation (reviewed in Gruden, Barutta, Kunos, & Pacher, 2016; Maccarrone et al., 2015; O'Sullivan, 2015; Pacher & Steffens, 2009). Furthermore, there is growing consensus that ECS dysregulation may contribute to pathophysiology, underscoring the importance of the ECS as a drugable target for multiple disease processes. This is particularly prescient with respect to the cardiovascular system. The cardiovascular actions of cannabinoids are complex, involving the CNS and peripheral nervous system, vasculature, cardiac muscles, and, particularly in pathophysiological conditions, immune cells. For instance, THC and eCBs have been reported to alter heart rate, vascular tone, and blood pressure in man and animals (Jones, 2002; O'Sullivan, 2015). With respect to cardiovascular pathophysiology, both potentially detrimental and beneficial roles have been attributed to eCB activities in pathological conditions, for instance hypertension, metabolic syndrome, heart failure, sepsis, stroke, and atherosclerosis (Pacher & Steffens, 2009). In this review, we examine some of the experimental and clinical research documenting the actions of cannabinoids in the cardiovascular system. In doing so, we aim to highlight both the local as well as systemic cardiovascular effects of cannabinoids and the important interaction between the immune system and the cardiovascular system. Given the breadth and depth of work on the cardiovascular effects of ECS, and due to space constraints, where relevant we have additionally cited other reviews that address material and topics not covered herein.

2. CARDIOVASCULAR EFFECTS OF CANNABINOIDS

Smoking or ingestion of cannabis has long been known to induce tachycardia with variable effects on blood pressure, although chronic users often experience bradycardia and prolonged reduction in blood pressure (Gorelick et al., 2006; Jones, 2002). This is due to a dose-dependent effects of the phytocannabinoid, THC, and modulation of the autonomic nervous system, at least partly via CB_1R activation (Benowitz, Rosenberg, Rogers, Bachman, & Jones, 1979; Fant, Heishman, Bunker, & Pickworth, 1998;

Gorelick et al., 2006). Since the identification of eCBs, extensive investigations have been carried out to examine their hemodynamic effects. In addition to neurons, both AEA and 2-AG are present in myocardium, vascular cells, circulating blood cells, platelets, and at lower levels in serum (Hillard et al., 2007; Ho, Barrett, & Randall, 2008; Ho, Hill, Miller, Gorzalka, & Hillard, 2012; Mukhopadhyay et al., 2011; Wagner, Hu, et al., 2001; Wagner et al., 1997).

2.1 In Vivo Effects of Endocannabinoids

Similar to THC, the effects of eCBs on arterial blood pressure are complex, but with a predominant hypotensive action. In anesthetized rodents, intravenous injection of AEA induces a triphasic response that is characterized by a transient drop (phase I) and then rise in blood pressure (phase II), followed by a prolonged hypotension (phase III). The initial hypotensive effect (phase I), which often requires high doses of AEA, is accompanied by bradycardia and decreased cardiac contractility, and is initiated by activation of TRPV1 receptors on vagal sensory nerves in the heart (Malinowska, Kwolek, & Gothert, 2001; Pacher, Bátkai, & Kunos, 2004; Varga, Lake, Martin, & Kunos, 1995). This is an example of the so-called Bezold–Jarisch reflex, which can also be activated by the TRPV1 agonist, capsaicin (McQueen, Bond, Smith, Balali-Mood, & Smart, 2004), but not synthetic CB_1 agonists that lack TRPV1 activity (Lake, Martin, Kunos, & Varga, 1997; Zygmunt et al., 1999). AEA, particularly at higher concentrations, directly activates TRPV1 receptors, which also mediate peripheral dilatory effects of AEA (Ho et al., 2008; Zygmunt et al., 1999). For phase III, activation of CB_1R by AEA underlies the prolonged hypotension and bradycardia, which are inhibited by selective CB_1 receptor antagonists, such as SR141716 (rimonabant), and absent in CB_1 receptor knockout mice (Járai et al., 1999; Ledent et al., 1999; Malinowska, Piszcz, Koneczny, Hryniewicz, & Schlicker, 2001; Wagner, Járai, Bátkai, & Kunos, 2001). This response is partly mediated by presynaptic CB_1 receptors in peripheral sympathetic nerves and subsequent inhibition of catecholamine release (Ishac et al., 1996; Kwolek et al., 2005; Malinowska, Piszcz, et al., 2001). Decreases in cardiac contractility via postsynaptic CB_1R in the myocardium and a direct vasodilator effect via multiple mechanisms also contribute to the hypotension induced by AEA or CB_1 agonists (Bátkai, Pacher, Osei-Hyiaman, et al., 2004; Bonz et al., 2003; Zakrzeska et al., 2010). It is, however, worth noting that the prolonged hypotensive effects of AEA, or CB_1R agonists, are more prominent in anesthetized compared to conscious animals (Gardiner, March, Kemp, & Bennett, 2002; Malinowska, Kwolek, et al., 2001), while the transient Bezold–Jarisch reflex in phase I is diminished under pentobarbitone anesthesia (Malinowska, Kwolek, et al., 2001; Pacher et al., 2004).

Although the hypotensive effects of cannabinoids and their peripheral sites of action have received more attention, synthetic CB_1 agonists can also induce centrally mediated sympathoexcitatory effects and subsequent hypertension, especially in conscious rats and rabbits (Gardiner et al., 2002; Malinowska et al., 2010; Niederhoffer & Szabo, 2000; Varga, Lake, Huangfu, Guyenet, & Kunos, 1996), which may contribute to the brief pressor response in phase II and explain the tachycardia induced by THC or synthetic cannabinoids. Indeed, eCBs have also been shown to modulate autonomic outflow in the brainstem via an action at the rostral ventrolateral medulla (Padley, Li, Pilowsky, & Goodchild, 2003), nucleus tractus solitaries (Herkenham et al., 1991; Seagard et al., 2004), and periaqueductal gray (Dean, 2011), where there is a high density of CB_1 receptors. Local production of eCBs in these regions could fine tune baroreflex response and buffer fluctuations in arterial blood pressure, perhaps particularly in stressful conditions (Dean, 2011; Guyenet, 2006; Seagard et al., 2004).

The tissue content of eCBs depends on the balance between production and degradation (Di Marzo, 2006), and their metabolism is thought to terminate receptor-mediated signaling. Specifically, the cardiovascular actions of AEA and 2-AG are regulated by their main degradation enzymes, FAAH (Cravatt et al., 1996) and MGL (Dinh et al., 2002), respectively. In anesthetized mice, 2-AG induces CB_1-mediated hypotension and bradycardia, but only if its rapid hydrolysis to arachidonic acid is inhibited (Járai et al., 2000). In addition, the cardiovascular effects of AEA, but not synthetic CB_1R agonists such as HU210, are potentiated by FAAH inhibitors (Gardiner, March, Kemp, & Bennett, 2009; Ho & Randall, 2007) or in FAAH knockout mice (Pacher et al., 2005). Despite tissue accumulation of AEA (Cravatt et al., 2001; Pacher et al., 2005), genetic deletion of FAAH has no significant effect on blood pressure, cardiac contractility, and baroreflex sensitivity (Pacher et al., 2005), suggestive of a limited role of FAAH in cardiovascular regulation under normal physiological conditions. CB_1R knockout mice also have normal blood pressure (Járai et al., 1999; Ledent et al., 1999), although tonic regulation of regional blood flow by AEA, especially through non-CB_1 mechanisms, cannot be excluded. Importantly, the hemodynamic effects of cannabinoids are increased under pathological conditions, such as hypertension and advanced liver cirrhosis, in which overactivation of ECS may either contribute to (Bátkai et al., 2001; Mukhopadhyay et al., 2011; Varga, Wagner, Bridgen, & Kunos, 1998; Wagner et al., 1997) or act as a compensatory mechanism against cardiovascular dysfunction (Bátkai, Pacher, Osei-Hyiaman, et al., 2004; Godlewski et al., 2010).

2.2 Local Vascular Tone Regulation

One of the most consistent cardiovascular effects of eCBs is vasodilation, which is key to regulation of regional blood flow with or without corresponding changes in blood pressure (Gardiner et al., 2002; Koura et al., 2004; Wagner, Járai, et al., 2001). This dilator response maybe partly mediated by CB_1-mediated inhibition of norepinephrine release from perivascular sympathetic nerves (Schultheiss, Flau, Kathmann, Göthert, & Schlicker, 2005), but direct actions on endothelial or smooth muscle cells are also important (Hillard, 2000). Diverse dilatory mechanisms have been reported in vessels from animals and humans, partly dependent on the vascular regions and species, and may be due to differences in the distribution and binding affinity of different receptor targets (Andersson, Adner, Högestätt, & Zygmunt, 2002). Fig. 1 summarizes the possible sites of vasodilatory actions of eCBs. Activation by AEA of CB_1 receptors in vascular smooth muscles is coupled to inhibition of voltage-gated calcium entry via $G_{i/o}$ proteins (Gebremedhin, Lange, Campbell, Hillard, & Harder, 1999), or AEA induces endothelium-dependent relaxation through endothelial CB_1 receptors and the subsequent activation of nitric oxide synthase and calcium-activated potassium channels (Deutsch et al., 1997; Koura et al., 2004; Romano & Lograno, 2006; Stanley, Hind, Tufarelli, & O'Sullivan, 2016). CB_2 receptors are also expressed in vascular cells (Rajesh et al., 2007), but so far there is no evidence for their involvement in acute vascular tone regulation (Járai et al., 1999; Stanley et al., 2016; Zygmunt et al., 1999) despite a report of hypotension to the synthetic CB_2R agonist, HU308 (Hanus et al., 1999).

In some vessels, AEA activates TRPV1 expressed in perivascular sensory nerves, leading to release of dilator neuropeptide, calcitonin gene-related peptide (CGRP), which in turn causes vasodilation through potassium channel activation (Ho et al., 2008; White, Ho, Bottrill, Ford, & Hiley, 2001; Zygmunt et al., 1999). For example, AEA increases forearm blood flow in humans via TRPV1 activation (Movahed et al., 2005). These AEA responses are largely blocked by TRPV1 antagonists or desensitization of the TRPV1/CGRP system by prolonged incubation with capsaicin, a

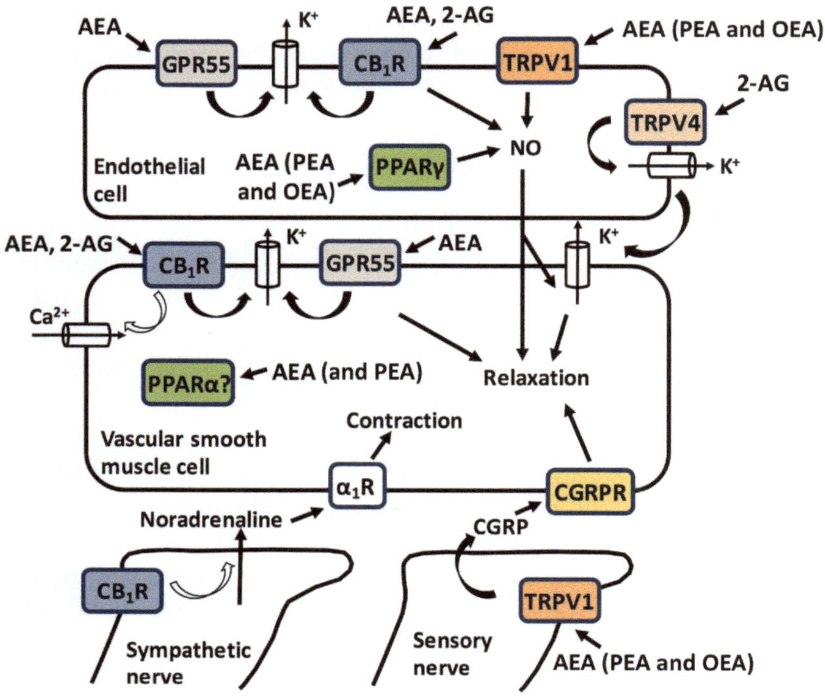

Fig. 1 Possible sites of vasodilatory actions of endocannabinoids. As detailed in the text, endocannabinoids induce dilation through multiple mechanisms of actions that are partly dependent on the vascular region. They include activation of CB_1R, which can lead to nitric oxide (NO) release from endothelial cells, inhibition of Ca^{2+} entry through voltage-gated Ca^{2+} channels in vascular smooth muscle cells, or reduced release of the vasoconstrictor norepinephrine from sympathetic nerve endings. AEA might also activate GPR55 receptor and then Ca^{2+}-activated K^+ channels in endothelial or vascular smooth muscle cells. AEA and 2-AG have also been shown to induce dilation through direct activation of TRPV1 and TRPV4, respectively. In perivascular sensory nerves, activation of TRPV1 by AEA induces the release of the vasodilator CGRP, whereas endothelial TRPV1/4 activity dilates arteries through subsequent NO release and/or activation of Ca^{2+}-activated K^+ channels. In addition to cell surface receptors, AEA is also known to activate the nuclear receptors, PPARα and PPARγ. In the endothelium, PPARγ activation might stimulate NO release.

potent TRPV1 agonist. TRPV receptors might also contribute to 2-AG-induced vasodilation. Data on the ability of 2-AG to activate TRPV1 receptors are conflicting (Stanley & O'Sullivan, 2014; Zygmunt et al., 2013, 1999), but 2-AG has recently been shown to activate endothelial TRPV4, which in turn activates calcium-activated potassium channels and subsequent smooth muscle relaxation (Ho, Zheng, & Zhang, 2015).

Additionally, it has been proposed that there is a novel AEA receptor, or receptors, in the vasculature (Begg et al., 2005; Járai et al., 1999; White et al., 2001), but their molecular identities remain contentious. For instance, in rodent mesenteric arteries, the endothelium-dependent component of AEA dilation is coupled to $G_{i/o}$ protein, but persists in CB_1R/CB_2R double-knockout mice, and is generally insensitive to CB receptor antagonists except for a high concentration of rimonabant (Járai et al., 1999). This response is also mimicked by abnormal-cannabidiol, a synthetic compound that is inactive at CB receptors, and antagonized by O-1918 (Ho & Hiley, 2003; Offertáler et al., 2003). These studies, therefore, provide a partial pharmacological profile of the purported novel AEA receptor, which is distinct from CB_1R, CB_2R, and TRPV1 and induces dilation via activation of calcium-activated potassium channels. The same, or a similar, receptor, is also suggested in other vascular regions (Kozłowska et al., 2007; Mukhopadhyay, Chapnick, & Howlett, 2002; White et al., 2001) and cardiac cells, although there are notable inconsistencies in the reported signaling mechanisms involved (Bondarenko, 2014).

Two G protein-coupled receptors, GPR55 and GPR18, which display sensitivity to eCBs, abnormal-cannabidiol, and O-1918 (Ross, 2009; Ryberg et al., 2007; Sharir & Abood, 2010), have been implicated as novel cannabinoid receptors. In human endothelial cells, GPR55 mediates AEA-induced Ca^{2+} signaling (Waldeck-Weiermair et al., 2008), which can potentially stimulate the production of relaxing factors or initiate endothelium-derived hyperpolarization. GPR55 has also been demonstrated in vascular smooth muscle (Daly et al., 2010), and in mouse mesenteric artery, endothelium-independent relaxation to AEA, but not abnormal-cannabidiol, is reduced in GPR55 knockout mice or reduced by a newly developed selective GPR55 antagonist (McNaughton, Choy, Sudlow, & Ho, 2016). GPR55 activity might also play a role in microvascular endothelial cell migration and wound healing (Kremshofer et al., 2015; Zhang, Maor, Wang, Kunos, & Groopman, 2010). However, accumulating evidence suggests that L-lysophosphatidylinositol, rather than AEA, is the likely the endogenous agonist for GPR55 (Marichal-Cancino et al., 2013; Ross, 2009; Sharir & Abood, 2010). It is also clear that O-1918 is not a selective GPR55 antagonist. Within the same concentration range, O-1918 also antagonizes GPR18-mediated responses (MacIntyre et al., 2014; McHugh et al., 2010), and inhibits cGMP signaling (Begg et al., 2003) or calcium-activated potassium channels (Godlewski et al., 2009; Parmar & Ho, 2012), all of which complicate interpretation of pharmacological evidence in vitro and in vivo

(Baranowska-Kuczko et al., 2014; Matouk, Taye, El-Moselhy, Heeba, & Abdel-Rahman, 2017; Penumarti & Abdel-Rahman, 2014). In retinal microvessels, activation of endothelial GPR18, which couples to $G_{i/o}$ proteins, may mediate dilation induced by abnormal-cannabidiol, but its relevance for eCB responses was not investigated (MacIntyre et al., 2014). Moving forward, further development of selective GPR55 and GPR18 ligands is much needed.

Adding to the pharmacological profile of eCBs, AEA and 2-AG can stimulate the transcription factor PPAR, which are relatively promiscuous (O'Sullivan, 2016). In some isolated arteries, AEA induces a time-dependent relaxation via endothelial PPARγ (O'Sullivan, Kendall, & Randall, 2009) or smooth muscle PPARα (Romano & Lograno, 2012). Some of the vascular effects of THC might also be mediated by PPAR (O'Sullivan, Tarling, Bennett, Kendall, & Randall, 2005). These PPAR-mediated dilator responses develop more slowly (over 2h or more) than those attributed to CB, TRPV, or GPR55 receptors. Since PPAR have been implicated in inflammatory, hypertrophic, and fibrotic responses (Calkin & Thomas, 2008), activation of PPAR by cannabinoids might be of particular significance in cardiometabolic diseases. Taken together, cannabinoids modulate vascular tone through a wide range of receptor targets and downstream signaling pathways, which can occur in parallel in vitro and in vivo (e.g., Járai et al., 1999; Mukhopadhyay et al., 2002).

An important aspect of vascular tone regulation by eCBs is their autocrine and paracrine function, acting as a crucial regulator of local blood flow. In isolated arteries, vasoconstrictors such as thromboxane analog or angiotensin II increase AEA and 2-AG levels in vascular smooth muscle, and their relaxant effects prevent excessive vasoconstriction (middle cerebral artery: Rademacher et al., 2005; Hillard et al., 2007; aorta: Szekeres et al., 2015). Vascular cells also express metabolizing enzymes of eCBs (Hillard et al., 2007; Ho et al., 2008). For the cerebral circulation, AEA derived from surrounding neurons can improve local cortical blood flow through activation of CB_1 receptors (Ho et al., 2010). In inflammatory conditions, large amounts of AEA and 2-AG can also be produced by leukocytes and platelets, which then act on vascular and cardiac cells leading to dilation, reduced cardiac contraction, and hypotension (Bátkai et al., 2001; Bátkai, Pacher, Járai, Wagner, & Kunos, 2004; Wagner, Hu, et al., 2001; Wagner et al., 1997). In addition to hemodynamic effects, the eCBs are also likely to participate in tissue remodeling seen in cardiovascular disorders (Hydock, Lien, & Hayward, 2009; Mukhopadhyay et al., 2011; Wenzel et al., 2013).

3. ENDOCANNABINOID METABOLITES

While catabolism has been shown to limit receptor-mediated actions of AEA and 2-AG, some of their breakdown products also exert cardiovascular effects, especially in specialized circulations. In coronary artery, hydrolysis to arachidonic acid and subsequent production of vasodilatory eicosanoids such as prostacyclin or epoxyeicosatrienoic acids underlies the dilation to AEA (Pratt, Hillard, Edgemond, & Campbell, 1998) and 2-AG (Gauthier et al., 2005). Due to a high lipase activity in serum, intravenously injected 2-AG is rapidly degraded, and the resulting arachidonic acid mediates part of its hypotensive effects (Járai et al., 2000). In pulmonary arteries, however, FAAH-mediated hydrolysis of AEA leads to prominent vasoconstrictions (Wahn, Wolf, Kram, Frantz, & Wagner, 2005; Wenzel et al., 2013). This contributes to pulmonary hypertension induced by hypoxia, which increases AEA generation from pulmonary smooth muscle cells (Wenzel et al., 2013). Similarly, 2-AG hydrolysis also results in pulmonary vasoconstriction that is independent of CB_1 receptors (Wahn et al., 2005). In addition to MGL, other enzymes, namely, FAAH, αβ-hydrolase domain-containing 6 (ABHD6), and αβ-hydrolase domain-containing 12 (ABHD12) also hydrolyze 2-AG to arachidonic acid and glycerol (Marrs et al., 2010), which underlie the labile properties of 2-AG. Moreover, AEA and 2-AG can also be directly oxidized by cyclooxygenase (COX-2), lipoxygenases (12-LOX and 15-LOX), and cytochrome P450 (Di Marzo, 2006; Urquhart, Nicolaou, & Woodward, 2015), but the cardiovascular actions of the resultant metabolites are unclear.

4. ENDOCANNABINOID CONGENERS

When considering the (patho)physiological role of eCBs, it is also important to recognize the presence of congeners alongside AEA and 2-AG, such as ethanolamines or glycerols derived from other fatty acids. These congeners are often inactive at CB receptors but can enhance the actions of eCBs (so-called entourage effect) and/or activate additional molecular targets (Schmid, Schmid, & Berdyshev, 2002). An entourage effect was first observed for 2-AG congeners, 2-linoleoylglycerol, and 2-palmitoylglycerol which protect 2-AG from hydrolysis and increase CB_1-mediated responses in vitro and in vivo (Ben-Shabat et al., 1998). Since then, AEA congeners *N*-oleoylethanolamine (OEA) and

N-palmitoylethanolamine (PEA) have also been shown to enhance AEA-induced TRPV1 activation, increasing mesenteric relaxation and hypotensive response to AEA (García Mdel, Adler-Graschinsky, & Celuch, 2009; Ho et al., 2008; Smart, Jonsson, Vandevoorde, Lambert, & Fowler, 2002). Given that OEA and PEA are also FAAH substrates, they can reduce AEA degradation through substrate competition and may contribute to the cardiovascular actions of FAAH inhibitors (García Mdel et al., 2009; Jonsson, Vandevoorde, Lambert, Tiger, & Fowler, 2001; Smart et al., 2002). Interestingly, OEA and PEA also activate GPR55, PPAR, as well as GPR119, which is closely associated with energy balance and diabetes (Overton, Fyfe, & Reynet, 2008). Of note, recent studies have reported that FAAH polymorphism and circulating levels of AEA, PEA, and OEA are correlated with impaired coronary dilation or cardiometabolic risk variables in humans (Martins et al., 2015; Quercioli et al., 2017), but causality and the underlying molecular mechanisms are yet to be established.

5. TARGETING THE ECS IN CARDIOVASCULAR DISEASES

Increasingly, eCBs and CB receptors have been implicated in cardiovascular diseases or disorders associated with inflammation and tissue injury (Bátkai, Pacher, Osei-Hyiaman, et al., 2004; Mukhopadhyay et al., 2011; summarized in Fig. 2). Modulators of ECS, such as FAAH inhibitors and CB receptor ligands, could therefore be used for therapeutic gains. In the context of cannabinoids as medicine, it is worth noting that there are concerns over possible increased cardiovascular risks in users of cannabis or synthetic cannabinoids, especially those with history of coronary artery disease (Heath, Burroughs, Thompson, & Tecklenburg, 2012; Jouanjus, Lapeyre-Mestre, & Micallef, 2014), although a definitive relationship has not been established.

5.1 Therapeutic Potential of CB_1 Antagonists

Overactivation of CB_1 receptors by eCBs derived from monocytes, macrophages, or platelets can lead to the vasodilation and hypotension associated with shock, myocardial infarction, and liver cirrhosis (Bátkai et al., 2001; Varga et al., 1998; Wagner, Hu, et al., 2001; Wagner et al., 1997). In these conditions, CB_1 antagonists might be beneficial (Kadoi, Hinohara, Kunimoto, Saito, & Goto, 2005). More recent studies have highlighted the proinflammatory, prooxidative, and profibrogenic effects of cardiac CB_1 activation in disease states. These include increasing formation of

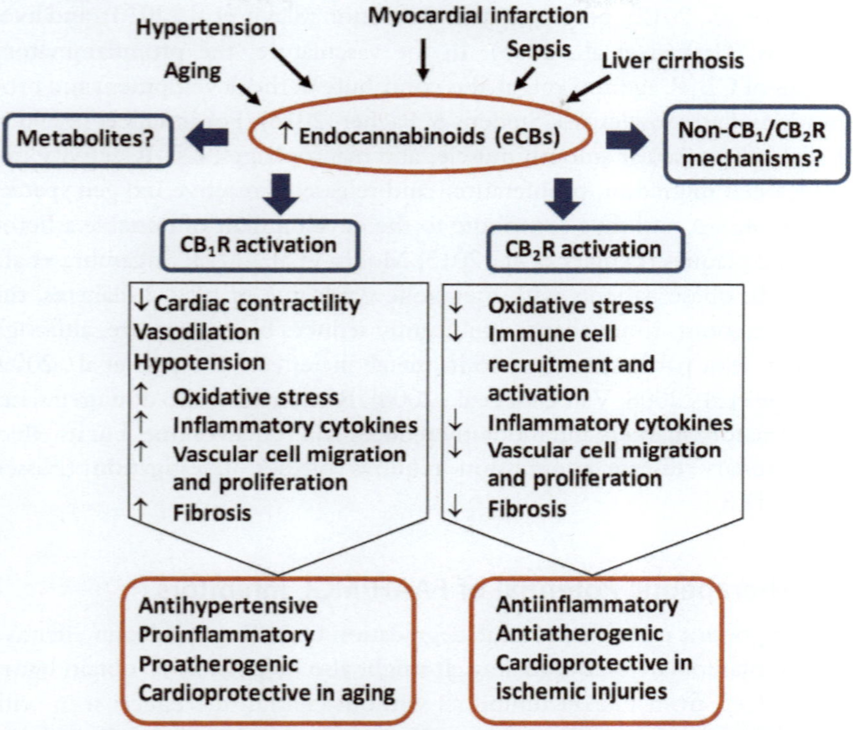

Fig. 2 Cardiovascular effects of cannabinoid receptor activation in pathophysiological conditions. In myocardial infarction, sepsis, and liver cirrhosis, the increases in endocannabinoid levels promote hypotension, inflammation, and tissue remodeling through CB_1R activation. On the other hand, activation of CB_2R has antiinflammation effects, reducing immune cell activation, and tissue remodeling. Interestingly, activation of either CB_1R or CB_2R might protect cardiac function depending on the precise context. It should be noted that endocannabinoids are also likely to exert cardiovascular effects through their metabolites. For instance, 2-AG metabolites generated by hydrolases and cyclooxygenases are known to induce increase regional blood flow and hypotension. In addition to cannabinoid receptors, endocannabinoids can also activate novel G protein-coupled receptors, although their involvement in cardiovascular disorders remains unclear.

reactive oxygen species, inflammatory cytokines, adhesion molecule expression, apoptotic signaling, and collagen accumulation (Montecucco & Di Marzo, 2012). The detrimental effects are amplified by increased local production of eCBs during oxidative stress and tissue injury (Gaskari, Liu, D'Mello, Kunos, & Lee, 2015; Mukhopadhyay et al., 2011). As a result, genetic deletion or pharmacological inhibition of CB_1 receptors partly restores cardiac contractile function in animal models of doxorubicin-induced toxicity (Mukhopadhyay et al., 2011), diabetic cardiomyopathy

(Rajesh et al., 2012), postmyocardial infarction (Slavic et al., 2013), and liver cirrhosis (Gaskari et al., 2015). In the vasculature, the proinflammatory actions of CB_1R agonists might also contribute to the development and progression of atherosclerosis (Steffens & Pacher, 2015). For instance, in endothelial cells, vascular smooth muscle, and macrophages, CB_1R activity can induce cell migration, proliferation, and release of reactive oxygen species and cytokines, and thus contribute to the development of unstable atherosclerotic plaques (Lenglet et al., 2013; Molica et al., 2013; Sugamura et al., 2009). In obese patients with metabolic syndrome or type 2 diabetes, the CB_1 antagonist, rimonabant, significantly reduces blood pressure, although this is at least partly secondary to its metabolic effects (Després et al., 2009; Ruilope et al., 2008; Van Gaal et al., 2008). Rimonabant also downregulates inflammatory markers and modestly reduces atheroma volume, but its effect on coronary disease progression requires further investigation (Nissen et al., 2008).

5.2 Therapeutic Potential of FAAH/MGL Inhibitors

The important role of enzymatic degradation of eCBs provides an effective way to manipulate eCB signaling. It might also be possible to obtain beneficial effects from FAAH inhibitors without central side effects seen with cannabis or synthetic CB_1 agonists (Kathuria et al., 2003). Preclinical data suggest that increases in AEA tone with FAAH inhibitors show larger hypotensive effects in various models of hypertension (Bátkai, Pacher, Osei-Hyiaman, et al., 2004; Godlewski et al., 2010; Lake et al., 1997; Toczek et al., 2016), indicating a protective role of AEA and potential use of FAAH inhibitors as antihypertensive agents. In young male volunteers, a gene variant of FAAH that has reduced enzymatic activity is associated with higher circulating AEA and lower blood pressure (Sarzani et al., 2008).

Based on the possible pathophysiological role of CB_1 receptors, reducing eCB degradation might be expected to exacerbate cardiovascular dysfunction, however, the effects of CB_2R activation in vascular and immune cells, which is often antiinflammatory and protective (Rajesh et al., 2007; Steffens & Pacher, 2015), and the involvement of non-CB receptors including TRPV1, GPR55, and PPAR receptors in eCB actions need to be considered. In particular, eCB congeners could contribute, or modify, the effects of FAAH or MGL inhibitors. PEA is antiinflammatory and reduces cytokine releases, whereas OEA might exert the opposite effects

(Berdyshev et al., 1997; Montecucco, Matias, et al., 2009). Inhibitors of FAAH have also been shown to elicit TRPV1- or PPAR-mediated responses (Sagar, Kendall, & Chapman, 2008; Starowicz et al., 2013).

Interestingly, FAAH deficiency improves cardiac contractility that is compromised by aging, by reducing oxidative stress, monocyte–endothelial cell adhesion, inflammatory cytokines, myocardial apoptosis (Bátkai et al., 2007). In addition to aging, anxiety and affective disorders may represent another example of context-dependent cardioprotective effects of FAAH inhibition. Tissue levels of AEA/2-AG and CB_1R signaling are often altered in anxiety and depression, which are in fact risk factors for cardiovascular diseases and predict poor prognosis for ischemic heart diseases (Carney, Freedland, Miller, & Jaffe, 2002; Roest, Martens, de Jonge, & Denollet, 2010). FAAH inhibitors not only act as anxiolytics and antidepressants (Hill et al., 2009) but also reduce ventricular tachyarrhythmia in anxious rats (Carnevali et al., 2015). Such an antiarrhythmic effect is partly mediated by CB_1 but not CB_2 receptors, although the contribution from central vs peripheral sites of action remains unclear (Carnevali et al., 2015). Serum levels of AEA and 2-AG are also correlated with higher blood pressure in depressed patients (Ho et al., 2012). One possible mechanistic link for the comorbidity between mood disorders and cardiovascular disease is autonomic dysfunction (Carney et al., 2002), which can be targeted by eCBs. On the other hand, atherosclerotic mice devoid of MGL have more stable atherosclerotic plagues as a result of CB_2R activation (Vujic et al., 2016). Overall, these data are supportive of FAAH/MGL inhibition as a therapeutic approach for some cardiovascular conditions. However, it should be noted that receptor desensitization may occur due to prolonged elevation of eCB levels, especially when MGL inhibitors or FAAH and MGL combined inhibitors are used (Schlosburg et al., 2010).

5.3 Therapeutic Potential of CB_2R Agonists

Localized expression of CB_2R is seen on immune cells, including neutrophils, monocytes (macrophage precursors), as well as CNS resident microglial cells (Chiurchiu, 2016; Chiurchiu, Battistini, & Maccarrone, 2015). Neutrophils, monocytes, and macrophages are key players in the innate immune responses and critical in host defense mediated via activation of Toll-like receptors (TLR) by pathogens or host-derived factors. TLR are also expressed by other tissues notably those of the cardiovascular system, and activation of TLR-mediated signaling contributes to the vascular and cardiac dysfunction associated with both the development and progression of cardiovascular diseases, including sepsis, septic shock, stroke, cardiac ischemia/reperfusion (I/R), as well as atherosclerosis (Frantz, Ertl, & Bauersachs, 2007; Vallejo, 2011). Activation of CB_2R attenuates TLR-mediated inflammatory responses by inhibiting production of proinflammatory mediators and decreasing neutrophil chemotaxis and extravasation into tissue (Chiurchiu, 2016; Chiurchiu et al., 2015). In injury models, levels of CB_2R expression, along with eCBs, are increased suggesting that this receptor may function in an "autoprotective role" to limit inflammation and slow disease progression (Pacher & Mechoulam, 2011).

Sepsis represents a dysregulated host immune response to infection and can progress to septic shock which is associated with high mortality risk and is characterized by massive circulatory, cellular, and metabolic abnormalities (Seymour et al., 2016; Singer et al., 2016). The time course of sepsis is complex and multiphasic with the initial hyperinflammatory stage of sepsis followed by immunosuppression in the latter stages of the disease. Decreased microvascular perfusion is an early event in the systemic inflammatory response and is accompanied by reduced functional capillary density (Miranda, Balarini, Caixeta, & Bouskela, 2016). Given the antiinflammatory actions of cannabinoids activating CB_2R, several experimental studies have now examined the potential for therapeutic targeting of CB_2R in experimental sepsis (reviewed in Kasten, Tschöp, Tschöp, & Caldwell, 2010; Maccarrone, Bari, Battista, & Finazzi-Agrò, 2002). Using an experimental abdominal sepsis model in CB_2R knockout mice, Tschöp et al. (2009) reported increased neutrophil recruitment and decreased p38 activity at the site of infection, consistent with an increased inflammatory response, while activation of CB_2R in this model was associated with a decrease in neutrophil recruitment, increased phagocytosis, and p38 activity (Tschöp et al., 2009). In contrast to this study, however, Csóka et al. (2009) also using a cecal ligation/puncture model of bacterial sepsis found that genetic knockout of CB_2R was associated with a decrease in sepsis-induced mortality and bacterial translocation into the bloodstream of septic animals. This was accompanied by suppression of splenic nuclear factor-kappaB and a decrease in the antiinflammatory cytokine, interleukin (IL)-10, as well as decreases in IL-6 and macrophage inflammatory protein-2 levels. CB_2R knockout in experimental abdominal sepsis also had a protective role against apoptosis in lymphoid organs and increased the leukocyte activity marker CD11b+, as well as CD19+ B cells (Csóka et al., 2009). The decrease in levels of IL-10 in both serum and peritoneal lavage in CB_2R knockout mice in this study by Csóka et al. (2009) is suggestive of a loss of constitutive CB_2R-mediated antiinflammatory activity during the early immune hyperactivation phase in sepsis. These findings are interesting given the increased inflammatory response and decrease in mortality reported by Tschöp et al. (2009) using a similar model of bacterial sepsis in CB_2R knockout mice and may be reflective of experimental differences such as puncture size and bacterial load, the complicated immune status changes that occur during sepsis and the timing and choice of biomarker assessment, coupled with compensatory mechanisms in knockout animals.

Gui et al. (2013) reported that CB_2R activation was protective against experimental sepsis in mice. This was consistent with a study by Sardinha, Kelly, Zhou, and Lehmann (2014) in which the authors examined leucocyte–endothelial interactions as marker of immune cell recruitment in the intestinal microvasculature during experimental endotoxemia. The results of this study showed that activation of CB_2R was antiinflammatory and associated with reduced leukocyte adherence to the endothelium within the intestinal microcirculation (Sardinha et al., 2014). Likewise, using a model of endotoxin-induced uveitis, Toguri et al. also confirmed decreased leukocyte recruitment in the ocular iridial microvasculature and improvements in capillary perfusion when animals were treated with a CB_2R agonist (Toguri et al., 2014, 2015). Taken together, these results indicate that activation of CB_2R is antiinflammatory in experimental models of sepsis. CB_2R agonists may be useful in patients during the acute hyperinflammatory phase of sepsis to inhibit innate immune response and mitigate progression to septic shock with the associated vascular dysfunction and organ failure. Given that the later stages of sepsis are characterized by immunosuppression, it is possible that use of CB_2R agonists during this phase of the disease may be counterproductive (Lehmann et al., 2014). While many sepsis studies have focussed on CB_2R as an immunosuppressive target, a few studies have indicated that CB_1R antagonism in experimental sepsis and septic shock models may improve microcirculatory function and systemic hemodynamics and may contribute to decreased mortality in these models (Kadoi et al., 2005; Kianian et al., 2014).

Interactions between the cardiovascular system and immune system also contribute to disease progression in cerebrovascular pathologies such as traumatic and ischemic brain injury. An acute ischemic stroke (the most frequent stroke etiology) results from arterial occlusion and leads to CNS neuronal apoptosis, as well as a myriad of focal neurological deficits (Ladecola & Anrather, 2011). In common with acute traumatic brain injury, the pathophysiology of stroke also includes secondary cell death caused by a release of cytotoxins in response to the initial ischemic onset and involvement of brain areas outside of the primary ischemic episode (Ladecola & Anrather, 2011; Weimar et al., 2002). The ECS, including CB_2R, contributes to the consequences of an acute CNS ischemic injury. CB_2R activation initiates immunosuppressive mechanisms and may limit neuroinflammation following ischemic brain injury (reviewed in Benyó, Ruisanchez, Leszl-Ishiguro, Sándor, & Pacher, 2016; Capettini et al., 2012; Fernández-Ruiz, Moro, & Martínez-Orgado, 2015).

While experimental data for the most part suggest beneficial CNS actions of CB_2R activity in acute traumatic brain injury and in the early poststroke time course (Amenta, Jallo, Tuma, Hooper, & Elliott, 2014), a study in rats with middle cerebral artery occlusion injury of stroke indicated a time-dependent neuroprotection using a CB_2R agonist; positive neuroprotection was obtained with early treatment with a CB_2R agonist but reduced benefit if treatment was delayed (Yu et al., 2015). This finding is important as less is known about the consequences of CB_2R modulation, particularly in the periphery, in the later stages after a brain injury. For example, immune suppression caused by peripheral CB_2R activation could contribute to CNS injury-induced immunodeficiency syndrome (CIDS) and negatively impact outcome after an acute CNS injury or stroke. CIDS is thought to arise as a compensatory homeostatic countermeasure against the initial CNS inflammatory response in order to prevent any further CNS damage (Dirnagl et al., 2007; Meisel, Schwab, Prass, Meisel, & Dirnagl, 2005). CIDS, unfortunately, also causes systemic susceptibility to infection with ensuing sepsis and septic shock and severe decrements in vascular function, including peripheral hypotension and decreased microvascular perfusion. Recent experimental evidence has suggested that use of cannabinoid therapy in concert with the patient's immune status may be useful during the aftermath of CNS ischemic injury particularly with risk of CIDS, i.e., use of CB_2R agonists during the early acute phase of CNS injury to reduce the CNS inflammatory response with pharmacologically inhibition of CB_2R activity, or use of adjunct immunostimulation, during the later disease stages when the patient is immunocompromised (Lehmann et al., 2014). A study by

Burkovskiy, Zhou, and Lehmann (2016) examined this premise experimentally in mice with CNS injury induced using a hypoxia–ischemia model. The results of this study indicated that animals that were given an immunochallenge following a prior CNS injury had a severely compromised immune response, confirming that CIDS was a preserved phenomenon in rodents. Inhibition of CB_2R with the antagonist, AM630, was able to reverse the immunosuppression associated with CIDS and restored some immune function (Burkovskiy et al., 2016). While data examining the use of CB receptor antagonism as a therapeutic strategy for immunostimulation is clearly warranted, this study highlights the importance of accounting for alterations in immune status in evaluating ECS drug regimens for acute traumatic brain injuries and stroke.

A number of experimental studies have examined the potential of cannabinoid receptor modulation in cardiac I/R injury. CB_2R expression has been reported in cardiac tissue including myocardium, cardiomyocytes, coronary artery endothelial, and smooth muscle cells, and experimental evidence from models of cardiac I/R supports potentially beneficial cardioprotective effects of endocannabinoids and cannabinoids that activate CB_2R (reviewed in Capettini et al., 2012; Carbone, Mach, Vuilleumier, & Montecucco, 2014; Maslov et al., 2016; Montecucco & Di Marzo, 2012; O'Sullivan, 2015; Pacher & Haskó, 2008; Zubrzycki, Liebold, Janecka, & Zubrzycka, 2014). Montecucco, Lenglet, et al. (2009) using a mouse model of left coronary artery ligation followed by reperfusion demonstrated that the CB_2R agonist, JWH-133, was able to decrease infarct size, as well as oxidative stress and neutrophil infiltration in the infarcted myocardium. JWH-133 was effective in reducing infarct size when administered either before, during, or after the ischemic period or even when given only during the reperfusion period (Lépicier, Bibeau-Poirier, Lagneux, Servant, & Lamontagne, 2006). The cardioprotective effects of CB_2R activation may involve signaling via protein kinase C (PKC) and mitogen-activated protein kinases (MAPKs) given that pharmacological inhibition of these pathways abrogates the protective effects of cannabinoids acting at CB_2R (Montecucco, Lenglet, et al., 2009; Lépicier et al., 2006). In another study of cardiac I/R injury in rat following left coronary artery occlusion, Li, Wang, Zhang, Zhou, and Zhang (2013) also reported that the CB_2R agonist, JWH-133, albeit at a relatively high dose (20 mg/kg i.v.), was cardioprotective and could reduce infarct size and prevent apoptosis during ischemia–reperfusion via mechanisms that involved inhibition of the intrinsic mitochondria-mediated apoptotic pathway and the PI3K/Akt signaling pathway (Li et al., 2013). Confirmation of the involvement of CB_2R in the cardioprotective effects of JWH-133 was obtained in this latter study using the CB_2R antagonist, AM630, which blocked the infarct reduction seen with the CB_2R agonist. Another study using wild-type (WT) and CB_2R knockout ($CB_2R^{-/-}$) mice further validated CB_2R as a target for the cardioprotection seen with JWH-133 (Defer et al., 2009). In this study, the authors used a lower dose of JWH-133 (3 mg/kg) at the end of a 1 h coronary artery occlusion and still obtained cardioprotection in WT animals. When hearts from WT animals were compared to $CB_2R^{-/-}$ hearts in this study, infarct size was greater and $CB_2R^{-/-}$ hearts had significantly more apoptosis and remodeling at 3 days after I/R injury together with enhanced fibrosis and left ventricular dysfunction.

Taken together, the results of these investigations provide promising experimental evidence that CB_2R is a useful target for the development of cardioprotective drugs and that CB_2R selective agonists may have utility in reducing cardiac pathology in ischemic cardiac disease (Fig. 2). However, significantly more studies are required to determine the dose-dependent effects of cannabinoids during the pre- and postischemic periods in cardiac I/R in order to clarify the mechanisms of action of CB_2R activation in reducing infarct size and cardiac remodeling and to optimize drug regimens during cardiac I/R injury.

Atherosclerosis falls under the umbrella of chronic inflammatory diseases and is the leading cause of mortality worldwide. It is a complex disease involving alterations in lipid metabolism with subsequent accumulation of cholesterol in the vessel wall together with plaque formation. Thrombolytic arterial blockage as a result of instability and rupture of atherosclerotic plaques results in cardiac infarct and stroke (Boudoulas, Triposciadis, Geleris, & Boudoulas, 2016). A greater understanding of the mechanisms giving rise to atherosclerosis has been aided by the generation of mouse models that mimic some of the aspects of the human disease. These include the apolipoprotein E (ApoE)-null and low-density lipoprotein receptor (LDLR)-null atherosclerosis mouse models (Getz & Reardon, 2015; Trusca, Fuior, & Gafencu, 2015).

A growing body of evidence suggests that alterations in the ECS may contribute to atherosclerosis (reviewed in Maccarrone et al., 2008; Steffens & Pacher, 2012); increased endocannabinoid levels and expression of CB_1R and CB_2R have been reported in atheromatous plaques in humans

(Meletta et al., 2017; Sugamura et al., 2009; Zhang et al., 2015) and in mouse models of atherosclerosis (Montecucco, Matias, et al., 2009). However, while activation of CB_1R in some experimental studies appears to be largely proatherosclerotic (Dol-Gleizes et al., 2009), CB_2R activation appears to contribute to antiinflammatory and antiatherosclerotic effects (reviewed in Carbone et al., 2014; O'Sullivan, 2015; Steffens & Pacher, 2015). In vitro studies of macrophage efferocytosis (the ability to clear apoptotic cells), a major contributer to atherosclerotic plaque stability, was improved when cells were treated with the CB_2R selective agonists, HU-308 or JWH-133 (Jiang et al., 2016). In a study of cultured human coronary artery smooth muscle cells, the selective CB_2R agonists, JWH-133 and HU-308, dose-dependently attenuated TNF-alpha-induced proliferation of smooth muscle cells and decreased TNF-alpha-induced Ras superfamily GTPases, MAPK, and Akt signaling (Rajesh et al., 2008).

In vivo, the experimental data examining cannabinoid actions between different mouse models of atherosclerosis has not always been consistent. The phytocannabinoid, THC, and the synthetic cannabinoid, WIN55212-2, both of which nonselectively activate CB_1R and CB_2R, were both able to reduce atherosclerosis in ApoE-null mice (Hoyer et al., 2011; Steffens et al., 2005; Zhao et al., 2010). These antiatherosclerotic effects were sensitive to CB_2R antagonism and mediated via a reduction in inflammation, monocyte recruitment, and adhesion factors. However, WIN55212-2 and the selective CB_2R agonist, JWH133, did not affect atherosclerotic lesion progression in LDLR-null mice, although activation of CB_2R in LDLR mice did reduce macrophage infiltration into plaques (Netherland-Van Dyke, Rodgers, Fulmer, Lahr, & Thewke, 2015). Increased neutrophil recruitment, reactive oxygen species production, and lesional macrophage and smooth muscle cells content, together with decreased endothelial cell dysfunction, was also seen with CB_2R gene deletion in ApoE-null and LDLR-null mice (Hoyer et al., 2011; Netherland, Pickle, Bales, & Thewke, 2010).

Overall, despite some variability between reported effects in mouse models of atherosclerosis, and taken together with in vitro data demonstrating that CB_2R activation improves macrophage efferocytosis, decreases proliferation of vascular smooth muscle cells, and reduces proinflammatory cytokine production, ROS, and neutrophil chemotaxis and adhesion, the data support a role for CB_2R, and cannabinoids that activate CB_2R, as a novel antiinflammatory treatment in atherosclerosis (Fig. 3).

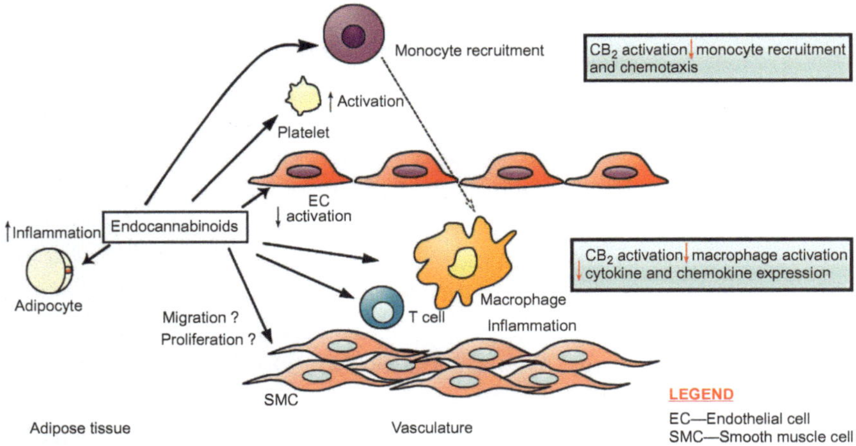

Fig. 3 An antiinflammatory role for CB_2R activation in atherosclerosis. Activation of CB_2R inhibits monocyte recruitment and chemotaxis and is associated with decreases in adhesion factors, proinflammatory chemokines, and cytokines and decreases in macrophage activation and infiltration into plaques. CB_2R expressed on T-cells may modulate T lymphocytes. Pathological increases in endocannabinoids (AEA, 2-AG) and activation of CB_2R-independent targets, including CB_1R, may contribute to disease progression, including adipose tissue inflammation, platelet activation, and proliferation of vascular cells. *Figure adapted from Mach F, Steffens, S. (2008). The role of the endocannabinoid system in atherosclerosis. Journal of Neuroendocrinology, 20(Suppl. 1), 53–57.*

6. CLINICAL TRIALS OF CB_1R ANTAGONISTS, CB_2R AGONISTS AND FAAH INHIBITORS

Rimonabant developed by Sanofi-Aventis was the first selective CB_1R antagonist to enter the clinic. Supporting by the strength of preclinical and clinical data on its ability to reduce food intake, improve cardiometabolic parameters, and promote weight loss, rimonabant was licensed as an antiobesity agent (Després, Golay, & Sjöström, 2005; Van Gaal et al., 2008). However, concerns over psychiatric side effects, specifically an increased risk of depression and thoughts of suicide, led to the subsequent market withdrawal of rimonabant in 2008 (Jones, 2008; Le Foll, Gorelick, & Goldberg, 2009). Sanofi-Aventis then discontinued all ongoing clinical development programmes on CB_1R antagonists, including those for smoking cessation. Other pharmaceutical companies also followed suit (Jones, 2008).

In terms of potential benefits of CB_1R antagonists on cardiovascular risks, rimonabant causes a modest reduction in arterial blood pressure in obese patients (Després et al., 2009). This hypotensive effect is likely limited by antagonism of CB_1R- or novel receptor-mediated reduction in cardiac contractility and vascular resistance, as described earlier. Thus far, clinical trials have only found minimal effects of rimonabant on atheroma volume and progression of atherosclerosis in obese patients (STRADIVARIUS trial: Nissen et al., 2008; AUDITOR trial: O′Leary et al., 2011). It also has no significant effect in the time to new cases of stroke, myocardial infarction, or cardiovascular death (AUDITOR: O′Leary et al., 2011). CRESCENDO is a larger double-blinded, multicentre trial that was designed to investigate if rimonabant improves major vascular event-free survival in patients with a history or an increased risk of vascular diseases (on almost 18,700 patients; Topol et al., 2010). Unfortunately, CRESCENDO was prematurely discontinued in 2008 (along with the marketing of rimonabant). Analysis of the initial results from CRESCENDO and another small but completed Phase IV trial, CARDIO-REDUSE appears to suggest that rimonabant has no overall effect on cardiovascular risks (Boesten, Kaper, Stoffers, Kroon, & van Schayck, 2012; Topol et al., 2010). It is, however, important to note that potential clinical benefit of peripherally restricted CB_1R antagonists has not been investigated.

At present, there are no available clinical data on the effects of CB_2R agonists or FAAH inhibitors on cardiovascular health. Several CB_2R agonists (Dhopeshwarkar & Mackie, 2014) and FAAH inhibitors have so far failed to demonstrate clinically meaningful analgesic effects (Huggins, Smart, Langman, Taylor, & Young, 2012; Pawsey et al., 2016). They are considered safe and devoid of psychiatric side effects but appear to lack efficacy in selected types of pain, such as osteoarthritic and neuropathic pain. However, in a recent first-in-human study, an unexpected fatal toxicity involving cerebral tissue damage and neurological symptoms with BIA10–2474, a FAAH inhibitor developed for neuropathic pain (Temporary Specialist Scientific Committee), has led to precautionary suspension of FAAH inhibitor trials for other indications including major depressive disorders. Although this tragedy is possibly due to an off-target action, which could have resulted from drug/metabolite accumulation—due to low drug clearance or saturated metabolitic pathways (Mallet, Dubray, & Dualé, 2016), it has implications for future development of FAAH inhibitors as a mechanistic class, and protocols of first-in-human trials with novel compounds (Eddleston, Cohen, & Webb, 2016).

7. CONCLUSION

To date, there is a wealth of preclinical evidence to indicate that the ECS plays a pivotal role in regulation of the cardiovascular system and could be an important therapeutic target for cardiovascular disease. Exogenous cannabinoids, including phytocannabinoids and synthetic cannabinoids, have chronotropic effects on heart rate and variable actions on blood pressure. We now know that eCBs, including AEA and 2-AG, are present in myocardium, vascular endothelial, and smooth muscle cells as well as circulating immune cells and exert their cardiovascular actions via both CB_1R and CB_2R as well as noncannabinoid receptors that may include TRPV1, PPARγ, and other cannabinoid-binding GPCRs such as GPR55 and GPR18. Given that eCBs are produced "on-demand" and that eCB tone reflects the balance of eCB production and degradation, it is not surprizing that alterations in local eCB production can occur under different physiological conditions or are altered in pathophysiology. This has lent a considerable degree of complexity to deciphering a comprehensive overview of ECS regulation of cardiovascular function. However, cumulative studies are starting to provide a clearer picture of the importance of the ECS, particularly in regulating vascular contractility, as well as identifying the links between ECS dysfunction, the immune system, and cardiovascular disease. For example, we now know that the ECS may have protective effects in the cardiovascular system during sepsis and septic shock and in cases of cardiac I/R as well as cerebrovascular ischemia (stroke). However, in many cases the situation with respect to ECS involvement and drug targeting is not clear in that activation of CB_1R and CB_2R results in opposing or conflicting outcomes. This is particularly so in the case of vascular inflammation and atherosclerotic plaque vulnerability in which activation of CB_1R appears to be proinflammatory, whereas CB_2R activation appears to reduce immune cell recruitment and production of proinflammatory mediators.

What is urgently needed now are preclinical studies of the most promising ECS modulating strategies for cardiovascular disease that are carried out by multiple independent laboratories using standardized approaches that consider disease stage, dosing and drug regimen, routes of delivery, and toxicology and that utilize animal models that closely mimic the human disease. Furthermore, additional human studies that explore in greater detail alterations in ECS components in disease pathology are an essential prerequisite to ensure that those ECS modulating agents that enter into clinical trials are successful and are able to move beyond the current trial failures of FAAH inhibitors and CB_1R inverse agonists/antagonists. That being said, the promise of modulating the ECS for alleviating human disease is enormous, and there is good evidence that ECS-targeted drugs, especially those that selectively activate CB_2R or antagonize peripheral CB_1R in a time- and disease stage-dependent manner, may show promise in mitigating the inflammation that is a part of many cardiovascular pathologies with resultant beneficial outcomes.

CONFLICT OF INTEREST

M.E.M.K. is a founder and Director of Panag Pharma Inc. Panag develops phytotherapeutics for local and regional treatment of pain and inflammation.

ACKNOWLEDGMENTS

M.E.M.K.'s research is funded by the Canadian Institutes of Health Research (Grant# MOP-97768). W.S.V.H. receives financial support from the Wellcome Trust and St George's University of London.

REFERENCES

Amenta, P. S., Jallo, J. I., Tuma, R. F., Hooper, D. C., & Elliott, M. B. (2014). Cannabinoid receptor type-2 stimulation, blockade, and deletion alter the vascular inflammatory responses to traumatic brain injury. *Journal of Neuroinflammation*, *11*, 191.

Andersson, D. A., Adner, M., Högestätt, E. D., & Zygmunt, P. M. (2002). Mechanisms underlying tissue selectivity of anandamide and other vanilloid receptor agonists. *Molecular Pharmacology*, *62*(3), 705–713.

Baranowska-Kuczko, M., Kozłowska, H., Kozłowski, M., Schlicker, E., Kloza, M., Surażyński, A., et al. (2014). Mechanisms of endothelium-dependent relaxation evoked by anandamide in isolated human pulmonary arteries. *Naunyn-Schmiedeberg's Archives of Pharmacology*, *387*(5), 477–486.

Bátkai, S., Járai, Z., Wagner, J. A., Goparaju, S. K., Varga, K., Liu, J., et al. (2001). Endocannabinoids acting at vascular CB1 receptors mediate the vasodilated state in advanced liver cirrhosis. *Nature Medicine*, 7, 82–832.

Bátkai, S., Pacher, P., Járai, Z., Wagner, J. A., & Kunos, G. (2004b). Cannabinoid antagonist SR-141716 inhibits endotoxic hypotension by a cardiac mechanism not involving CB1 or CB2 receptors. *American Journal of Physiology. Heart and Circulatory Physiology*, *287*(2), H595–H600.

Bátkai, S., Pacher, P., Osei-Hyiaman, D., Radaeva, S., Liu, J., Harvey-White, J., et al. (2004a). Endocannabinoids acting at cannabinoid-1 receptors regulate cardiovascular function in hypertension. *Circulation*, *110*(14), 1996–2002.

Bátkai, S., Rajesh, M., Mukhopadhyay, P., Haskó, G., Liaudet, L., Cravatt, B. F., et al. (2007). Decreased age-related cardiac dysfunction, myocardial nitrative stress, inflammatory gene expression, and apoptosis in mice lacking fatty acid amide hydrolase. *American Journal of Physiology. Heart and Circulatory Physiology*, *293*(2), H909–H918.

Begg, M., Mo, F. M., Offertaler, L., Bátkai, S., Pacher, P., Razdan, R. K., et al. (2003). G protein-coupled endothelial receptor for atypical cannabinoid ligands modulates a Ca2+-dependent K+ current. *The Journal of Biological Chemistry*, *278*(46), 46188–46194.

Begg, M., Pacher, P., Bátkai, S., Osei-Hyiaman, D., Offertáler, L., Mo, F. M., et al. (2005). Evidence for novel cannabinoid receptors. *Pharmacology & Therapeutics*, *106*(2), 133–145.

Benowitz, N. L., Rosenberg, J., Rogers, W., Bachman, J., & Jones, R. T. (1979). Cardiovascular effects of intravenous delta-9-tetrahydrocannabinol: Autonomic nervous mechanisms. *Clinical Pharmacology and Therapeutics*, *25*, 440–446.

Ben-Shabat, S., Fride, E., Sheskin, T., Tamiri, T., Rhee, M. H., Vogel, Z., et al. (1998). An entourage effect: Inactive endogenous fatty acid glycerol esters enhance 2-arachidonoyl-glycerol cannabinoid activity. *European Journal of Pharmacology*, *353*(1), 23–31.

Benyó, Z., Ruisanchez, É., Leszl-Ishiguro, M., Sándor, P., & Pacher, P. (2016). Endocannabinoids in cerebrovascular regulation. *American Journal of Physiology. Heart and Circulatory Physiology*, *310*(7), H785–H801.

Berdyshev, E. V., Boichot, E., Germain, N., Allain, N., Anger, J. P., & Lagente, V. (1997). Influence of fatty acid ethanolamides and delta9-tetrahydrocannabinol on cytokine and arachidonate release by mononuclear cells. *European Journal of Pharmacology*, *330*(2–3), 231–240.

Boesten, J. E., Kaper, J., Stoffers, H. E., Kroon, A. A., & van Schayck, O. C. (2012). Rimonabant improves obesity but not the overall cardiovascular risk and quality of life; results from CARDIO-REDUSE (CArdiometabolic risk reDuctIOn by Rimonabant: The effectiveness in daily practice and its USE). *Family Practice*, *29*(5), 521–527.

Bondarenko, A. I. (2014). Endothelial atypical cannabinoid receptor: Do we have enough evidence? *British Journal of Pharmacology*, *171*(24), 5573–5588.

Bonz, A., Laser, M., Küllmer, S., Kniesch, S., Babin-Ebell, J., Popp, V., et al. (2003). Cannabinoids acting on CB1 receptors decrease contractile performance in human atrial muscle. *Journal of Cardiovascular Pharmacology*, *41*(4), 657–664.

Boudoulas, K. D., Triposciadis, F., Geleris, P., & Boudoulas, H. (2016). Coronary atherosclerosis: Pathophysiologic basis for diagnosis and management. *Progress in Cardiovascular Diseases*, *58*(6), 676–692.

Burkovskiy, I., Zhou, J., & Lehmann, C. (2016). Experimental cannabinoid 2 receptor in CNS injury-induced immunodeficiency syndrome. *Microcirculation*, *23*(4), 283–292.

Calkin, A. C., & Thomas, M. C. (2008). PPAR agonists and cardiovascular disease in diabetes. *PPAR Research*, *2008*, 245410.

Capettini, L. S., Savergnini, S. Q., da Silva, R. F., Stergiopulos, N., Santos, R. A., Mach, F., et al. (2012). Update on the role of cannabinoid receptors after ischemic stroke. *Mediators of Inflammation*, *2012*, 824093.

Carbone, F., Mach, F., Vuilleumier, N., & Montecucco, F. (2014). Cannabinoid receptor type 2 activation in atherosclerosis and acute cardiovascular diseases. *Current Medicinal Chemistry*, *21*(35), 4046–4058.

Carnevali, L., Vacondio, F., Rossi, S., Macchi, E., Spadoni, G., Bedini, A., et al. (2015). Cardioprotective effects of fatty acid amide hydrolase inhibitor URB694, in a rodent model of trait anxiety. *Scientific Reports*, *5*, 18218.

Carney, R. M., Freedland, K. E., Miller, G. E., & Jaffe, A. S. (2002). Depression as a risk factor for cardiac mortality and morbidity: A review of potential mechanisms. *Journal of Psychosomatic Research*, *53*(4), 897–902.

Chiurchiu, V. (2016). Endocannabinoids and immunity. *Cannabis and Cannabinoid Research*, *1*(1), 59–66.

Chiurchiu, V., Battistini, L., & Maccarrone, M. (2015). Endocannabinoid signaling in innate and adaptive immunity. *Immunology*, *144*(3), 352–364.

Cravatt, B. F., Demarest, K., Patricelli, M. P., Bracey, M. H., Giang, D. K., Martin, B. R., et al. (2001). Supersensitivity to anandamide and enhanced endogenous cannabinoid signaling in mice lacking fatty acid amide hydrolase. *Proceedings of the National Academy of Sciences of the United States of America*, *98*(16), 9371–9376.

Cravatt, B. F., Giang, D. K., Mayfield, S. P., Boger, D. L., Lerner, R. A., & Gilula, N. B. (1996). Molecular characterization of an enzyme that degrades neuromodulatory fatty-acid amides. *Nature, 384*(6604), 83–87.

Csóka, B., Németh, Z. H., Mukhopadhyay, P., Spolarics, Z., Rajesh, M., Federici, S., et al. (2009). CB2 cannabinoid receptors contribute to bacterial invasion and mortality in polymicrobial sepsis. *PloS One, 4*(7), e6409.

Daly, C. J., Ross, R. A., Whyte, J., Henstridge, C. M., Irving, A. J., & McGrath, J. C. (2010). Fluorescent ligand binding reveals heterogeneous distribution of adrenoceptors and 'cannabinoid-like' receptors in small arteries. *British Journal of Pharmacology, 159*(4), 787–796.

Dean, C. (2011). Cannabinoid and GABA modulation of sympathetic nerve activity and blood pressure in the dorsal periaqueductal gray of the rat. *American Journal of Physiology. Regulatory, Integrative and Comparative Physiology, 301*(6), R1765–R1772.

Defer, N., Wan, J., Souktani, R., Escoubet, B., Perier, M., Caramelle, P., et al. (2009). The cannabinoid receptor type 2 promotes cardiac myocyte and fibroblast survival and protects against ischemia/reperfusion-induced cardiomyopathy. *The FASEB Journal, 23*(7), 2120–2130.

Després, J. P., Golay, A., & Sjöström, L. (2005). Effects of rimonabant on metabolic risk factors in overweight patients with dyslipidemia. *The New England Journal of Medicine, 353*, 2121–2134.

Després, J. P., Ross, R., Boka, G., Alméras, N., Lemieux, I., & ADAGIO-Lipids Investigators (2009). Effect of rimonabant on the high-triglyceride/ low-HDL-cholesterol dyslipidemia, intraabdominal adiposity, and liver fat: The ADAGIO-lipids trial. *Arteriosclerosis, Thrombosis, and Vascular Biology, 29*(3), 416–423.

Deutsch, D. G., Goligorsky, M. S., Schmid, P. C., Krebsbach, R. J., Schmid, H. H., Das, S. K., et al. (1997). Production and physiological actions of anandamide in the vasculature of the rat kidney. *The Journal of Clinical Investigation, 100*, 1538–1546.

Devane, W. A., Hanus, L., Breuer, A., Pertwee, R. G., Stevenson, L. A., Griffin, G., et al. (1992). Isolation and structure of a brain constituent that binds to the cannabinoid receptor. *Science, 258*(5090), 1946–1949.

Dhopeshwarkar, A., & Mackie, K. (2014). CB2 cannabinoid receptors as a therapeutic target—What does the future hold? *Molecular Pharmacology, 86*(4), 430–437.

Di Marzo, V. (2006). Endocannabinoids: Synthesis and degradation. In S. G. Amara, et al. (Eds.), *Review of physiology biochemistry and pharmacology: Vol. 160* (pp. 1–24). Berlin/Heidelberg: Springer.

Dinh, T. P., Carpenter, D., Leslie, F. M., Freund, T. F., Katona, I., Sensi, S. L., et al. (2002). Brain monoglyceride lipase participating in endocannabinoid inactivation. *Proceedings of the National Academy of Sciences of the United States of America, 99*(16), 10819–10824.

Dirnagl, U., Klehmet, J., Braun, J. S., Harms, H., Meisel, C., Ziemssen, T., et al. (2007). Stroke-induced immunodepression: Experimental evidence and clinical relevance. *Stroke, 38*(Suppl. 2), 770–773.

Dol-Gleizes, F., Paumelle, R., Visentin, V., Marés, A. M., Desitter, P., Hennuyer, N., et al. (2009). Rimonabant, a selective cannabinoid CB1 receptor antagonist, inhibits atherosclerosis in LDL receptor-deficient mice. *Arteriosclerosis, Thrombosis, and Vascular Biology, 29*, 12–18.

Eddleston, M., Cohen, A. F., & Webb, D. J. (2016). Implications of the BIA-102474-101 study for review of first-into-human clinical trials. *British Journal of Clinical Pharmacology, 81*(4), 582–586.

Fant, R. V., Heishman, S. J., Bunker, E. B., & Pickworth, W. B. (1998). Acute and residual effects of marijuana in humans. *Pharmacology, Biochemistry, and Behavior, 60*(4), 777–784.

Fernández-Ruiz, J., Moro, M. A., & Martínez-Orgado, J. (2015). Cannabinoids in neurodegenerative disorders and stroke/brain trauma: From preclinical models to clinical applications. *Neurotherapeutics, 12*, 793–806.

Frantz, S., Ertl, G., & Bauersachs, J. (2007). Mechanisms of disease: Toll-like receptors in cardiovascular disease. *Nature Clinical Practice Cardiovascular Medicine*, *4*(8), 444–454.
Gaoni, Y., & Mechoulam, R. (1964). Isolation, structure and partial synthesis if an active constituent of hashish. *Journal of the American Chemical Society*, *86*, 1646–1647.
García Mdel, C., Adler-Graschinsky, E., & Celuch, S. M. (2009). Enhancement of the hypotensive effects of intrathecally injected endocannabinoids by the entourage compound palmitoylethanolamide. *European Journal of Pharmacology*, *610*(1–3), 75–80.
Gardiner, S. M., March, J. E., Kemp, P. A., & Bennett, T. (2002). Complex regional haemodynamic effects of anandamide in conscious rats. *British Journal of Pharmacology*, *135*(8), 1889–1896.
Gardiner, S. M., March, J. E., Kemp, P. A., & Bennett, T. (2009). Factors influencing the regional haemodynamic responses to methanandamide and anandamide in conscious rats. *British Journal of Pharmacology*, *158*(4), 1143–1152.
Gaskari, S. A., Liu, H., D'Mello, C., Kunos, G., & Lee, S. S. (2015). Blunted cardiac response to hemorrhage in cirrhotic rats is mediated by local macrophage-released endocannabinoids. *Journal of Hepatology*, *62*(6), 1272–1277.
Gauthier, K. M., Baewer, D. V., Hittner, S., Hillard, C. J., Nithipatikom, K., Reddy, D. S., et al. (2005). Endothelium-derived 2-arachidonylglycerol: An intermediate in vasodilatory eicosanoid release in bovine coronary arteries. *American Journal of Physiology. Heart and Circulatory Physiology*, *288*(3), H1344–H1351.
Gebremedhin, D., Lange, A. R., Campbell, W. B., Hillard, C. J., & Harder, D. R. (1999). Cannabinoid CB1 receptor of cat cerebral arterial muscle functions to inhibit L-type Ca2+ channel current. *The American Journal of Physiology*, *266*, H2085–H2093.
Gerard, C. M., Mollereau, C., Vassart, G., & Parmentier, M. (1991). Molecular cloning of a human cannabinoid receptor which is also expressed in testis. *Biochemical Journal*, *279*, 129–134.
Getz, G. S., & Reardon, C. A. (2015). Use of mouse models in atherosclerosis research. *Methods in Molecular Biology*, *1339*, 1–16.
Godlewski, G., Alapafuja, S. O., Bátkai, S., Nikas, S. P., Cinar, R., Offertáler, L., et al. (2010). Inhibitor of fatty acid amide hydrolase normalizes cardiovascular function in hypertension without adverse metabolic effects. *Chemistry & Biology*, *17*(11), 1256–1266.
Godlewski, G., Offertáler, L., Osei-Hyiaman, D., Mo, F. M., Harvey-White, J., Liu, J., et al. (2009). The endogenous brain constituent N-arachidonoyl L-serine is an activator of large conductance Ca2+-activated K+ channels. *The Journal of Pharmacology and Experimental Therapeutics*, *328*(1), 351–361.
Gorelick, D. A., Heishman, S. J., Preston, K. L., Nelson, R. A., Moolchan, E. T., & Huestis, M. A. (2006). The cannabinoid CB1 receptor antagonist rimonabant attenuates the hypotensive effect of smoked marijuana in male smokers. *American Heart Journal*, *151*(3), 754.e1–754.e5.
Gruden, G., Barutta, F., Kunos, G., & Pacher, P. (2016). Role of the endocannabinoid system in diabetes and diabetic complications. *British Journal of Pharmacology*, *173*(7), 1116–1127.
Gui, H., Sun, Y., Luo, Z. M., Su, D. F., Dai, S. M., & Liu, X. (2013). Cannabinoid receptor 2 protects against acute experimental sepsis in mice. *Mediators of Inflammation*, *2013*, 741303.
Guyenet, P. G. (2006). The sympathetic control of blood pressure. *Nature Reviews Neuroscience*, 7, 335–346.
Hanus, L., Breuer, A., Tchilibon, S., Shiloah, S., Goldenberg, D., Horowitz, M., et al. (1999). HU-308: A specific agonist for CB2, a peripheral cannabinoid receptor. *Proceedings of the National Academy of Sciences of the United States of America*, *96*(25), 14228–14233.
Heath, T. S., Burroughs, Z., Thompson, A. J., & Tecklenburg, F. W. (2012). Acute intoxication caused by a synthetic cannabinoid in two adolescents. *Journal of Pediatric Pharmacology and Therapeutics*, *17*(2), 177–181.

Herkenham, M., Lynn, A. B., Johnson, M. R., Melvin, L. S., De Costa, B. R., & Rice, K. C. (1991). Characterisation and localisation of cannabinoid receptors in rat brain: A quantitative in vitro autoradiographic study. *The Journal of Neuroscience*, *11*, 563–583.

Hill, M. N., Hillard, C. J., Bambico, F. R., Patel, S., Gorzalka, B. B., & Gobbi, G. (2009). The therapeutic potential of the endocannabinoid system for the development of a novel class of antidepressants. *Trends in Pharmacological Sciences*, *30*(9), 484–493.

Hillard, C. J. (2000). Endocannabinoids and vascular function. *The Journal of Pharmacology and Experimental Therapeutics*, *294*(1), 27–32.

Hillard, C. J. (2015). The endocannabinoid signaling system in the CNS: A primer. *International Review of Neurobiology*, *125*, 1–47.

Hillard, C. J., Ho, W. S., Thompson, J., Gauthier, K. M., Wheelock, C. E., Huang, H., et al. (2007). Inhibition of 2-arachidonoylglycerol catabolism modulates vasoconstriction of rat middle cerebral artery by the thromboxane mimetic, U-46619. *British Journal of Pharmacology*, *152*(5), 691–698.

Ho, W. S., Barrett, D. A., & Randall, M. D. (2008). 'Entourage' effects of N-palmitoylethanolamide and N-oleoylethanolamide on vasorelaxation to anandamide occur through TRPV1 receptors. *British Journal of Pharmacology*, *155*(6), 837–846.

Ho, W. S., & Hiley, C. R. (2003). Vasodilator actions of abnormal-cannabidiol in rat isolated small mesenteric artery. *British Journal of Pharmacology*, *138*(7), 1320–1332.

Ho, W. S., Hill, M. N., Miller, G. E., Gorzalka, B. B., & Hillard, C. J. (2012). Serum contents of endocannabinoids are correlated with blood pressure in depressed women. *Lipids in Health and Disease*, *11*, 32.

Ho, W. S., Patel, S., Thompson, J. R., Roberts, C. J., Stuhr, K. L., & Hillard, C. J. (2010). Endocannabinoid modulation of hyperaemia evoked by physiologically relevant stimuli in the rat primary somatosensory cortex. *British Journal of Pharmacology*, *160*(3), 736–746.

Ho, W. S., & Randall, M. D. (2007). Endothelium-dependent metabolism by endocannabinoid hydrolases and cyclooxygenases limits vasorelaxation to anandamide and 2-arachidonoylglycerol. *British Journal of Pharmacology*, *150*(5), 641–651.

Ho, W. S., Zheng, X., & Zhang, D. X. (2015). Role of endothelial TRPV4 channels in vascular actions of the endocannabinoid, 2-arachidonoylglycerol. *British Journal of Pharmacology*, *172*(22), 5251–5264.

Howlett, A. C. (1984). Inhibition of neuroblastoma adenylate cyclase by cannabinoid and nantradol compounds. *Life Sciences*, *35*(17), 1803–1810.

Howlett, A. C., Barth, F., Bonner, T. I., Cabral, G., Casellas, P., Devane, W. A., et al. (2002). International union of pharmacology. XXVII. Classification of cannabinoid receptors. *Pharmacological Reviews*, *54*(2), 161–202.

Hoyer, F. F., Steinmetz, M., Zimmer, S., Becker, A., Lütjohann, D., Buchalla, R., et al. (2011). Atheroprotection via cannabinoid receptor-2 is mediated by circulating and vascular cells in vivo. *Journal of Molecular and Cellular Cardiology*, *51*(6), 1007–1014.

Huggins, J. P., Smart, T. S., Langman, S., Taylor, L., & Young, T. (2012). An efficient randomised, placebo-controlled clinical trial with the irreversible fatty acid amide hydrolase-1 inhibitor PF-04457845, which modulates endocannabinoids but fails to induce effective analgesia in patients with pain due to osteoarthritis of the knee. *Pain*, *153*(9), 1837–1846.

Hydock, D. S., Lien, C. Y., & Hayward, R. (2009). Anandamide preserves cardiac function and geometry in an acute doxorubicin cardiotoxicity rat model. *Pharmacology & Therapeutics*, *106*(2), 133–145.

Ishac, E. J., Jiang, L., Lake, K. D., Varga, K., Abood, M. E., & Kunos, G. (1996). Inhibition of exocytotic noradrenaline release by presynaptic cannabinoid CB1 receptors on peripheral sympathetic nerves. *British Journal of Pharmacology*, *118*(8), 2023–2028.

Járai, Z., Wagner, J. A., Goparaju, S. K., Wang, L., Razdan, R. K., Sugiura, T., et al. (2000). Cardiovascular effects of 2-arachidonoyl glycerol in anesthetized mice. *Hypertension*, *35*(2), 679–684.

Járai, Z., Wagner, J. A., Varga, K., Lake, K. D., Compton, D. R., Martin, B. R., et al. (1999). Cannabinoid-induced mesenteric vasodilation through an endothelial site distinct from CB1 or CB2 receptors. *Proceedings of the National Academy of Sciences of the United States of America, 96*, 14136–14141.

Jiang, L., Chen, Y., Huang, X., Yuan, A., Shao, Q., Pu, J., et al. (2016). Selective activation of CB2 receptor improves efferocytosis in cultured macrophages. *Life Sciences, 161*, 10–18.

Jones, R. T. (2002). Cardiovascular system effects of marijuana. *Journal of Clinical Pharmacology, 42*(Suppl. 11), 58S–63S.

Jones, D. (2008). End of the line for cannabinoid receptor 1 as an anti-obesity target? *Nature Reviews. Drug Discovery, 7*, 961–962.

Jonsson, K. O., Vandevoorde, S., Lambert, D. M., Tiger, G., & Fowler, C. J. (2001). Effects of homologues and analogues of palmitoylethanolamide upon the inactivation of the endocannabinoid anandamide. *British Journal of Pharmacology, 133*(8), 1263–1275.

Jouanjus, E., Lapeyre-Mestre, M., & Micallef, J. (2014). Cannabis use: Signal of increasing risk of serious cardiovascular disorders. *Journal of the American Heart Association, 3*(2), e000638.

Kadoi, Y., Hinohara, H., Kunimoto, F., Saito, S., & Goto, F. (2005). Cannabinoid antagonist AM 281 reduces mortality rate and neurologic dysfunction after cecal ligation and puncture in rats. *Critical Care Medicine, 33*(11), 2629–2636.

Kasten, K. R., Tschöp, J., Tschöp, M. H., & Caldwell, C. C. (2010). The cannabinoid 2 receptor as a potential therapeutic target for sepsis. *Endocrine, Metabolic & Immune Disorders Drug Targets, 10*(3), 224–234.

Kathuria, S., Gaetani, S., Fegley, D., Valiño, F., Duranti, A., Tontini, A., et al. (2003). Modulation of anxiety through blockade of anandamide hydrolysis. *Nature Medicine, 9*(1), 76–81.

Kianian, M., Kelly, M. E., Zhou, J., Hung, O., Cerny, V., Rowden, G., et al. (2014). Cannabinoid receptor 1 inhibition improves the intestinal microcirculation in experimental endotoxemia. *Clinical Hemorheology and Microcirculation, 58*(2), 333–342.

Koura, Y., Ichihara, A., Tada, Y., Kaneshiro, Y., Okada, H., Temm, C. J., et al. (2004). Anandamide decreases glomerular filtration rate through predominant vasodilation of efferent arterioles in rat kidneys. *Journal of the American Society of Nephrology, 15*(6), 1488–1494.

Kozłowska, H., Baranowska, M., Schlicker, E., Kozłowski, M., Laudański, J., & Malinowska, B. (2007). Identification of the vasodilatory endothelial cannabinoid receptor in the human pulmonary artery. *Journal of Hypertension, 25*, 2240–2248.

Kremshofer, J., Siwetz, M., Berghold, V. M., Lang, I., Huppertz, B., & Gauster, M. (2015). A role for GPR55 in human placental venous endothelial cells. *Histochemistry and Cell Biology, 144*(1), 49–58.

Kwolek, G., Zakrzeska, A., Schlicker, E., Göthert, M., Godlewski, G., & Malinowska, B. (2005). Central and peripheral components of the pressor effect of anandamide in urethane-anaesthetized rats. *British Journal of Pharmacology, 145*(5), 567–575.

Ladecola, C., & Anrather, J. (2011). The immunology of stroke: From mechanisms to translation. *Nature Medicine, 17*, 796–808.

Lake, K. D., Martin, B. R., Kunos, G., & Varga, K. (1997). Cardiovascular effects of anandamide in anesthetized and conscious normotensive and hypertensive rats. *Hypertension, 29*, 1204–1210.

Le Foll, B., Gorelick, D. A., & Goldberg, S. R. (2009). The future of endocannabinoid-oriented clinical research after CB1 antagonists. *Psychopharmacology (Berl), 205*(1), 171–174.

Ledent, C., Valverde, O., Cossu, G., Petitet, F., Aubert, J. F., Beslot, F., et al. (1999). Unresponsiveness to cannabinoids and reduced addictive effects of opiates in CB1 receptor knockout mice. *Science, 283*, 401–404.

Lehmann, C., Burkovskiy, I., Kuethe, J., Zhou, J., Caldwell, C., & Kelly, M. E. (2014). Inhibition of the cannabinoid 2 receptor in CNS-injury induced immunodeficiency syndrome. *Medical Hypotheses*, *82*(6), 736–739.

Lenglet, S., Thomas, A., Soehnlein, O., Montecucco, F., Burger, F., Pelli, G., et al. (2013). Fatty acid amide hydrolase deficiency enhances intraplaque neutrophil recruitment in atherosclerotic mice. *Arteriosclerosis, Thrombosis, and Vascular Biology*, *33*(2), 215–223.

Lépicier, P., Bibeau-Poirier, A., Lagneux, C., Servant, M. J., & Lamontagne, D. (2006). Signaling pathways involved in the cardioprotective effects of cannabinoids. *Journal of Pharmacological Sciences*, *102*(2), 155–166.

Li, Q., Wang, F., Zhang, Y. M., Zhou, J. J., & Zhang, Y. (2013). Activation of cannabinoid type 2 receptor by JWH133 protects heart against ischemia/reperfusion-induced apoptosis. *Cellular Physiology and Biochemistry*, *31*(4–5), 693–702.

Maccarrone, M., Bab, I., Bíró, T., Cabral, G. A., Dey, S. K., Di Marzo, V., et al. (2008). Cannabinoid receptors in acute and chronic complications of atherosclerosis. *British Journal of Pharmacology*, *153*(2), 290–298.

Maccarrone, M., Bab, I., Bíró, T., Cabral, G. A., Dey, S. K., Di Marzo, V., et al. (2015). Endocannabinoid signaling at the periphery: 50 years after THC. *Trends in Pharmacological Sciences*, *36*(5), 277–296.

Maccarrone, M., Bari, M., Battista, N., & Finazzi-Agrò, A. (2002). Endocannabinoid degradation, endotoxic shock and inflammation. *Current Drug Targets. Inflammation and Allergy*, *1*(1), 53–63.

MacIntyre, J., Dong, A., Straiker, A., Zhu, J., Howlett, S. E., Bagher, A., et al. (2014). Cannabinoid and lipid-mediated vasorelaxation in retinal microvasculature. *European Journal of Pharmacology*, *735*, 105–114.

Malinowska, B., Kwolek, G., & Gothert, M. (2001a). Anandamide and methanandamide induce both vanilloid VR1- and cannabinoids CB1 receptor-mediated changes in heart rate and blood pressure in anaesthetized rats. *Naunyn-Schmiedeberg's Archives of Pharmacology*, *364*, 562–569.

Malinowska, B., Piszcz, J., Koneczny, B., Hryniewicz, A., & Schlicker, E. (2001b). Modulation of the cardiac autonomic transmission of pithed rats by presynaptic opioid OP4 and cannabinoid CB1 receptors. *Naunyn-Schmiedeberg's Archives of Pharmacology*, *364*(3), 233–241.

Malinowska, B., Zakrzeska, A., Kurz, C. M., Göthert, M., Kwolek, G., Wielgat, P., et al. (2010). Involvement of central beta2-adrenergic, NMDA and thromboxane A2 receptors in the pressor effect of anandamide in rats. *Naunyn-Schmiedeberg's Archives of Pharmacology*, *381*(4), 349–360.

Mallet, C., Dubray, C., & Dualé, C. (2016). FAAH inhibitors in the limelight, but regrettably. *International Journal of Clinical Pharmacology and Therapeutics*, *54*(7), 498–501.

Marichal-Cancino, B. A., Manrique-Maldonado, G., Altamirano-Espinoza, A. H., Ruiz-Salinas, I., González-Hernández, A., Maassenvandenbrink, A., et al. (2013). Analysis of anandamide- and lysophosphatidylinositol-induced inhibition of the vasopressor responses produced by sympathetic stimulation or noradrenaline in pithed rats. *European Journal of Pharmacology*, *721*, 168–177.

Marrs, W. R., Blankman, J. L., Horne, E. A., Thomazeau, A., Lin, Y. H., Coy, J., et al. (2010). The serine hydrolase ABHD6 controls the accumulation and efficacy of 2-AG at cannabinoid receptors. *Nature Neuroscience*, *13*(8), 951–957.

Martins, C. J., Genelhu, V., Pimentel, M. M., Celoria, B. M., Mangia, R. F., Aveta, T., et al. (2015). Circulating endocannabinoids and the polymorphism 385C>a in fatty acid amide hydrolase (FAAH) gene may identify the obesity phenotype related to cardiometabolic risk: A study conducted in a Brazilian population of complex interethnic admixture. *PloS One*, *10*(11), e0142728.

Maslov, L. N., Khaliulin, I., Zhang, Y., Krylatov, A. V., Naryzhnaya, N. V., Mechoulam, R., et al. (2016). Prospects for creation of cardioprotective drugs based on cannabinoid receptor agonists. *Journal of Cardiovascular Pharmacology and Therapeutics, 21*(3), 262–272.

Matouk, A. I., Taye, A., El-Moselhy, M. A., Heeba, G. H., & Abdel-Rahman, A. A. (2017). The effect of chronic activation of the novel endocannabinoid receptor GPR18 on myocardial function and blood pressure in conscious rats. *Journal of Cardiovascular Pharmacology, 69*(1), 23–33.

Matsuda, L. A., Lolait, S. J., Brownstein, M. J., Young, A. C., & Bonner, T. I. (1990). Structure of a cannabinoid receptor and functional expression of the cloned cDNA. *Nature, 346*(6284), 561–564.

McHugh, D., Hu, S. S., Rimmerman, N., Juknat, A., Vogel, Z., Walker, J. M., et al. (2010). N-Arachidonoyl glycine potently drives directed BV-2 microglial migration through GPR18, the putative abnormal cannabidiol receptor. *BMC Neuroscience, 11*, 44.

McNaughton, E. M., Choy, C. T., Sudlow, C. E., & Ho, W. S. V. (2016). In *Role of gpr55 and gpr18 receptors in the vascular actions of endocannabinoids and related lipids. Proceedings of 26th annual symposium of the international cannabinoid research society, Bukovina, Poland, 2016.*

McQueen, D. S., Bond, S. M., Smith, P. J., Balali-Mood, K., & Smart, D. (2004). Cannabidiol lacks the vanilloid VR1-mediated vasorespiratory effects of capsaicin and anandamide in anaesthetised rats. *European Journal of Pharmacology, 491*(2–3), 181–189.

Mechoulam, R., Ben-Shabat, S., Hanus, L., Ligumsky, M., Kaminski, N. E., Schatz, A. R., et al. (1995). Identification of an endogenous 2-monoglyceride, present in canine gut, that binds to cannabinoid receptors. *Biochemical Pharmacology, 50*(1), 83–90.

Mechoulam, R., Feigenbaum, J. J., Lander, N., Segal, M., Järbe, T. U., Hiltunen, A. J., et al. (1988). Enantiomeric cannabinoids: Stereospecificity of psychotropic activity. *Experientia, 44*(9), 762–764.

Mechoulam, R., Hanuš, L. O., Pertwee, R., & Howlett, A. C. (2014). Early phytocannabinoid chemistry to endocannabinoids and beyond. *Nature Reviews Neuroscience, 15*(11), 757–764.

Meisel, C., Schwab, J. M., Prass, K., Meisel, A., & Dirnagl, U. (2005). Central nervous system injury-induced immune deficiency syndrome. *Nature Reviews. Neuroscience, 6*, 775–786.

Meletta, R., Slavik, R., Mu, L., Rancic, Z., Borel, N., Schibli, R., et al. (2017). Cannabinoid receptor type 2 (CB2) as one of the candidate genes in human carotid plaque imaging: Evalu1ation of the novel radiotracer [(11)C]RS-016 targeting CB2 in atherosclerosis. *Nuclear Medicine and Biology, 47*, 31–43.

Miranda, M., Balarini, M., Caixeta, D., & Bouskela, E. (2016). Microcirculatory dysfunction in sepsis: Pathophysiology, clinical monitoring, and potential therapies. *American Journal of Physiology. Heart and Circulatory Physiology, 311*(1), H24–H35.

Molica, F., Burger, F., Thomas, A., Staub, C., Tailleux, A., Staels, B., et al. (2013). Endogenous cannabinoid receptor CB1 activation promotes vascular smooth-muscle cell proliferation and neointima formation. *Journal of Lipid Research, 54*(5), 1360–1368.

Montecucco, F., & Di Marzo, V. (2012). At the heart of the matter: The endocannabinoid system in cardiovascular function and dysfunction. *Trends in Pharmacological Sciences, 33*(6), 331–340.

Montecucco, F., Lenglet, S., Braunersreuther, V., Burger, F., Pelli, G., Bertolotto, M., et al. (2009b). CB(2) cannabinoid receptor activation is cardioprotective in a mouse model of ischemia/reperfusion. *Journal of Molecular and Cellular Cardiology, 46*(5), 612–620.

Montecucco, F., Matias, I., Lenglet, S., Petrosino, S., Burger, F., Pelli, G., et al. (2009a). Regulation and possible role of endocannabinoids and related mediators in hypercholesterolemic mice with atherosclerosis. *Atherosclerosis, 205*(2), 433–441.

Movahed, P., Evilevitch, V., Andersson, T. L. G., Jönsson, B. A. G., Wollmer, P., Zygmunt, P. M., et al. (2005). Vascular effects of anandamide and N-acylvanillylamines in the human forearm and skin microcirculation. *British Journal of Pharmacology*, *146*, 171–179.

Mukhopadhyay, S., Chapnick, B. M., & Howlett, A. C. (2002). Anandamide-induced vasorelaxation in rabbit aortic rings has two components: G protein dependent and independent. *American Journal of Physiology. Heart and Circulatory Physiology*, *282*(6), H2046–H2054.

Mukhopadhyay, P., Horváth, B., Rajesh, M., Matsumoto, S., Saito, K., Bátkai, S., et al. (2011). Fatty acid amide hydrolase is a key regulator of endocannabinoid-induced myocardial tissue injury. *Free Radical Biology & Medicine*, *50*(1), 179–195.

Netherland, C. D., Pickle, T. G., Bales, A., & Thewke, D. P. (2010). Cannabinoid receptor type 2 (CB2) deficiency alters atherosclerotic lesion formation in hyperlipidemic LDLR-null mice. *Atherosclerosis*, *213*(1), 102–108.

Netherland-Van Dyke, C., Rodgers, W., Fulmer, M., Lahr, Z., & Thewke, D. (2015). Cannabinoid receptor type 2 (cb2) dependent and independent effects of WIN55, 212-2 on atherosclerosis in LDLR-null mice. *Journal of Cardiology and Therapeutics*, *3*(2), 53–63.

Niederhoffer, N., & Szabo, B. (2000). Cannabinoids cause central sympathoexcitation and bradycardia in rabbits. *The Journal of Pharmacology and Experimental Therapeutics*, *294*, 707–713.

Nissen, S. E., Nicholls, S. J., Wolski, K., Rodés-Cabau, J., Cannon, C. P., Deanfield, J. E., et al. (2008). Effect of rimonabant on progression of atherosclerosis in patients with abdominal obesity and coronary artery disease: The STRADIVARIUS randomized controlled trial. *Journal of the American Medical Association*, *299*(13), 1547–1560.

Offertáler, L., Mo, F. M., Bátkai, S., Liu, J., Begg, M., Razdan, R. K., et al. (2003). Selective ligands and cellular effectors of a G protein-coupled endothelial cannabinoid receptor. *Molecular Pharmacology*, *63*, 699–705.

O'Leary, D. H., Reuwer, A. Q., Nissen, S. E., Després, J. P., Deanfield, J. E., Brown, M. W., et al. (2011). Effect of rimonabant on carotid intima-media thickness (CIMT) progression in patients with abdominal obesity and metabolic syndrome: The AUDITOR trial. *Heart*, *97*(14), 1143–1150.

O'Sullivan, S. E. (2015). Endocannabinoids and the cardiovascular system in health and disease. *Handbook of Experimental Pharmacology*, *231*, 393–422.

O'Sullivan, S. E. (2016). An update on PPAR activation by cannabinoids. *British Journal of Pharmacology*, *173*(12), 1899–1910.

O'Sullivan, S. E., Kendall, D. A., & Randall, M. D. (2009). Time-dependent vascular effects of endocannabinoids mediated by peroxisome proliferator-activated receptor gamma (PPARγ). *PPAR Research*, *2009*, 425289.

O'Sullivan, S. E., Tarling, E. J., Bennett, A. J., Kendall, D. A., & Randall, M. D. (2005). Novel time-dependent vascular actions of Δ9-tetrahydrocannabinol mediated by peroxisome proliferator-activated receptor gamma. *Biochemical and Biophysical Research Communications*, *337*(3), 824–831.

Overton, H. A., Fyfe, M. C. T., & Reynet, C. (2008). GPR119, a novel G protein-coupled receptor target for the treatment of type 2 diabetes and obesity. *British Journal of Pharmacology*, *153*(Suppl. 1), S76–S81.

Pacher, P., Bátkai, S., & Kunos, G. (2004). Haemodynamic profile and responsiveness to anandamide of TRPV1 receptor knock-out mice. *The Journal of Physiology*, *558*(Pt. 2), 647–657.

Pacher, P., Bátkai, S., Osei-Hyiaman, D., Offertáler, L., Liu, J., Harvey-White, J., et al. (2005). Hemodynamic profile, responsiveness to anandamide, and baroreflex sensitivity of mice lacking fatty acid amide hydrolase. *American Journal of Physiology. Heart and Circulatory Physiology*, *289*(2), H533–H541.

Pacher, P., & Haskó, G. (2008). Endocannabinoids and cannabinoid receptors in ischaemia-reperfusion injury and preconditioning. *British Journal of Pharmacology, 153*(2), 252–262.

Pacher, P., & Mechoulam, R. (2011). Is lipid signaling through cannabinoid 2 receptors part of a protective system? *Progress in Lipid Research, 50*(2), 193–211.

Pacher, P., & Steffens, S. (2009). The emerging role of the endocannabinoid system in cardiovascular disease. *Seminars in Immunopathology, 31*(1), 63–77.

Padley, J. R., Li, Q., Pilowsky, P. M., & Goodchild, A. K. (2003). Cannabinoid receptor activation in the rostral ventrolateral medulla oblongata evokes cardiorespiratory effects in anaesthetised rats. *British Journal of Pharmacology, 140*(2), 384–394.

Parmar, N., & Ho, W. S. (2012). N-arachidonoyl glycine, an endogenous lipid that acts as a vasorelaxant via nitric oxide and large conductance calcium-activated potassium channels. *British Journal of Pharmacology, 160*, 594–603.

Pawsey, S., Wood, M., Browne, H., Donaldson, K., Christie, M., & Warrington, S. (2016). Safety, tolerability and pharmacokinetics of FAAH inhibitor V158866: A double-blind, randomised, placebo-controlled phase I study in healthy volunteers. *Drugs in R&D, 16*(2), 181–191.

Penumarti, A., & Abdel-Rahman, A. A. (2014). Neuronal nitric oxide synthase-dependent elevation in adiponectin in the rostral ventrolateral medulla underlies g protein-coupled receptor 18-mediated hypotension in conscious rats. *The Journal of Pharmacology and Experimental Therapeutics, 351*(1), 44–53.

Pertwee, R. G. (2006). Cannabinoid pharmacology: The first 66 years. *British Journal of Pharmacology, 147*(Suppl. 1), S163–S171.

Pertwee, R. G. (2015). Endocannabinoids and their pharmacological actions. *Handbook of Experimental Pharmacology, 231*, 1–37.

Pertwee, R. G., Howlett, A. C., Abood, M. E., Alexander, S. P., Di Marzo, V., Elphick, M. R., et al. (2010). International Union of Basic and Clinical Pharmacology. LXXIX. Cannabinoid receptors and their ligands: Beyond CB_1 and CB_2. *Pharmacological Reviews, 62*(4), 588–631.

Pisanti, S., & Bifulco, M. (2017). Modern history of medical cannabis: From widespread use to prohibitionism and back. *Trends in Pharmacological Sciences, 38*, 195–198. pii: S0165-6147(16)30184-5.

Pratt, P. F., Hillard, C. J., Edgemond, W. S., & Campbell, W. B. (1998). N-Arachidonylethanolamide relaxation of bovine coronary artery is not mediated by CB1 cannabinoid receptor. *The American Journal of Physiology, 274*(1 Pt. 2), H375–H381.

Quercioli, A., Carbone, F., Bonaventura, A., Liberale, L., Pataky, Z., Thomas, A., et al. (2017). Plasma palmitoylethanolamide (PEA) as a potential biomarker for impaired coronary function. *International Journal of Cardiology, 231*, 1–5. pii: S0167-5273(16) 32953-9.

Rademacher, D. J., Patel, S., Ho, W. S., Savoie, A. M., Rusch, N. J., Gauthier, K. M., et al. (2005). U-46619 but not serotonin increases endocannabinoid content in middle cerebral artery: Evidence for functional relevance. *American Journal of Physiology. Heart and Circulatory Physiology, 288*(6), H2694–H2701.

Rajesh, M., Bátkai, S., Kechrid, M., Mukhopadhyay, P., Lee, W. S., Horváth, B., et al. (2012). Cannabinoid 1 receptor promotes cardiac dysfunction, oxidative stress, inflammation, and fibrosis in diabetic cardiomyopathy. *Diabetes, 61*(3), 716–727.

Rajesh, M., Mukhopadhyay, P., Bátkai, S., Haskó, G., Liaudet, L., Huffman, J. W., et al. (2007). CB2-receptor stimulation attenuates TNF-alpha-induced human endothelial cell activation, transendothelial migration of monocytes, and monocyte-endothelial adhesion. *American Journal of Physiology. Heart and Circulatory Physiology, 293*(4), H2210–H2218.

Rajesh, M., Mukhopadhyay, P., Haskó, G., Huffman, J. W., Mackie, K., & Pacher, P. (2008). CB2 cannabinoid receptor agonists attenuate TNF-alpha-induced human vascular smooth muscle cell proliferation and migration. *British Journal of Pharmacology, 153*(2), 347–357.

Roest, A. M., Martens, E. J., de Jonge, P., & Denollet, J. (2010). Anxiety and risk of incident coronary heart disease: A meta-analysis. *Journal of the American College of Cardiology*, *56*(1), 38–46.

Rom, S., & Persidsky, Y. (2013). Cannabinoid receptor 2: Potential role in immunomodulation and neuroinflammation. *Journal of Neuroimmune Pharmacology*, *8*(3), 608–620.

Romano, M. R., & Lograno, M. D. (2006). Cannabinoid agonists induce relaxation in the bovine ophthalmic artery: Evidences for CB1 receptors, nitric oxide and potassium channels. *British Journal of Pharmacology*, *147*(8), 917–925.

Romano, M. R., & Lograno, M. D. (2012). Involvement of the peroxisome proliferator-activated receptor (PPAR) alpha in vascular response of endocannabinoids in the bovine ophthalmic artery. *European Journal of Pharmacology*, *683*(1–3), 197–203.

Ross, R. A. (2009). The enigmatic pharmacology of GPR55. *Trends in Pharmacological Sciences*, *30*(3), 156–163.

Ruilope, L. M., Després, J. P., Scheen, A., Pi-Sunyer, X., Mancia, G., Zanchetti, A., et al. (2008). Effect of rimonabant on blood pressure in overweight/obese patients with/without co-morbidities: Analysis of pooled RIO study results. *Journal of Hypertension*, *26*(2), 357–367.

Russo, E. B. (2011). Taming THC: Potential cannabis synergy and phytocannabinoid-terpenoid entourage effects. *British Journal of Pharmacology*, *163*(7), 1344–1364.

Russo, E. B. (2017). Cannabis and epilepsy: An ancient treatment returns to the fore. *Epilepsy & Behavior*, *70*(Pt B), 292–297. pii: S1525-5050(16)30412-7.

Ryberg, E., Larsson, N., Sjögren, S., Hjorth, S., Hermansson, N. O., Leonova, J., et al. (2007). The orphan receptor GPR55 is a novel cannabinoid receptor. *British Journal of Pharmacology*, *152*(7), 1092–1101.

Sagar, D. R., Kendall, D. A., & Chapman, V. (2008). Inhibition of fatty acid amide hydrolase produces PPAR-alpha-mediated analgesia in a rat model of inflammatory pain. *British Journal of Pharmacology*, *155*(8), 1297–1306.

Sardinha, J., Kelly, M. E., Zhou, J., & Lehmann, C. (2014). Experimental cannabinoid 2 receptor-mediated immune modulation in sepsis. *Mediators of Inflammation*, *2014*, 978678.

Sarzani, R., Bordicchia, M., Salvi, F., Cola, G., Franchi, E., Battistoni, I., et al. (2008). A human fatty acid amide hydrolase (FAAH) functional gene variant is associated with lower blood pressure in young males. *American Journal of Hypertension*, *21*(8), 960–963.

Schlosburg, J. E., Blankman, J. L., Long, J. Z., Nomura, D. K., Pan, B., Kinsey, S. G., et al. (2010). Chronic monoacylglycerol lipase blockade causes functional antagonism of the endocannabinoid system. *Nature Neuroscience*, *13*(9), 1113–1119.

Schmid, H. H., Schmid, P. C., & Berdyshev, E. V. (2002). Cell signaling by endocannabinoids and their congeners: Questions of selectivity and other challenges. *Chemistry and Physics of Lipids*, *121*(1–2), 111–134.

Schultheiss, T., Flau, K., Kathmann, M., Göthert, M., & Schlicker, E. (2005). Cannabinoid CB1 receptor-mediated inhibition of noradrenaline release in guinea-pig vessels, but not in rat and mouse aorta. *Naunyn-Schmiedeberg's Archives of Pharmacology*, *372*(2), 139–146.

Seagard, J. L., Dean, C., Patel, S., Rademacher, D. J., Hopp, F. A., Schmeling, W. T., et al. (2004). Anandamide conent, and interaction of endocannabinoid/GABA modulatory effects in the NTS on baroreflex-evoked sympathoinhibition. *American Journal of Physiology Heart and Circulatory Physiology*, *286*, H992–H1000.

Seymour, C. W., Liu, V. X., Iwashyna, T. J., Brunkhorst, F. M., Rea, T. D., Scherag, A., et al. (2016). Assessment of clinical criteria for sepsis: For the third international consensus definitions for sepsis and septic shock (sepsis-3). *JAMA*, *315*(8), 762–774.

Sharir, H., & Abood, M. E. (2010). Pharmacological characterization of GPR55, a putative cannabinoid receptor. *Pharmacology and Therapeutics*, *126*, 301–313.

Singer, M., Deutschman, C. S., Seymour, C. W., Shankar-Hari, M., Annane, D., Bauer, M., et al. (2016). The third international consensus definitions for sepsis and septic shock (sepsis-3). *Journal of the American Medical Association, 315*(8), 801–810.

Slavic, S., Lauer, D., Sommerfeld, M., Kemnitz, U. R., Grzesiak, A., Trappiel, M., et al. (2013). Cannabinoid receptor 1 inhibition improves cardiac function and remodelling after myocardial infarction and in experimental metabolic syndrome. *Journal of Molecular Medicine, 91*(7), 811–823.

Smart, D., Jonsson, K. O., Vandevoorde, S., Lambert, D. M., & Fowler, C. J. (2002). 'Entourage' effects of N-acyl ethanolamines at human vanilloid receptors. Comparison of effects upon anandamide-induced vanilloid receptor activation and upon anandamide metabolism. *British Journal of Pharmacology, 136*(3), 452–458.

Stanley, C. P., Hind, W. H., Tufarelli, C., & O'Sullivan, S. E. (2016). The endocannabinoid anandamide causes endothelium-dependent vasorelaxation in human mesenteric arteries. *Pharmacological Research, 113*(Pt. A), 356–363.

Stanley, C. P., & O'Sullivan, S. E. (2014). Cyclooxygenase metabolism mediates vasorelaxation to 2-arachidonoylglycerol (2-AG) in human mesenteric arteries. *Pharmacological Research, 81*, 74–82.

Starowicz, K., Makuch, W., Korostynski, M., Malek, N., Slezak, M., Zychowska, M., et al. (2013). Full inhibition of spinal FAAH leads to TRPV1-mediated analgesic effects in neuropathic rats and possible lipoxygenase-mediated remodeling of anandamide metabolism. *PloS One, 8*(4), e60040.

Steffens, S., & Pacher, P. (2012). Targeting cannabinoid receptor CB(2) in cardiovascular disorders: Promises and controversies. *British Journal of Pharmacology, 167*(2), 313–323.

Steffens, S., & Pacher, P. (2015). The activated endocannabinoid system in atherosclerosis: Driving force or protective mechanism? *Current Drug Targets, 16*(4), 334–341.

Steffens, S., Veillard, N. R., Arnaud, C., Pelli, G., Burger, F., Staub, C., et al. (2005). Low dose oral cannabinoid therapy reduces progression of atherosclerosis in mice. *Nature, 434*(7034), 782–786.

Sugamura, K., Sugiyama, S., Nozaki, T., Matsuzawa, Y., Izumiya, Y., Miyata, K., et al. (2009). Activated endocannabinoid system in coronary artery disease and anti-inflammatory effects of cannabinoid 1 receptor blockade on macrophages. *Circulation, 119*(1), 28–36.

Sugiura, T., Kondo, S., Sukagawa, A., Nakane, S., Shinoda, A., Itoh, K., et al. (1995). 2-Arachidonoylglycerol: A possible endogenous cannabinoid receptor ligand in brain. *Biochemical and Biophysical Research Communications, 215*(1), 89–97.

Szekeres, M., Nádasy, G. L., Turu, G., Soltész-Katona, E., Benyó, Z., Offermanns, S., et al. (2015). Endocannabinoid-mediated modulation of Gq/11 protein-coupled receptor signaling-induced vasoconstriction and hypertension. *Molecular and Cellular Endocrinology, 403*, 46–56.

Temporary Specialist Scientific Committee (TSSC), & FAAH (Fatty Acid Amide Hydrolase). Report on the Causes of the Accident during a Phase 1 Clinical Trial in Rennes in January 2016. Available from http://www.ansm.sante.fr/var/ansm_site/storage/original/application/744c7c6daf96b141bc9509e2f85c227e.pdf.

Toczek, M., Baranowska-Kuczko, M., Grzęda, E., Pędzińska-Betiuk, A., Weresa, J., & Malinowska, B. (2016). Age-specific influences of chronic administration of the fatty acid amide hydrolase inhibitor URB597 on cardiovascular parameters and organ hypertrophy in DOCA-salt hypertensive rats. *Pharmacological Reports, 68*(2), 363–369.

Toguri, J. T., Lehmann, C., Laprairie, R. B., Szczesniak, A. M., Zhou, J., Denovan-Wright, E. M., et al. (2014). Anti-inflammatory effects of cannabinoid CB(2) receptor activation in endotoxin-induced uveitis. *British Journal of Pharmacology, 171*(6), 1448–1461.

Toguri, J. T., Moxsom, R., Szczesniak, A. M., Zhou, J., Kelly, M. E., & Lehmann, C. (2015). Cannabinoid 2 receptor activation reduces leukocyte adhesion and improves capillary perfusion in the iridial microvasculature during systemic inflammation. *Clinical Hemorheology and Microcirculation*, *61*(2), 237–249.

Topol, E. J., Bousser, M. G., Fox, K. A., Creager, M. A., Despres, J. P., Easton, J. D., et al. (2010). Rimonabant for prevention of cardiovascular events (CRESCENDO): A randomised, multicentre, placebo-controlled trial. *Lancet*, *376*(9740), 517–523.

Trusca, V. G., Fuior, E. V., & Gafencu, A. V. (2015). Beyond lipoprotein receptors: Learning from receptor knockouts mouse models about new targets for reduction of the atherosclerotic plaque. *Current Molecular Medicine*, *15*(10), 905–931.

Tschöp, J., Kasten, K. R., Nogueiras, R., Goetzman, H. S., Cave, C. M., England, L. G., et al. (2009). The cannabinoid receptor 2 is critical for the host response to sepsis. *Journal of Immunology*, *183*(1), 499–505.

Urquhart, P., Nicolaou, A., & Woodward, D. F. (2015). Endocannabinoids and their oxygenation by cyclo-oxygenases, lipoxygenases and other oxygenases. *Biochimica et Biophysica Acta*, *1851*(4), 366–376.

Vallejo, J. G. (2011). Role of toll-like receptors in cardiovascular diseases. *Clinical Science (London, England)*, *121*(1), 1–10.

Van Gaal, L. F., Scheen, A. J., Rissanen, A. M., Rössner, S., Hanotin, C., & Ziegler, O. (2008). Long-term effect of CB1 blockade with rimonabant on cardiometabolic risk factors: Two year results from the RIO-Europe study. *European Heart Journal*, *29*(14), 1761–1771.

Van Sickle, M. D., Duncan, M., Kingsley, P. J., Mouihate, A., Urbani, P., Mackie, K., et al. (2005). Identification and functional characterization of brainstem cannabinoid CB2 receptors. *Science*, *310*(5746), 329–332.

Varga, K., Lake, K. D., Huangfu, D., Guyenet, P. G., & Kunos, G. (1996). Mechanism of the hypotensive action of anandamide in anesthetized rats. *Hypertension*, *28*, 682–686.

Varga, K., Lake, K., Martin, B. R., & Kunos, G. (1995). Novel antagonist implicates the CB1 cannabinoid receptor in the hypotensive action of anandamide. *European Journal of Pharmacology*, *278*, 279–283.

Varga, K., Wagner, J. A., Bridgen, D. T., & Kunos, G. (1998). Platelet- and macrophage-derived endogenous cannabinoids are involved in endotoxin-induced hypotension. *The FASEB Journal*, *12*(11), 1035–1044.

Vujic, N., Schlager, S., Eichmann, T. O., Madreiter-Sokolowski, C. T., Goeritzer, M., Rainer, S., et al. (2016). Monoglyceride lipase deficiency modulates endocannabinoid signaling and improves plaque stability in ApoE-knockout mice. *Atherosclerosis*, *244*, 9–21.

Wagner, J. A., Hu, K., Bauersachs, J., Karcher, J., Wiesler, M., Goparaju, S. K., et al. (2001a). Endogenous cannabinoids mediate hypotension after experimental myocardial infarction. *American College of Cardiology*, *38*(7), 2048–2054.

Wagner, J. A., Járai, Z., Bátkai, S., & Kunos, G. (2001b). Hemodynamic effects of cannabinoids: Coronary and cerebral vasodilation mediated by cannabinoid CB(1) receptors. *European Journal of Pharmacology*, *423*, 203–210.

Wagner, J. A., Varga, K., Ellis, E. F., Rzigalinski, B. A., Martin, B. R., & Kunos, G. (1997). Activation of peripheral CB1 cannabinoid receptors in haemorrhagic shock. *Nature*, *390*(6659), 518–521.

Wahn, H., Wolf, J., Kram, F., Frantz, S., & Wagner, J. A. (2005). The endocannabinoid arachidonyl ethanolamide (anandamide) increases pulmonary arterial pressure via cyclooxygenase-2 products in isolated rabbit lungs. *American Journal of Physiology. Heart and Circulatory Physiology*, *289*(6), H2491–H2496.

Waldeck-Weiermair, M., Zoratti, C., Osibow, K., Balenga, N., Goessnitzer, E., Waldhoer, M., et al. (2008). Integrin clustering enables anandamide-induced Ca2+

signaling in endothelial cells via GPR55 by protection against CB1-receptor-triggered repression. *Journal of Cell Science, 121*(Pt. 10), 1704–1717.

Weimar, C., Roth, M. P., Zillessen, G., Glahn, J., Wimmer, M. L., Busse, O., et al. (2002). Complications following acute ischemic stroke. *European Neurology, 48*(3), 133–140.

Wenzel, D., Matthey, M., Bindila, L., Lerner, R., Lutz, B., Zimmer, A., et al. (2013). Endocannabinoid anandamide mediates hypoxic pulmonary vasoconstriction. *Proceedings of the National Academy of Sciences of the United States of America, 110*(46), 18710–18715.

White, R., Ho, W. S., Bottrill, F. E., Ford, W. R., & Hiley, C. R. (2001). Mechanisms of anandamide-induced vasorelaxation in rat isolated coronary arteries. *British Journal of Pharmacology, 134*, 921–929.

Xiong, W., Cui, T., Cheng, K., Yang, F., Chen, S. R., Willenbring, D., et al. (2012). Cannabinoids suppress inflammatory and neuropathic pain by targeting α3 glycine receptors. *The Journal of Experimental Medicine, 209*(6), 1121–1134.

Yu, S. J., Reiner, D., Shen, H., Wu, K. J., Liu, Q. R., & Wang, Y. (2015). Time-dependent protection of CB2 receptor agonist in stroke. *PloS One, 10*(7), e0132487.

Zakrzeska, A., Schlicker, E., Baranowska, M., Kozłowska, H., Kwolek, G., & Malinowska, B. (2010). A cannabinoid receptor, sensitive to O-1918, is involved in the delayed hypotension induced by anandamide in anaesthetized rats. *British Journal of Pharmacology, 160*(3), 574–584.

Zhang, X., Maor, Y., Wang, J. F., Kunos, G., & Groopman, J. E. (2010). Endocannabinoid-like N-arachidonoyl serine is a novel pro-angiogenic mediator. *British Journal of Pharmacology, 160*(7), 1583–1594.

Zhang, S., Shao, P., Ling, X., Yang, L., Hou, W., Thorne, S. H., et al. (2015). In vivo inflammation imaging using a CB2R-targeted near infrared fluorescent probe. *American Journal of Nuclear Medicine and Molecular Imaging, 5*(3), 246–258.

Zhao, Y., Liu, Y., Zhang, W., Xue, J., Wu, Y. Z., Xu, W., et al. (2010). WIN55212-2 ameliorates atherosclerosis associated with suppression of pro-inflammatory responses in ApoE-knockout mice. *European Journal of Pharmacology, 649*, 285–292.

Zubrzycki, M., Liebold, A., Janecka, A., & Zubrzycka, M. (2014). A new face of endocannabinoids in pharmacotherapy. Part I: Protective role of endocannabinoids in hypertension and myocardial infarction. *Journal of Physiology and Pharmacology, 65*(2), 171–181.

Zygmunt, P. M., Ermund, A., Movahed, P., Andersson, D. A., Simonsen, C., Jönsson, B. A., et al. (2013). Monoacylglycerols activate TRPV1—A link between phospholipase C and TRPV1. *PloS One, 8*(12), e81618.

Zygmunt, P. M., Petersson, J., Andersson, D. A., Chuang, H., Sørgård, M., Di Marzo, V., et al. (1999). Vanilloid receptors on sensory nerves mediate the vasodilator action of anandamide. *Nature, 400*(6743), 452–457.

CHAPTER ELEVEN

Is the Cannabinoid CB_2 Receptor a Major Regulator of the Neuroinflammatory Axis of the Neurovascular Unit in Humans?

Dan T. Kho*, Michelle Glass†, Euan S. Graham*,[1]

*School of Medical Sciences, Faculty of Medical and Health Sciences, University of Auckland, Auckland, New Zealand

†Faculty of Medical and Health Sciences, University of Auckland, Auckland, New Zealand

[1]Corresponding author: e-mail address: s.graham@auckland.ac.nz

Contents

Abstract

The central nervous system (CNS) is an immune privileged site where the neurovascular unit (NVU) and the blood–brain barrier (BBB) act as a selectively permeable interface to control the passage of nutrients and inflammatory cells into the brain parenchyma. However, in response to injury, infection, or disease, CNS cells become activated, and release inflammatory mediators to recruit immune cells to the site of inflammation. Increasing evidence suggests that cannabinoids may have a neuroprotective role in CNS inflammatory conditions. For many years, it was widely accepted that cannabinoid receptor type 1 (CB_1) modulates neurological function centrally, while peripheral cannabinoid receptor type 2 (CB_2) modulates immune function. As knowledge about the physiology and pharmacology of the endocannabinoid system advances, there is increasing interest in targeting CB_2 as a potential treatment for inflammation-dependent CNS diseases (Ashton & Glass, 2007), where recent rodent and human

Advances in Pharmacology, Volume 80
ISSN 1054-3589
http://dx.doi.org/10.1016/bs.apha.2017.03.009

studies have implicated intervention at the level of the NVU and BBB. These are incredibly important in brain health and disease. Therefore, this review begins by explaining the cellular and molecular components of these systems, highlighting important molecules potentially regulated by cannabinoid ligands and then takes an unbiased look at the evidence in support (or otherwise) of cannabinoid receptor expression and control of the NVU and BBB function in humans.

ABBREVIATIONS

BBB blood–brain barrier
CB cannabinoid receptor
CD cluster of differentiation
CNS central nervous system
EAE experimental autoimmune encephalomyelitis
FAAH fatty acid amide hydrolase
GPCRs G-protein-coupled receptors
ICAM-1 intercellular adhesion molecule-1
JAM junctional adhesion molecule
K_i inhibitory constant
LFA-1 lymphocyte function-associated antigen 1
MCAO middle cerebral artery occlusion
MS multiple sclerosis
NAPE *N*-acylphosphatidylethanolamine
NVU neurovascular unit
PPAR peroxisome proliferator-activated receptors
VCAM-1 vascular cell adhesion molecule 1
VLA-4 very late antigen 4
ZO zonula occludens

1. INTRODUCTION

1.1 The Endocannabinoid System in Brief

The endocannabinoid system, including endocannabinoids, cannabinoid receptors (CBs), and synthesizing/metabolizing enzymes, is an endogenous system conserved from plants to mammals. *Cannabis sativa*, or marijuana, is the most widely used recreational drug in Western societies, and medicinal use of the plant was recorded over 3000 years ago as pain relief and antianxiety (Pacher, Bátkai, & Kunos, 2006). The field of cannabinoid research took a great leap forward in the 1960s when Gaoni and Mechoulam isolated and identified the active constituent of marijuana, $(-)\Delta^9$ tetrahydrocannabinol (THC) (Gaoni & Mechoulam, 1964,

1971). Despite advancements in the knowledge of the physiological effects of THC, the mode of action for this substance remained a mystery until the elucidation of the "brain" cannabinoid receptor (CB_1). CB_1 was discovered in the brain in 1988 (Devane, Dysarz, Johnson, Melvin, & Howlett, 1988) and was cloned 2 years later (Matsuda, Lolait, Brownstein, Young, & Bonner, 1990). Soon after, the second CB was discovered in splenic immune cells (Munro, Thomas, & Abu-Shaar, 1993). These two G-protein-coupled receptors (GPCRs), which are now termed CB_1 and CB_2, respectively, are activated by highly lipophilic arachidonate-based endogenous ligands collectively called endocannabinoids. The endocannabinoids *N*-arachidonyl ethanolamine (anandamide) and 2-arachidonyl glycerol (2-AG) are the two most studied endocannabinoids. Recent studies have suggested relatively similar affinities for both endocannabinoids at human CB_1 and CB_2 receptors (pK_i 2-AG 6.9 at CB_1, 7.2 at CB_2; AEA 6.9 at CB_1 and 7.0 at CB_2), and only subtle differences in their signaling pathways (Soethoudt et al., 2017). Anandamide is produced from the hydrolysis of the *N*-acylphosphatidylethanolamine (NAPE) by NAPE-selective phospholipase D (NAPE-PLD) enzyme in a one step or multiple steps process (Liu et al., 2008). On the other hand, 2-AG is formed from the hydrolysis of diacylglycerol (DAG) by either diacylglycerol lipase α or diacylglycerol lipase β (Bisogno et al., 2003). These endocannabinoids are inactivated by enzymatic metabolism. Anandamide is hydrolyzed by fatty acid amide hydrolase (FAAH), whereas 2-AG is mainly metabolized by monoacylglycerol lipase, and to a smaller extent by α,β-hydrolase 6 and 12 (Cravatt et al., 1996; Dinh et al., 2002; Marrs et al., 2010).

1.2 CB Locale

The CB_1 (encoded by *CNR1* gene) is most abundant in the brain, in regions such as hippocampus, cortex, basal ganglia, amygdala, and cerebellum (Mackie, 2005). CB_1 are expressed on neurons, particularly on axons and presynaptic terminals of both excitatory and inhibitory neurons, highlighting the role of this receptor in modulating neurotransmission (Mackie, 2005). Owing to the central distribution of CB_1, it is now known to be liable for the psychoactive effects of cannabinoids.

In contrast, CB_2 (encoded by *CNR2* gene) was first recognized as a peripheral CB predominantly expressed by immune cells (Galiègue et al., 1995;

Munro et al., 1993). The peripheral expression of CB_2 and its immune-modulatory role has attracted attention as a possible therapeutic target without psychoactive side effects. Human CB_1 and CB_2 share 44% homology in amino acid structure, and the sequence of CB_2 is conserved between species: 82% similarity between human and mouse, 81% similarity between human and rat, and 90% similarity between mouse and rat (Griffin, Tao, & Abood, 2000; Munro et al., 1993; Shire et al., 1996). Being a member of the GPCR family, CB_2 has the characteristic seven transmembrane α-helices, an extracellular N-terminus, and an intracellular C-terminus (Fig. 1) (Xie, Chen, & Billings, 2003).

There are other candidate CBs that can either be activated by synthetic or phytocannabinoids or endocannabinoids, or both. Currently, there is debate around three candidate GPCRs, namely, GPR18, GPR55, and GPR119, which have emerged as potential members of the CB family (Brown, 2007; Console-Bram, Brailoiu, Brailoiu, Sharir, & Abood, 2014; Ryberg et al., 2007). Despite the lack of structural homology with the classical CBs, CB_1 and CB_2, the cannabinoid activation of peroxisome proliferator-activated receptors (PPARs) and transient receptor potential

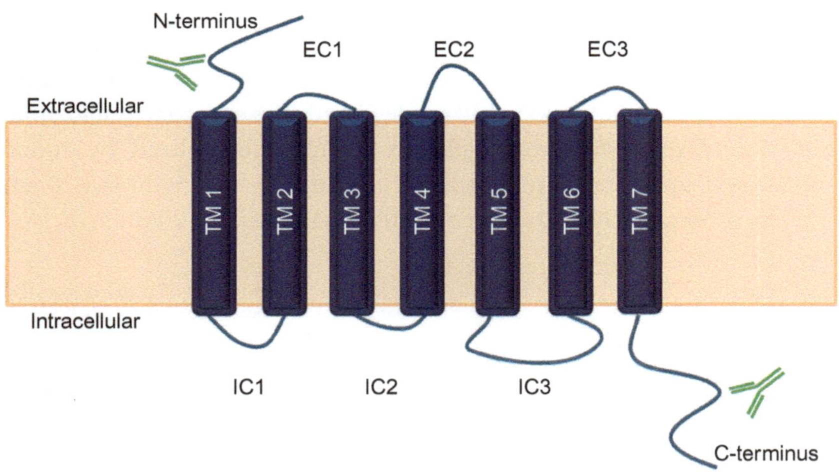

Fig. 1 A schematic representation of the two-dimensional model of cannabinoid receptor CB_2. CB_2 is a GPCR, consists of an extracellular N-terminus, intracellular C-terminus, seven-transmembrane domains (TM 1–7), three extracellular loops (EC1–3), and three intracellular loops (IC1–3). The commonly used polyclonal anti-CB_2 antibodies are raised either against amino acids 20–33 at the N-terminus, or against the C-terminal region surrounding the nonphosphorylated serine 352. *Image drawn by Dan Kho.*

vanilloid type 1 have also been established (Patwardhan et al., 2006; Sun & Bennett, 2007).

1.3 CB_2 Expression in the Peripheral Immune System

Messenger RNA studies reveal that the CB_2 encoding gene (*CNR2*) is expressed by all hematopoietic cells at different levels (Galiègue et al., 1995). *CNR2* mRNA expression level in human immune cell populations is highest in B cells, followed by NK cells, monocytes, neutrophils, $CD8^+$ T cells, and the expression is lowest in $CD4^+$ T cells (Galiègue et al., 1995). In conjunction with CB_2 mRNA expression, protein expression of CB_2 was also detected in circulating blood-derived immune cells using the N-terminal (see Fig. 1) anti-CB_2 polyclonal antibody-based flow analysis (Graham, Angel, Schwarcz, Dunbar, & Glass, 2010). CB_2 protein expression in human peripheral blood immune cells is higher in NK cells, B cells, and monocytes than in $CD4^+$ or $CD8^+$ T cells (Graham et al., 2010). CB_2 protein expression in mouse peripheral blood immune cells differ slightly from the human profile, where B cells and monocytes express a much higher level of CB_2 than T cells and NK cells (Schmöle et al., 2015).

Immunohistochemical analysis using a C-terminal anti-CB_2 polyclonal antibody (see Fig. 1), which detects inactive nonphosphorylated CB_2 isoform at serine 352, reveals that CB_2 expression in human lymph nodes is restricted to resting B cells in the mantle zones, marginal zones of secondary follicles, and in the primary follicles (Rayman et al., 2004). On the other hand, the N-terminal anti-CB_2 antibody, demonstrates high levels of CB_2 expression in the germinal centers of secondary follicles, particularly in B cells that coexpress CD40, indicating active B cells (Rayman et al., 2004). Furthermore, CB_2 expression in $CD23^+$ follicular dendritic cells and a subpopulation of $CD68^+$ macrophages is also detected in human lymphoid tissues using a N-terminal specific anti-CB_2 antibody (Rayman et al., 2007). Abnormally high CB_2 expression is also seen in T cell from non-Hodgkin's lymphomas, which is not observed in normal lymphoid tissues. These data collectively indicate that active CB_2 is constitutively expressed in various subsets of immune cells.

Due to the wide and abundant expression of CB_2 receptors in many subsets of leukocytes, it is widely accepted that CB_2 is a mediator of the immune-suppressive and antiinflammatory effects of cannabinoids. Pharmacological studies have suggested that CB_2 agonists alter leukocyte functions such as splenocyte proliferation, B cell and T cell differentiation, and neutrophil migration (McKallip, Lombard, Martin, Nagarkatti, & Nagarkatti, 2002; Nilsson, Fowler, & Jacobsson, 2006; Ziring et al., 2006). The CB_2 agonist, JWH-015, also modulates human monocyte/macrophage migration through ERK and phosphoinositide 3-kinase pathways (Montecucco, Burger, Mach, & Steffens, 2008). Additionally, ex vivo and in vitro studies reveal that CB_2 could attenuate monocyte/macrophage-endothelium engagement and migration across the blood–brain barrier (BBB) by downregulating the active form of integrins, lymphocyte function-associated antigen 1 (LFA-1), and very late antigen 4 (VLA-4) (Buch, 2013; Rom et al., 2013) expressed by the myeloid cells. Furthermore, CB_2 is implicated in the regulation of human macrophage differentiation where CB_2 activation during differentiation reduced the expression of CD4, CCR5, and CXCR4 in monocyte-derived macrophages, which are receptors involved in HIV-1 infection (Williams et al., 2014). Additionally, CB_2 is upregulated in monocytes and monocyte-derived macrophages in human encephalitis in vitro (Ramirez et al., 2013). CB_2 activation negatively modulates inflammatory responses in human macrophages in vitro by inhibiting macrophage proliferation, phagocytosis, and release of proinflammatory cytokines (Chiurchiù et al., 2014; Chuchawankul, Shima, Buckley, Hartmann, & McCoy, 2004). In vitro CB_2 activation in human macrophages is also thought to suppress the upregulation of genes induced by lipopolysaccharide (LPS; TLR4 ligand) (Persidsky et al., 2015). However, a study using mouse macrophages demonstrated that several "selective" CB_2 agonists mediated chemotaxis independent of CB_2 receptor involvement, indicating that some CB_2 agonists have off-target effects/pharmacology (Taylor et al., 2015). For much of the history of CB_2, there has been good agreement that CB_2 is primarily a peripheral CB and is absent from the central nervous system (CNS). However, this view has been increasingly challenged in the past 10–15 years and is a topic of substantial debate between researchers. The spectrum of views spans complete absence of brain expression to the other extreme where all cell types in the brain express CB_2. The human data supports some limited brain expression and will be discussed after we have introduced the neurovascular unit (NVU), and the BBB.

2. THE NVU AND THE BBB

What is the NVU? The brain vasculature forms the interface between the peripheral circulatory system and the CNS to maintain the neural microenvironment. The brain vasculature is a multicellular unit with cerebral endothelial cells interacting with neural components such as the pericytes, glial cells (astrocytes), neurons, and the basal lamina membrane to form the NVU (Fig. 2). The term BBB is often used interchangeably with the NVU. However, the BBB is the specific property conferred by the vascular endothelium due to the very high density of junctional proteins, solute transporters, and molecular pumps expressed by these cells to form a strong tight cellular and molecular barrier.

This BBB is selectively permeable and controls movement of substances between the brain and periphery. The control of ion movement across the BBB is crucial for maintaining homeostasis in the CNS. The BBB restricts transport of toxins and cells from the periphery to brain by (a) the

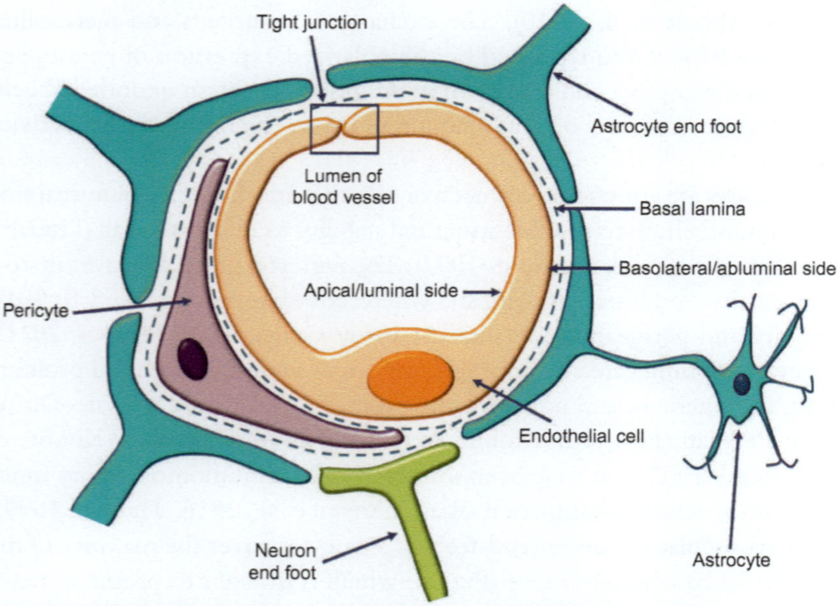

Fig. 2 Components of the neurovascular unit at the blood–brain barrier. Specialized cerebral endothelial cells lining the blood vasculature are capable of forming tight junctions to reduce permeability. The endothelium is attached to the pericytes and is embedded in the basal lamina. The astrocyte end-feet ensheath majority of the endothelium on the abluminal side. Neuronal projections are in close proximity to regulate blood flow. *Image drawn by Dan Kho based on the concept from Abbott, N. J., Patabendige, A. A. K., Dolman, D. E. M., Yusof, S. R., & Begley, D. J. (2010). Structure and function of the blood–brain barrier.* Neurobiology of Disease, *37(1), 13–25. http://dx.doi.org/10.1016/j.nbd.2009.07.030.*

paracellular barrier formed by the junctions of two adjacent endothelial cells; (b) the transcellular barrier formed by the low endocytosis and transcytosis of brain endothelial cells; and (c) the enzymatic barrier where a variety of enzymes degrade different molecules. Additionally, BBB efflux transporters such as ATP-binding cassette (ABC) transporters actively deliver selected nutrients and remove metabolites across the BBB (Abbott, Patabendige, Dolman, Yusof, & Begley, 2010).

Cerebral endothelial cells have different properties when compared to endothelial cells originating from the periphery. The low paracellular permeability of the BBB is due to the epithelial-like continuous expression of intercellular tight junctions, which reduces the fenestration seen in noncerebral endothelial cells (Obermeier, Daneman, & Ransohoff, 2013). The transcellular permeability is also low in brain endothelial cells owing to low level of pinocytosis and restricted diffusion of hydrophilic compounds (Abbott et al., 2010). The exchange of nutrients and metabolites across the BBB is also regulated by the polarized expression of endothelial membrane receptors and transporters. Additionally, brain endothelial cells have higher number of mitochondria, hence high metabolic activity (Abbott et al., 2010).

Pericytes are contractile connective cells that attach to the abluminal side of the endothelium to provide structural stability to the vessel wall (Lindahl, Johansson, Levéen, & Betsholtz, 1997). The pericytes normally cover up to a third of the endothelium (Fig. 2), where coverage is correlated to BBB integrity and permeability (Dalkara, Gursoy-Ozdemir, & Yemisci, 2011). Pericytes are implicated in vasoregulatory roles such as endothelial proliferation, angiogenesis, and inflammatory processes (Balabanov & Dore-Duffy, 1998; Peppiatt, Howarth, Mobbs, & Attwell, 2006; Ramsauer, Krause, & Dermietzel, 2002) and have been shown to have immunomodulatory functions during neuroinflammation (Rustenhoven et al., 2016; Thomas, 1999). The perivascular processes (end-feet) of astrocytes cover the majority of the endothelial basolateral surface (Fig. 2), which is thought to promote metabolic exchange between blood vessels and nerve terminals (Kacem, Lacombe, Seylaz, & Bonvento, 1998). These glial cells are the source of various important regulatory factors such as transforming growth factor β and glial cell-derived neurotrophic factor (Tran, Correale, Schreiber, & Fisher, 1999; Utsumi et al., 2000). In addition to pericytes and astrocytes, the basal lamina is another key component of the NVU that provides structural anchorage. The pericytes and endothelial cells are embedded in the ~40-nm thick basal lamina, which is contiguous with the astrocyte end-feet

(Abbott et al., 2010). The matrix of the basal lamina is composed of various types of laminin, collagen, glycoproteins, and proteoglycans produced by endothelial cells, pericytes, and astrocytes (Kalluri, 2003). Neurons do not contribute greatly to the physical structure of the NVU but are involved in innervation of some vessels to control vascular contraction. This occurs through noradrenergic, serotonergic, cholinergic, and GABA-ergic regulation of cerebral blood flow (Hawkins & Davis, 2005).

2.1 Key BBB Junctional Structures

Ever since Lewamdowsky coined the term *bluthirnschranke* (BBB) over a century ago (Lewandowsky, 1900), it has been known that brain vessels have very different barrier properties to peripheral vessels. This is due in part to the presence of junctional molecules including adherens junctions (Schulze & Firth, 1993), tight junctions (Wolburg & Lippoldt, 2002), and gap junctions (Simard, Arcuino, Takano, Liu, & Nedergaard, 2003). Both adherens and tight junctions (Fig. 3) are essential regulators of BBB permeability (Bazzoni & Dejana, 2004), while gap junctions mediate intercellular communication and do not contribute directly to barrier function

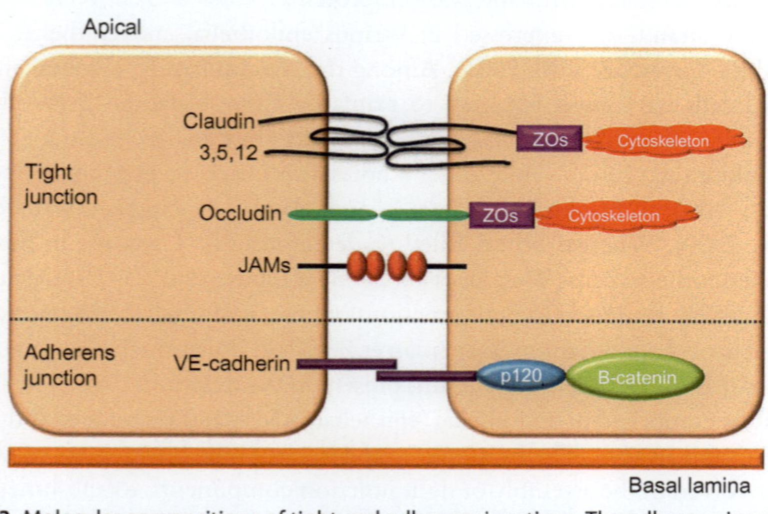

Fig. 3 Molecular compositions of tight and adherens junctions. The adherens junctions maintain the cell–cell adhesion between adjacent endothelial cells. The homophilic binding of VE-cadherin is coupled with cytoskeleton via catenin. The tight junction consists of the transmembrane proteins claudins, occludin, and junction adhesion molecules (JAMs), as well as intracellular scaffolding proteins zonula occludens (ZOs) is responsible for the low intercellular permeability. *Image drawn by Dan Kho.*

(Simard et al., 2003). It is important to understand the complexity of this system as it is known to be compromised in a range of human neurological diseases and is an obvious target for any drug hitting the NVU including cannabinoids.

Adherens junctions in the vasculature mediate endothelial cell–cell adhesion, regulate vascular growth, endothelial cell polarity and contribute to paracellular permeability (Bazzoni & Dejana, 2004). The adherens junction protein, VE-cadherin (CD144), clusters at the intercellular junction and facilitates adjacent endothelial cell–cell adhesion by calcium-dependent, homophilic interactions at the extracellular domains (Vincent, Xiao, Buckley, & Kowalczyk, 2004). Tight junctions are intermembranous network of strands at the apical region of the endothelial intercellular cleft, and the strands on the protoplasmic side of the membrane associate like a zip with the neighboring cell to seal the intercellular space. Tight junctions separate the apical domain from the basolateral membrane, leading to polarization of endothelial cells. They consist of three transmembrane proteins, namely, claudins, occludin, and junction adhesion molecules. In addition, tight junctions also contain the intracellular scaffolding proteins, zonula occludens-1, -2, and -3 (ZO-1, -2, and -3). Claudins constitute a large family of over 20 transmembrane phosphoproteins localized exclusively at tight junction strands and expressed in various endothelial and epithelial cells (Tsukita, Furuse, & Itoh, 2001). Among the claudin family, cerebral endothelial cells have been reported to primarily express claudin-3 (Wolburg et al., 2003) and claudin-5 (Morita, Sasaki, Furuse, & Tsukita, 1999; Ohtsuki et al., 2007), while other studies also observed claudin-12 (Nitta et al., 2003; Ohtsuki et al., 2007) and claudin-1 expression (Liebner et al., 2000). Whereas others failed to detect claudin-1 epitope in human brain endothelial cells (Weksler et al., 2005; Wolburg et al., 2003). Occludin is selectively expressed in tight junctions of brain endothelial cells but not in nonneuronal endothelium (Daneman et al., 2010). Junctional adhesion molecules (JAMs) are immunoglobulins present in the tight junctions. The JAM family is comprised of endothelial/epithelial JAM-1 and vascular endothelial JAM-2 and JAM-3. The homophilic and heterophilic interactions of JAMs are involved in the assembly of tight junction components, establishment of cell polarity and in leukocyte diapedesis (Bazzoni, 2011; Del Maschio et al., 1999). The ZO-1, -2, and -3 belong to the family of membrane-associated guanylate kinases (MAGUK). These intracellular scaffolding proteins play a major role in anchoring transmembrane tight junction proteins to the cytoskeleton.

Tight junction opening is a common cause of BBB integrity loss, which would lead to the influx of toxins, loss of ion and neurotransmitter homeostasis, and neuroinflammation (Vendel & de Lange, 2014). Neuroinflammation is also a cause of BBB disruption and can aggravate the loss of barrier function at the BBB. CB_2 agonists have been implicated in maintaining the BBB integrity at the molecular level in inflamed brain endothelial cells (Lu et al., 2008; Ramirez et al., 2012). This will be discussed further later.

2.2 Transport Across the BBB

The BBB utilizes transmembrane protein carrier/transporter as routes for permeation across the BBB. Nutrients such as glucose and amino acids are unable to diffuse freely across the BBB and rely on specific solute carriers to enter the CNS from the periphery. Expression of the protein carriers may be polarized on either the luminal or abluminal membrane to facilitate the transport of substrate in one orientation, i.e., from blood to brain or brain to blood (Abbott et al., 2010). The human BBB has a density of active efflux carriers, ABC transporter such as multidrug resistance protein (ABCB1), multidrug resistance-associated proteins (MRPs), and breast cancer resistance protein (BRCP). These effectively prevent brain penetration of a range of drugs and toxins. There is a dearth of research into the cannabinoid-mediated regulation of these aspects of NVU and BBB function. However, as these transporters are also very important during disease pathogenesis, it is interesting to speculate that altered CB function or expression during states of neuroinflammation could adversely affects these key controllers of brain homeostasis.

3. EVIDENCE FOR THE EXPRESSION OF CB2 BY THE NVU AND BBB

Historically, the expression of many genes (including CB_2) was conducted via the assessment of the respective mRNA and when this was detected, followed up by the analysis of the protein where good antibodies were available. In the case of receptors, this can also be done using radioligand binding as has been done extensively for CB_1. All of the early studies looking for CB_2 mRNA expression in the healthy brain (Galiègue et al., 1995; Griffin et al., 1999; Lynn & Herkenham, 1994; Munro et al., 1993; Schatz, Lee, Condie, Pulaski, & Kaminski, 1997) concluded that

CB2 was largely absent. However, some years later, various CB_2 antibodies were used for the histological analysis of CB_2 in diseased neurological tissue and inflamed brain tissue. Cerebral blood vessels stained positively for CB_2 in these immunohistochemical studies of the human and rodent brains (Ashton, Friberg, Darlington, & Smith, 2006; Núñez et al., 2004). Abundant CB_2 expression was also revealed in human brain tumors and was localized to the vascular endothelial cells, indicating a possible role of CB_2 in tumor growth or vascularization (Schley et al., 2009). A later study demonstrated coexpression of CB_2 and CD31 in blood vessel endothelium and vascular smooth muscle in human brain using double-labeled immunohistochemistry (Dowie, Grimsey, Hoffman, Faull, & Glass, 2014). Dowie and colleagues also revealed higher CB_2 expression in Huntington's disease compared to control brains. Contrary to previous findings that described microglial CB_2 expression (Benito et al., 2003), no CB_2 immunolabeling of microglia was detected in the brain in this study (Dowie et al., 2014). Interestingly, endothelial CB_2 expression in multiple sclerosis (MS) brain is highest in chronic active plaques, which are regions of extensive immune infiltration and tissue inflammation (Zhang, Hilton, Hanemann, & Zajicek, 2011). Similarly, elevated endothelial CB_2 has been reported in the HIV-encephalitis human brain (Ramirez et al., 2012). Evidence for endothelial CB_2 expression in the CNS is largely based on immunohistochemical analysis using polyclonal CB_2 antibodies (Ashton et al., 2006; Schley et al., 2009). Several independent studies have evaluated the specificity of commercially and academically used αCB_2 antibodies in rodent brain and retina (Baek, Darlington, Smith, & Ashton, 2013; Cécyre, Thomas, Ptito, Casanova, & Bouchard, 2014). Both studies concluded a lack of antibody specificity for use in immunohistochemistry (Baek et al., 2013; Cécyre et al., 2014).

An additional consideration, which is particularly relevant to inflamed tissue, is the binding of IgG to Fc-gamma receptors (e.g., CD16, CD32, and CD64). These are typically elevated in inflamed tissue. Generally, control steps to block binding of IgGs to elevated Fc receptors (e.g., TruStain FcX™ Fc blocker from BioLegend) were not considered in these studies (Schmöle et al., 2015). It is also important to note that basic groups in basal lamina collagen fibers of human blood vessels are prone to nonspecific binding of the Fc portion of IgG (Honig, Rieger, Kapp, Dietl, & Kämmerer, 2005). Therefore, as the sole proof of CB_2 expression, reports of antibody-based endothelial CB_2 expression should be interpreted with some caution and future studies should consider additional means of definitive proof.

Multiple studies have reported the presence of CB_2 in inflamed human brains (Benito et al., 2003, 2007, 2008; Gómez-Gálvez, Palomo-Garo, Fernández-Ruiz, & García, 2015; Núñez et al., 2004; Solas, Francis, Franco, & Ramirez, 2013), where some of the staining associates with the location of microglial cells. Benito and colleagues first reported the presence of CB_2 and the anandamide metabolizing enzyme FAAH in neuritic plaque-associated microglia in Alzheimer's disease brains (Benito et al., 2003). The study described an elevated level of CB_2 antibody-labeling in microglial cells of diseased brains when compared to healthy brains (Benito et al., 2003). This finding was supported by an immunohistochemistry-based study that indicated the presence of CB_2 in perivascular microglia but not in parenchymal microglia within the white matter area of human cerebellum (Núñez et al., 2004). CB_2 has also been noted in activated microglial cells in lesion sites of MS, amyotrophic lateral sclerosis spinal cord, and Parkinson's disease (Gómez-Gálvez et al., 2015; Yiangou et al., 2006). The neuroprotective role of microglial CB_2 has also been indicated in mouse models of Huntington's disease excitotoxicity (Palazuelos et al., 2009). Targeting the elevated microglial CB_2 expression in CNS injury and inflammatory conditions as a therapeutic potential to modulate disease progress has been previously reviewed (Ashton & Glass, 2007; Cabral & Griffin-Thomas, 2009).

Recently, immunohistochemical studies have also described widespread distribution of CB_2 in uninjured rodent brains (Gong et al., 2006; Suárez et al., 2008, 2009). Abundant CB_2 immunolabeling was observed in neurons, endothelium, microglia, and Purkinje cells of the rodent brain (Ashton et al., 2006; Gong et al., 2006; Onaivi et al., 2006; Suárez et al., 2008). Contrary to this, a study in mouse brain reported that CB_2 mRNA and protein were detected specifically in the dopaminergic neurons of the ventral tegmental area and CB_2 agonists inhibited dopaminergic neuronal firing in vivo and ex vivo (Zhang et al., 2014). More recently, studies have suggested CB_2 expression in mouse hippocampal principle neurons that contribute to neuronal plasticity (Stempel et al., 2016). The latter studies demonstrate that some strains of rodent may have CB_2 located in certain brain regions but the same expression has not been detected in human brain tissue to the best of our knowledge.

CB_2 mRNA has also been identified in peripheral mouse neurons, and functional studies have shown that CB_2 agonists JWH-015 and JWH-051 were capable of inhibiting electrically evoked contractions in mouse vas deferens tissues (Griffin et al., 1997). However, the use of CB_2 antagonist

AM630 could not block JWH-015- and JWH-051-mediated effects (Griffin et al., 1997). This is possibly due to the fact that JWH-051 has high and almost equal affinity for both CB_1 ($K_i = 1.2$ nM) and CB_2 ($K_i = 0.2$ nM), while JWH-015 is more selective toward CB_2 ($K_i = 13.8$ nM), it could still bind to CB_1 ($K_i = 383$ nM) at high concentrations (Huffman, 2005). It is noteworthy that these agonists are also ligands for GPR55, indicating a possibility that CB_2 receptors might not be involved in JWH-015- and JWH-051-induced effects in peripheral neurons as reported by Griffin and colleagues (Griffin et al., 1997; Ryberg et al., 2007). Meanwhile, there is evidence of a functional role for CB_2 in sensory neurons, where the CB_2 agonist JWH-133 inhibited nerve depolarizations in rodent vagus nerve which was abolished by the CB_2 antagonist SR144528 but not by the CB_1 antagonist (Patel et al., 2003).

Many researchers have remained skeptical with regards to neuronal CB_2 expression (Atwood & Mackie, 2010). Contrary to the immunohistochemical studies reporting high neuronal CB_2, only very low levels of *CNR2* mRNA were detected in the mouse CNS using the more sensitive real-time PCR technique (Maresz, Carrier, Ponomarev, Hillard, & Dittel, 2005). In addition, the GFP-reporter study by Schmöle et al. revealed very low CB_2 expression levels in the mouse hippocampus that colocalized only with the $Iba1^+$ microglial cells but not with the $NeuN^+$ neurons (Schmöle et al., 2015). It is hoped that a clearer picture of CB_2 expression and function in the CNS will emerge as more selective ligands and a greater awareness of the limitations of immunohistochemistry become more prevalent.

4. EVIDENCE OF THE REGULATION OF NVU FUNCTIONS BY CANNABINOIDS

The key functions of the NVU are nutrient supply to the brain and maintaining a molecular, cellular, and immune barrier. There are a range of rodent-based studies that show that cannabinoid ligands influence various key NVU functions, but there are substantially fewer studies using human cells and tissues. Here, we will summarize the findings of the rodent studies and look closely at the human studies, which have mostly investigated cannabinoid-mediated effects on barrier integrity and immune cell migration.

Immune cell migration across the BBB during neuroinflammation (diapedesis) is a highly complex and coordinated process which requires key molecules to be upregulated by the vascular endothelium and activation of the interacting molecules by the migratory immune cells (Muller, 2011) following receipt of the correct signals. The leukocyte diapedesis cascade is characterized by capture and slow rolling of leukocytes, adhesion strengthening, intraluminal crawling, paracellular and transcellular migration, and migration through the basement membrane (Ley, Laudanna, Cybulsky, & Nourshargh, 2007). Inflammatory mediators stimulate acute expression of P-selectin (CD62P) followed by E-selectin (CD62E) at the apical surface of endothelial cells. These molecules mediate the early steps of leukocyte tethering to the apical face of the endothelium. Then chemokine receptor activation of leukocytes leads to activation of leukocyte β2 integrin (CD18) in the macrophage receptor 1 (MAC1, also known as CD11b-CD18) and LFA-1 (also known as CD11a-CD18). The activated β2 integrin firmly adheres to the endothelium by interacting with endothelial intercellular adhesion molecule-1 (ICAM-1) (Miller & Stella, 2008). Meanwhile, lymphocytes and monocytes also interact with endothelial cells through VLA-4 (Berlin et al., 1995; Chan, Hyduk, & Cybulsky, 2001). The endothelial ligand of VLA-4 is vascular cell adhesion molecule 1 (VCAM-1). Both ICAM-1 and VCAM-1 are transiently upregulated by brain endothelial cells during proinflammatory activation (O'Carroll et al., 2015; Weksler et al., 2005). All of these aforementioned molecules are critically involved in leukocyte capture and firm adhesion prior to the event of migration. Disruption of these interactions by CB_2 agonists is most likely responsible for the reduction of leukocyte recruitment in the majority of rodent brain injury models where cannabinoid/CB_2 agonists have shown efficacy (Fig. 4). These rodent models include the (i) experimental autoimmune encephalomyelitis (EAE) mouse model (Kong, Li, Tuma, & Ganea, 2014; Maresz et al., 2007; Ni et al., 2004); (ii) the transient middle cerebral artery occlusion (MCAO) mouse model (Zhang et al., 2008); (iii) the LPS-induced encephalitis mouse model (Ramirez et al., 2012); and (vi) the traumatic brain injury model (Amenta, Jallo, Tuma, & Elliott, 2012; Amenta, Jallo, Tuma, Hooper, & Elliott, 2014). These and other rodent studies have clearly suggested involvement of CB_2 in the prevention of the inflammation induced damage. Most of these studies have pharmacologically confirmed the involvement of CB_2 with the coapplication of the CB_2 antagonist SR144528, and some have used CB_2 knockout mice (Ramirez et al., 2012), which typically have poorer neurological function compared to wild-type mice following MCAO (Murikinati et al., 2010; Zhang, Adler, et al., 2009). CB_1 and CB_2 receptors have both been implicated in EAE (Maresz et al., 2007) with CB_1-deficient and CB_2-deficient mice developing

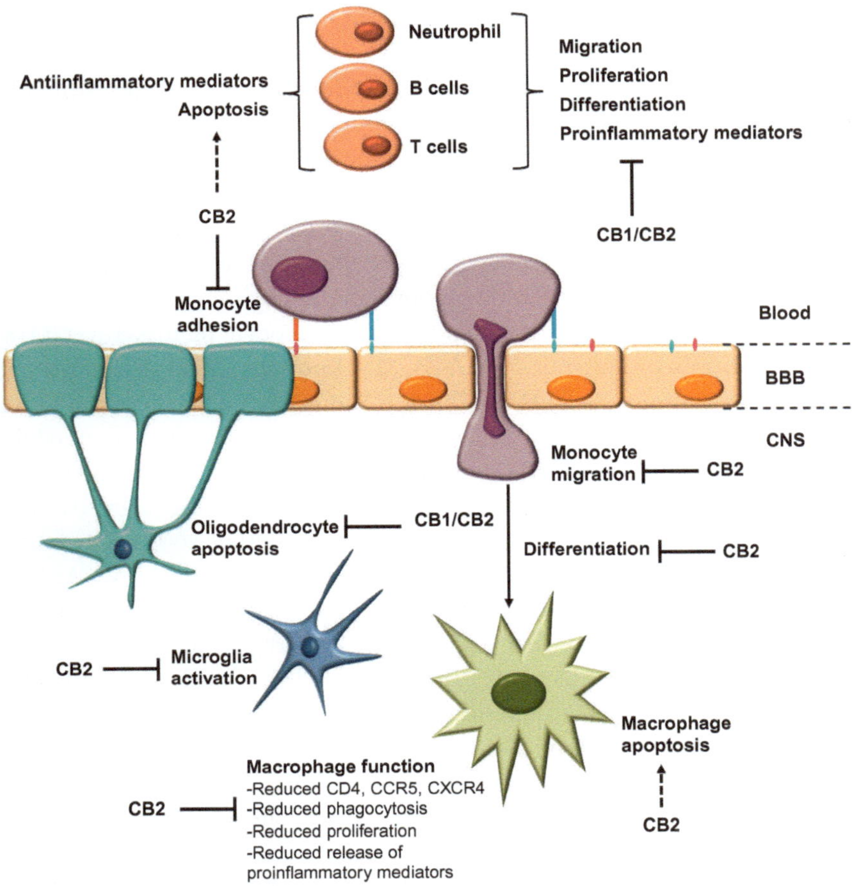

Fig. 4 The complex role of the cannabinoid system in modulating immune response during (neuro)-inflammatory conditions. Cannabinoids may dampen inflammatory reaction by suppressing peripheral blood leukocytes proliferation, differentiation, migration, expression of adhesion molecules, and the secretion of proinflammatory cytokines. Cannabinoid could also regulate endothelial cells at the blood–brain barrier by inhibiting the expression of cell adhesion molecules such as ICAM-1 and VCAM-1 to prevent monocyte transendothelial migration. Within the brain parenchyma, cannabinoids could suppress microglial activation, and also modulate macrophage function to prevent brain injury elicited by these immune cells. *Image drawn by Dan Kho.*

more severe symptoms compared to control EAE mice (Kubajewska & Constantinescu, 2010; Maresz et al., 2007; Pryce et al., 2003). The non-selective cannabinoid WIN55212-2 ameliorates disease progression in the mouse model of chronic-progressive MS characterized by Th1-mediated CNS demyelination and spastic hind limb paralysis (Croxford & Miller,

2003). In chronic and remitting relapsing EAE, systemic administration of selective CB_2 agonist reduces rolling and adhesion of leukocytes to pial microvasculature and reduces infiltration of $CD4^+$ T cells into the spinal cord, potentially through CB_2-mediated apoptosis of cells (Arévalo-Martin, Vela, Molina-Holgado, Borrell, & Guaza, 2003; Lombard, Nagarkatti, & Nagarkatti, 2007; Sánchez, González-Pérez, Galve-Roperh, & García-Merino, 2006; Zhang, Martin, et al., 2009). CB_2 is also implicated in remyelination through modulation of inflammatory responses by astrocytes and microglia in order to protect myelin-producing oligodendrocytes from apoptosis (Molina-Holgado et al., 2002). Recently, administration of the putative highly selective CB_2 agonist, GP1a, in EAE facilitated recovery in conjunction with reduction in demyelination and axonal loss by inhibiting Th1/Th17 differentiation and reduced expression of chemokines, chemokine receptors, and some of the aforementioned adhesion molecules involved in leukocyte diapedesis into the CNS (Kong et al., 2014). However, studies using GP1a should be interpreted with some caution as it has recently been shown to be only 20-fold selective for mouse CB_2 over CB_1, and to act as an inverse agonist in a range of functional studies (Soethoudt et al., 2017).

These studies have clearly highlighted the potential of targeting CB_2 in rodent models of neurological diseases. Direct suppression of leukocyte effector functions by CB_2 is clearly evident (Adhikary, Kocieda, Yen, Tuma, & Ganea, 2012; Kong et al., 2014; Maresz et al., 2007) as is the improvement in BBB integrity (Amenta et al., 2012, 2014). However, it is most challenging to prove the cellular target and actual mechanism of action in the BBB protection using in vivo models as the CB_2 agonist effects could be mediated by a range of leukocyte subsets, brain vascular endothelial cells, and/or resident innate glial cells. In addition, humans and rodents differ greatly in terms of immune complexity and this lesson is well known in the stroke field where hundreds of drug candidates that "cure" stroke in rodents have failed abysmally in human clinical trials (Kwiecien, Sy, & Ding, 2014). This issue has not generally been due to incompatible pharmacology, but more related to an under appreciation of the simplicity of the rodent models compared to human disease and the significant differences in immune regulation (Kwiecien et al., 2014).

The expression or function of CB_2 has been reported in human brain endothelial cultures (Golech et al., 2004; Persidsky et al., 2015; Ramirez et al., 2012). The first of these studies demonstrated that the CB_2 receptor mediates 2-AG-induced calcium influx in human brain endothelial cells in vitro that can be abolished by the CB_2 antagonist, SR144528 (Golech et al., 2004). Several reports also suggested a role for CB_2 in modulating leukocyte–endothelial interactions at the BBB (Ramirez et al., 2012; Rom et al., 2013). In addition, CB_2 activation in primary human brain vascular endothelial cells has been shown to diminish the proinflammatory activation of the brain endothelial cells by TNFα, which is a very potent proinflammatory mediator (Persidsky et al., 2015). The latter study conducted by Yuri Persidsky's group at Temple used two highly selective CB2 agonists (JWH133 and O-1966) in a battery of state-of-the-art assays to demonstrate the antiinflammatory effects of these agonists on the brain endothelial cells. However, a major concern of this and other studies (Ramirez et al., 2012; Rom et al., 2013) is the micromolar concentrations required to mediate the effects shown. For agonists with published nanomolar potency in heterologous signaling assays, why is 10 μM required to drive the effects in these cells? In addition, the authors do not confirm CB_2 expression in these primary cultures, which are obtained from patients with retractable epilepsy. As there is a possibility that CB_2 expression may vary between donors who are not healthy controls, CB_2 expression should be shown for each and every donor. In contrast to the aforementioned studies, a study by Saoirse O′Sullivan's group reported a lack of CB_2 mRNA expression in primary human brain microvascular endothelial cells (Hind et al., 2015).

Some studies have also suggested that cannabinoid agonist suppression of endothelial ICAM-1 and VCAM-1 is independent of CB receptors, where the inhibitory effects of WIN-55212-2 are exerted through the activation PPARγ (Mestre et al., 2009). PPAR receptor activation is thought to modulate monocyte–endothelial interactions by inhibiting downstream signaling following ICAM-1 cross-linking in human brain endothelial cells (Ramirez et al., 2008). Historically, the pharmacological selectivity of cannabinoid compounds has usually been assessed in the context of binding or activation of CB_1 vs CB_2. However, given the new candidate receptors for cannabinoids, perhaps this selectivity needs to be broadened and redefined, indeed a recent analysis of selectivity of a wide range of cannabinoid ligands showed significant off-target activity (Soethoudt et al., 2017).

A key step in leukocyte diapedesis is the transmigration of leukocytes through the NVU into the inflamed brain. Leukocytes face three physical hurdles while crossing the NVU, namely, the endothelium, the endothelial-cell basement membrane, and pericytes (Ley et al., 2007). The migration across the endothelial cell barrier *can* occur through paracellular and transcellular routes. Paracellular movement requires the rearrangement of endothelial cell junctions (tight junctions and adherens junctions), whereas transcellular migration involves entry into the endothelial cells rather than through the paracellular space. Persidsky and colleagues have shown in epileptogenic brain endothelial cultures that JWH133 and O-1966 both increase the basal barrier strength (TEER) and suggest that this is mediated by increased expression of Occludin and Claudin 5 (Ramirez et al., 2012). Logically increased tight junction expression would confer a stronger endothelial barrier and reduce the ability of immune cells to migrate through the tight junction strengthened cleft. This may however occur as a consequence of subverting the migration route from paracellular to transcellular effectively blocking the paracellular route. In this study (Ramirez et al., 2012), the CB_2 agonists were used at concentrations of 10–25 μM. JWH133 has a reported K_i of 3.4 nM and is approximately 200-fold more selective for CB_2 over CB_1. Thus at the concentrations used, could it be acting at CB_1 receptors?

5. CONCLUSION

Improving BBB or NVU integrity has broad appeal for a range of neuroinflammatory conditions in the context of stabilizing the barrier, reducing inflammation, and preventing vascular bleeds. There is also considerable interest in exploiting these pathways in order to traffic drugs into the brain (Sanchez-Covarrubias, Slosky, Thompson, Davis, & Ronaldson, 2014; Upadhyay, 2014) especially with regard to neurodegenerative diseases or active immune cells into the brain in the context of brain tumors. Although there have been some very interesting observations in the high caliber publications discussed throughout this review, there are still important questions that need addressing and suggestions for the future. These include:

(i) Is the CB_2 expression by these primary endothelial cells influenced by their dissociation from the brain tissue or the health of the donor? If, for example, the CB_2 expression is a function of the patient's epilepsy then could this be exploited to traffic drugs to that particular brain region?

(ii) If these CB_2 agonists are mediating their effects through CB_2 expressed by the brain endothelial cells, why are such high concentrations required? Do the brain endothelial cells give different responses if the agonists are used in the lower nanomolar range closer to their reported K_i? If the responses are not mediated by CB_2 what is the molecular target?

(iii) If the CB_2 gene is globally expressed in the human brain vasculature why have most mRNA-based studies failed to detect it given the abundance of blood vessels in the CNS? Perhaps with the development of high-affinity specific CB_2 agonists this can be investigated using ligand-binding studies on normal and disease tissue.

(iv) Antibodies are clearly useful when used correctly. The problem with assessment of human tissues, however, is the lack of suitable controls or the lack of consideration of what controls actual prove antibody specificity. We need to consider this more carefully especially where inflamed tissue is used as there will be increased Fc receptors (CD16a, CD16b, CD32, and CD64) expressed by innate immune infiltrates that will nonspecifically bind to antibodies.

(v) Advances are being made continually with technologies such as Nanostrings and Digital Droplet PCR for the analysis of mRNA. It is hoped that the sensitivity and specificity of such platforms will advance our understanding of CB expression in diseased tissues.

(vi) Pericytes are key structural and immunological cells of the human NVU but have been largely ignored in the cannabinoid literature. It is plausible that some CB_2 expression detected histologically may be due to pericytes under inflammatory conditions but detailed analysis of their functional regulation has not been conducted to date.

(vii) Species differences in expression or function. Key differences in receptor pharmacology have recently been described (Soethoudt et al., 2017). In addition, physiology, immunology (neuroinflammation mechanisms), or neurodegeneration is vastly different between the models and humans. There are some stunningly eloquent rodent studies showing various cannabinoid responses (e.g., the mouse ventral tegmental region); however, this expression is not currently supported from human studies. Therefore, if the expensive lessons are to be learned from the drug failures of the past (e.g., in the stroke field), this needs to be addressed from an ethical, biological, and pharmacological perspective.

(viii) Development of PET tracers for real-time CB_2 imaging in humans. Rawaha Ahmad's group has developed (Slavik, Grether, et al., 2015; Slavik, Herde, et al., 2015) and conducted the first-in-man CB_2 PET tracer study in healthy volunteers (Slavik, Herde, et al., 2015). This brief safety study reported rapid brain signals followed by rapid washout consistent with very limited binding sites in brain tissue (Slavik, Herde, et al., 2015). This promising study potentially paves the way to assess these ligands under inflammatory and neuroinflammatory conditions. There is a huge amount of development and interest in the PET ligands and this is clearly an emergent "hot" topic in clinical cannabinoid research.

CONFLICT OF INTEREST

The authors have no conflicts of interest to declare.

REFERENCES

Abbott, N. J., Patabendige, A. A. K., Dolman, D. E. M., Yusof, S. R., & Begley, D. J. (2010). Structure and function of the blood–brain barrier. *Neurobiology of Disease*, *37*(1), 13–25. http://dx.doi.org/10.1016/j.nbd.2009.07.030.

Adhikary, S., Kocieda, V. P., Yen, J. H., Tuma, R. F., & Ganea, D. (2012). Signaling through cannabinoid receptor 2 suppresses murine dendritic cell migration by inhibiting matrix metalloproteinase 9 expression. *Blood*, *120*(18), 3741–3749. http://dx.doi.org/10.1182/blood-2012-06-435362.

Amenta, P. S., Jallo, J. I., Tuma, R. F., & Elliott, M. B. (2012). A cannabinoid type 2 receptor agonist attenuates blood-brain barrier damage and neurodegeneration in a murine model of traumatic brain injury. *Journal of Neuroscience Research*, *90*(12), 2293–2305. http://dx.doi.org/10.1002/jnr.23114.

Amenta, P. S., Jallo, J. I., Tuma, R. F., Hooper, D. C., & Elliott, M. B. (2014). Cannabinoid receptor type-2 stimulation, blockade, and deletion alter the vascular inflammatory responses to traumatic brain injury. *Journal of Neuroinflammation*, *11*, 191. http://dx.doi.org/10.1186/s12974-014-0191-6.

Arévalo-Martin, A., Vela, J. M., Molina-Holgado, E., Borrell, J., & Guaza, C. (2003). Therapeutic action of cannabinoids in a murine model of multiple sclerosis. *The Journal of Neuroscience*, *23*(7), 2511–2516.

Ashton, J. C., Friberg, D., Darlington, C. L., & Smith, P. F. (2006). Expression of the cannabinoid CB2 receptor in the rat cerebellum: An immunohistochemical study. *Neuroscience Letters*, *396*(2), 113–116. http://dx.doi.org/10.1016/j.neulet.2005.11.038.

Ashton, J. C., & Glass, M. (2007). The cannabinoid CB2 receptor as a target for inflammation-dependent neurodegeneration. *Current Neuropharmacology*, *5*(2), 73–80.

Atwood, B. K., & Mackie, K. (2010). CB2: A cannabinoid receptor with an identity crisis. *British Journal of Pharmacology*, *160*(3), 467–479. http://dx.doi.org/10.1111/j.1476-5381.2010.00729.x.

Baek, J.-H., Darlington, C. L., Smith, P. F., & Ashton, J. C. (2013). Antibody testing for brain immunohistochemistry: Brain immunolabeling for the cannabinoid CB2 receptor. *Journal of Neuroscience Methods*, *216*(2), 87–95. http://dx.doi.org/10.1016/j.jneumeth.2013.03.021.

Balabanov, R., & Dore-Duffy, P. (1998). Role of the CNS microvascular pericyte in the blood-brain barrier. *Journal of Neuroscience Research*, *53*(6), 637–644. http://dx.doi.org/10.1002/(SICI)1097-4547(19980915)53:6<637::AID-JNR1>3.0.CO;2-6.

Bazzoni, G. (2011). Pathobiology of junctional adhesion molecules. *Antioxidants & Redox Signaling*, *15*(5), 1221–1234. http://dx.doi.org/10.1089/ars.2010.3867.

Bazzoni, G., & Dejana, E. (2004). Endothelial cell-to-cell junctions: Molecular organization and role in vascular homeostasis. *Physiological Reviews*, *84*(3), 869–901. http://dx.doi.org/10.1152/physrev.00035.2003.

Benito, C., Núñez, E., Tolón, R. M., Carrier, E. J., Rábano, A., Hillard, C. J., et al. (2003). Cannabinoid CB2 receptors and fatty acid amide hydrolase are selectively overexpressed in neuritic plaque-associated glia in Alzheimer's disease brains. *The Journal of Neuroscience, 23*(35), 11136–11141.

Benito, C., Romero, J. P., Tolón, R. M., Clemente, D., Docagne, F., Hillard, C. J., et al. (2007). Cannabinoid CB1 and CB2 receptors and fatty acid amide hydrolase are specific markers of plaque cell subtypes in human multiple sclerosis. *The Journal of Neuroscience, 27*(9), 2396–2402. http://dx.doi.org/10.1523/jneurosci.4814-06.2007.

Benito, C., Tolón, R. M., Pazos, M. R., Núñez, E., Castillo, A. I., & Romero, J. (2008). Cannabinoid CB2 receptors in human brain inflammation. *British Journal of Pharmacology, 153*(2), 277–285. http://dx.doi.org/10.1038/sj.bjp.0707505.

Berlin, C., Bargatze, R. F., Campbell, J. J., von Andrian, U. H., Szabo, M. C., Hasslen, S. R., et al. (1995). α4 Integrins mediate lymphocyte attachment and rolling under physiologic flow. *Cell, 80*(3), 413–422. http://dx.doi.org/10.1016/0092-8674(95)90491-3.

Bisogno, T., Howell, F., Williams, G., Minassi, A., Cascio, M. G., Ligresti, A., et al. (2003). Cloning of the first sn1-DAG lipases points to the spatial and temporal regulation of endocannabinoid signaling in the brain. *The Journal of Cell Biology, 163*(3), 463–468. http://dx.doi.org/10.1083/jcb.200305129.

Brown, A. J. (2007). Novel cannabinoid receptors. *British Journal of Pharmacology, 152*(5), 567–575. http://dx.doi.org/10.1038/sj.bjp.0707481.

Buch, S. J. (2013). Cannabinoid receptor 2 activation: A means to prevent monocyte–endothelium engagement. *The American Journal of Pathology, 183*(5), 1375–1377. http://dx.doi.org/10.1016/j.ajpath.2013.08.003.

Cabral, G. A., & Griffin-Thomas, L. (2009). Emerging role of the cannabinoid receptor CB2 in immune regulation: Therapeutic prospects for neuroinflammation. *Expert Reviews in Molecular Medicine, 11*. http://dx.doi.org/10.1017/S1462399409000957.

Cécyre, B., Thomas, S., Ptito, M., Casanova, C., & Bouchard, J.-F. (2014). Evaluation of the specificity of antibodies raised against cannabinoid receptor type 2 in the mouse retina. *Naunyn-Schmiedeberg's Archives of Pharmacology, 387*(2), 175–184. http://dx.doi.org/10.1007/s00210-013-0930-8.

Chan, J. R., Hyduk, S. J., & Cybulsky, M. I. (2001). Chemoattractants induce a rapid and transient upregulation of monocyte α4 integrin affinity for vascular cell adhesion molecule 1 which mediates arrest: An early step in the process of emigration. *The Journal of Experimental Medicine, 193*(10), 1149–1158. http://dx.doi.org/10.1084/jem.193.10.1149.

Chiurchiù, V., Lanuti, M., Catanzaro, G., Fezza, F., Rapino, C., & Maccarrone, M. (2014). Detailed characterization of the endocannabinoid system in human macrophages and foam cells, and anti-inflammatory role of type-2 cannabinoid receptor. *Atherosclerosis, 233*(1), 55–63. http://dx.doi.org/10.1016/j.atherosclerosis.2013.12.042.

Chuchawankul, S., Shima, M., Buckley, N. E., Hartmann, C. B., & McCoy, K. L. (2004). Role of cannabinoid receptors in inhibiting macrophage costimulatory activity. *International Immunopharmacology, 4*(2), 265–278. http://dx.doi.org/10.1016/j.intimp.2003.12.011.

Console-Bram, L., Brailoiu, E., Brailoiu, G. C., Sharir, H., & Abood, M. E. (2014). Activation of GPR18 by cannabinoid compounds: A tale of biased agonism. *British Journal of Pharmacology, 171*(16), 3908–3917. http://dx.doi.org/10.1111/bph.12746.

Cravatt, B. F., Giang, D. K., Mayfield, S. P., Boger, D. L., Lerner, R. A., & Gilula, N. B. (1996). Molecular characterization of an enzyme that degrades neuromodulatory fatty-acid amides. *Nature, 384*(6604), 83–87.

Croxford, J. L., & Miller, S. D. (2003). Immunoregulation of a viral model of multiple sclerosis using the synthetic cannabinoid R(+)WIN55,212. *The Journal of Clinical Investigation, 111*(8), 1231–1240. http://dx.doi.org/10.1172/JCI17652.

Dalkara, T., Gursoy-Ozdemir, Y., & Yemisci, M. (2011). Brain microvascular pericytes in health and disease. *Acta Neuropathologica*, *122*(1), 1–9. http://dx.doi.org/10.1007/s00401-011-0847-6.

Daneman, R., Zhou, L., Agalliu, D., Cahoy, J. D., Kaushal, A., & Barres, B. A. (2010). The mouse blood-brain barrier transcriptome: A new resource for understanding the development and function of brain endothelial cells. *PloS One*, *5*(10), e13741. http://dx.doi.org/10.1371/journal.pone.0013741.

Del Maschio, A., De Luigi, A., Martin-Padura, I., Brockhaus, M., Bartfai, T., Fruscella, P., et al. (1999). Leukocyte recruitment in the cerebrospinal fluid of mice with experimental meningitis is inhibited by an antibody to junctional adhesion molecule (Jam). *The Journal of Experimental Medicine*, *190*(9), 1351–1356. http://dx.doi.org/10.1084/jem.190.9.1351.

Devane, W. A., Dysarz, F. A., Johnson, M. R., Melvin, L. S., & Howlett, A. C. (1988). Determination and characterization of a cannabinoid receptor in rat brain. *Molecular Pharmacology*, *34*(5), 605–613.

Dinh, T. P., Carpenter, D., Leslie, F. M., Freund, T. F., Katona, I., Sensi, S. L., et al. (2002). Brain monoglyceride lipase participating in endocannabinoid inactivation. *Proceedings of the National Academy of Sciences of the United States of America*, *99*(16), 10819–10824. http://dx.doi.org/10.1073/pnas.152334899.

Dowie, M. J., Grimsey, N. L., Hoffman, T., Faull, R. L. M., & Glass, M. (2014). Cannabinoid receptor CB2 is expressed on vascular cells, but not astroglial cells in the post-mortem human Huntington's disease brain. *Journal of Chemical Neuroanatomy*, *59–60*, 62–71. http://dx.doi.org/10.1016/j.jchemneu.2014.06.004.

Galiègue, S., Mary, S., Marchand, J., Dussossoy, D., Carrière, D., Carayon, P., et al. (1995). Expression of central and peripheral cannabinoid receptors in human immune tissues and leukocyte subpopulations. *European Journal of Biochemistry*, *232*(1), 54–61. http://dx.doi.org/10.1111/j.1432-1033.1995.tb20780.x.

Gaoni, Y., & Mechoulam, R. (1964). Isolation, structure, and partial synthesis of an active constituent of hashish. *Journal of the American Chemical Society*, *86*(8), 1646–1647. http://dx.doi.org/10.1021/ja01062a046.

Gaoni, Y., & Mechoulam, R. (1971). The isolation and structure of delta-1-tetrahydrocannabinol and other neutral cannabinoids from hashish. *Journal of the American Chemical Society*, *93*(1), 217–224.

Golech, S. A., McCarron, R. M., Chen, Y., Bembry, J., Lenz, F., Mechoulam, R., et al. (2004). Human brain endothelium: Coexpression and function of vanilloid and endocannabinoid receptors. *Molecular Brain Research*, *132*(1), 87–92. http://dx.doi.org/10.1016/j.molbrainres.2004.08.025.

Gómez-Gálvez, Y., Palomo-Garo, C., Fernández-Ruiz, J., & García, C. (2015). Potential of the cannabinoid CB2 receptor as a pharmacological target against inflammation in Parkinson's disease. *Progress in Neuro-Psychopharmacology and Biological Psychiatry*, *64*, 200–208. http://dx.doi.org/10.1016/j.pnpbp.2015.03.017.

Gong, J.-P., Onaivi, E. S., Ishiguro, H., Liu, Q.-R., Tagliaferro, P. A., Brusco, A., et al. (2006). Cannabinoid CB2 receptors: Immunohistochemical localization in rat brain. *Brain Research*, *1071*(1), 10–23. http://dx.doi.org/10.1016/j.brainres.2005.11.035.

Graham, E. S., Angel, C. E., Schwarcz, L. E., Dunbar, P. R., & Glass, M. (2010). Detailed characterisation of CB2 receptor protein expression in peripheral blood immune cells from healthy human volunteers using flow cytometry. *International Journal of Immunopathology and Pharmacology*, *23*(1), 25–34. http://dx.doi.org/10.1177/039463201002300103.

Griffin, G., Fernando, S. R., Ross, R. A., McKay, N. G., Ashford, M. L. J., Shire, D., et al. (1997). Evidence for the presence of CB2-like cannabinoid receptors on peripheral nerve terminals. *European Journal of Pharmacology*, *339*(1), 53–61. http://dx.doi.org/10.1016/S0014-2999(97)01336-8.

Griffin, G., Tao, Q., & Abood, M. E. (2000). Cloning and pharmacological characterization of the rat CB2 cannabinoid receptor. *Journal of Pharmacology and Experimental Therapeutics, 292*(3), 886–894.

Griffin, G., Wray, E. J., Tao, Q., McAllister, S. D., Rorrer, W. K., Aung, M., et al. (1999). Evaluation of the cannabinoid CB2 receptor-selective antagonist, SR144528: Further evidence for cannabinoid CB2 receptor absence in the rat central nervous system. *European Journal of Pharmacology, 377*(1), 117–125. http://dx.doi.org/10.1016/S0014-2999(99)00402-1.

Hawkins, B. T., & Davis, T. P. (2005). The blood-brain barrier/neurovascular unit in health and disease. *Pharmacological Reviews, 57*(2), 173–185. http://dx.doi.org/10.1124/pr.57.2.4.

Hind, W. H., Tufarelli, C., Neophytou, M., Anderson, S. I., England, T. J., & O'Sullivan, S. E. (2015). Endocannabinoids modulate human blood-brain barrier permeability in vitro. *British Journal of Pharmacology, 172*, 3015–3027. http://dx.doi.org/10.1111/bph.13106.

Honig, A., Rieger, L., Kapp, M., Dietl, J., & Kämmerer, U. (2005). Immunohistochemistry in human placental tissue—Pitfalls of antigen detection. *Journal of Histochemistry & Cytochemistry, 53*(11), 1413–1420. http://dx.doi.org/10.1369/jhc.5A6664.2005.

Huffman, J. W. (2005). CB2 receptor ligands. *Mini Reviews in Medicinal Chemistry, 5*(7), 641–649. http://dx.doi.org/10.2174/1389557054368844.

Kacem, K., Lacombe, P., Seylaz, J., & Bonvento, G. (1998). Structural organization of the perivascular astrocyte endfeet and their relationship with the endothelial glucose transporter: A confocal microscopy study. *Glia, 23*(1), 1–10. http://dx.doi.org/10.1002/(SICI)1098-1136(199805)23:1<1::AID-GLIA1>3.0.CO;2-B.

Kalluri, R. (2003). Basement membranes: Structure, assembly and role in tumour angiogenesis. *Nature Reviews. Cancer, 3*(6), 422–433.

Kong, W., Li, H., Tuma, R. F., & Ganea, D. (2014). Selective CB2 receptor activation ameliorates EAE by reducing Th17 differentiation and immune cell accumulation in the CNS. *Cellular Immunology, 287*(1), 1–17. http://dx.doi.org/10.1016/j.cellimm.2013.11.002.

Kubajewska, I., & Constantinescu, C. S. (2010). Cannabinoids and experimental models of multiple sclerosis. *Immunobiology, 215*(8), 647–657. http://dx.doi.org/10.1016/j.imbio.2009.08.004.

Kwiecien, T. D., Sy, C., & Ding, Y. (2014). Rodent models of ischemic stroke lack translational relevance... are baboon models the answer? *Neurological Research, 36*(5), 417–422. http://dx.doi.org/10.1179/1743132814Y.0000000358.

Lewandowsky, M. (1900). Zur lehre von der cerebrospinalflüssigkeit. *Zeitschrift für Klinische Medizin, 40*, 480–494.

Ley, K., Laudanna, C., Cybulsky, M. I., & Nourshargh, S. (2007). Getting to the site of inflammation: The leukocyte adhesion cascade updated. *Nature Reviews. Immunology*, 7(9), 678–689. http://www.nature.com/nri/journal/v7/n9/suppinfo/nri2156_S1.html.

Liebner, S., Fischmann, A., Rascher, G., Duffner, F., Grote, E. H., Kalbacher, H., et al. (2000). Claudin-1 and claudin-5 expression and tight junction morphology are altered in blood vessels of human glioblastoma multiforme. *Acta Neuropathologica, 100*(3), 323–331. http://dx.doi.org/10.1007/s004010000180.

Lindahl, P., Johansson, B. R., Levéen, P., & Betsholtz, C. (1997). Pericyte loss and microaneurysm formation in PDGF-B-deficient mice. *Science, 277*(5323), 242–245. http://dx.doi.org/10.1126/science.277.5323.242.

Liu, J., Wang, L., Harvey-White, J., Huang, B. X., Kim, H.-Y., Luquet, S., et al. (2008). Multiple pathways involved in the biosynthesis of anandamide. *Neuropharmacology, 54*(1), 1–7. http://dx.doi.org/10.1016/j.neuropharm.2007.05.020.

Lombard, C., Nagarkatti, M., & Nagarkatti, P. (2007). CB2 cannabinoid receptor agonist, JWH-015, triggers apoptosis in immune cells: Potential role for CB2-selective ligands as immunosuppressive agents. *Clinical Immunology*, *122*(3), 259–270. http://dx.doi.org/10.1016/j.clim.2006.11.002.

Lu, T.-S., Avraham, H. K., Seng, S., Tachado, S. D., Koziel, H., Makriyannis, A., et al. (2008). Cannabinoids inhibit HIV-1 Gp120-mediated insults in brain microvascular endothelial cells. *The Journal of Immunology*, *181*(9), 6406–6416.

Lynn, A. B., & Herkenham, M. (1994). Localization of cannabinoid receptors and non-saturable high-density cannabinoid binding sites in peripheral tissues of the rat: Implications for receptor-mediated immune modulation by cannabinoids. *Journal of Pharmacology and Experimental Therapeutics*, *268*(3), 1612–1623.

Mackie, K. (2005). Distribution of cannabinoid receptors in the central and peripheral nervous system. In R. G. Pertwee (Ed.), *Cannabinoids* (pp. 299–325). Berlin, Heidelberg: Springer Berlin Heidelberg.

Maresz, K., Carrier, E. J., Ponomarev, E. D., Hillard, C. J., & Dittel, B. N. (2005). Modulation of the cannabinoid CB2 receptor in microglial cells in response to inflammatory stimuli. *Journal of Neurochemistry*, *95*(2), 437–445. http://dx.doi.org/10.1111/j.1471-4159.2005.03380.x.

Maresz, K., Pryce, G., Ponomarev, E. D., Marsicano, G., Croxford, J. L., Shriver, L. P., et al. (2007). Direct suppression of CNS autoimmune inflammation via the cannabinoid receptor CB1 on neurons and CB2 on autoreactive T cells. *Nature Medicine*, *13*(4), 492–497. http://www.nature.com/nm/journal/v13/n4/suppinfo/nm1561_S1.html.

Marrs, W. R., Blankman, J. L., Horne, E. A., Thomazeau, A., Lin, Y. H., Coy, J., et al. (2010). The serine hydrolase ABHD6 controls the accumulation and efficacy of 2-AG at cannabinoid receptors. *Nature Neuroscience*, *13*(8), 951–957. http://dx.doi.org/10.1038/nn.2601.

Matsuda, L. A., Lolait, S. J., Brownstein, M. J., Young, A. C., & Bonner, T. I. (1990). Structure of a cannabinoid receptor and functional expression of the cloned cDNA. *Nature*, *346*(6284), 561–564.

McKallip, R. J., Lombard, C., Martin, B. R., Nagarkatti, M., & Nagarkatti, P. S. (2002). Δ9-Tetrahydrocannabinol-induced apoptosis in the thymus and spleen as a mechanism of immunosuppression in vitro and in vivo. *Journal of Pharmacology and Experimental Therapeutics*, *302*(2), 451–465. http://dx.doi.org/10.1124/jpet.102.033506.

Mestre, L., Docagne, F., Correa, F., Loría, F., Hernangómez, M., Borrell, J., et al. (2009). A cannabinoid agonist interferes with the progression of a chronic model of multiple sclerosis by downregulating adhesion molecules. *Molecular and Cellular Neuroscience*, *40*(2), 258–266. http://dx.doi.org/10.1016/j.mcn.2008.10.015.

Miller, A. M., & Stella, N. (2008). CB2 receptor-mediated migration of immune cells: It can go either way. *British Journal of Pharmacology*, *153*(2), 299–308. http://dx.doi.org/10.1038/sj.bjp.0707523.

Molina-Holgado, E., Vela, J. M., Arévalo-Martín, A., Almazán, G., Molina-Holgado, F., Borrell, J., et al. (2002). Cannabinoids promote oligodendrocyte progenitor survival: Involvement of cannabinoid receptors and phosphatidylinositol-3 kinase/Akt signaling. *The Journal of Neuroscience*, *22*(22), 9742–9753.

Montecucco, F., Burger, F., Mach, F., & Steffens, S. (2008). CB2 cannabinoid receptor agonist JWH-015 modulates human monocyte migration through defined intracellular signaling pathways. *American Journal of Physiology—Heart and Circulatory Physiology*, *294*(3), H1145–H1155.

Morita, K., Sasaki, H., Furuse, M., & Tsukita, S. (1999). Endothelial claudin: Claudin-5/Tmvcf constitutes tight junction strands in endothelial cells. *The Journal of Cell Biology, 147*(1), 185–194. http://dx.doi.org/10.1083/jcb.147.1.185.

Muller, W. A. (2011). Mechanisms of leukocyte transendothelial migration. *Annual Review of Pathology, 6*, 323–344. http://dx.doi.org/10.1146/annurev-pathol-011110-130224.

Munro, S., Thomas, K. L., & Abu-Shaar, M. (1993). Molecular characterization of a peripheral receptor for cannabinoids. *Nature, 365*(6441), 61–65.

Murikinati, S., Jüttler, E., Keinert, T., Ridder, D. A., Muhammad, S., Waibler, Z., et al. (2010). Activation of cannabinoid 2 receptors protects against cerebral ischemia by inhibiting neutrophil recruitment. *The FASEB Journal, 24*(3), 788–798. http://dx.doi.org/10.1096/fj.09-141275.

Ni, X., Geller, E. B., Eppihimer, M. J., Eisenstein, T. K., Adler, M. W., & Tuma, R. F. (2004). Win 55212-2, a cannabinoid receptor agonist, attenuates leukocyte/endothelial interactions in an experimental autoimmune encephalomyelitis model. *Multiple Sclerosis, 10*(2), 158–164. http://dx.doi.org/10.1191/1352458504ms1009oa.

Nilsson, O., Fowler, C. J., & Jacobsson, S. O. P. (2006). The cannabinoid agonist WIN 55,212-2 inhibits TNF-α-induced neutrophil transmigration across ECV304 cells. *European Journal of Pharmacology, 547*(1–3), 165–173. http://dx.doi.org/10.1016/j.ejphar.2006.07.016.

Nitta, T., Hata, M., Gotoh, S., Seo, Y., Sasaki, H., Hashimoto, N., et al. (2003). Size-selective loosening of the blood-brain barrier in claudin-5–deficient mice. *The Journal of Cell Biology, 161*(3), 653–660. http://dx.doi.org/10.1083/jcb.200302070.

Núñez, E., Benito, C., Pazos, M. R., Barbachano, A., Fajardo, O., González, S., et al. (2004). Cannabinoid CB2 receptors are expressed by perivascular microglial cells in the human brain: An immunohistochemical study. *Synapse, 53*(4), 208–213. http://dx.doi.org/10.1002/syn.20050.

Obermeier, B., Daneman, R., & Ransohoff, R. M. (2013). Development, maintenance and disruption of the blood-brain barrier. *Nature Medicine, 19*(12), 1584–1596. http://dx.doi.org/10.1038/nm.3407.

O'Carroll, S. J., Kho, D. T., Wiltshire, R., Nelson, V., Rotimi, O., Johnson, R., et al. (2015). Pro-inflammatory TNFalpha and IL-1beta differentially regulate the inflammatory phenotype of brain microvascular endothelial cells. *Journal of Neuroinflammation, 12*, 131. http://dx.doi.org/10.1186/s12974-015-0346-0.

Ohtsuki, S., Sato, S., Yamaguchi, H., Kamoi, M., Asashima, T., & Terasaki, T. (2007). Exogenous expression of claudin-5 induces barrier properties in cultured rat brain capillary endothelial cells. *Journal of Cellular Physiology, 210*(1), 81–86. http://dx.doi.org/10.1002/jcp.20823.

Onaivi, E. S., Ishiguro, H., Gong, J.-P., Patel, S., Perchuk, A., Meozzi, P. A., et al. (2006). Discovery of the presence and functional expression of cannabinoid CB2 receptors in brain. *Annals of the New York Academy of Sciences, 1074*(1), 514–536. http://dx.doi.org/10.1196/annals.1369.052.

Pacher, P., Bátkai, S., & Kunos, G. (2006). The endocannabinoid system as an emerging target of pharmacotherapy. *Pharmacological Reviews, 58*(3), 389–462. http://dx.doi.org/10.1124/pr.58.3.2.

Palazuelos, J., Aguado, T., Pazos, M. R., Julien, B., Carrasco, C., Resel, E., et al. (2009). Microglial CB2 cannabinoid receptors are neuroprotective in Huntington's disease excitotoxicity. *Brain, 132*(11), 3152–3164. http://dx.doi.org/10.1093/brain/awp239.

Patel, H. J., Birrell, M. A., Crispino, N., Hele, D. J., Venkatesan, P., Barnes, P. J., et al. (2003). Inhibition of guinea-pig and human sensory nerve activity and the cough reflex in guinea-pigs by cannabinoid (CB2) receptor activation. *British Journal of Pharmacology, 140*(2), 261–268. http://dx.doi.org/10.1038/sj.bjp.0705435.

Patwardhan, A. M., Jeske, N. A., Price, T. J., Gamper, N., Akopian, A. N., & Hargreaves, K. M. (2006). The cannabinoid WIN 55,212-2 inhibits transient receptor potential vanilloid 1 (TRPV1) and evokes peripheral antihyperalgesia via calcineurin. *Proceedings of the National Academy of Sciences of the United States of America, 103*(30), 11393–11398. http://dx.doi.org/10.1073/pnas.0603861103.

Peppiatt, C. M., Howarth, C., Mobbs, P., & Attwell, D. (2006). Bidirectional control of CNS capillary diameter by pericytes. *Nature, 443*(7112), 700–704. http://www.nature.com/nature/journal/v443/n7112/suppinfo/nature05193_S1.html.

Persidsky, Y., Fan, S., Dykstra, H., Reichenbach, N., Rom, S., & Ramirez, S. (2015). Activation of cannabinoid type two receptors (CB2) diminish inflammatory responses in macrophages and brain endothelium. *Journal of Neuroimmune Pharmacology, 10*, 302–308. http://dx.doi.org/10.1007/s11481-015-9591-3.

Pryce, G., Ahmed, Z., Hankey, D. J. R., Jackson, S. J., Croxford, J. L., Pocock, J. M., et al. (2003). Cannabinoids inhibit neurodegeneration in models of multiple sclerosis. *Brain, 126*(10), 2191–2202. http://dx.doi.org/10.1093/brain/awg224.

Ramirez, S. H., Hasko, J., Skuba, A., Fan, S., Dykstra, H., McCormick, R., et al. (2012). Activation of cannabinoid receptor 2 attenuates leukocyte-endothelial cell interactions and blood-brain barrier dysfunction under inflammatory conditions. *The Journal of Neuroscience: The Official Journal of the Society for Neuroscience, 32*(12), 4004–4016. 32/12/4004 [pii]. http://dx.doi.org/10.1523/JNEUROSCI.4628-11.2012.

Ramirez, S. H., Heilman, D., Morsey, B., Potula, R., Haorah, J., & Persidsky, Y. (2008). Activation of peroxisome proliferator-activated receptor γ (PPARγ) suppresses rho GTPases in human brain microvascular endothelial cells and inhibits adhesion and Transendothelial migration of HIV-1 infected monocytes. *The Journal of Immunology, 180*(3), 1854–1865. http://dx.doi.org/10.4049/jimmunol.180.3.1854.

Ramirez, S. H., Reichenbach, N. L., Fan, S., Rom, S., Merkel, S. F., Wang, X., et al. (2013). Attenuation of HIV-1 replication in macrophages by cannabinoid receptor 2 agonists. *Journal of Leukocyte Biology, 93*(5), 801–810. http://dx.doi.org/10.1189/jlb.1012523.

Ramsauer, M., Krause, D., & Dermietzel, R. (2002). Angiogenesis of the blood–brain barrier in vitro and the function of cerebral pericytes. *The FASEB Journal, 16*(10), 1274–1276. http://dx.doi.org/10.1096/fj.01-0814fje.

Rayman, N., Lam, K. H., Laman, J. D., Simons, P. J., Löwenberg, B., Sonneveld, P., et al. (2004). Distinct expression profiles of the peripheral cannabinoid receptor in lymphoid tissues depending on receptor activation status. *The Journal of Immunology, 172*(4), 2111–2117. http://dx.doi.org/10.4049/jimmunol.172.4.2111.

Rayman, N., Lam, K. H., Van Leeuwen, J., Mulder, A. H., Budel, L. M., Löwenberg, B., et al. (2007). The expression of the peripheral cannabinoid receptor on cells of the immune system and non-Hodgkin's lymphomas. *Leukemia & Lymphoma, 48*(7), 1389–1399. http://dx.doi.org/10.1080/10428190701377030.

Rom, S., Zuluaga-Ramirez, V., Dykstra, H., Reichenbach, N. L., Pacher, P., & Persidsky, Y. (2013). Selective activation of cannabinoid receptor 2 in leukocytes suppresses their engagement of the brain endothelium and protects the blood-brain barrier. *The American Journal of Pathology, 183*(5), 1548–1558. http://dx.doi.org/10.1016/j.ajpath.2013.07.033.

Rustenhoven, J., Aalderink, M., Scotter, E. L., Oldfield, R. L., Bergin, P. S., Mee, E. W., et al. (2016). TGF-beta1 regulates human brain pericyte inflammatory processes involved in neurovasculature function. *Journal of Neuroinflammation, 13*(1), 1–15. http://dx.doi.org/10.1186/s12974-016-0503-0.

Ryberg, E., Larsson, N., Sjögren, S., Hjorth, S., Hermansson, N. O., Leonova, J., et al. (2007). The orphan receptor GPR55 is a novel cannabinoid receptor. *British Journal of Pharmacology, 152*(7), 1092–1101. http://dx.doi.org/10.1038/sj.bjp.0707460.

Sánchez, A. J., González-Pérez, P., Galve-Roperh, I., & García-Merino, A. (2006). R-(+)-[2,3-Dihydro-5-methyl-3-(4-morpholinylmethyl)-pyrrolo-[1,2,3-de]-1,4-

benzoxazin-6-yl]-1-naphtalenylmethanone (WIN-2) ameliorates experimental autoimmune encephalomyelitis and induces encephalitogenic T cell apoptosis: Partial involvement of the CB2 receptor. *Biochemical Pharmacology*, *72*(12), 1697–1706. http://dx.doi.org/10.1016/j.bcp.2006.08.018.

Sanchez-Covarrubias, L., Slosky, L. M., Thompson, B. J., Davis, T. P., & Ronaldson, P. T. (2014). Transporters at CNS barrier sites: Obstacles or opportunities for drug delivery? *Current Pharmaceutical Design*, *20*(10), 1422–1449.

Schatz, A. R., Lee, M., Condie, R. B., Pulaski, J. T., & Kaminski, N. E. (1997). Cannabinoid receptors CB1 and CB2: A characterization of expression and adenylate cyclase modulation within the immune system. *Toxicology and Applied Pharmacology*, *142*(2), 278–287. http://dx.doi.org/10.1006/taap.1996.8034.

Schley, M., Ständer, S., Kerner, J., Vajkoczy, P., Schüpfer, G., Dusch, M., et al. (2009). Predominant CB2 receptor expression in endothelial cells of glioblastoma in humans. *Brain Research Bulletin*, *79*(5), 333–337. http://dx.doi.org/10.1016/j.brainresbull.2009.01.011.

Schmöle, A.-C., Lundt, R., Gennequin, B., Schrage, H., Beins, E., Krämer, A., et al. (2015). Expression analysis of CB2-GFP BAC transgenic mice. *PloS One*, *10*(9), e0138986. http://dx.doi.org/10.1371/journal.pone.0138986.

Schulze, C., & Firth, J. A. (1993). Immunohistochemical localization of adherens junction components in blood-brain barrier microvessels of the rat. *Journal of Cell Science*, *104*(3), 773–782.

Shire, D., Calandra, B., Rinaldi-Carmona, M., Oustric, D., Pessègue, B., Bonnin-Cabanne, O., et al. (1996). Molecular cloning, expression and function of the murine CB2 peripheral cannabinoid receptor. *Biochimica et Biophysica Acta (BBA)—Gene Structure and Expression*, *1307*(2), 132–136. http://dx.doi.org/10.1016/0167-4781(96)00047-4.

Simard, M., Arcuino, G., Takano, T., Liu, Q. S., & Nedergaard, M. (2003). Signaling at the gliovascular interface. *The Journal of Neuroscience*, *23*(27), 9254–9262.

Slavik, R., Grether, U., Muller Herde, A., Gobbi, L., Fingerle, J., Ullmer, C., et al. (2015a). Discovery of a high affinity and selective pyridine analog as a potential positron emission tomography imaging agent for cannabinoid type 2 receptor. *Journal of Medicinal Chemistry*, *58*(10), 4266–4277. http://dx.doi.org/10.1021/acs.jmedchem.5b00283.

Slavik, R., Herde, A. M., Bieri, D., Weber, M., Schibli, R., Kramer, S. D., et al. (2015b). Synthesis, radiolabeling and evaluation of novel 4-oxo-quinoline derivatives as PET tracers for imaging cannabinoid type 2 receptor. *European Journal of Medicinal Chemistry*, *92*, 554–564. http://dx.doi.org/10.1016/j.ejmech.2015.01.028.

Soethoudt, M., Grether, U., Fingerle, J., Grim, T. W., Fezza, F., de Petrocellis, L., et al. (2017). Cannabinoid CB2 receptor ligand profiling reveals biased signalling and off-target activity. *Nature Communications*, *8*, 13958. http://dx.doi.org/10.1038/ncomms13958.

Solas, M., Francis, P. T., Franco, R., & Ramirez, M. J. (2013). CB2 receptor and amyloid pathology in frontal cortex of Alzheimer's disease patients. *Neurobiology of Aging*, *34*(3), 805–808. http://dx.doi.org/10.1016/j.neurobiolaging.2012.06.005.

Stempel, A. V., Stumpf, A., Zhang, H. Y., Ozdogan, T., Pannasch, U., Theis, A. K., et al. (2016). Cannabinoid type 2 receptors mediate a cell type-specific plasticity in the hippocampus. *Neuron*, *90*(4), 795–809. http://dx.doi.org/10.1016/j.neuron.2016.03.034.

Suárez, J., Bermúdez-Silva, F. J., Mackie, K., Ledent, C., Zimmer, A., Cravatt, B. F., et al. (2008). Immunohistochemical description of the endogenous cannabinoid system in the rat cerebellum and functionally related nuclei. *The Journal of Comparative Neurology*, *509*(4), 400–421. http://dx.doi.org/10.1002/cne.21774.

Suárez, J., Llorente, R., Romero-Zerbo, S. Y., Mateos, B., Bermúdez-Silva, F. J., de Fonseca, F. R., et al. (2009). Early maternal deprivation induces gender-dependent changes on the expression of hippocampal CB1 and CB2 cannabinoid receptors of neonatal rats. *Hippocampus*, *19*(7), 623–632. http://dx.doi.org/10.1002/hipo.20537.

Sun, Y., & Bennett, A. (2007). Cannabinoids: A new group of agonists of PPARs. *PPAR Research*, *2007*, 23513. http://dx.doi.org/10.1155/2007/23513.

Taylor, L., Christou, I., Kapellos, T. S., Buchan, A., Brodermann, M. H., Gianella-Borradori, M., et al. (2015). Primary macrophage chemotaxis induced by cannabinoid receptor 2 agonists occurs independently of the CB2 receptor. *Scientific Reports*, *5*, 10682. http://dx.doi.org/10.1038/srep10682. http://www.nature.com/srep/2015/150602/srep10682/abs/srep10682.html#supplementary-information.

Thomas, W. E. (1999). Brain macrophages: On the role of pericytes and perivascular cells. *Brain Research Reviews*, *31*(1), 42–57. http://dx.doi.org/10.1016/S0165-0173(99)00024-7.

Tran, N. D., Correale, J., Schreiber, S. S., & Fisher, M. (1999). Transforming growth factor-β mediates astrocyte-specific regulation of brain endothelial anticoagulant factors. *Stroke*, *30*(8), 1671–1678. http://dx.doi.org/10.1161/01.str.30.8.1671.

Tsukita, S., Furuse, M., & Itoh, M. (2001). Multifunctional strands in tight junctions. *Nature Reviews. Molecular Cell Biology*, *2*(4), 285–293.

Upadhyay, R. K. (2014). Transendothelial transport and its role in therapeutics. *International Scholarly Research Notices*, *2014*, 309404. http://dx.doi.org/10.1155/2014/309404.

Utsumi, H., Chiba, H., Kamimura, Y., Osanai, M., Igarashi, Y., Tobioka, H., et al. (2000). Expression of GFRα-1, receptor for GDNF, in rat brain capillary during postnatal development of the BBB. *American Journal of Physiology—Cell Physiology*, *279*(2), C361–C368.

Vendel, E., & de Lange, E. M. (2014). Functions of the CB1 and CB2 receptors in neuroprotection at the level of the blood–brain barrier. *Neuromolecular Medicine*, *16*(3), 620–642. http://dx.doi.org/10.1007/s12017-014-8314-x.

Vincent, P. A., Xiao, K., Buckley, K. M., & Kowalczyk, A. P. (2004). VE-cadherin: Adhesion at arm's length. *American Journal of Physiology—Cell Physiology*, *286*(5), C987–C997. http://dx.doi.org/10.1152/ajpcell.00522.2003.

Weksler, B. B., Subileau, E. A., Perrière, N., Charneau, P., Holloway, K., Leveque, M., et al. (2005). Blood-brain barrier-specific properties of a human adult brain endothelial cell line. *The FASEB Journal*, *19*(13), 1872–1874. http://dx.doi.org/10.1096/fj.04-3458fje.

Williams, J., Appelberg, S., Goldberger, B., Klein, T., Sleasman, J., & Goodenow, M. (2014). Δ9-tetrahydrocannabinol treatment during human monocyte differentiation reduces macrophage susceptibility to HIV-1 infection. *Journal of Neuroimmune Pharmacology*, *9*(3), 369–379. http://dx.doi.org/10.1007/s11481-014-9527-3.

Wolburg, H., & Lippoldt, A. (2002). Tight junctions of the blood–brain barrier: Development, composition and regulation. *Vascular Pharmacology*, *38*(6), 323–337. http://dx.doi.org/10.1016/S1537-1891(02)00200-8.

Wolburg, H., Wolburg-Buchholz, K., Kraus, J., Rascher-Eggstein, G., Liebner, S., Hamm, S., et al. (2003). Localization of claudin-3 in tight junctions of the blood-brain barrier is selectively lost during experimental autoimmune encephalomyelitis and human glioblastoma multiforme. *Acta Neuropathologica*, *105*(6), 586–592. http://dx.doi.org/10.1007/s00401-003-0688-z.

Xie, X.-Q., Chen, J.-Z., & Billings, E. M. (2003). 3D structural model of the G-protein-coupled cannabinoid CB2 receptor. *Proteins: Structure, Function, and Bioinformatics*, *53*(2), 307–319. http://dx.doi.org/10.1002/prot.10511.

Yiangou, Y., Facer, P., Durrenberger, P., Chessell, I. P., Naylor, A., Bountra, C., et al. (2006). COX-2, CB2 and P2X7-immunoreactivities are increased in activated microglial cells/macrophages of multiple sclerosis and amyotrophic lateral sclerosis spinal cord. *BMC Neurology*, *6*(1), 1–14. http://dx.doi.org/10.1186/1471-2377-6-12.

Zhang, M., Adler, M. W., Abood, M. E., Ganea, D., Jallo, J., & Tuma, R. F. (2009a). CB2 receptor activation attenuates microcirculatory dysfunction during cerebral ischemic/reperfusion injury. *Microvascular Research*, *78*(1), 86–94. http://dx.doi.org/10.1016/j.mvr.2009.03.005.

Zhang, H.-Y., Gao, M., Liu, Q.-R., Bi, G.-H., Li, X., Yang, H.-J., et al. (2014). Cannabinoid CB2 receptors modulate midbrain dopamine neuronal activity and dopamine-related behavior in mice. *Proceedings of the National Academy of Sciences of the United States of America*, *111*(46), E5007–E5015. http://dx.doi.org/10.1073/pnas.1413210111.

Zhang, H., Hilton, D. A., Hanemann, C. O., & Zajicek, J. (2011). Cannabinoid receptor and N-acyl phosphatidylethanolamine phospholipase D—Evidence for altered expression in multiple sclerosis. *Brain Pathology*, *21*(5), 544–557. http://dx.doi.org/10.1111/j.1750-3639.2011.00477.x.

Zhang, M., Martin, B. R., Adler, M. W., Razdan, R. K., Ganea, D., & Tuma, R. F. (2008). Modulation of the balance between cannabinoid CB1 and CB2 receptor activation during cerebral ischemic/reperfusion injury. *Neuroscience*, *152*(3), 753–760. http://dx.doi.org/10.1016/j.neuroscience.2008.01.022.

Zhang, M., Martin, B., Adler, M., Razdan, R., Kong, W., Ganea, D., et al. (2009b). Modulation of cannabinoid receptor activation as a neuroprotective strategy for EAE and stroke. *Journal of Neuroimmune Pharmacology*, *4*(2), 249–259. http://dx.doi.org/10.1007/s11481-009-9148-4.

Ziring, D., Wei, B., Velazquez, P., Schrage, M., Buckley, N. E., & Braun, J. (2006). Formation of B and T cell subsets require the cannabinoid receptor CB2. *Immunogenetics*, *58*(9), 714–725. http://dx.doi.org/10.1007/s00251-006-0138-x.

CHAPTER TWELVE

Cannabinoids as Anticancer Drugs

Robert Ramer, Burkhard Hinz[1]
Institute of Pharmacology and Toxicology, Rostock University Medical Center, Rostock, Germany
[1]Corresponding author: e-mail address: burkhard.hinz@med.uni-rostock.de

Contents

Abstract

The endocannabinoid system encompassing cannabinoid receptors, endogenous receptor ligands (endocannabinoids), as well as enzymes conferring the synthesis and degradation of endocannabinoids has emerged as a considerable target for pharmacotherapeutical approaches of numerous diseases. Besides palliative effects of cannabinoids used in cancer treatment, phytocannabinoids, synthetic agonists, as well as substances that increase endogenous endocannabinoid levels have gained interest as potential agents for systemic cancer treatment. Accordingly, cannabinoid compounds have been reported to inhibit tumor growth and spreading in numerous rodent models. The underlying mechanisms include induction of apoptosis, autophagy, and cell cycle arrest in tumor cells as well as inhibition of tumor cell invasion and angiogenic features of endothelial cells. In addition, cannabinoids have been shown to suppress epithelial-to-mesenchymal transition, to enhance tumor immune surveillance, and to support chemotherapeutics' effects on drug-resistant cancer cells. However, unwanted side effects include psychoactivity and possibly pathogenic effects on liver health. Other cannabinoids such as the nonpsychoactive cannabidiol exert a comparatively good safety profile while exhibiting considerable anticancer properties. So far experience with

Advances in Pharmacology, Volume 80
ISSN 1054-3589
http://dx.doi.org/10.1016/bs.apha.2017.04.002

anticarcinogenic effects of cannabinoids is confined to in vitro studies and animal models. Although a bench-to-bedside conversion remains to be established, the current knowledge suggests cannabinoid compounds to serve as a group of drugs that may offer significant advantages for patients suffering from cancer diseases. The present review summarizes the role of the endocannabinoid system and cannabinoid compounds in tumor progression.

ABBREVIATIONS

2-AG 2-arachidonoylglycerol
AA-5HT *N*-arachidonoyl serotonin
ABCG ATP-binding cassette, subfamily G
ACPA arachidonoyl cyclopropylamide
AEA *N*-arachidonoylethanolamine, arachidonoylethanolamide, anandamide
CB_1 cannabinoid receptor 1
CB_2 cannabinoid receptor 2
CBD cannabidiol
CBN cannabinol
CD cluster of differentiation
Cdc25A cell division cycle 25 homolog A
Cdk2 cyclin-dependent kinase 2
JNK c-Jun NH_2-terminal kinase
DAG lipase diacylglycerol lipase
DAG diacylglycerol
EGF epidermal growth factor
EMT epithelial-to-mesenchymal transition
FAAH fatty acid amide hydrolase
GPR G protein-coupled receptor
HER human epidermal growth factor receptor
HUVEC human umbilical vein endothelial cells
ICAM-1 intercellular adhesion molecule-1
Id inhibitor of DNA binding
LAK lymphokine-activated killer cells
LFA-1 lymphocyte function-associated antigen-1
MAGL monoacylglycerol lipase
MAPK mitogen-activated protein kinase
Met-F-AEA 2-methyl-2′-F-anandamide
MMP matrix metalloproteinase
mRNA messenger RNA
NAPE *N*-acyl-phosphatidylethanolamine
NGF nerve growth factor
OEA *N*-oleoylethanolamine, oleoylethanolamide
PAI-1 plasminogen activator inhibitor-1
PEA *N*-palmitoylethanolamine, palmitoylethanolamide
p-GP p-glycoprotein
PLD phospholipase D
PPAR peroxisome proliferator-activated receptor

ROS reactive oxygen species
SDF1α stromal cell-derived factor-1α
SEA *N*-stearoylethanolamine, stearoylethanolamide
siRNA small interfering RNA
THC Δ^9-tetrahydrocannabinol
TIMP-1 tissue inhibitor of matrix metalloproteinases-1
TRPM8 transient receptor potential melastatin type-8
TRPV transient receptor potential vanilloid
VEGF vascular endothelial growth factor

1. INTRODUCTION

The first study aiming at cannabinoid compounds as possible anticancer agents was published in the 1970s far before the discovery of cannabinoid receptors. With their initial experiments, Munson et al. were able to demonstrate that Δ^8-tetrahydrocannabinol, Δ^9-tetrahydrocannabinol (THC), and cannabinol (CBN) suppress tumor growth and prolong the survival of mice in a Lewis lung adenocarcinoma model (Munson, Harris, Friedman, Dewey, & Carchman, 1975). Three years later, the same research group presented data that suggested cannabinoids to exhibit stereospecific binding to biological materials (Harris, Carchman, & Martin, 1978). Notably, at that time cannabinoids were rather supposed to interact with steroid-binding sites than having their own specific cannabinoid target structures. Accordingly, THC was found to interfere with estrogen receptor activation (Rawitch, Schultz, Ebner, & Vardaris, 1977). From the current point of view, the interference of cannabinoids with estrogen action may at least partly be explained by an estrogen response element in exon 1 of the gene encoding the cannabinoid receptor 1 (CB_1) and a cannabinoid-induced upregulation of estrogen receptor-β (Proto et al., 2012; Zhang et al., 2004). However, some investigators also found several cannabinoid compounds to lack interference with estrogen receptors (Ruh, Taylor, Howlett, & Welshons, 1997).

In the 1990s, the Gi/o-coupled cannabinoid receptors, referred to as CB_1 and CB_2 (Matsuda, Lolait, Brownstein, Young, & Bonner, 1990; Munro, Thomas, & Abu-Shaar, 1993), as well as endogenously synthesized fatty acid derivatives acting at these receptors, i.e., arachidonoylethanolamide (anandamide, AEA) and 2-arachidonoylglycerol (2-AG), have been identified (Devane et al., 1992; Mechoulam et al., 1995). Further investigations unraveled the formation of AEA by enzymatic turnover of *N*-arachidonoyl-phosphatidylethanolamine by phospholipase D (PLD) (Di Marzo et al., 1994) and of 2-AG by cleavage of membrane phospholipids via phospholipase C as well as by turnover of diacylglycerol (DAG) via diacylglycerol lipase (DAG lipase) (Stella, Schweitzer, & Piomelli, 1997). In this context, the serine hydrolase fatty acid amide hydrolase (FAAH) has been demonstrated as catabolic enzyme for the degradation of AEA (Deutsch & Chin, 1993) as well as of 2-AG (Di Marzo, Bisogno, Sugiura, Melck, & De Petrocellis, 1998; Goparaju, Ueda, Yamaguchi, & Yamamoto, 1998). Although lacking affinity to cannabinoid receptors, the endocannabinoid-like substances oleoylethanolamide (OEA) and palmitoylethanolamide (PEA) are likewise hydrolyzed by FAAH (Saghatelian et al., 2004). Later, the monoacylglycerol lipase (MAGL) was discovered as the major enzyme of 2-AG degradation (Blankman, Simon, & Cravatt, 2007).

In addition to the specific cannabinoid receptors CB_1 and CB_2, the cation channel transient receptor potential vanilloid 1 (TRPV1) has been reported as additional receptor activated by AEA (Zygmunt et al., 1999) and by the phytocannabinoid cannabidiol (CBD) (Bisogno et al., 2001). Another receptor of the TRP family triggered by the phytocannabinoid cannabigerol is the transient receptor potential melastatin type-8 (TRPM8) (Borrelli et al., 2014). Additionally, CBD has been demonstrated to elicit apoptosis in prostate cancer cells partly via antagonism at the TRPM8 (De Petrocellis et al., 2013).

Meanwhile, several studies have suggested additional G protein-coupled receptors (GPR) to be involved in cannabinoid action such as GPR55 which is antagonized by CBD and activated by abnormal-CBD (synthetic regioisomer of CBD), the specific GPR55 agonist O-1602, R(+)-methanandamide (hydrolysis-stable analog of AEA), JWH-015 (CB_2 receptor agonist), as well as THC (Johns et al., 2007; Lauckner et al., 2008; Ryberg et al., 2007). As a further orphan receptor implicated in cannabinoid action, GPR119 was shown to be triggered by the endocannabinoid-like substances OEA and PEA (Overton et al., 2006). In addition, these endocannabinoid-like substances have been described as ligands at the intracellular receptor peroxisome proliferator-activated receptor-α (PPARα) (Artmann et al., 2008; Fu et al., 2003; Tellez et al., 2013). In this context, OEA was shown to induce satiety and to reduce body weight gain via PPARα activation (Fu et al., 2003).

Recently, TRPV2 was described as additional cannabinoid target. Accordingly, CBD was shown to enhance the sensitivity of glioblastoma and blood cancer cells toward chemotherapeutics via TRPV2 activation (Morelli et al., 2014; Nabissi, Morelli, Santoni, & Santoni, 2013). Moreover, TRPV2 has been demonstrated to mediate CBD-induced autophagy of glioblastoma cells (Nabissi et al., 2015).

The first comprehensive study that addressed cannabinoid receptors as platform for a growth-inhibitory action on cancer cells was published in 1998 (De Petrocellis et al., 1998). In subsequent years anticancer effects of cannabinoids were confirmed by in vitro and in vivo studies using glioblastoma cells (Galve-Roperh et al., 2000; Gomez del Pulgar, Velasco, Sanchez, Haro, & Guzman, 2002; Guzmán, Sanchez, & Galve-Roperh, 2001), followed by an avalanche of publications on anticarcinogenic effects of diverse cannabinoid compounds on various cancer entities.

Noteworthy, R(+)-methanandamide has also been reported to induce apoptosis in cancer cells via enhanced intracellular ceramide levels without involvement of cannabinoid receptors (Hinz, Ramer, Eichele, Weinzierl, & Brune, 2004a). In context with such receptor-independent effects lipid raft microdomains were demonstrated as initial platforms for the toxic impact of R(+)-methanandamide on neuroglioma cells (Hinz, Ramer, Eichele, Weinzierl, & Brune, 2004b). Other studies reported cannabinoids such as AEA to confer toxic effects toward head and neck squamous cell carcinoma cells via production of reactive oxygen species (ROS) regardless of cannabinoid receptor activation (Park et al., 2015). In this context, particularly CBD has been described as anticancer drug due to its capacity to act as a redox modulator thereby conferring inhibition of glioma cell proliferation (Singer et al., 2015) as well as of breast cancer growth and spreading (McAllister et al., 2011).

The main shortcoming and challenge with reference to bench-to-bedside conversion today, however, is the lack of clinical knowledge concerning the safety and efficacy of the cannabinoid dosing regimes that may yield systemic anticancer effects. Until today, merely a single clinical pilot study published in 2006 was carried out that indicated intracranially administered THC to be safe in glioblastoma patients (Guzmán et al., 2006). Other observations were only case reports that suggested, e.g., cannabinoid administration to be associated with a regression of septum pellucidum/forniceal pilocytic astrocytoma tumors in two children (Foroughi, Hendson, Sargent, & Steinbok, 2011) or to elicit beneficial effects on treatment of terminal acute lymphoblastic leukemia with a Philadelphia chromosome mutation of a 14-year-old girl (Singh & Bali, 2013).

As a matter of fact, the clinical use of cannabinoid compounds may be limited by their property to activate central CB_1 receptors being associated with psychoactive effects. In addition, recent findings suggested activation of peripheral CB_1 receptors to confer a risk for the development of liver fibrosis (Teixeira-Clerc et al., 2006). In line with their psychoactive effects, a recent meta-analysis revealed nervous system disorders as most common adverse effects of cannabinoids. However, the authors of this study did not explicitly record liver diseases as serious adverse effect, probably due to the lack of larger studies required to characterize safety issues under conditions of long-term exposure (Wang, Collet, Shapiro, & Ware, 2008).

With respect to central adverse effects, the scientific focus was set on nonpsychoactive cannabinoids. Of particular interest in this context are CB_2 agonists that spare psychoactive effects and may further elicit beneficial effects on the liver by virtue of their antifibrotic action (Julien et al., 2005; Muñoz-Luque et al., 2008). JWH-133, a CB_2 receptor agonist, has been reported to exert tumor-regressive effects in glioblastoma (Sanchez et al., 2001) and skin cancer (Blazquez et al., 2003).

A further anticancerogenic cannabinoid with considerable efficacy in preclinical studies is the nonpsychoactive phytocannabinoid CBD that has been shown to confer a broad array of tumor-blocking properties such as inhibition of cancer cell proliferation (De Petrocellis et al., 2013; Ligresti et al., 2006), cancer cell invasion, and metastasis (Ramer, Merkord, Rohde, & Hinz, 2010; Ramer et al., 2012), as well as tumor angiogenesis (Ramer, Fischer, Haustein, Manda, & Hinz, 2014; Solinas et al., 2012). In addition, CBD has been described to cause apoptosis (Ramer et al., 2013), to enhance immune responses toward tumor cells (Haustein, Ramer, Linnebacher, Manda, & Hinz, 2014), and to sensitize cancer cells toward chemotherapeutics (Holland et al., 2006; Morelli et al., 2014; Nabissi et al., 2013). Finally, CBD was recently found to downregulate markers of epithelial-to-mesenchymal transition (EMT) (Soroceanu et al., 2013). Noteworthy in this context, inhibition of EMT was likewise presented for the cannabinoids WIN 55,212-2 (Xian et al., 2016) and AEA (Laezza, d'Alessandro, Malfitano, & Bifulco, 2013).

Taken together, the current knowledge suggests the endocannabinoid system as considerable target for pharmacological intervention conferring antineoplastic effects that cancer patients might benefit from. The following sections summarize the role of the endocannabinoid system in tumor progression and highlight the options and risks of cannabinoid compounds as anticancer drugs.

2. MODULATION OF THE ENDOCANNABINOID SYSTEM IN TUMOR PROGRESSION

In past years, a number of studies were carried out to address the regulation of endocannabinoids, cannabinoid receptors, and endocannabinoid-degrading enzymes in cancer tissue. Data obtained from these investigations have raised several contradictory interpretations concerning the impact of the endocannabinoid system on cancer progression. The following section provides an overview on data obtained in this field.

2.1 Regulation of Endocannabinoids in Cancer Tissue

In agreement with the hypothesis of endocannabinoids as tumor growth-limiting endogenous substances, an early investigation found AEA and other acylethanolamides such as OEA, PEA, and stearoylethanolamide (SEA) at lower concentrations in meningiomas and gliomas as compared to healthy tissues (Maccarrone, Attinà, Cartoni, Bari, & Finazzi-Agrò, 2001). This finding was further substantiated by a study that reported decreased AEA levels in gliomas vs nontumor tissue (Wu et al., 2012). However, in the latter investigation, tissues of high-grade gliomas were found to contain more AEA than low-grade sections, and 2-AG appeared to be upregulated in glioma vs healthy tissue. Increased levels of AEA were observed in hepatocellular carcinoma vs tumor-free tissue (Mukhopadhyay et al., 2015). In addition, AEA and 2-AG concentrations were found to be upregulated in human meningiomas vs noncancerous brain tissue (Petersen et al., 2005) as well as in adenomatous polyps and colorectal carcinomas as compared to the healthy mucosa (Ligresti et al., 2003). Moreover, analyses of lipid extracts from endometrial carcinomas revealed an upregulation of 2-AG compared to biopsies from healthy patients, whereas AEA and PEA remained virtually unaltered (Guida et al., 2010). Finally, upregulation of endocannabinoids in cancer vs healthy tissue has been substantiated for prostate cancer (Nithipatikom et al., 2004; Schmid, Wold, Krebsbach, Berdyshev, & Schmid, 2002), pituitary adenomas (Pagotto et al., 2001), and colorectal cancer tissue (Chen et al., 2015).

On the other hand, the abovementioned pattern of AEA down-regulation and increased 2-AG levels in cancer tissue as published for gliomas (Wu et al., 2012) could be confirmed in analyses addressing circulating endocannabinoids. Accordingly, patients with different kinds of cancers had lower AEA and higher 2-AG plasma concentrations when compared to a control group (Sailler et al., 2014). The latter study further found increasing OEA levels to correlate with higher numbers of metastases. Another investigation substantiated this notion by detecting elevated serum 2-AG levels to be associated with diffuse large B-cell lymphoma. Here, serum 2-AG levels were significantly higher in cases with late stage disease (Zhang et al., 2016).

2.2 FAAH and MAGL Expression in Cancerous Lesions

The majority of studies that evaluated levels of FAAH and MAGL in cancer patients, revealed an even higher expression of these endocannabinoid-degrading enzymes in cancer vs healthy tissue.

Thus, higher expression levels of FAAH have been reported for biopsies obtained from patients with prostate cancer (Endsley et al., 2008). Another investigation found a correlation between FAAH expression and disease severity using a midrange, but not a high CB_1 level cutoff value (Thors et al., 2010).

Higher expression levels have been also reported for MAGL in ductal breast tumors when compared to less malignant medullary breast tumors (Gjerstorff et al., 2006). Furthermore, an increase of MAGL expression could be confirmed for high-grade primary ovarian tumors (Nomura et al., 2010) as well as for colorectal cancer compared to normal tissue (Ye et al., 2011).

However, some publications have contradicted the assumption of elevated FAAH and MAGL levels as tumor-promoting functional hallmarks. Accordingly, high levels of both enzymes were reported to positively correlate with the prognosis in terms of pancreatic ductal adenocarcinomas (Michalski et al., 2008).

In contrast to endocannabinoid-degrading enzymes, data on the expression levels of endocannabinoid-synthesizing enzymes are rare. In one report, evidence was provided for lower expression levels of *N*-acyl-phosphatidylethanolamine-hydrolyzing phospholipase D (NAPE-PLD), the main enzyme for AEA synthesis, in gliomas vs nontumor controls

(Wu et al., 2012). The same study further found FAAH and MAGL to be downregulated in glioma tissue, while the expression of the 2-AG-synthesizing enzyme DAG lipase remained unchanged, resulting in a decrease of AEA and an increase of 2-AG, respectively. Another investigation reported elevated messenger RNA (mRNA) levels of NAPE-PLD as well as of FAAH in colorectal cancer tissue (Chen et al., 2015). Finally, a downregulation of MAGL was found in endometrial carcinoma (Guida et al., 2010).

Taken together, the data concerning the regulation of endocannabinoids and their degrading enzymes cannot be considered as reliable tumor markers and do not provide consistent information regarding their functional role in tumor progression.

2.3 Cannabinoid Receptor Expression in Cancerous Lesions

Several studies addressing the regulation of cannabinoid receptors in cancerous lesions reported higher cannabinoid receptor expression levels in cancer cells or tissues as compared to healthy counterparts. Accordingly, an early investigation revealed CB_2 receptor upregulation to be directly related to tumor malignancy (Sanchez et al., 2001). Later, the CB_2 receptor was shown to be expressed in a high percentage of human acute myeloid leukemias (Alberich Jorda et al., 2004) and to be elevated in breast cancer (Caffarel, Sarrio, Palacios, Guzman, & Sanchez, 2006), in endometrial carcinoma (Guida et al., 2010), and in bladder tumors (Bettiga et al., 2017). Recent investigations reported a correlation between high levels of CB_2 receptor expression and reduction of disease-specific survival of patients suffering from head and neck squamous cell carcinoma (Klein Nulent et al., 2013) and human epidermal growth factor receptor 2 (HER2)-positive breast cancer (Pérez-Gómez et al., 2015).

The CB_1 receptor was found to be upregulated in mantle cell lymphoma compared to reactive lymphoid tissue (Islam et al., 2003). An increased CB_1 receptor expression has been shown to be associated with poor prognosis in pancreatic cancer (Michalski et al., 2008) and with disease severity and worse outcome in prostate cancer (Chung et al., 2009). The latter finding was substantiated by investigations showing CB_1 upregulation to correlate with Gleason score in prostate cancer (Fowler, 2015). CB_1 receptor expression levels were furthermore demonstrated as marker for adverse outcome in ovarian cancer (Messalli, Grauso, Luise, Angelini, & Rossiello, 2014) as well as advanced stage colorectal cancer (Jung et al., 2013). In human hepatocellular carcinomas, CB_1 receptors were recently reported to appear increased relative to tumor-free areas (Mukhopadhyay et al., 2015). In contrast, another study indicated CB_1 receptor downregulation in clear cell renal carcinoma (Larrinaga et al., 2010). In agreement with this finding, analyses of mRNA obtained from human grade II–III colon carcinomas revealed a downregulation of the CB_1 receptor in 18 of 19 cancer specimens as compared to adjacent healthy mucosa, whereas the CB_2 receptor here remained virtually unaltered (Wang, Wang, Ning, Backlund, Dey, & DuBois, 2008).

Concerning an implication of cannabinoid receptors in hepatocellular carcinoma, overexpression of both cannabinoid receptors was found to be associated with improved prognosis (Xu et al., 2006). On the other hand, a correlation between cannabinoid receptor levels and malignancy was not found in glioblastoma patients (Held-Feindt, Dorner, Sahan, Mehdorn, & Mentlein, 2006).

Collectively, cannabinoid receptor upregulation seems to exhibit a tendency to adverse outcome in terms of some cancer entities. However, cannabinoid receptors do not serve as reliable markers or predictor for cancer development.

3. THE ROLE OF THE ENDOCANNABINOID SYSTEM IN CANCER PROGRESSION AND POTENTIAL PHARMACOLOGICAL OPTIONS OF CANNABINOID COMPOUNDS

The currently available data concerning the effects of the endocannabinoid system on cancer progression provide promising results that suggest cannabinoids as potential antineoplastic agents. With reference to the mechanisms of action, a modulation of several factors has been reported to be associated with suppression of angiogenesis and tumor cell invasion. These facts will be discussed in the following sections.

3.1 Cannabinoids as Anticancer Drugs

Despite the lack of comprehensive clinical data, a large number of in vitro and in vivo studies found cannabinoids to elicit a broad array of anticancer effects with anticarcinogenic effects on cancers of different origin. Probably most comprehensively investigated are effects of cannabinoids on glioblastoma, initiated by experiments that revealed a tumor-regressive action of THC and WIN 55,212-2 to be associated with cannabinoid receptor activation and intracellular ceramide accumulation (Galve-Roperh et al., 2000). Other tumor entities for which cannabinoids were preclinically demonstrated as effective antineoplastic agents include pheochromocytomas (Sarker, Obara, Nakata, Kitajima, & Maruyama, 2000), thyroid epitheliomas (Bifulco et al., 2001), skin carcinomas (Casanova et al., 2002, 2003; Glodde, Jakobs, Bald, Tüting, & Gaffal, 2015), prostate cancers (Nithipatikom et al., 2004), leukemias (McKallip et al., 2006), mantle cell lymphomas (Gustafsson, Christensson, Sander, & Flygare, 2006), pancreatic cancers (Carracedo et al., 2006; Fogli et al., 2006), breast cancers (McAllister et al., 2011; Qamri et al., 2009), rhabdomyosarcomas (Oesch et al., 2009), cervical cancers (Lukhele & Motadi, 2016; Ramer & Hinz, 2008), cholangiocarcinomas (Leelawat, Leelawat, Narong, & Matangkasombut, 2010), colon cancers (Patsos et al., 2010), gastric cancers (Ortega et al., 2016; Xian et al., 2010), neuroblastomas (Hamtiaux et al., 2011), nonsmall cell lung cancers (Ramer et al., 2013), hepatocarcinomas (Pourkhalili et al., 2013), head and neck squamous cell carcinomas (Park et al., 2015), bladder carcinomas (Bettiga et al., 2017; Gasperi et al., 2015), and multiple myeloma (Barbado et al., 2017).

The spectrum of anticarcinogenic impacts of cannabinoids encompass antiproliferative effects (De Petrocellis et al., 1998) as well as induction of apoptosis (Galve-Roperh et al., 2000) and autophagy (Hernández-Tiedra et al., 2016; Salazar et al., 2009; Shrivastava, Kuzontkoski, Groopman, & Prasad, 2011; Vara et al., 2011). Additionally, cannabinoids were shown to enhance the tumor-immune surveillance system as shown in Fig. 1A (Haustein et al., 2014; Kishimoto et al., 2005). Some studies even suggested cannabinoids as possible adjuvants due to their virtue to reduce chemoresistance as has been shown for THC and CBD combined with vinblastine in leukemia cells (Holland et al., 2006) as well as for combinations of CBN, CBD, or THC with mitoxantrone in fibroblasts (Holland, Lau, Allen, & Arnold, 2007). In agreement with this notion, a recent report was able to demonstrate WIN 55,212-2 to support the antimyeloma activity of dexamethasone and melphalan thereby overcoming the resistance to melphalan in cell culture experiments (Barbado et al., 2017). Other studies found CBD to enhance the sensitivity of glioblastoma cells toward the chemotherapeutics carmustine, temozolomide, doxorubicin, and cisplatin (Deng, Ng, Ozawa, & Stella, 2017; Nabissi et al., 2013) as well as of multiple

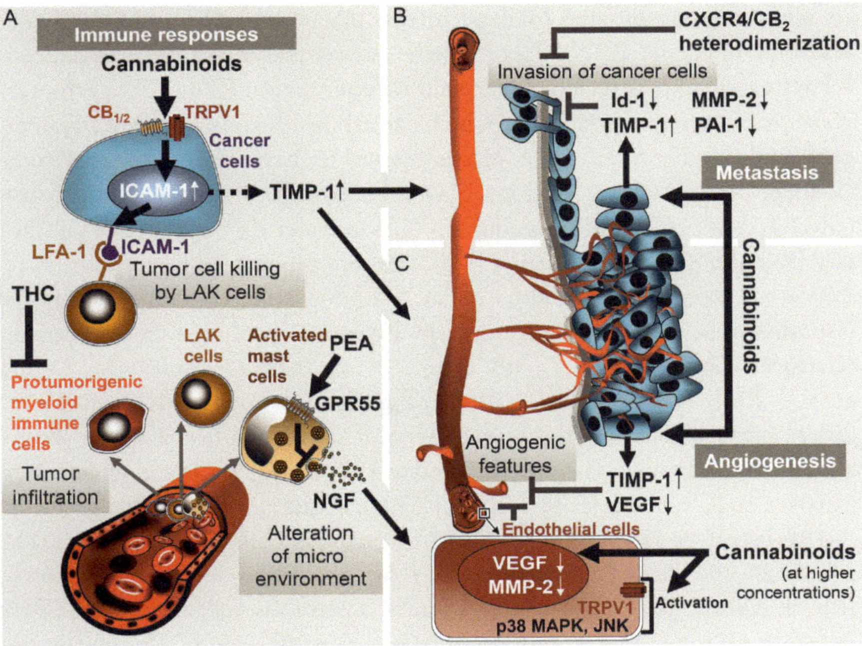

Fig. 1 Selected antineoplastic mechanisms by cannabinoids besides induction of cancer cell apoptosis. (A) Cannabinoids induce expression of intercellular adhesion molecule-1 (ICAM-1) in lung cancer cells via activation of the cannabinoid receptors CB_1 and CB_2 as well as the nonselective cation-channel transient receptor potential vanilloid 1 (TRPV1). ICAM-1 subsequently acts as counter receptor at the lymphocyte function-associated antigen-1 (LFA-1) on the surface of lymphokine-activated killer (LAK) cells conferring LAK cell-induced tumor cell killing. The endocannabinoid-like substance PEA inhibits the release of nerve growth factor (NGF) from mast cells via activation of the orphan receptor GPR55. Endothelial cells exposed to culture media of PEA-treated mast cells exhibit reduction of angiogenic features. ICAM-1 further acts as intracellular signaling molecule that induces enhanced release of tissue inhibitor of matrix metalloproteinases-1 (TIMP-1). THC inhibits the infiltration of protumorigenic myeloid immune cells into skin cancer tissue thereby conferring a less fruitful microenvironment for cancer cell growth. (B) Cannabinoid-induced TIMP-1 release inhibits lung and cervical cancer cell invasion. Further antiinvasive mechanisms of cannabinoids include decrease of matrix metalloproteinase-2 (MMP-2; gastric, breast cancer, glioblastomas), plasminogen activator inhibitor-1 (PAI-1; lung cancer) as well as reduction of inhibitor of DNA binding-1 (Id-1; glioblastomas, breast cancer). Furthermore, a CXCR4/CB_2 receptor heterodimerization was found to inhibit breast cancer cell invasion induced by the CXCR4 chemokine receptor ligand, stromal cell-derived factor-1α (SDF1α). (C) Inhibition of tumor neovascularization by cannabinoids is associated with decrease of vascular endothelial growth factor (VEGF) in experimental glioblastomas, skin, thyroid, and lung cancers. Conditioned media from lung cancer cells challenged with cannabinoids contain increased amounts of TIMP-1 that cause inhibition of angiogenic capacities of endothelial cells. Higher concentrations of cannabinoids that directly inhibit angiogenic features of endothelial cells such as proliferation and migration are associated with downregulation of VEGF, MMP-2, as well as activation of TRPV1, c-Jun NH_2-terminal kinase (JNK), and p38 mitogen-activated protein kinase (MAPK).

myeloma cells toward the proteasome inhibitor bortezomib via activation of TRPV2 (Morelli et al., 2014). Furthermore, a CBD/THC combination was shown to synergistically increase cell death and inhibition of migration induced upon treatment of multiple myeloma cells with the proteasome inhibitor carfilzomib (Nabissi et al., 2016). THC alone has further been demonstrated to support the apoptotic impact of the cytotoxic drugs cytarabine, doxorubicin, and vincristine on leukemia cells via downregulation of p42/44 MAPK (Liu, Scott, Shamash, Joel, & Powles, 2008). In addition, the cannabinoid compounds arachidonoyl cyclopropylpamide (ACPA, CB_1 agonist) and GW405833 (CB_2 agonist) have been reported to enhance chemosensitivity of pancreatic cancer cells toward gemcitabine by an enhanced ROS-dependent induction of autophagy (Donadelli et al., 2011). A synergistic proapoptotic action was further described for the combination of AEA and paclitaxel when using gastric cancer cells (Miyato et al., 2009).

Meanwhile there are several studies that provide evidence for a synergistic action of CB_1 receptor antagonists with chemotherapeutics. As such, one investigation reported an antiproliferative synergism on pancreatic cancer cells between gemcitabine and the CB_1 receptor antagonist SR141716 via enhanced ROS production and autophagy. In this study, SR141716 and gemcitabine further caused a drastic growth inhibition of pancreatic cancer xenograft (Donadelli et al., 2011). Interestingly, the CB_1 antagonist AM-251 has also been shown to gain the toxic impact of 5-fluorouracil on pancreatic cancer cells (Fogli et al., 2006). On the basis of gene expression profile analyses, the authors of the latter study assumed modulation of JAK/STAT and MAPK signaling network as underlying mechanism. This synergism was here discussed as a result of AM-251's diarylpyrazole structure exhibiting substantial structural similarity to the selective COX-2 inhibitor celecoxib rather than specific modulation of the endocannabinoid system. In line with this notion, AM-251 has been demonstrated to induce a synergistic antitumor activity on melanoma cells when combined with celecoxib (Carpi et al., 2015).

An overview of preclinical data on combinations of cannabinoids and chemotherapeutics is provided in Table 1. Here, results from studies that evaluated a synergistic action of cannabinoids combined with chemotherapeutics on the viability of cancer cells were included.

Finally, a recent study observed the combinational treatment of THC/CBD to even enhance the radiosensitivity of cancer cells in an orthotopic murine glioma model (Scott, Dalgleish, & Liu, 2014).

Table 1 Cannabinoids That Enhance Chemosensitivity in Combination With Currently Used Anticancer Drugs

Cannabinoid	Anticancer Drug	Mechanism	Cell Type	Reference
ACPA GW405833 SR141716	Gemcitabine	Autophagy ↑ ROS ↑ NF-κB ↑	Pancreatic cancer	Donadelli et al. (2011)
AEA	Paclitaxel	Caspase-3, -8, and -9 ↑	Gastric cancer	Miyato et al. (2009)
AM-251	Celecoxib	n.d.	Melanoma	Carpi et al. (2015)
	5-Fluorouracil	n.d.	Pancreatic cancer	Fogli et al. (2006)
CBD	Bortezomib	TRPV2 activation	Multiple myeloma	Morelli et al. (2014)
	Carmustine Doxorubicin Temozolomide	TRPV2 activation	Glioblastoma	Nabissi et al. (2013)
	Carmustine Cisplatin Temozolomide	n.d.	Glioblastoma	Deng et al. (2017)
CBD/THC	Carfilzomib	Adducts with the β5i subunit ↑	Multiple myeloma	Nabissi et al. (2016)
CBD THC	Vinblastine	p-GP expression ↓	Leukemia	Holland et al. (2006)
CBD CBN THC	Mitoxantrone	ABCG2 inhibition	Murine embryonic fibroblast	Holland et al. (2007)
THC	Cytarabine Doxorubicin Vincristine	p42/44 MAPK ↓	Leukemia	Liu et al. (2008)
WIN 55,212-2	Dexamethasone Melphalan	n.d.	Multiple myeloma	Barbado et al. (2017)

Arrows (third column) specify cannabinoid-induced upregulation (↑) or downregulation (↓) of the indicated intracellular parameter/mechanism involved in the toxic effects that result from combination of the respective cannabinoid (first column) with the anticancer drug (second column). The fourth column specifies the cell types affected by the combination indicated in the respective line. *Abbreviations*: *ABCG2*, ATP-binding cassette, subfamily G2; *ACPA*, arachidonoyl cyclopropamide; *AEA*, *N*-arachidonoylethanolamine, anandamide; *CBD*, cannabidiol; *CBN*, cannabinol; *GW405833*, CB_2 agonist; *MAPK*, mitogen-activated protein kinase; *n. d.*, not determined; *p-GP*, p-glycoprotein; *ROS*, reactive oxygen species; *SR141716*, CB_1 antagonist; *THC*, Δ^9-tetrahydrocannabinol; *TRPV2*, transient receptor potential vanilloid 2; *WIN 55,212-2*, potent non-selective cannabinoid receptor agonist; *β5i subunit*, catalytic subunit of the proteasome.

3.2 Effects of Cannabinoids on Tumor Angiogenesis

3.2.1 In Vivo Effects of Cannabinoids on Tumor Angiogenesis

The knowledge obtained from animal experiments using immunodeficient mice suggests cannabinoids to inhibit neovascularization in several different cancer types. Accordingly, inhibition of tumor angiogenesis has been reported for epidermal tumors (Casanova et al., 2003), melanomas (Blazquez et al., 2006), breast (Caffarel et al., 2010; Qamri et al., 2009), and lung cancer (Preet et al., 2011) when mice were treated with WIN 55,212-2 or JWH-133. JWH-133 was further demonstrated to be effective against neovascularization of glioma xenografts (Blazquez et al., 2003). Additionally, THC was found to inhibit tumor angiogenesis in models of lung (Preet, Ganju, & Groopman, 2008) and breast cancer (Caffarel et al., 2010) as well as in glioblastomas (Hernán Pérez de la et al., 2013). Furthermore, CBD was proven to inhibit tumor angiogenesis in experimental lung cancer tissue (Ramer et al., 2013). HU-311, a chinone derivative of CBD with topoisomerase II inhibitory properties, was successfully tested for antiangiogenic action in colon carcinomas (Kogan et al., 2006).

Although the antiangiogenic effects of cannabinoids in murine tumor xenograft systems appear undoubtful, the general mechanisms by which cannabinoids elicit their antiangiogenic impact are still a matter of debate. The following parts will address the different cellular aspects of cannabinoids' impact on angiogenesis.

3.2.2 Inhibition of Angiogenic Capacities of Endothelial Cells by Cannabinoids

Several studies revealed cannabinoids to directly inhibit angiogenic capacities of endothelial cells. Thus, the cannabinoids WIN 55,212-2 and JWH-133 were found to suppress migration and survival of human umbilical vein endothelial cells (HUVEC) associated with decrease of vascular endothelial growth factor (VEGF) and matrix metalloproteinase-2 (MMP-2) expression (Blazquez et al., 2003). Another investigation addressing a probable involvement of endocannabinoids in endothelial injuries and shock conditions revealed AEA to exhibit toxic effects toward HUVEC via TRPV1 (Yamaji et al., 2003). As pivotal events conferring this toxic impact, phoshorylations of p38 mitogen-activated protein kinase (MAPK) and c-Jun NH_2-terminal kinase (JNK) were identified. Later, the stable AEA analog, 2-methyl-2′-F-anandamide (Met-F-AEA), was found to inhibit basic fibroblast growth factor-induced proliferation of pig aortic endothelial cells and HUVEC associated with decreased MMP-2 expression (Pisanti et al., 2007). The latter study further revealed Met-F-AEA to inhibit vascular formation in the chick chorioallantoic membrane assays. Furthermore, the CBD chinone HU-331 was found to directly inhibit angiogenic features of endothelial cells (Kogan et al., 2006). Additionally, CBD has been attributed to suppress angiogenic features of endothelial cells (Solinas et al., 2012). Further cannabinoid compounds that were found to act antiangiogenically toward endothelial cells are the hexahydrocannabinol analogs LYR-7 and LYR-8 (Thapa et al., 2011), HU-210, and AEA (Rajesh et al., 2010).

However, some contradictory results have been reported concerning effects of cannabinoids on several types of endothelial cells. Accordingly, knockdown of the CB_1 receptor or pharmacological inhibition of CB_1 was associated with decreased migration, proliferation, and tube formation of growth factor-challenged HUVEC (Pisanti et al., 2011). In agreement with this notion, AEA was here found to even enhance angiogenic capacities. Notably, in other reports AEA was observed to act proapoptotic on the same type of endothelial cells (Yamaji et al., 2003). A simple explanation for this discrepancy may be given by the different concentrations used in the respective studies. Whereas higher concentrations of AEA (10 μM) elicit apoptosis and inhibition of endothelial activation (Yamaji et al., 2003), lower submicromolar concentrations of AEA (0.1 nM–0.1 μM) induce angiogenic features of endothelial cells (Pisanti et al., 2011). Noteworthy, *N*-arachidonoyl serine, another arachidonic acid derivative implicated in endocannabinoid-like action, was shown to elicit proangiogenic effects via activation of GPR55 (Zhang, Maor, Wang, Kunos, & Groopman, 2010). However, a probable proangiogenic impact restricted to the group of endocannabinoids at lower concentrations seems unlikely due to recent findings demonstrating modest proangiogenic effects when HUVEC were directly exposed to 3 μM concentrations of either CBD, THC, R(+)-methanandamide, or JWH-133 (Ramer et al., 2014). Taken into further account an earlier report demonstrating THC and CBD to confer proangiogenic effects when tested at a concentration of 50 nM (Kogan et al., 2006), it is tempting to speculate that cannabinoids may act in a proangiogenic manner toward endothelial cells at pharmacologically relevant concentrations. Accordingly, an analysis of plasma concentrations in patients treated with CBD yielded plasma peaks of 36 nM (Consroe, Kennedy, & Schram, 1991). Moreover, oral doses of 15 and 20 mg THC resulted in average peak plasma concentrations of 30 and 46 nM, respectively (Wall, Sadler, Brine, Taylor, & Perez-Reyes, 1983). Thus, these in vitro findings partly contradict the large number of preclinical in vivo findings demonstrating inhibition of angiogenesis in cancer tissue by cannabinoids. The antiangiogenic actions of cannabinoids tested at higher concentrations are depicted in Fig. 1C.

3.2.3 *Suppression of Tumor Angiogenesis by Cannabinoid-Modulated Intercellular Cross Talks*

Taken into further consideration various factors modulated by cannabinoids in cancer or immune cells, cannabinoid-induced anti-angiogenesis in cancer tissue may likewise arise from tumor-to-endothelial or immune-to-endothelial cell communications finally leading to reduced neovascularization.

As depicted in Fig. 1C, diverse cannabinoids (i.e., CBD, THC, R(+)-methanandamide, and JWH-133) were demonstrated to alter the microenvironment of lung cancer cells thereby conferring inhibition of angiogenic capacities of endothelial cells. As mechanism of action, the aforementioned cannabinoids were demonstrated to inhibit angiogenesis via stimulating the release of tissue inhibitor of matrix metalloproteinases-1 (TIMP-1) from cancer cells (Ramer et al., 2014). TIMP-1 acting as an endogenous inhibitor of MMPs exhibits antiangiogenic effects (Oh et al., 2004), although some data likewise support an MMP-independent effect on endothelial cells (Akahane, Akahane, Shah, Connor, & Thorgeirsson, 2004). The assumption of a cannabinoid-induced tumor-to-endothelial communication resulting in attenuation of cancer-related angiogenesis is further substantiated by a study that found conditioned media from AEA-treated breast cancer cells to inhibit endothelial cell proliferation (Picardi, Ciaglia, Proto, & Pisanti, 2014). In this study, inhibition of HUVEC proliferation was associated with downregulation of several angiogenesis-related factors such as VEGF, leptin, interferon-γ, and thrombopoietin. Other studies have suggested a modulation of inflammatory immune cells to contribute to cannabinoids' antiangiogenic responses. Accordingly, the endocannabinoid-like substance PEA was found to reduce the release of nerve growth factor (NGF) into conditioned media from activated mast cells via GPR55 thereby eliciting inhibition of endothelial cell proliferation (Fig. 1A) (Cantarella et al., 2011). Concerning further effects of cannabinoids on immune responses, a recent study reported THC to decrease the number of inflammatory immune cells in the microenvironment of experimental melanomas (Glodde et al., 2015). Interestingly, in this investigation the authors did not observe a toxic impact of THC on skin cancer cells in vitro. Nevertheless, THC was found to inhibit the recruitment of protumorigenic myeloid immune cells in vivo thereby producing a less fruitful microenvironment for cancer cell growth without alteration of tumor angiogenesis (Fig. 1A).

The main factors expected to be modulated in an intercellular communication resulting in antiangiogenic effects of cannabinoids include growth factors such as VEGF as well as members of the MMP family. In fact, a downregulation of MMP-2 by several cannabinoid compounds in different tumor types was found to be associated with the antiangiogenic and antiinvasive action of the respective substances (Blazquez et al., 2003; Caffarel et al., 2010; Ramer & Hinz, 2008; see also Section 3.3). Using murine glioma and human astrocytoma xenograft models, an early investigation reported JWH-133 to decrease the levels of VEGF and MMP-2 (Blazquez et al., 2003). Later, the authors found JWH-133 to downregulate the upstream mediator of VEGF expression, hypoxia-inducible factor-1α on the transcriptional level (Blázquez et al., 2004). A cannabinoid-induced downregulation of VEGF was also confirmed for experimental skin tumors following treatment with the cannabinoids JWH-133 and WIN 55,212-2 (Casanova et al., 2003), for rat thyroid cancer cells exposed to Met-F-AEA (Portella et al., 2003), as well as for lung cancer cells treated with THC (Preet et al., 2008).

The complex interaction of different cell types involved in angiogenic responses affected by cannabinoid compounds is illustrated in Fig. 1A and C.

3.3 Effects of Cannabinoids on Metastasis

A number of reports found cannabinoids to elicit antiinvasive effects in vitro as well as a reduction of metastasis in rodent models. In an early work published in this field, 2-AG was demonstrated to suppress invasion of prostate cancer cells in a CB_1-dependent manner (Nithipatikom et al., 2004). As intracellular antiinvasive mechanisms, cannabinoids were found to downregulate inhibitors of DNA binding (Ids), among which Id-1 was described to support progression of metastasis of breast cancer cells into the lung by inhibiting basic helix-loop-helix transcription factors (Minn et al., 2005). In this context, the decrease of breast cancer cell invasion by CBD was associated with downregulation of Id-1 (McAllister, Christian, Horowitz, Garcia, & Desprez, 2007). An Id-1-dependent antiinvasive property of CBD was later substantiated by experiments using brain cancer as well as primary glioblastoma cells (Soroceanu et al., 2013). Recently, O-1663, a bicyclic resorcinol with selective affinity to the CB_2 receptor, was discovered as another cannabinoid with antiinvasive properties dependent on Id-1 inhibition (Murase et al., 2014).

As further important metastasis-related factors that facilitate cancer spreading by virtue of their proteolytic action but also independent thereof (for review, see Ramer & Hinz, 2016), members of the MMP family have been described to be modulated by cannabinoids on the level of expression (Curran & Murray, 2000; Stamenkovic, 2000). In this context, MMP-2 has been shown to be downregulated by cannabinoid compounds in several reports. As such, the selective CB_2 agonist JWH-133 conferred MMP-2 decrease in glioma cells in vitro and in xenograft tissue (Blazquez et al., 2003). MMP-2 downregulation was further associated with decreased invasion of glioma cells challenged with THC (Blázquez et al., 2008), of cervical cancer cells treated with R(+)-methanandamide or THC (Ramer & Hinz, 2008), of gastric cancer cells treated with WIN 55,212-2 (Xian et al., 2010), and of hepatocarcinoma cells treated with the CB_1 receptor agonist arachidonoyl 2′-chloroethylamide or the high affinity and selective CB_2 agonist CB65, respectively (Pourkhalili et al., 2013). The antiinvasive and MMP-2-downregulating properties of arachidonoyl 2′-chloroethylamide and R(+)-methanandamide were further substantiated in experiments using breast cancer cells (Farsandaj, Ghahremani, & Ostad, 2012). Remarkably and in contrast to the observed antiinvasive and MMP-2-attenuating effects caused by CB65 in liver cancer cells (Pourkhalili et al., 2013), the authors here found CB65 to increase both invasiveness and MMP-2 expression of breast cancer cells. Noteworthy in this context, in another study CBD did not alter MMP-2 expression in cervical cancer cells (Ramer, Merkord, et al., 2010). Thus, MMP-2 downregulation by cannabinoids may appear in a cancer cell type-dependent manner.

Considering further members of the MMP family modulated upon cannabinoid treatment, the regulation of the endogenous inhibitor of MMP, TIMP-1, was focused on as key regulator of cannabinoid-modulated cancer cell invasion in past years. In previous studies, TIMP-1 was shown to negatively correlate with metastatic promotion in athymic mice (Khokha et al., 1989) and to exhibit an antiinvasive impact on cancer cells in vitro (Cattaneo, Fontanella, Canton, Delia, & Biunno, 2005; Ramer, Eichele, & Hinz, 2007). TIMP-1 becomes induced by THC, R(+)-methanandamide and CBD in cervical and lung cancer cells (Ramer & Hinz, 2008; Ramer, Merkord, et al., 2010; Ramer et al., 2012). Using small interfering (si) RNA approaches, evidence was provided to suggest a causal relation between TIMP-1 upregulation and the antiinvasive properties of

THC and R(+)-methanandamide (Ramer & Hinz, 2008) as well as CBD (Ramer, Merkord, et al., 2010; Ramer et al., 2012). The intercellular adhesion molecule-1 (ICAM-1) was later identified as upstream regulator of cannabinoid-induced TIMP-1 expression in lung cancer cells (Ramer et al., 2012). In addition, ICAM-1, upregulated upon treatment of lung cancer cells with diverse cannabinoids, has recently been further found to act as counter receptor for the lymphocyte function-associated antigen-1 (LFA-1) on the surface of lymphokine-activated killer cells (LAK), thereby conferring enhanced killing of cannabinoid-challenged cancer cells (Haustein et al., 2014). The diverse actions of ICAM-1 are presented in Fig. 1A and B.

A recent publication revealed the FAAH inhibitors URB597 and *N*-arachidonoyl serotonin (AA-5HT) as well as the FAAH substrates AEA and OEA to likewise block lung cancer cell invasion by virtue of their TIMP-1-inducing properties (Winkler et al., 2016). Moreover, a contribution of 2-AG turnover to tumor cell invasion was shown by findings indicating the MAGL inhibitor JZL184 and small interfering RNA (siRNA) targeting MAGL to inhibit invasion of colorectal cancer cell lines associated with downregulation of cyclin D1 and B-cell lymphoma 2 (Bcl-2) (Ye et al., 2011).

Searching for further antiinvasive mechanisms of CBD, plasminogen activator inhibitor-1 (PAI-1) was found to be downregulated in CBD-treated lung cancer cells. In this study, CBD's antiinvasive properties were partly reversed in the presence of recombinant PAI-1 at concentrations not eliciting a basal proinvasive action. Thus, a suppression of PAI-1 may contribute, at least in part, to the antiinvasive action of CBD (Ramer, Rohde, Merkord, Rohde, & Hinz, 2010).

THC has been found to modulate several downstream targets of epidermal growth factor (EGF) signaling such as Akt, p42/44 MAPK, and JNK resulting in decreased invasiveness of EGF-activated cancer cells (Preet et al., 2008). Antiinvasive effects were also reported for the selective CB_2 receptor agonists AM-1241 and JWH-015 with both compounds inhibiting the migration of breast cancer cells activated by the agonist at the chemokine receptor CXCR4, stromal cell-derived factor-1α (SDF1α). The authors postulated a CXCR4/CB_2 receptor heterodimerization to be responsible for reduced cancer cell migration as presented in Fig. 1B (Coke et al., 2016). An interference of cannabinoid compounds with CXCR4 signaling was likewise found in multiple myeloma cells (Nabissi et al., 2016). In this study, CBD, THC, a combination of both cannabinoids as well as a combination of both cannabinoids with carfilzomib were shown to inhibit SDF1α-induced migration of a multiple myeloma cell line. This study additionally found treatment with CBD and THC combined with carfilzomib to inhibit chemotaxis of these cells challenged with eCyPA, an agonist at the CD147 receptor, that triggers myeloma bone marrow homing. The data concerning cannabinoids' antiinvasive mechanisms are presented in Fig. 1B.

In case of CBD acid, an enzymatic product of cannabigerolic acid, a downregulation of c-fos has been discussed as a further mechanism involved in inhibition of breast cancer cell migration (Takeda et al., 2017). Moreover, the antiinvasive action of Met-F-AEA was reported to include activation of the wingless/integrated (Wnt) signaling pathway via downregulation of Id-1. AEA-induced increase of glycogen synthase kinase 3β conferred subsequent decrease of β-catenin thereby inhibiting β-catenin-dependent oncogenes such as the markers of EMT, Snail1, Slug, and Twist (Laezza et al., 2013). The suppression of EMT by the endocannabinoid is presented in Fig. 2.

In vitro findings on antiinvasive properties of cannabinoids were confirmed in vivo by numerous reports using rodent models. Thus, inhibition of metastasis was observed in a mouse model of Lewis lung carcinoma metastasis in Met-F-AEA-treated animals (Portella et al., 2003). Additionally, WIN 55,212-2 was described to inhibit melanoma metastasis (Blazquez et al., 2006). In a murine cancer metastasis model, using a nonsmall cell lung cancer cell line, the antimetastatic impact of CBD was repeatedly confirmed (Ramer, Merkord, et al., 2010; Ramer et al., 2012). As underlying mechanism, the CBD-induced ICAM-1 expression by lung cancer cells could be proven as key signaling event. Accordingly, suppression of ICAM-1 by use of a neutralizing antibody partly reversed the inhibitory impact of CBD on lung cancer metastasis (Ramer et al., 2012). CBD has also been found to block breast cancer (McAllister et al., 2011) and glioblastoma metastasis (Soroceanu et al., 2013) with both effects being associated with downregulation of Id-1. The key role of Id-1 reduction within the antimetastatic mechanism of cannabinoids toward breast cancer was later also confirmed for the cannabinoid O-1663 (Murase et al., 2014). WIN 55,212-2 and JWH-133 were further approved as cannabinoid-based drugs conferring inhibition of breast cancer spreading in vivo (Qamri et al., 2009). Inhibition of lung cancer metastasis was also confirmed for THC (Preet et al., 2008). Finally, a recent investigation found the endocannabinoid-elevating FAAH inhibitors URB597 and AA-5HT to inhibit lung cancer metastasis in vivo (Winkler et al., 2016). In line with this data, the latter study likewise revealed antimetastatic properties for intraperitoneally applied AEA, 2-AG, OEA, and PEA.

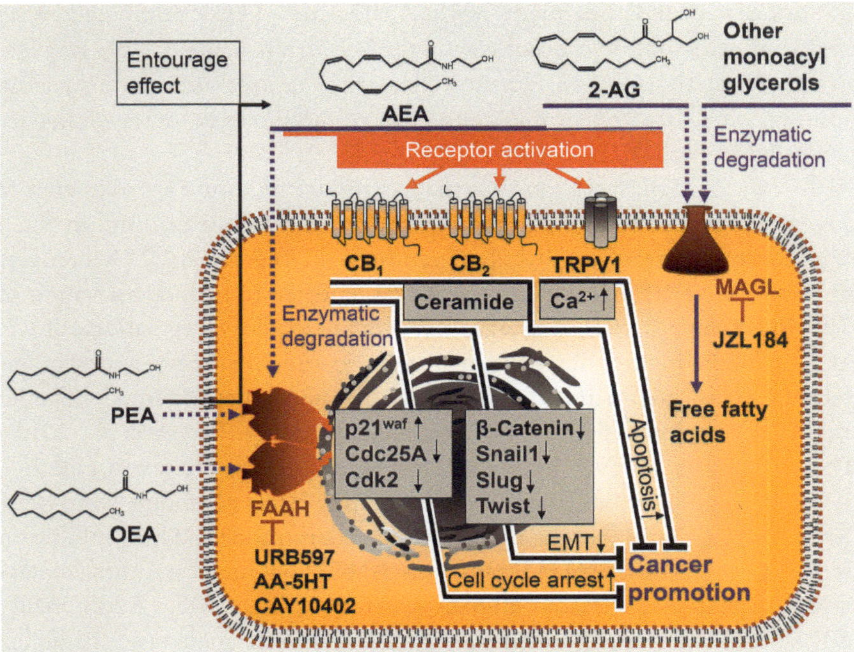

Fig. 2 Involvement of the endocannabinoid system in cancer progression. Fatty acid amide hydrolase (FAAH) confers hydrolysis of the endocannabinoids anandamide (AEA) and 2-arachidonoylglycerol (2-AG) as well as of the endocannabinoid-like substances oleoylethanolamide (OEA) and palmitoylethanolamide (PEA) that do not exhibit affinity to cannabinoid receptors CB_1 and CB_2. Levels of AEA, 2-AG, OEA, and PEA are increased upon inhibition of FAAH by URB597, arachidonoyl-serotonin (AA-5HT), and CAY10402. PEA enhances effects of AEA at cannabinoid receptors via downregulation of FAAH and support of calcium (Ca^{2+}) conductance, assigned as entourage effect. Endocannabinoids in turn may inhibit cancer growth and induce apoptosis via cannabinoid receptor-triggered intracellular ceramide accumulation or TRPV1-dependent Ca^{2+} influx. AEA further inhibits cell cycle checkpoint response via upregulation of $p21^{waf}$, degradation of the dual specificity phosphatase Cdc25A converging on suppression of cyclin-dependent kinase 2 (Cdk2) activity. Transformation of cancer cells into invasive phenotypes is further suppressed by AEA via downregulation of the EMT markers β-catenin, Snail1, Slug, and Twist. Monoacylglycerol lipase (MAGL) is the major degrading enzyme for 2-AG but also for other monoacylglycerols. Inhibition of MAGL by JZL184 suppresses cancer growth via prolonged activation of cannabinoid receptors by 2-AG or by decrease of cancer-promoting free fatty acids. Factors written in *gray font* indicate transcriptionally modulated genes.

4. INHIBITION OF ENDOCANNABINOID-DEGRADING ENZYMES AS ANTICANCER STRATEGY

According to several research groups, the endocannabinoid system may pose an endogenous anticancer system (for review, see Petrosino & Di Marzo, 2010; Ramer & Hinz, 2016). This view is mainly based on findings that indicate endocannabinoids to act anticancerogenic and on experiments that clearly provide evidence for antineoplastic effects of drugs that inhibit endocannabinoid turnover.

With respect to anticancer properties of endocannabinoids, AEA was reported to inhibit proliferation of NGF- (De Petrocellis et al., 1998) and EGF-stimulated prostate cancer cells (Mimeault, Pommery, Wattez, Bailly, & Hénichart, 2003) as well as of mantle cell lymphoma cell lines (Gustafsson et al., 2006) and thyroid cancer cells (Bifulco et al., 2004). Antiproliferative effects of AEA and 2-AG were further confirmed in murine glioma (Jacobsson, Wallin, & Fowler, 2001) and colorectal cancer cells (Ligresti et al., 2003). As mechanism of action, AEA was found to modulate cell cycle arrest via upregulation of $p21^{waf}$, degradation of Cdc25A, and inhibition of the cyclin *E*–Cdk2 kinase complex activation in a CB_1 receptor-dependent manner (Fig. 2) (Laezza, Pisanti, Crescenzi, & Bifulco, 2006). Furthermore, AEA was found to elicit apoptosis of human gastric adenocarcinoma (Ortega et al., 2016), prostate cancer (Orellana-Serradell et al., 2015), colorectal cancer (Patsos et al., 2010), and melanoma cells (Adinolfi et al., 2013).

In agreement with the data obtained with AEA, inhibition of the AEA-degrading enzyme, FAAH, revealed similar anticancer effects (Ligresti et al., 2003). Most of these experiments were performed using the FAAH inhibitors AA-5HT (Bisogno et al., 1998) and URB597 (Alexander & Cravatt, 2005). An antiproliferative effect of AA-5HT was confirmed in thyroid cancer cells in vitro and in vivo (Bifulco et al., 2004). Noteworthy, antiproliferative effects of AA-5HT and AEA observed in the latter investigation were shown to involve a CB_1-dependent pathway. On the other hand, AA-5HT was found to completely reverse the formation of aberrant crypt foci regardless of the genotype (CB_1 knockout vs wild-type mice) in a rodent model with azoxymethane-induced colonic aberrant crypt foci (Izzo et al., 2008).

Using neuroblastoma cells, AEA was proven to elicit an antiproliferative action that became even enhanced in the presence of URB597 (Hamtiaux et al., 2011). Similar results were obtained from experiments that addressed the effect of combinational treatment of inhibitors of endocannabinoid-degrading enzymes and PEA in melanoma cells (Hamtiaux et al., 2012). In this study, the FAAH inhibitors URB597 and CAY10402 as well as the unspecific FAAH/MAGL inhibitors MAFP and CAY10499 potentiated the cytotoxic impact of PEA toward melanoma cells. By use of a melanoma xenograft model, the latter study could further confirm a growth-inhibitory action of URB597 when combined with PEA, but not when administered alone. In contrast to the cytotoxic action of PEA shown by Hamtiaux et al. (2012), earlier reports found PEA to act as an entourage agent that enhances the cytostatic impact of AEA without causing a cytotoxic action on cancer cells per se (Fig. 2) (Di Marzo et al., 2001). Furthermore, a combination of URB597 with Met-F-AEA was demonstrated to confer a growth-inhibitory action via interference with EGF signaling in vitro and in vivo (Ravi, Sneh, Shilo, Nasser, & Ganju, 2014). As likewise demonstrated for melanoma cells (Hamtiaux et al., 2012), URB597 was later found to lack a tumor growth-inhibitory action in xenografts derived from lung cancer cells (Ravi et al., 2014; Winkler et al., 2016).

An overview of the connection between FAAH inhibition, prolonged action of endocannabinoids at their cognate receptors and the subsequent growth-inhibitory action is presented in Fig. 2.

A further target of endocannabinoid turnover, the 2-AG-degrading MAGL, has attracted considerable scientific interest as modulator of cancer growth. Accordingly, a recent study found knockdown of MAGL and treatment with the MAGL inhibitor JZL184 to elicit suppression of proliferation and induction of apoptosis in colorectal cancer cells (Ye et al., 2011). The latter report provided first-time proof for a tumor-regressive action of MAGL siRNA and JZL184 in vivo using a colon cancer xenograft model. In agreement with the tumor-regressive impact of MAGL inhibition, the MAGL substrate 2-AG was demonstrated to inhibit cell invasion of androgen-independent prostate carcinoma cells in a CB_1 receptor-dependent manner (Nithipatikom et al., 2004). The latter study further found inhibition of 2-AG synthesis by the DAG lipase inhibitor RHC-80267 to increase cancer cell invasion, vice versa. Additionally, MAGL inhibition by a small hairpin RNA approach or by treatment with JZL184 was associated with decreased invasion in vitro as well as with a growth-inhibitory action toward prostate carcinoma xenografts (Nomura et al., 2011). Here, the authors presented a dual mechanism underlying the antiinvasive and growth-inhibitory action of MAGL inhibition that partially involved CB_1 receptor activation. In addition to CB_1 receptor activation, free fatty acids conferred a partial suppression of this antiinvasive action. Therefore, these products of MAGL activity were supposed to act as procancerogenic lipid precursors for synthesis of lysophosphatidic acid and prostaglandins. This hypothesis was substantiated using breast, ovarian, and melanoma cancer cells (Nomura et al., 2010). MAGL was additionally described as integral component of the EMT and cancer cell stemness according to a large-scale transcriptional analysis that monitored gene expression signatures of aggressive vs nonaggressive cancer cells (Nomura et al., 2011). The abovementioned facts concerning the role of the endocannabinoid system in cancer progression are summarized in Fig. 2.

5. CONCLUSION

When almost four decades ago Harris et al. (1978) were presenting the first data suggesting cannabinoids to stereospecifically bind to cell fractions, they stated that it remained to be determined "whether such binding has any relevance to the pharmacological effects of this interesting class of drugs." From the current point of view, it has to be concluded that far above this assumption, cannabinoid receptor modulation represents an integral component of ubiquitous physiological processes and appears as attractive target for treatment of neoplastic diseases. However, at present, it still remains to be unraveled whether cannabinoids may reach any clinical relevance for systemic cancer treatment.

Despite many beneficial effects, several studies have raised doubts concerning anticancer effects of cannabinoids with findings suggesting cannabinoids to even support cancer growth and spreading. As such, early investigations found mitotic effects of THC in prostate cancer (Sánchez, Ruiz-Llorente, Sánchez, & Díaz-Laviada, 2003) and glioblastoma cells (Hart, Fischer, & Ullrich, 2004). Furthermore, R(+)-methanandamide and THC were shown to increase tumor growth in immunocompetent mice (Gardner, Zhu, Sharma, Tashkin, & Dubinett, 2003; Zhu et al., 2000). Moreover, high cannabinoid receptor levels were demonstrated to confer mitotic effects by coupling to prosurvival pathways in astrocytoma cells (Cudaback, Marrs, Moeller, & Stella, 2010). A recent investigation even reported CB_1 receptor knockout mice or wild-type mice treated with a peripheral CB_1 receptor antagonist to develop fewer and smaller tumors in a chemically induced hepatocellular carcinoma model (Mukhopadhyay et al., 2015). Another study showed knockdown of CB_2 receptors in

HER-overexpressing breast cancer cells to be associated with decreased growth of xenografts and metastasis (Pérez-Gómez et al., 2015). In agreement with these findings, the CB_1 receptor antagonist SR141716 was found to act antineoplastic in some studies (Ciaglia et al., 2015; Sarnataro et al., 2006). However, these reports are in contrast to the vast majority of preclinical data that support cannabinoids or substances that enhance the endocannabinoid levels as option for anticancer treatment.

Established cannabinoid effects that cancer patients may benefit from result from reduction of severe side effects of currently used chemotherapeutics. Accordingly, cannabinoids are currently already used in cancer patients to suppress emesis and nausea (Tramèr et al., 2001), and to relieve cancer pain (Khasabova et al., 2012). A previous meta-analysis revealed cannabinoids as considerable option for the treatment of cancer-related pain (Martin-Sanchez, Furukawa, Taylor, & Martin, 2009). Another recently published meta-analysis assessed 28 studies (including 1772 participants) that addressed cannabinoid effects on nausea and vomiting due to chemotherapy. Here, benefits of cannabinoid treatments were recorded vs comparator (mostly prochlorperazine) or placebo without yielding statistical significance (Whiting et al., 2015).

Additionally, several protective effects were proven for cannabinoid compounds suggesting, e.g., benefits for cancer patients with chemotherapy-induced peripheral neuropathy (Gingerich, Wadhwa, Lemanski, Krahn, & Daeninck, 2009). Cannabinoids were furthermore demonstrated to palliate adverse effects of the chemotherapeutic agent cisplatin. In this context, the CB_2 agonist LEI-101 was found to decrease the nephrotoxicity of cisplatin in a murine model (Mukhopadhyay et al., 2016). With respect to systemic anticancer effects of cannabinoids, their synergistic interaction with a number of cytostatic drugs as well as their property to suppress metastasis and tumor-associated neovascularization is of particular interest.

Concerning putative combinational treatments in cancer therapies, cannabinoids seem to elicit a synergistic increase of the antitumorigenic action of conventional chemotherapeutics, while counteracting some of their adverse effects. Indeed, several recently published studies demonstrated THC and CBD to boost the cytostatic effects of a considerable number of chemotherapeutic drugs (Table 1). With respect to some reports that demonstrated cannabinoids to alter transport capacities of chemotherapeutic drugs via inhibition of efflux transporters such as p-glycoprotein (p-GP) (Holland et al., 2006; Molnár et al., 2000; Nieri et al., 2006), however, possible adverse drug interactions have to be taken into consideration.

The significance of drugs that elicit inhibition of metastasis arises from the fact that almost all fatal progressions of malignant diseases are associated with metastasis. Unfortunately, specific options to counteract metastasis are currently barely available. Hence, there is an urgent need for novel therapeutic approaches that specifically target metastatic processes. Based on the preclinical findings summarized here, cannabinoids may serve as "antimetastatics" to improve the clinical prospects of treating advance stage cancer diseases. In addition, cannabinoids may provide an option as anti-angiogenic drugs. In this context, various innovative pharmacotherapeutical approaches currently pursue this strategy such as an antibody against VEGF, bevacizumab, that has been proven to provide benefits in metastatic renal cell cancer (Yang et al., 2003), colorectal cancer (Hurwitz et al., 2004), non-small cell lung cancer (Sandler et al., 2006), and ovarian cancer (Perren et al., 2011). Small molecules targeting tumor angiogenesis currently used are sunitinib, sorafenib, and pazopanib (Iacovelli et al., 2014). Thus, cannabinoid compounds may offer an attractive small molecule supplement for antiangiogenic treatments of solid tumors.

Unfortunately, data concerning efficacy and safety of cannabinoids are currently not available from clinical studies that address systemic effects on cancer progression beyond palliative use. In this context, it is tempting to speculate that, according to anecdotal reports, high-dose applications are favorable (Abrams, 2016). Concerning the safety and efficacy of cannabinoids, the recently published largest multicenter observational study (1615 patients from 30 centers) specified nabiximols (Sativex™), a combination of THC and CBD, as an effective and safe treatment for patients with multiple sclerosis with moderate to severe spasticity (Patti et al., 2016).

According to such clinical evaluations, the major therapy-limiting unwanted side effect of cannabinoids lies in the psychoactive properties of compounds such as THC that exert high affinity to the CB_1 receptor and pass the blood–brain barrier. As considerable alternatives for systemic cancer treatment, nonpsychoactive cannabinoids such as CBD or JWH-133 have been demonstrated to exert remarkable anticancer properties with respect to the existing preclinical expertise. In this context, CBD was demonstrated to exert high safety even when applied chronically with high doses up to 1.5 g/day (Bergamaschi, Queiroz, Zuardi, & Crippa, 2011). Thus, the anticarcinogenic effects of cannabinoids are not obligatory associated with psychoactivity. This particular fact favors nonpsychoactive cannabinoids for systemic cancer therapies.

Taken together, cannabinoids may support the future armamentarium for treatment of cancer diseases beyond their palliative use, as inhibitors of cancer growth, as cytostatic boosters, as antimetastatics, and as inhibitors of tumor neovascularization, given that clinical studies will exceed case reports and will provide evidence for considerable systemic benefits.

CONFLICT OF INTEREST

The authors state no conflict of interest.

REFERENCES

Abrams, D. I. (2016). Integrating cannabis into clinical cancer care. *Current Oncology, 23*, 8–14.

Adinolfi, B., Romanini, A., Vanni, A., Martinotti, E., Chicca, A., Fogli, S., et al. (2013). Anticancer activity of anandamide in human cutaneous melanoma cells. *European Journal of Pharmacology, 718*, 154–159.

Akahane, T., Akahane, M., Shah, A., Connor, C. M., & Thorgeirsson, U. P. (2004). TIMP-1 inhibits microvascular endothelial cell migration by MMP-dependent and MMP-independent mechanisms. *Experimental Cell Research, 301*, 158–167.

Alberich Jorda, M., Rayman, N., Tas, M., Verbakel, S. E., Battista, N., van Lom, K., et al. (2004). The peripheral cannabinoid receptor Cb2, frequently expressed on AML blasts, either induces a neutrophilic differentiation block or confers abnormal migration properties in a ligand dependent manner. *Blood, 104*, 526–534.

Alexander, J. P., & Cravatt, B. F. (2005). Mechanism of carbamate inactivation of FAAH: Implications for the design of covalent inhibitors and in vivo functional probes for enzymes. *Chemistry & Biology, 12*, 1179–1187.

Artmann, A., Petersen, G., Hellgren, L. I., Boberg, J., Skonberg, C., Nellemann, C., et al. (2008). Influence of dietary fatty acids on endocannabinoid and N-acylethanolamine levels in rat brain, liver and small intestine. *Biochimica et Biophysica Acta, 1781*, 200–212.

Barbado, M. V., Medrano, M., Caballero-Velázquez, T., Álvarez-Laderas, I., Sánchez-Abarca, L. I., García-Guerrero, E., et al. (2017). Cannabinoid derivatives exert a potent anti-myeloma activity both in vitro and in vivo. *International Journal of Cancer, 140*, 674–685.

Bergamaschi, M. M., Queiroz, R. H., Zuardi, A. W., & Crippa, J. A. (2011). Safety and side effects of cannabidiol, a Cannabis sativa constituent. *Current Drug Safety, 6*, 237–249.

Bettiga, A., Aureli, M., Colciago, G., Murdica, V., Moschini, M., Lucianò, R., et al. (2017). Bladder cancer cell growth and motility implicate cannabinoid 2 receptor-mediated modifications of sphingolipids metabolism. *Scientific Reports*, 7, 42157. http://dx.doi.org/10.1038/srep42157.

Bifulco, M., Laezza, C., Portella, G., Vitale, M., Orlando, P., De Petrocellis, L., et al. (2001). Control by the endogenous cannabinoid system of ras oncogene-dependent tumor growth. *The FASEB Journal, 15*, 2745–2747.

Bifulco, M., Laezza, C., Valenti, M., Ligresti, A., Portella, G., & Di Marzo, V. (2004). A new strategy to block tumor growth by inhibiting endocannabinoid inactivation. *The FASEB Journal, 18*, 1606–1608.

Bisogno, T., Hanus, L., De Petrocellis, L., Tchilibon, S., Ponde, D. E., Brandi, I., et al. (2001). Molecular targets for cannabidiol and its synthetic analogues: Effect on vanilloid VR1 receptors and on the cellular uptake and enzymatic hydrolysis of anandamide. *British Journal of Pharmacology, 134*, 845–852.

Bisogno, T., Melck, D., De Petrocellis, L., Bobrov, M. Y., Gretskaya, N. M., Bezuglov, V. V., et al. (1998). Arachidonoylserotonin and other novel inhibitors of fatty acid amide hydrolase. *Biochemical and Biophysical Research Communications, 248*, 515–522.

Blankman, J. L., Simon, G. M., & Cravatt, B. F. (2007). A comprehensive profile of brain enzymes that hydrolyze the endocannabinoid 2-arachidonoylglycerol. *Chemistry & Biology, 14*, 1347–1356.

Blazquez, C., Carracedo, A., Barrado, L., Real, P. J., Fernandez-Luna, J. L., Velasco, G., et al. (2006). Cannabinoid receptors as novel targets for the treatment of melanoma. *The FASEB Journal, 20*, 2633–2635.

Blazquez, C., Casanova, M. L., Planas, A., Gomez Del Pulgar, T., Villanueva, C., Fernandez-Acenero, M. J., et al. (2003). Inhibition of tumor angiogenesis by cannabinoids. *The FASEB Journal, 17*, 529–531.

Blázquez, C., González-Feria, L., Alvarez, L., Haro, A., Casanova, M. L., & Guzmán, M. (2004). Cannabinoids inhibit the vascular endothelial growth factor pathway in gliomas. *Cancer Research, 64*, 5617–5623.

Blázquez, C., Salazar, M., Carracedo, A., Lorente, M., Egia, A., González-Feria, L., et al. (2008). Cannabinoids inhibit glioma cell invasion by down-regulating matrix metalloproteinase-2 expression. *Cancer Research, 68*, 1945–1952.

Borrelli, F., Pagano, E., Romano, B., Panzera, S., Maiello, F., Coppola, D., et al. (2014). Colon carcinogenesis is inhibited by the TRPM8 antagonist cannabigerol, a cannabis-derived non-psychotropic cannabinoid. *Carcinogenesis, 35*, 2787–2797.

Caffarel, M. M., Andradas, C., Mira, E., Pérez-Gómez, E., Cerutti, C., Moreno-Bueno, G., et al. (2010). Cannabinoids reduce ErbB2-driven breast cancer progression through Akt inhibition. *Molecular Cancer, 9*, 196.

Caffarel, M. M., Sarrio, D., Palacios, J., Guzman, M., & Sanchez, C. (2006). Delta9-tetrahydrocannabinol inhibits cell cycle progression in human breast cancer cells through Cdc2 regulation. *Cancer Research, 66*, 6615–6621.

Cantarella, G., Scollo, M., Lempereur, L., Saccani-Jotti, G., Basile, F., & Bernardini, R. (2011). Endocannabinoids inhibit release of nerve growth factor by inflammation-activated mast cells. *Biochemical Pharmacology, 82*, 380–388.

Carpi, S., Fogli, S., Romanini, A., Pellegrino, M., Adinolfi, B., Podestà, A., et al. (2015). AM251 induces apoptosis and G2/M cell cycle arrest in A375 human melanoma cells. *Anti-Cancer Drugs, 26*, 754–762.

Carracedo, A., Lorente, M., Egia, A., Blázquez, C., García, S., Giroux, V., et al. (2006). The stress-regulated protein p8 mediates cannabinoid-induced apoptosis of tumor cells. *Cancer Cell, 9*, 301–312.

Casanova, M. L., Blazquez, C., Martinez-Palacio, J., Villanueva, C., Fernandez-Acenero,-M. J., Huffman, J. W., et al. (2003). Inhibition of skin tumor growth and angiogenesis in vivo by activation of cannabinoid receptors. *The Journal of Clinical Investigation, 111*, 43–50.

Casanova, M. L., Larcher, F., Casanova, B., Murillas, R., Fernandez-Acenero, M. J., Villanueva, C., et al. (2002). A critical role for ras-mediated, epidermal growth factor receptor-dependent angiogenesis in mouse skin carcinogenesis. *Cancer Research, 62*, 3402–3407.

Cattaneo, M., Fontanella, E., Canton, C., Delia, D., & Biunno, I. (2005). SEL1L affects human pancreatic cancer cell cycle and invasiveness through modulation of PTEN and genes related to cell-matrix interactions. *Neoplasia, 7*, 1030–1038.

Chen, L., Chen, H., Li, Y., Li, L., Qiu, Y., & Ren, J. (2015). Endocannabinoid and ceramide levels are altered in patients with colorectal cancer. *Oncology Reports, 34*, 447–454.

Chung, S. C., Hammarsten, P., Josefsson, A., Stattin, P., Granfors, T., Egevad, L., et al. (2009). A high cannabinoid CB_1 receptor immunoreactivity is associated with disease severity and outcome in prostate cancer. *European Journal of Cancer, 45*, 174–182.

Ciaglia, E., Torelli, G., Pisanti, S., Picardi, P., D'Alessandro, A., Laezza, C., et al. (2015). Cannabinoid receptor CB1 regulates STAT3 activity and its expression dictates the responsiveness to SR141716 treatment in human glioma patients' cells. *Oncotarget*, *6*, 15464–15481.

Coke, C. J., Scarlett, K. A., Chetram, M. A., Jones, K. J., Sandifer, B. J., Davis, A. S., et al. (2016). Simultaneous activation of induced heterodimerization between CXCR4 chemokine receptor and cannabinoid receptor 2 (CB2) reveal a mechanism for regulation of tumor progression. *The Journal of Biological Chemistry*, *291*, 9991–10005.

Consroe, P., Kennedy, K., & Schram, K. (1991). Assay of plasma cannabidiol by capillary gas chromatography/ion trap mass spectroscopy following high-dose repeated daily oral administration in humans. *Pharmacology, Biochemistry, and Behavior*, *40*, 517–552.

Cudaback, E., Marrs, W., Moeller, T., & Stella, N. (2010). The expression level of CB_1 and CB_2 receptors determines their efficacy at inducing apoptosis in astrocytomas. *PloS One*, *5*. e8702.

Curran, S., & Murray, G. I. (2000). Matrix metalloproteinases: Molecular aspects of their roles in tumour invasion and metastasis. *European Journal of Cancer*, *36*, 1621–1630.

De Petrocellis, L., Ligresti, A., Schiano Moriello, A., Iappelli, M., Verde, R., Stott, C. G., et al. (2013). Non-THC cannabinoids inhibit prostate carcinoma growth in vitro and in vivo: Pro-apoptotic effects and underlying mechanisms. *British Journal of Pharmacology*, *168*, 79–102.

De Petrocellis, L., Melck, D., Palmisano, A., Bisogno, T., Laezza, C., Bifulco, M., et al. (1998). The endogenous cannabinoid anandamide inhibits human breast cancer cell proliferation. *Proceedings of the National Academy of Sciences of the United States of America*, *95*, 8375–8380.

Deng, L., Ng, L., Ozawa, T., & Stella, N. (2017). Quantitative analyses of synergistic responses between cannabidiol and DNA-damaging agents on the proliferation and viability of glioblastoma and neural progenitor cells in culture. *The Journal of Pharmacology and Experimental Therapeutics*, *360*, 215–224.

Deutsch, D. G., & Chin, S. A. (1993). Enzymatic synthesis and degradation of anandamide, a cannabinoid receptor agonist. *Biochemical Pharmacology*, *46*, 791–796.

Devane, W. A., Hanus, L., Breuer, A., Pertwee, R. G., Stevenson, L. A., Griffin, G., et al. (1992). Isolation and structure of a brain constituent that binds to the cannabinoid receptor. *Science*, *258*, 1946–1949.

Di Marzo, V., Bisogno, T., Sugiura, T., Melck, D., & De Petrocellis, L. (1998). The novel endogenous cannabinoid 2-arachidonoylglycerol is inactivated by neuronal- and basophil-like cells: Connections with anandamide. *The Biochemical Journal*, *331*, 15–19.

Di Marzo, V., Fontana, A., Cadas, H., Schinelli, S., Cimino, G., Schwartz, J. C., et al. (1994). Formation and inactivation of endogenous cannabinoid anandamide in central neurons. *Nature*, *372*, 686–691.

Di Marzo, V., Melck, D., Orlando, P., Bisogno, T., Zagoory, O., Bifulco, M., et al. (2001). Palmitoylethanolamide inhibits the expression of fatty acid amide hydrolase and enhances the anti-proliferative effect of anandamide in human breast cancer cells. *The Biochemical Journal*, *358*, 249–255.

Donadelli, M., Dando, I., Zaniboni, T., Costanzo, C., Dalla Pozza, E., Scupoli, M. T., et al. (2011). Gemcitabine/cannabinoid combination triggers autophagy in pancreatic cancer cells through a ROS-mediated mechanism. *Cell Death & Disease*, *2*. e152.

Endsley, M. P., Thill, R., Choudhry, I., Williams, C. L., Kajdacsy-Balla, A., Campbell, W. B., et al. (2008). Expression and function of fatty acid amide hydrolase in prostate cancer. *International Journal of Cancer*, *123*, 1318–1326.

Farsandaj, N., Ghahremani, M. H., & Ostad, S. N. (2012). Role of cannabinoid and vanilloid receptors in invasion of human breast carcinoma cells. *Journal of Environmental Pathology, Toxicology and Oncology*, *31*, 377–387.

Fogli, S., Nieri, P., Chicca, A., Adinolfi, B., Mariotti, V., Iacopetti, P., et al. (2006). Cannabinoid derivatives induce cell death in pancreatic MIA PaCa-2 cells via a receptor-independent mechanism. *FEBS Letters*, *580*, 1733–1739.

Foroughi, M., Hendson, G., Sargent, M. A., & Steinbok, P. (2011). Spontaneous regression of septum pellucidum/forniceal pilocytic astrocytomas—Possible role of cannabis inhalation. *Child's Nervous System*, *27*, 671–679.

Fowler, C. J. (2015). Delta^9-tetrahydrocannabinol and cannabidiol as potential curative agents for cancer: A critical examination of the preclinical literature. *Clinical Pharmacology and Therapeutics*, *97*, 587–596.

Fu, J., Gaetani, S., Oveisi, F., Lo Verme, J., Serrano, A., de Fonseca, F. R., et al. (2003). Oleylethanolamide regulates feeding and body weight through activation of the nuclear receptor PPAR-alpha. *Nature*, *425*, 90–93.

Galve-Roperh, I., Sanchez, C., Cortes, M. L., Gomez del Pulgar, T., Izquierdo, M., & Guzman, M. (2000). Anti-tumoral action of cannabinoids: Involvement of sustained ceramide accumulation and extracellular signal-regulated kinase activation. *Nature Medicine*, *6*, 313–319.

Gardner, B., Zhu, L. X., Sharma, S., Tashkin, D. P., & Dubinett, S. M. (2003). Methanandamide increases COX-2 expression and tumor growth in murine lung cancer. *The FASEB Journal*, *17*, 2157–2159.

Gasperi, V., Evangelista, D., Oddi, S., Florenzano, F., Chiurchiù, V., Avigliano, L., et al. (2015). Regulation of inflammation and proliferation of human bladder carcinoma cells by type-1 and type-2 cannabinoid receptors. *Life Sciences*, *138*, 41–51.

Gingerich, J., Wadhwa, D., Lemanski, L., Krahn, M., & Daeninck, P. J. (2009). The use of cannabinoids (CBs) for the treatment of chemotherapy-induced peripheral neuropathy (CIPN): A retrospective review. *Journal of Clinical Oncology*, *27*. e20743.

Gjerstorff, M. F., Benoit, V. M., Laenkholm, A. V., Nielsen, O., Johansen, L. E., & Ditzel, H. J. (2006). Identification of genes with altered expression in medullary breast cancer vs. ductal breast cancer and normal breast epithelia. *International Journal of Oncology*, *28*, 1327–1335.

Glodde, N., Jakobs, M., Bald, T., Tüting, T., & Gaffal, E. (2015). Differential role of cannabinoids in the pathogenesis of skin cancer. *Life Sciences*, *138*, 35–40.

Gomez del Pulgar, T., Velasco, G., Sanchez, C., Haro, A., & Guzman, M. (2002). De novo-synthesized ceramide is involved in cannabinoid-induced apoptosis. *The Biochemical Journal*, *363*, 183–188.

Goparaju, S. K., Ueda, N., Yamaguchi, H., & Yamamoto, S. (1998). Anandamide amidohydrolase reacting with 2-arachidonoylglycerol, another cannabinoid receptor ligand. *FEBS Letters*, *422*, 69–73.

Guida, M., Ligresti, A., De Filippis, D., D'Amico, A., Petrosino, S., Cipriano, M., et al. (2010). The levels of the endocannabinoid receptor CB2 and its ligand 2-arachidonoylglycerol are elevated in endometrial carcinoma. *Endocrinology*, *151*, 921–928.

Gustafsson, K., Christensson, B., Sander, B., & Flygare, J. (2006). Cannabinoid receptor-mediated apoptosis induced by R(+)-methanandamide and Win55,212 is associated with ceramide accumulation and p38 activation in mantle cell lymphoma. *Molecular Pharmacology*, *70*, 1612–1620.

Guzmán, M., Duarte, M. J., Blázquez, C., Ravina, J., Rosa, M. C., Galve-Roperh, I., et al. (2006). A pilot study of Delta-9-tetrahydrocannabinol in patients with recurrent glioblastoma multiforme. *British Journal of Cancer*, *95*, 197–203.

Guzmán, M., Sanchez, C., & Galve-Roperh, I. (2001). Control of the cell survival/death decision by cannabinoids. *Journal of Molecular Medicine (Berlin, Germany)*, *78*, 613–625.

Hamtiaux, L., Hansoulle, L., Dauguet, N., Muccioli, G. G., Gallez, B., & Lambert, D. M. (2011). Increasing antiproliferative properties of endocannabinoids in N1E-115 neuroblastoma cells through inhibition of their metabolism. *PloS One*, *6*. e26823.

Hamtiaux, L., Masquelier, J., Muccioli, G. G., Bouzin, C., Feron, O., Gallez, B., et al. (2012). The association of N-palmitoylethanolamine with the FAAH inhibitor URB597 impairs melanoma growth through a supra-additive action. *BMC Cancer*, *12*, 92.
Harris, L. S., Carchman, R. A., & Martin, B. R. (1978). Evidence for the existence of specific cannabinoid binding sites. *Life Sciences*, *22*, 1131–1137.
Hart, S., Fischer, O., & Ullrich, A. (2004). Cannabinoids induce cancer cell proliferation via tumor necrosis factor a-converting enzyme (TACE/ADAM17)-mediated trans-activation of the epidermal growth factor. *Cancer Research*, *64*, 1943–1950.
Haustein, M., Ramer, R., Linnebacher, M., Manda, K., & Hinz, B. (2014). Cannabinoids increase lung cancer cell lysis by lymphokine-activated killer cells via upregulation of ICAM-1. *Biochemical Pharmacology*, *92*, 312–325.
Held-Feindt, J., Dorner, L., Sahan, G., Mehdorn, H. M., & Mentlein, R. (2006). Cannabinoid receptors in human astroglial tumors. *Journal of Neurochemistry*, *98*, 886–893.
Hernán Pérez de la Ossa, D., Lorente, M., Gil-Alegre, M. E., Torres, S., García-Taboada, E., Aberturas Mdel, R., et al. (2013). Local delivery of cannabinoid-loaded microparticles inhibits tumor growth in a murine xenograft model of glioblastoma multiforme. *PloS One*, *8*. e54795.
Hernández-Tiedra, S., Fabriàs, G., Dávila, D., Salanueva, Í. J., Casas, J., Montes, L. R., et al. (2016). Dihydroceramide accumulation mediates cytotoxic autophagy of cancer cells via autolysosome destabilization. *Autophagy*, *12*, 2213–2229.
Hinz, B., Ramer, R., Eichele, K., Weinzierl, U., & Brune, K. (2004a). Up-regulation of cyclooxygenase-2 expression is involved in R(+)-methanandamide-induced apoptotic death of human neuroglioma cells. *Molecular Pharmacology*, *66*, 1643–1651.
Hinz, B., Ramer, R., Eichele, K., Weinzierl, U., & Brune, K. (2004b). R(+)-methanandamide-induced cyclooxygenase-2 expression in H4 human neuroglioma cells: Possible involvement of membrane lipid rafts. *Biochemical and Biophysical Research Communications*, *324*, 621–626.
Holland, M. L., Lau, D. T., Allen, J. D., & Arnold, J. C. (2007). The multidrug transporter ABCG2 (BCRP) is inhibited by plant-derived cannabinoids. *British Journal of Pharmacology*, *152*, 815–824.
Holland, M. L., Panetta, J. A., Hoskins, J. M., Bebawy, M., Roufogalis, B. D., Allen, J. D., et al. (2006). The effects of cannabinoids on P-glycoprotein transport and expression in multidrug resistant cells. *Biochemical Pharmacology*, *71*, 1146–1154.
Hurwitz, H., Fehrenbacher, L., Novotny, W., Cartwright, T., Hainsworth, J., Heim, W., et al. (2004). Bevacizumab plus irinotecan, fluorouracil, and leucovorin for metastatic colorectal cancer. *The New England Journal of Medicine*, *350*, 2335–2342.
Iacovelli, R., Alesini, D., Palazzo, A., Trenta, P., Santoni, M., De Marchis, L., et al. (2014). Targeted therapies and complete responses in first line treatment of metastatic renal cell carcinoma. A meta-analysis of published trials. *Cancer Treatment Reviews*, *40*, 271–275.
Islam, T. C., Asplund, A. C., Lindvall, J. M., Nygren, L., Liden, J., Kimby, E., et al. (2003). High level of cannabinoid receptor 1, absence of regulator of G protein signalling 13 and differential expression of cyclin D1 in mantle cell lymphoma. *Leukemia*, *17*, 1880–1890.
Izzo, A. A., Aviello, G., Petrosino, S., Orlando, P., Marsicano, G., Lutz, B., et al. (2008). Increased endocannabinoid levels reduce the development of precancerous lesions in the mouse colon. *Journal of Molecular Medicine (Berlin, Germany)*, *86*, 89–98.
Jacobsson, S. O., Wallin, T., & Fowler, C. J. (2001). Inhibition of rat C6 glioma cell proliferation by endogenous and synthetic cannabinoids. Relative involvement of cannabinoid and vanilloid receptors. *The Journal of Pharmacology and Experimental Therapeutics*, *299*, 951–959.
Johns, D. G., Behm, D. J., Walker, D. J., Ao, Z., Shapland, E. M., Daniels, D. A., et al. (2007). The novel endocannabinoid receptor GPR55 is activated by atypical

cannabinoids but does not mediate their vasodilator effects. *British Journal of Pharmacology, 152*, 825–831.

Julien, B., Grenard, P., Teixeira-Clerc, F., Van Nhieu, J. T., Li, L., Karsak, M., et al. (2005). Antifibrogenic role of the cannabinoid receptor CB2 in the liver. *Gastroenterology, 128*, 742–755.

Jung, C. K., Kang, W. K., Park, J. M., Ahn, H. J., Kim, S. W., Taek Oh, S., et al. (2013). Expression of the cannabinoid type I receptor and prognosis following surgery in colorectal cancer. *Oncology Letters, 5*, 870–876.

Khasabova, I. A., Khasabov, S., Paz, J., Harding-Rose, C., Simone, D. A., & Seybold, V. S. (2012). Cannabinoid type-1 receptor reduces pain and neurotoxicity produced by chemotherapy. *The Journal of Neuroscience, 32*, 7091–7101.

Khokha, R., Waterhouse, P., Yagel, S., Lala, P. K., Overall, C. M., Norton, G., et al. (1989). Antisense RNA-induced reduction in murine TIMP levels confers oncogenicity on Swiss 3T3 cells. *Science, 243*, 947–950.

Kishimoto, S., Muramatsu, M., Gokoh, M., Oka, S., Waku, K., & Sugiura, T. (2005). Endogenous cannabinoid receptor ligand induces the migration of human natural killer cells. *Journal of Biochemistry, 137*, 217–223.

Klein Nulent, T. J., Van Diest, P. J., van der Groep, P., Leusink, F. K., Kruitwagen, C. L., Koole, R., et al. (2013). Cannabinoid receptor-2 immunoreactivity is associated with survival in squamous cell carcinoma of the head and neck. *The British Journal of Oral & Maxillofacial Surgery, 1*, 604–609.

Kogan, N. M., Blázquez, C., Alvarez, L., Gallily, R., Schlesinger, M., Guzmán, M., et al. (2006). A cannabinoid quinone inhibits angiogenesis by targeting vascular endothelial cells. *Molecular Pharmacology, 70*, 51–59.

Laezza, C., d'Alessandro, A., Malfitano, A. M., & Bifulco, M. (2013). Anandamide inhibits the Wnt/β-catenin signalling pathway in human breast cancer MDA MB 231 cells. *European Journal of Cancer, 48*, 3112–3122.

Laezza, C., Pisanti, S., Crescenzi, E., & Bifulco, M. (2006). Anandamide inhibits Cdk2 and activates Chk1 leading to cell cycle arrest in human breast cancer cells. *FEBS Letters, 580*, 6076–6082.

Larrinaga, G., Sanz, B., Pérez, I., Blanco, L., Cándenas, M. L., Pinto, F. M., et al. (2010). Cannabinoid CB_1 receptor is downregulated in clear cell renal cell carcinoma. *The Journal of Histochemistry and Cytochemistry, 58*, 1129–1134.

Lauckner, J. E., Jensen, J. B., Chen, H. Y., Lu, H. C., Hille, B., & Mackie, K. (2008). GPR55 is a cannabinoid receptor that increases intracellular calcium and inhibits M current. *Proceedings of the National Academy of Sciences of the United States of America, 105*, 2699–2704.

Leelawat, S., Leelawat, K., Narong, S., & Matangkasombut, O. (2010). The dual effects of delta(9)-tetrahydrocannabinol on cholangiocarcinoma cells: Anti-invasion activity at low concentration and apoptosis induction at high concentration. *Cancer Investigation, 28*, 357–363.

Ligresti, A., Bisogno, T., Matias, I., De Petrocellis, L., Cascio, M. G., Cosenza, V., et al. (2003). Possible endocannabinoid control of colorectal cancer growth. *Gastroenterology, 125*, 677–687.

Ligresti, A., Moriello, A. S., Starowicz, K., Matias, I., Pisanti, S., De Petrocellis, L., et al. (2006). Antitumor activity of plant cannabinoids with emphasis on the effect of cannabidiol on human breast carcinoma. *The Journal of Pharmacology and Experimental Therapeutics, 318*, 1375–1387.

Liu, W. M., Scott, K. A., Shamash, J., Joel, S., & Powles, T. B. (2008). Enhancing the in vitro cytotoxic activity of Delta9-tetrahydrocannabinol in leukemic cells through a combinatorial approach. *Leukemia & Lymphoma, 49*, 1800–1809.

Lukhele, S. T., & Motadi, L. R. (2016). Cannabidiol rather than Cannabis sativa extracts inhibit cell growth and induce apoptosis in cervical cancer cells. *BMC Complementary and Alternative Medicine, 16*, 335.

Maccarrone, M., Attinà, M., Cartoni, A., Bari, M., & Finazzi-Agrò, A. (2001). Gas chromatography–mass spectrometry analysis of endogenous cannabinoids in healthy and tumoral human brain and human cells in culture. *Journal of Neurochemistry*, *76*, 594–601.

Martin-Sanchez, E., Furukawa, T. A., Taylor, J., & Martin, J. L. (2009). Systematic review and meta-analysis of cannabis treatment for chronic pain. *Pain Medicine*, *10*, 1353.

Matsuda, L. A., Lolait, S. J., Brownstein, M. J., Young, A. C., & Bonner, T. I. (1990). Structure of a cannabinoid receptor and functional expression of the cloned cDNA. *Nature*, *346*, 561–564.

McAllister, S. D., Christian, R. T., Horowitz, M. P., Garcia, A., & Desprez, P. Y. (2007). Cannabidiol as a novel inhibitor of Id-1 gene expression in aggressive breast cancer cells. *Molecular Cancer Therapeutics*, *6*, 2921–2927.

McAllister, S. D., Murase, R., Christian, R. T., Lau, D., Zielinski, A. J., Allison, J., et al. (2011). Pathways mediating the effects of cannabidiol on the reduction of breast cancer cell proliferation, invasion, and metastasis. *Breast Cancer Research and Treatment*, *129*, 37–47.

McKallip, R. J., Jia, W., Schlomer, J., Warren, J. W., Nagarkatti, P. S., & Nagarkatti, M. (2006). Cannabidiol-induced apoptosis in human leukemia cells: A novel role of cannabidiol in the regulation of p22phox and Nox4 expression. *Molecular Pharmacology*, *70*, 897–908.

Mechoulam, R., Ben-Shabat, S., Hanus, L., Ligumsky, M., Kaminski, N. E., Schatz, A. R., et al. (1995). Identification of an endogenous 2-monoglyceride, present in canine gut, that binds to cannabinoid receptors. *Biochemical Pharmacology*, *50*, 83–90.

Messalli, E. M., Grauso, F., Luise, R., Angelini, A., & Rossiello, R. (2014). Cannabinoid receptor type 1 immunoreactivity and disease severity in human epithelial ovarian tumors. *American Journal of Obstetrics and Gynecology*, *211*, 234.e1–234.e6.

Michalski, C. W., Oti, F. E., Erkan, M., Sauliunaite, D., Bergmann, F., Pacher, P., et al. (2008). Cannabinoids in pancreatic cancer: Correlation with survival and pain. *International Journal of Cancer*, *122*, 742–750.

Mimeault, M., Pommery, N., Wattez, N., Bailly, C., & Hénichart, J. P. (2003). Antiproliferative and apoptotic effects of anandamide in human prostatic cancer cell lines: Implication of epidermal growth factor receptor downregulation and ceramide production. *Prostate*, *56*, 1–12.

Minn, A. J., Gupta, G. P., Siegel, P. M., Bos, P. D., Shu, W., Giri, D. D., et al. (2005). Genes that mediate breast cancer metastasis to lung. *Nature*, *436*, 518–524.

Miyato, H., Kitayama, J., Yamashita, H., Souma, D., Asakage, M., Yamada, J., et al. (2009). Pharmacological synergism between cannabinoids and paclitaxel in gastric cancer cell lines. *The Journal of Surgical Research*, *155*, 40–47.

Molnár, J., Szabó, D., Pusztai, R., Mucsi, I., Berek, L., Ocsovszki, I., et al. (2000). Membrane associated antitumor effects of crocine-, ginsenoside- and cannabinoid derivates. *Anticancer Research*, *20*, 861–867.

Morelli, M. B., Offidani, M., Alesiani, F., Discepoli, G., Liberati, S., Olivieri, A., et al. (2014). The effects of cannabidiol and its synergism with bortezomib in multiple myeloma cell lines. A role for transient receptor potential vanilloid type-2. *International Journal of Cancer*, *134*, 2534–2546.

Mukhopadhyay, P., Baggelaar, M., Erdelyi, K., Cao, Z., Cinar, R., Fezza, F., et al. (2016). The novel, orally available and peripherally restricted selective cannabinoid CB_2 receptor agonist LEI-101 prevents cisplatin-induced nephrotoxicity. *British Journal of Pharmacology*, *173*, 446–458.

Mukhopadhyay, B., Schuebel, K., Mukhopadhyay, P., Cinar, R., Godlewski, G., Xiong, K., et al. (2015). Cannabinoid receptor 1 promotes hepatocellular carcinoma initiation and progression through multiple mechanisms. *Hepatology*, *61*, 1615–1626.

Muñoz-Luque, J., Ros, J., Fernández-Varo, G., Tugues, S., Morales-Ruiz, M., Alvarez, C. E., et al. (2008). Regression of fibrosis after chronic stimulation of cannabinoid CB2 receptor in cirrhotic rats. *The Journal of Pharmacology and Experimental Therapeutics*, *324*, 475–483.

Munro, S., Thomas, K. L., & Abu-Shaar, M. (1993). Molecular characterization of a peripheral receptor for cannabinoids. *Nature*, *365*, 61–65.

Munson, A. E., Harris, L. S., Friedman, M. A., Dewey, W. L., & Carchman, R. A. (1975). Antineoplastic activity of cannabinoids. *Journal of the National Cancer Institute*, *55*, 597–602.

Murase, R., Kawamura, R., Singer, E., Pakdel, A., Sarma, P., Judkins, J., et al. (2014). Targeting multiple cannabinoid antitumor pathways with a resorcinol derivate leads to inhibition of advanced stages of breast cancer. *British Journal of Pharmacology*, *171*, 4464–4477.

Nabissi, M., Morelli, M. B., Amantini, C., Liberati, S., Santoni, M., et al. (2015). Cannabidiol stimulates Aml-1a-dependent glial differentiation and inhibits glioma stem like cells proliferation by inducing autophagy in a TRPV2-dependent manner. *International Journal of Cancer*, *137*, 1855–1869.

Nabissi, M., Morelli, M. B., Offidani, M., Amantini, C., Gentili, S., Soriani, A., et al. (2016). Cannabinoids synergize with carfilzomib, reducing multiple myeloma cells viability and migration. *Oncotarget*, *7*, 77543–77557.

Nabissi, M., Morelli, M. B., Santoni, M., & Santoni, G. (2013). Triggering of the TRPV2 channel by cannabidiol sensitizes glioblastoma cells to cytotoxic chemotherapeutic agents. *Carcinogenesis*, *34*, 48–57.

Nieri, P., Romiti, N., Adinolfi, B., Chicca, A., Massarelli, I., & Chieli, E. (2006). Modulation of P glycoprotein activity by cannabinoid molecules in HK-2 renal cells. *British Journal of Pharmacology*, *148*, 682–687.

Nithipatikom, K., Endsley, M. P., Isbell, M. A., Falck, J. R., Iwamoto, Y., Hillard, C. J., et al. (2004). 2-arachidonoylglycerol: A novel inhibitor of androgen-independent prostate cancer cell invasion. *Cancer Research*, *64*, 8826–8830.

Nomura, D. K., Lombardi, D. P., Chang, J. W., Niessen, S., Ward, A. M., Long, J. Z., et al. (2011). Monoacylglycerol lipase exerts dual control over endocannabinoid and fatty acid pathways to support prostate cancer. *Chemistry & Biology*, *18*, 846–856.

Nomura, D. K., Long, J. Z., Niessen, S., Hoover, H. S., Ng, S. W., & Cravatt, B. F. (2010). Monoacylglycerol lipase regulates a fatty acid network that promotes cancer pathogenesis. *Cell*, *140*, 49–61.

Oesch, S., Walter, D., Wachtel, M., Pretre, K., Salazar, M., Guzman, M., et al. (2009). Cannabinoid receptor 1 is a potential drug target for treatment of translocation-positive rhabdomyosarcoma. *Molecular Cancer Therapeutics*, *8*, 1838–1845.

Oh, J., Seo, D. W., Diaz, T., Wei, B., Ward, Y., Ray, J. M., et al. (2004). Tissue inhibitors of metalloproteinase 2 inhibits endothelial cell migration through increased expression of RECK. *Cancer Research*, *64*, 9062–9069.

Orellana-Serradell, O., Poblete, C. E., Sanchez, C., Castellón, E. A., Gallegos, I., Huidobro, C., et al. (2015). Proapoptotic effect of endocannabinoids in prostate cancer cells. *Oncology Reports*, *2015*(33), 1599–1608.

Ortega, A., García-Hernández, V. M., Ruiz-García, E., Meneses-García, A., Herrera-Gómez, A., Aguilar-Ponce, J. L., et al. (2016). Comparing the effects of endogenous and synthetic cannabinoid receptor agonists on survival of gastric cancer cells. *Life Sciences*, *165*, 56–62.

Overton, H. A., Babbs, A. J., Doel, S. M., Fyfe, M. C., Gardner, L. S., Griffin, G., et al. (2006). Deorphanization of a G protein-coupled receptor for oleoylethanolamide and its use in the discovery of small molecule hypophagic agents. *Cell Metabolism*, *3*, 167–175.

Pagotto, U., Marsicano, G., Fezza, F., Theodoropoulou, M., Grübler, Y., Stalla, J., et al. (2001). Normal human pituitary gland and pituitary adenomas express cannabinoid receptor type 1 and synthesize endogenous cannabinoids: First evidence for a direct role of cannabinoids on hormone modulation at the human pituitary level. *The Journal of Clinical Endocrinology and Metabolism*, *86*, 2687–2696.

Park, S. W., Kim, J. E., Oh, S. M., Cha, W. J., Hah, J. H., & Sung, M. W. (2015). Anticancer effects of anandamide on head and neck squamous cell carcinoma cells via the production of receptor-independent reactive oxygen species. *Head & Neck*, *37*, 1187–1192.

Patsos, H. A., Greenhough, A., Hicks, D. J., Al Kharusi, M., Collard, T. J., Lane, J. D., et al. (2010). The endogenous cannabinoid, anandamide, induces COX-2-dependent cell death in apoptosis-resistant colon cancer cells. *International Journal of Oncology*, *37*, 187–193.

Patti, F., Messina, S., Solaro, C., Amato, M. P., Bergamaschi, R., Bonavita, S., et al. (2016). Efficacy and safety of cannabinoid oromucosal spray for multiple sclerosis spasticity. *Journal of Neurology, Neurosurgery, and Psychiatry*, *87*, 944–951.

Pérez-Gómez, E., Andradas, C., Blasco-Benito, S., Caffarel, M. M., García-Taboada, E., Villa-Morales, M., et al. (2015). Role of cannabinoid receptor CB_2 in HER_2 pro-oncogenic signaling in breast cancer. *Journal of the National Cancer Institute*, *107*. djv077.

Perren, T. J., Swart, A. M., Pfisterer, J., Ledermann, J. A., Pujade-Lauraine, E., Kristensen, G., et al. (2011). A phase 3 trial of bevacizumab in ovarian cancer. *The New England Journal of Medicine*, *365*, 2484–2496.

Petersen, G., Moesgaard, B., Schmid, P. C., Schmid, H. H., Broholm, H., Kosteljanetz, M., et al. (2005). Endocannabinoid metabolism in human glioblastomas and meningiomas compared to human non-tumour brain tissue. *Journal of Neurochemistry*, *93*, 299–309.

Petrosino, S., & Di Marzo, V. (2010). FAAH and MAGL inhibitors: Therapeutic opportunities from regulating endocannabinoid levels. *Current Opinion in Investigational Drugs*, *11*, 51–62.

Picardi, P., Ciaglia, E., Proto, M., & Pisanti, S. (2014). Anandamide inhibits breast tumor-induced angiogenesis. *Translational Medicine @ UniSa*, *10*, 8–12.

Pisanti, S., Borselli, C., Oliviero, O., Laezza, C., Gazzerro, P., & Bifulco, M. (2007). Anti-angiogenic activity of the endocannabinoid anandamide: Correlation to its tumor-suppressor efficacy. *Journal of Cellular Physiology*, *211*, 495–503.

Pisanti, S., Picardi, P., Prota, L., Proto, M. C., Laezza, C., McGuire, P., et al. (2011). Genetic and pharmacologic inactivation of cannabinoid CB1 receptor inhibits angiogenesis. *Blood*, *117*, 5541–5550.

Portella, G., Laezza, C., Laccetti, P., De Petrocellis, L., Di Marzo, V., & Bifulco, M. (2003). Inhibitory effects of cannabinoid CB_1 receptor stimulation on tumor growth and metastatic spreading: Actions on signals involved in angiogenesis and metastasis. *The FASEB Journal*, *17*, 1771–1773.

Pourkhalili, N., Ghahremani, M. H., Farsandaj, N., Tavajohi, S., Majdzadeh, M., Parsa, M., et al. (2013). Evaluation of anti-invasion effect of cannabinoids on human hepatocarcinoma cells. *Toxicology Mechanisms and Methods*, *23*, 120–126.

Preet, A., Ganju, R. K., & Groopman, J. E. (2008). Delta9-tetrahydrocannabinol inhibits epithelial growth factor-induced lung cancer cell migration in vitro as well as its growth and metastasis in vivo. *Oncogene*, *27*, 339–346.

Preet, A., Qamri, Z., Nasser, M. W., Prasad, A., Shilo, K., Zou, X., et al. (2011). Cannabinoid receptors, CB1 and CB2, as novel targets for inhibition of non-small cell lung cancer growth and metastasis. *Cancer Prevention Research (Philadelphia, Pa.)*, *4*, 65–75.

Proto, M. C., Gazzerro, P., Di Croce, L., Santoro, A., Malfitano, A. M., Pisanti, S., et al. (2012). Interaction of endocannabinoid system and steroid hormones in the control of colon cancer cell growth. *Journal of Cellular Physiology*, *227*, 250–258.

Qamri, Z., Preet, A., Nasser, M. W., Bass, C. E., Leone, G., Barsky, S. H., et al. (2009). Synthetic cannabinoid receptor agonists inhibit tumor growth and metastasis of breast cancer. *Molecular Cancer Therapeutics*, *8*, 3117–3129.

Rajesh, M., Mukhopadhyay, P., Haskó, G., Liaudet, L., Mackie, K., & Pacher, P. (2010). Cannabinoid-1 receptor activation induces reactive oxygen species-dependent and -independent mitogen-activated protein kinase activation and cell death in human coronary artery endothelial cells. *British Journal of Pharmacology*, *160*, 688–700.

Ramer, R., Bublitz, K., Freimuth, N., Merkord, J., Rohde, H., Haustein, M., et al. (2012). Cannabidiol inhibits lung cancer cell invasion and metastasis via intercellular adhesion molecule-1. *The FASEB Journal*, *26*, 1535–1548.

Ramer, R., Eichele, K., & Hinz, B. (2007). Upregulation of tissue inhibitor of matrix metalloproteinases-1 confers the anti-invasive action of cisplatin on human cancer cells. *Oncogene*, *26*, 5822–5827.

Ramer, R., Fischer, S., Haustein, M., Manda, K., & Hinz, B. (2014). Cannabinoid inhibit angiogenic capacities of endothelial cells via release of tissue inhibitor of matrix metalloproteinases-1 from lung cancer cells. *Biochemical Pharmacology*, *91*, 202–216.

Ramer, R., Heinemann, K., Merkord, J., Rohde, H., Salamon, A., Linnebacher, M., et al. (2013). COX-2 and PPAR-gamma confer cannabidiol-induced apoptosis of human lung cancer cells. *Molecular Cancer Therapeutics*, *12*, 69–82.

Ramer, R., & Hinz, B. (2008). Inhibition of cancer cell invasion by cannabinoids via increased expression of tissue inhibitor of matrix metalloproteinases-1. *Journal of the National Cancer Institute*, *100*, 59–69.

Ramer, R., & Hinz, B. (2016). Antitumorigenic targets of cannabinoids—Current status and implications. *Expert Opinion on Therapeutic Targets*, *20*, 1219–1235.

Ramer, R., Merkord, J., Rohde, H., & Hinz, B. (2010). Cannabidiol inhibits cancer cell invasion via upregulation of tissue inhibitor of matrix metalloproteinases-1. *Biochemical Pharmacology*, *79*, 955–966.

Ramer, R., Rohde, A., Merkord, J., Rohde, H., & Hinz, B. (2010). Decrease of plasminogen activator inhibitor-1 may contribute to the anti-invasive action of cannabidiol on human lung cancer cells. *Pharmaceutical Research*, *27*, 2162–2174.

Ravi, J., Sneh, A., Shilo, K., Nasser, M. W., & Ganju, R. K. (2014). FAAH inhibition enhances anandamide mediated anti-tumorigenic effects in non-small cell lung cancer by downregulating the EGF/EGFR pathway. *Oncotarget*, *5*, 2475–2486.

Rawitch, A. B., Schultz, G. S., Ebner, K. E., & Vardaris, R. M. (1977). Competition of delta 9-tetrahydrocannabinol with estrogen in rat uterine estrogen receptor binding. *Science*, *197*, 1189–1191.

Ruh, M. F., Taylor, J. A., Howlett, A. C., & Welshons, W. V. (1997). Failure of cannabinoid compounds to stimulate estrogen receptors. *Biochemical Pharmacology*, *53*, 35–41.

Ryberg, E., Larsson, N., Sjogren, S., Hjorth, S., Hermansson, N. O., Leonova, J., et al. (2007). The orphan receptor GPR55 is a novel cannabinoid receptor. *British Journal of Pharmacology*, *152*, 1092–1101.

Saghatelian, A., Trauger, S. A., Want, E. J., Hawkins, E. G., Siuzdak, G., & Cravatt, B. F. (2004). Assignment of endogenous substrates to enzymes by global metabolite profiling. *Biochemistry*, *43*, 14332–14339.

Sailler, S., Schmitz, K., Jäger, E., Ferreiros, N., Wicker, S., Zschiebsch, K., et al. (2014). Regulation of circulating endocannabinoids associated with cancer and metastases in mice and humans. *Oncoscience*, *1*, 272–282. eCollection 2014.

Salazar, M., Carracedo, A., Salanueva, I. J., Hernandez-Tiedra, S., Lorente, M., Egia, A., et al. (2009). Cannabinoid action induces autophagy-mediated cell death through stimulation of ER stress in human glioma cells. *The Journal of Clinical Investigation*, *119*, 1359–1372.

Sanchez, C., de Ceballos, M. L., Gomez del Pulgar, T., Rueda, D., Corbacho, C., Velasco, G., et al. (2001). Inhibition of glioma growth in vivo by selective activation of the CB_2 cannabinoid receptor. *Cancer Research, 61*, 5784–5789.

Sánchez, M. G., Ruiz-Llorente, L., Sánchez, A. M., & Díaz-Laviada, I. (2003). Activation of phosphoinositide 3-kinase/PKB pathway by CB_1 and CB_2 cannabinoid receptors expressed in prostate PC-3 cells. Involvement in Raf-1 stimulation and NGF induction. *Cellular Signalling, 15*, 851–859.

Sandler, A., Gray, R., Perry, M. C., Brahmer, J., Schiller, J. H., Dowlati, A., et al. (2006). Paclitaxel-carboplatin alone or with bevacizumab for non-small cell lung cancer. *The New England Journal of Medicine, 355*, 2542–2550.

Sarker, K. P., Obara, S., Nakata, M., Kitajima, I., & Maruyama, I. (2000). Anandamide induces apoptosis of PC-12 cells: Involvement of superoxide and caspase-3. *FEBS Letters, 472*, 39–44.

Sarnataro, D., Pisanti, S., Santoro, A., Gazzerro, P., Malfitano, A. M., Laezza, C., et al. (2006). The cannabinoid CB1 receptor antagonist Rimonabant (SR141716) inhibits human breast cancer cell proliferation through a lipid raft-mediated mechanism. *Molecular Pharmacology, 70*, 1298–1306.

Schmid, P. C., Wold, L. E., Krebsbach, R. J., Berdyshev, E. V., & Schmid, H. H. (2002). Anandamide and other N-acylethanolamines in human tumors. *Lipids, 37*, 907–912.

Scott, K. A., Dalgleish, A. G., & Liu, W. M. (2014). The combination of cannabidiol and Δ9-tetrahydrocannabinol enhances the anticancer effects of radiation in an orthotopic murine glioma model. *Molecular Cancer Therapeutics, 13*, 2955–2967.

Shrivastava, A., Kuzontkoski, P. M., Groopman, J. E., & Prasad, A. (2011). Cannabidiol induces programmed cell death in breast cancer cells by coordinating the cross talk between apoptosis and autophagy. *Molecular Cancer Therapeutics, 10*, 1161–1172.

Singer, E., Judkins, J., Salomonis, N., Matlaf, L., Soteropoulos, P., McAllister, S., et al. (2015). Reactive oxygen species-mediated therapeutic response and resistance in glioblastoma. *Cell Death & Disease, 6*. e1601.

Singh, Y., & Bali, C. (2013). Cannabis extract treatment for terminal acute lymphoblastic leukemia with a Philadelphia chromosome mutation. *Case Reports in Oncology, 6*, 585–592.

Solinas, M., Massi, P., Cantelmo, A. R., Cattaneo, M. G., Cammarota, R., Bartolini, D., et al. (2012). Cannabidiol inhibits angiogenesis by multiple mechanisms. *British Journal of Pharmacology, 167*, 1218–1231.

Soroceanu, L., Murase, R., Limbad, C., Singer, E., Allison, J., Adrados, I., et al. (2013). Id-1 is a key transcriptional regulator of glioblastoma aggressiveness and a novel therapeutic target. *Cancer Research, 73*, 1559–1569.

Stamenkovic, I. (2000). Matrix metalloproteinases in tumor invasion and metastasis. *Seminars in Cancer Biology, 10*, 415–433.

Stella, N., Schweitzer, P., & Piomelli, D. (1997). A second endogenous cannabinoid that modulates long-term potentiation. *Nature, 388*, 773–778.

Takeda, S., Himeno, T., Kakizoe, K., Okazaki, H., Okada, T., Watanabe, K., et al. (2017). Cannabidiolic acid-mediated selective down-regulation of c-fos in highly aggressive breast cancer MDA-MB-231 cells: Possible involvement of its down-regulation in the abrogation of aggressiveness. *Journal of Natural Medicines, 71*, 286–291.

Teixeira-Clerc, F., Julien, B., Grenard, P., Tran Van Nhieu, J., Deveaux, V., Li, L., et al. (2006). CB1 cannabinoid receptor antagonism: A new strategy for the treatment of liver fibrosis. *Nature Medicine, 12*, 671–676.

Tellez, L. A., Medina, S., Han, W., Ferreira, J. G., Licona-Limón, P., Ren, X., et al. (2013). A gut lipid messenger links excess dietary fat to dopamine deficiency. *Science, 341*, 800–802.

Thapa, D., Lee, J. S., Heo, S. W., Lee, Y. R., Kang, K. W., Kwak, M. K., et al. (2011). Novel hexahydrocannabinol analogs as potential anti-cancer agents inhibit cell proliferation and tumor angiogenesis. *European Journal of Pharmacology, 650*, 64–71.

Thors, L., Bergh, A., Persson, E., Hammarsten, P., Stattin, P., Egevad, L., et al. (2010). Fatty acid amide hydrolase in prostate cancer: Association with disease severity and outcome, CB1 receptor expression and regulation by IL-4. *PloS One*, 5. e12275.

Tramèr, M. R., Carroll, D., Campbell, F. A., Reynolds, D. J., Moore, R. A., & McQuay, H. J. (2001). Cannabinoids for control of chemotherapy-induced nausea and vomiting: Quantitative systematic review. *BMJ, 323*, 16–21.

Vara, D., Salazar, M., Olea-Herrero, N., Guzmán, M., Velasco, G., & Díaz-Laviada, I. (2011). Anti-tumoral action of cannabinoids on hepatocellular carcinoma: Role of AMPK-dependent activation of autophagy. *Cell Death and Differentiation, 18*, 1099–1111.

Wall, M. E., Sadler, B. M., Brine, D., Taylor, H., & Perez-Reyes, M. (1983). Metabolism, disposition, and kinetics of delta-9-tetrahydrocannabinol in men and women. *Clinical Pharmacology and Therapeutics, 34*, 352–363.

Wang, T., Collet, J. P., Shapiro, S., & Ware, M. A. (2008). Adverse effects of medical cannabinoids: A systematic review. *CMAJ, 178*, 1669–1678.

Wang, D., Wang, H., Ning, W., Backlund, M. G., Dey, S. K., & DuBois, R. N. (2008). Loss of cannabinoid receptor 1 accelerates intestinal tumor growth. *Cancer Research, 68*, 6468–6476.

Whiting, P. F., Wolff, R. F., Deshpande, S., Di Nisio, M., Duffy, S., Hernandez, A. V., et al. (2015). Cannabinoids for medical use: A systematic review and meta-analysis. *JAMA, 313*, 2456–2473.

Winkler, K., Ramer, R., Dithmer, S., Ivanov, I., Merkord, J., & Hinz, B. (2016). Fatty acid amide hydrolase inhibitors confer anti-invasive and antimetastatic effects on lung cancer cells. *Oncotarget*, 7, 15047–15064.

Wu, X., Han, L., Zhang, X., Li, L., Jiang, C., Qiu, Y., et al. (2012). Alteration of endocannabinoid system in human gliomas. *Journal of Neurochemistry, 120*, 842–849.

Xian, X., Huang, L., Zhang, B., Wu, C., Cui, J., & Wang, Z. (2016). WIN 55,212-2 inhibits the epithelial mesenchymal transition of gastric cancer cells via COX-2 signals. *Cellular Physiology and Biochemistry, 39*, 2149–2157.

Xian, X. S., Park, H., Cho, Y. K., Lee, I. S., Kim, S. W., Choi, M. G., et al. (2010). Effect of a synthetic cannabinoid agonist on the proliferation and invasion of gastric cancer cells. *Journal of Cellular Biochemistry, 110*, 321–332.

Xu, X., Liu, Y., Huang, S., Liu, G., Xie, C., Zhou, J., et al. (2006). Overexpression of cannabinoid receptors CB1 and CB2 correlates with improved prognosis of patients with hepatocellular carcinoma. *Cancer Genetics and Cytogenetics, 171*, 31–38.

Yamaji, K., Sarker, K. P., Kawahara, K., Iino, S., Yamakuchi, M., Abeyama, K., et al. (2003). Anandamide induces apoptosis in human endothelial cells: Its regulation system and clinical implications. *Thrombosis and Haemostasis, 89*, 875–884.

Yang, J. C., Haworth, L., Sherry, R. M., Hwu, P., Schwartzentruber, D. J., Topalian, S. L., et al. (2003). A randomized trial of bevacizumab, an anti-vascular endothelial growth factor antibody, for metastatic renal cancer. *The New England Journal of Medicine, 349*, 427–434.

Ye, L., Zhang, B., Seviour, E. G., Tao, K. X., Liu, X. H., Ling, Y., et al. (2011). Monoacylglycerol lipase (MAGL) knockdown inhibits tumor cells growth in colorectal cancer. *Cancer Letters, 307*, 6–17.

Zhang, P.-W., Ishiguro, H., Ohtsuki, T., Hess, J., Carillo, F., Walther, D., et al. (2004). Human cannabinoid receptor 1: 5 exons, candidate regulatory regions, polymorphisms, haplotypes and association with polysubstance abuse. *Molecular Psychiatry, 9*, 916–931.

Zhang, X., Maor, Y., Wang, J. F., Kunos, G., & Groopman, J. E. (2010). Endocannabinoid-like N-arachidonoyl serine is a novel pro-angiogenic mediator. *British Journal of Pharmacology*, *160*, 1583–1594.

Zhang, J., Medina-Cleghorn, D., Bernal-Mizrachi, L., Bracci, P. M., Hubbard, A., Conde, L., et al. (2016). The potential relevance of the endocannabinoid, 2-arachidonoylglycerol, in diffuse large B-cell lymphoma. *Oncoscience*, *3*, 31–41.

Zhu, L. X., Sharma, S., Stolina, M., Gardner, B., Roth, M. D., Tashkin, D. P., et al. (2000). Delta-9-tetrahydrocannabinol inhibits antitumor immunity by a CB2 receptor-mediated, cytokine-dependent pathway. *Journal of Immunology*, *165*, 373–380.

Zygmunt, P. M., Petersson, J., Andersson, D. A., Chuang, H., Sorgard, M., Di Marzo, V., et al. (1999). Vanilloid receptors on sensory nerves mediate the vasodilator action of anandamide. *Nature*, *400*, 452–457.

CHAPTER THIRTEEN

Cannabinoids and Pain: Sites and Mechanisms of Action

Katarzyna Starowicz*, David P. Finn†,1

*Institute of Pharmacology, Polish Academy of Sciences, Laboratory of Pain Pathophysiology, Krakow, Poland
†Pharmacology and Therapeutics, School of Medicine, Galway Neuroscience Centre and Centre for Pain Research, NCBES, National University of Ireland, Galway, Ireland
[1]Corresponding author: e-mail address: david.finn@nuigalway.ie

Contents

Abstract

The endocannabinoid system, consisting of the cannabinoid$_1$ receptor (CB$_1$R) and cannabinoid$_2$ receptor (CB$_2$R), endogenous cannabinoid ligands (endocannabinoids), and metabolizing enzymes, is present throughout the pain pathways. Endocannabinoids, phytocannabinoids, and synthetic cannabinoid receptor agonists have antinociceptive effects in animal models of acute, inflammatory, and neuropathic pain. CB$_1$R and CB$_2$R located at peripheral, spinal, or supraspinal sites are important targets mediating these antinociceptive effects. The mechanisms underlying the analgesic effects of

Advances in Pharmacology, Volume 80
ISSN 1054-3589
http://dx.doi.org/10.1016/bs.apha.2017.05.003

cannabinoids likely include inhibition of presynaptic neurotransmitter and neuropeptide release, modulation of postsynaptic neuronal excitability, activation of the descending inhibitory pain pathway, and reductions in neuroinflammatory signaling. Strategies to dissociate the psychoactive effects of cannabinoids from their analgesic effects have focused on peripherally restricted CB_1R agonists, CB_2R agonists, inhibitors of endocannabinoid catabolism or uptake, and modulation of other non-CB_1R/non-CB_2R targets of cannabinoids including TRPV1, GPR55, and PPARs. The large body of preclinical evidence in support of cannabinoids as potential analgesic agents is supported by clinical studies demonstrating their efficacy across a variety of pain disorders.

ABBREVIATIONS

2-AG 2-arachidonoyl glycerol
AEA anandamide
BLA basolateral nucleus of the amygdala
CB_1R cannabinoid receptor type 1
CB_2R cannabinoid receptor type 2
CCI chronic constriction injury
CeA central nucleus of the amygdala
CFA complete Freund's adjuvant
CGRP calcitonin gene-related peptide
DRG dorsal root ganglia
FAAH fatty acid amide hydrolase
GPR55 G protein-coupled receptor 55
i.p. intraperitoneal
i.t. intrathecal
MAGL monoacylglycerol lipase
PAG periaqueductal gray
PEA *N*-palmitoylethanolamide
PPARs peroxisome proliferator-activated receptors
RVM rostral ventromedial medulla
SNI spared nerve injury
SNL spinal nerve ligation
TRPV1 transient receptor potential subfamily V member 1
Δ^9-THC Δ^9-tetrahydrocannabinol

1. INTRODUCTION

Cannabis sativa has been used for medicinal purposes, including relief of pain, for thousands of years (Grinspoon & Bakalar, 1993). The isolation and identification of the principal psychoactive constituent of cannabis,

Δ^9-tetrahydrocannabinol (Δ^9-THC), in the 1960s (Mechoulam & Gaoni, 1967), sparked a search for its mechanism of action which in turn led to the discovery of two cannabinoid receptors, the cannabinoid$_1$ receptor (CB_1R) (Devane, Dysarz, Johnson, Melvin, & Howlett, 1988; Matsuda, Lolait, Brownstein, Young, & Bonner, 1990) and cannabinoid$_2$ receptor (CB_2R) (Munro, Thomas, & Abu-Shaar, 1993). Endogenous ligands (endocannabinoids) which exert their effects upon binding to these cannabinoid receptors were also discovered, the two best characterized being arachidonoyl ethanolamide (anandamide, AEA) (Devane et al., 1992) and 2-arachidonoyl glycerol (2-AG) (Mechoulam et al., 1995; Sugiura et al., 1995). The receptors, endocannabinoids, transport proteins, and enzymes that synthesize or degrade the endocannabinoids together comprise the endocannabinoid system. A large body of preclinical and clinical research indicates that this lipid signaling system modulates a broad range of physiological processes and behaviors including, but not limited to, pain, mood, appetite, emesis, neuronal activity, memory, immunity, cell development and cell fate, and the cardiovascular system. In particular, the antinociceptive effects of cannabinoids and endocannabinoid signaling have received a lot of attention over the past 30 years, with thousands of peer-reviewed publications reporting antinociceptive/analgesic effects in preclinical and clinical studies and elucidating the sites and mechanisms of action. The impact of this research has started to be seen in clinical practice with the introduction of the Δ^9-THC/Cannabidiol buccal spray nabiximols (Sativex®) for the adjunctive treatment of neuropathic pain in multiple sclerosis patients and severe cancer pain in Canada, and with many US states and countries around the world relaxing their laws to allow patients to use cannabis or cannabinoids for a range of conditions including chronic pain. The present review will focus primarily on the evidence from preclinical studies utilizing animal models of acute, inflammatory, and neuropathic pain with an emphasis on the sites and mechanisms underlying cannabinoid-mediated antinociception. For excellent recent reviews and meta-analyses of clinical studies in this area, please see Barnes (2006), Boychuk, Goddard, Mauro, and Orellana (2015), Canadian Agency for Drugs and Technologies in Health (2016), Iskedjian, Bereza, Gordon, Piwko, and Einarson (2007), Lynch and Ware (2015), McCormick et al. (2017), Russo (2016), Vermersch (2011), and Whiting et al. (2015).

With regards preclinical studies in rodents, both genetic and pharmacological (Table 1) approaches have been used to demonstrate and understand

Table 1 Compounds Referred to in the Text and Used to Elucidate the Role of Cannabinoids and the Endocannabinoid System in Pain Modulation

Pharmacological Substance	IUPAC Name	Target
THC	(−)-(6*aR*,10*aR*)-6,6,9-Trimethyl-3-pentyl-6*a*,7,8,10*a*-tetrahydro-6*H*-benzo[*c*]chromen-1-ol; Δ^9-tetrahydrocannabinol	The main psychotropic constituent of cannabis, CB_1/CB_2 receptor partial agonist
ACEA	*N*-(2-Chloroethyl)-5*Z*,8*Z*,11*Z*,14*Z*-eicosatetraenamide	Potent and highly selective synthetic CB_1 receptor agonist has low affinity for CB_2
2-AG	(5*Z*,8*Z*,11*Z*,14*Z*)-5,8,11,14-Eicosatetraenoic acid, 2-hydroxy-1-(hydroxymethyl)ethyl ester; 2-arachidonoyl glycerol	Endogenous CB_1 and CB_2 receptor agonists without any marked selectivity for either subtype. AEA is also an agonist at TRPV1
AEA	*N*-(2-Hydroxyethyl)-5*Z*,8*Z*,11*Z*,14*Z*-eicosatetraenamide; anandamide	
WIN55,212-2	{(*R*)-(+)-[2,3-Dihydro-5-methyl-3-[(4-morpholino)methyl]pyrrolo-[1,2,3-de]-1,4-benzoxazin-6-yl](1-naphthyl)methanone}	Mixed CB_1/CB_2 receptor agonist
CP-55,940	{(−)-3-[2-Hydroxy-4-(1,1-dimethylheptyl)phenyl]-4-(3-hydroxypropyl)cyclohexan-1-ol}	
HU210	3-(1,1′-Dimethylheptyl)-6*aR*,7,10,10*aR*-tetrahydro-1-hydroxy-6,6-dimethyl-6*H*-dibenzo[*b*,*d*]pyran-9-methanol	
AM251	*N*-(Piperidin-1-yl)-5-(4-iodophenyl)-1-(2,4-dichlorophenyl)-4-methyl-1*H*-pyrazole-3-carboxamide	CB_1-selective antagonists
AM281	1-(2,4-Dichlorophenyl)-5-(4-iodophenyl)-4-methyl-*N*-4-morpholinyl-1*H*-pyrazole-3-carboxamide	
SR141716A (rimonabant)	[*N*-(Piperidin-1-yl)-5-(4-chlorophenyl)-1-(2,4-dichlorophenyl)-4-methyl-1*H*-pyrazole-3-carboxamide hydrochloride] (rimonabant)	

A-836339	[*N*(*Z*)]-*N*-[3-(2-Methoxyethyl)-4,5-dimethyl-2(3*H*)-thiazolylidene]-2,2,3,3-tetramethyl-cyclopropanecarboxamide	CB_2-selective agonists
AM1241	(2-Iodo-5-nitrophenyl)-(1-(1-methylpiperidin-2-ylmethyl)-1*H*-indol-3-yl)methanone	
GW-405,833	1-(2,3-Dichlorobenzoyl)-5-methoxy-2-methyl-3-[2-(4-morpholinyl) ethyl]-1*H*-indole	
JTE-907	*N*-(1,3-Benzodioxol-5-ylmethyl)-7-methoxy-2-oxo-8-pentoxy-1*H*-quinoline-3-carboxamide	
JWH-015	(2-Methyl-1-propylindol-3-yl)-naphthalen-1-ylmethanone	
JWH-133	(6*aR*,10*aR*)-6,6,9-Trimethyl-3-(2-methylpentan-2-yl)-6*a*,7,10,10*a*-tetrahydrobenzo[*c*]chromene	
NESS400	1-(2′,4′-Dichlorophenyl)-6-methyl-*N*-cyclohexylamine-1,4-dihydroindeno[1,2-*c*]pyrazole-3-carboxamide	
O-3223	(6*aR*,10*aR*)-6,6,9-Trimethyl-3-(2-methylpentan-2-yl)-6*a*,7,10,10*a*-tetrahydrobenzo[*c*]chromene	
AM630	6-Iodopravadoline	CB_2-selective antagonists
SR144528	5-(4-Chloro-3-methylphenyl)-1-[(4-methylphenyl)methyl]-*N*-[(1*R*,3*S*,4*S*)-2,2,4-trimethyl-3-bicyclo[2.2.1]heptanyl]pyrazole-3-carboxamide	
OL-135	7-Phenyl-1-(5-pyridin-2-yl-1,3-oxazol-2-yl)heptan-1-one	FAAH inhibitor
PF-3845	*N*-Pyridin-3-yl-4-[[3-[5-(trifluoromethyl)pyridin-2-yl]oxyphenyl] methyl]piperidine-1-carboxamide	
URB597	(3-Phenylphenyl) *N*-(4-methoxyphenyl)carbamate	

Continued

Table 1 Compounds Referred to in the Text and Used to Elucidate the Role of Cannabinoids and the Endocannabinoid System in Pain Modulation—cont'd

Pharmacological Substance	IUPAC Name	Target
JZL184	4-Nitrophenyl-4-[bis(1,3-benzodioxol-5-yl)(hydroxy)methyl] piperidine-1-carboxylate	MAGL inhibitor
URB602	[1,1′-Biphenyl]-3-yl-carbamic acid, cyclohexyl ester	
I-RTX	6,7-Deepoxy-6,7-didehydro-5-deoxy-21-dephenyl-21-(phenylmethyl)-daphnetoxin,20-(4-hydroxy-5-iodo-3-methoxybenzeneacetate); iodoresiniferatoxin	Potent TRPV1 antagonist
AA-5-HT	(5*Z*,8*Z*,11*Z*,14*Z*)-*N*-(2-(5-Hydroxy-1*H*-indol-3-yl)ethyl)icosa-5,8,11,14-tetraenamide; *N*-arachidonoyl-serotonin	FAAH inhibitor and TRPV1 antagonist
ML-193 (alternative name CID 1261822)	*N*-[4-[[(3,4-Dimethyl-5-isoxazolyl)amino]sulfonyl]phenyl]-6,8-dimethyl-2-(2-pyridinyl)-4-quinolinecarboxamide	Potent and selective GPR55 antagonist

the modulation of pain by cannabinoids and the endocannabinoid system. Enhanced thermal analgesia and reduced nociceptive behavior in the formalin and carrageenan models were observed in mice lacking the enzyme fatty acid amide hydrolase (FAAH) which catabolizes AEA and other *N*-acylethanolamines including *N*-palmitoylethanolamide (PEA) and *N*-oleoylethanolamide, compared with wild-type controls (Carey et al., 2016; Cravatt et al., 2001; Lichtman, Shelton, Advani, & Cravatt, 2004). These results suggest that one or more FAAH substrates exert antinociceptive actions in these models. FAAH knockout mice, and mice that express FAAH exclusively in nervous tissue, have also been shown to display antiinflammatory and antihyperalgesic effects in both the carrageenan and collagen-induced arthritis models, effects prevented by administration of a CB_2R, but not CB_1R, antagonist (Kinsey, Naidu, Cravatt, Dudley, & Lichtman, 2011; Lichtman et al., 2004). Thus, the augmented levels of AEA in these mice appear to exert tonic analgesia via CB_2R. However, a pronociceptive phenotype of FAAH knockout mice can be unmasked following intradermal injection of the transient receptor potential subfamily V member 1 (TRPV1) agonist capsaicin (Carey et al., 2016). Similarly, mice lacking the 2-AG-catabolizing enzyme monoacylglycerol lipase (MAGL) exhibited significantly augmented nociceptive behavior in the formalin and acetic acid tests and no alterations in thermal tail-withdrawal latency, effects that were likely due to desensitization of CB_1R (Petrenko, Yamazaki, Sakimura, Kano, & Baba, 2014; Schlosburg et al., 2010). In a recent study, nitroglycerin-induced mechanical allodynia and neuronal activation of the trigeminal nucleus to model migraine were abolished in FAAH-deficient mice, results also seen in mice administered FAAH inhibitors (Nozaki, Markert, & Zimmer, 2015). These effects were shown to be CB_1R mediated and they infer that one or more FAAH substrates mediate antinociception via CB_1R. Knockouts of the CB_1R have also been generated and exhibit hypoalgesia in the hot plate, tail immersion, and formalin tests (Valverde, Karsak, & Zimmer, 2005; Zimmer, Zimmer, Hohmann, Herkenham, & Bonner, 1999), suggesting, somewhat paradoxically, a pronociceptive role for CB_1R. However, a different $CB_1^{-/-}$ mouse line displayed similar basal responses to noxious stimuli compared to wild-type animals (Castane et al., 2006; Ledent et al., 1999). Development of mechanical hypersensitivity following partial sciatic nerve ligation was unaltered in CB_1R knockout mice (Castane et al., 2006; Racz, Nent, Erxlebe, & Zimmer, 2015); however, these mice did exhibit more pronounced behavioral manifestations of anxiety-related behaviors compared to wild-type mice (Racz et al., 2015), suggesting an anxiolytic role for CB_1R. Mice lacking the CB_2R have also been generated as have CB_1/CB_2 double knockouts (Buckley, 2008; Buckley et al., 2000) and mice overexpressing the CB_2R (La Porta, Bura, Aracil-Fernandez, Manzanares, & Maldonado, 2013). The affective manifestations of osteoarthritis pain in the monosodium iodoacetate model were enhanced in CB_1R knockout mice and absent in CB_2R knockouts, suggesting that the presence of CB_1R attenuates the affective component in this model, while CB_2R is required for expression of the affective component. Both the CB_1R agonist ACEA and the CB_2R agonist JWH-133 ameliorated the nociceptive and affective alterations, with ACEA also improving the associated memory impairment (La Porta et al., 2015). It had previously been shown that development of mechanical allodynia in this model was unaltered in CB_1R and CB_2R knockout mice, but attenuated in those overexpressing CB_2R, compared with wild-type mice (La Porta et al., 2013). In another recent study, paclitaxel-induced mechanical and cold allodynia developed to an equivalent degree in mice lacking CB_1R, CB_2R, and wild-type mice (Deng et al., 2015), suggesting that CB_1R and CB_2R do not impact on the development of the pain-related phenotype in this model. Following intraplantar administration of complete Freund's adjuvant (CFA), or partial nerve ligation, mechanical hyperalgesia was absent in mice lacking GPR55 (Staton et al., 2008), a receptor sensitive to some cannabinoids. However, another study reported thermal hyperalgesia in GPR55 knockout mice (Bjursell et al., 2016) and, most recently, it was shown that genetic deletion of GPR55 did not alter the development of pain-related behavior in a number of mechanistically distinct models of inflammatory and neuropathic pain (Carey et al., 2017).

Shortly after its discovery, Bicher and Mechoulam (1968) showed that Δ^9-THC was antinociceptive in rabbits (Bicher & Mechoulam, 1968). Since then, many studies have shown that cannabinoids are antinociceptive following systemic administration (for comprehensive review, see Pertwee, 2001). The animal (usually rodent) models used can be divided into three broad groups: (1) acute pain, (2) inflammatory pain involving tissue injury, and (3) neuropathic pain involving peripheral nerve injury. Cannabinoid receptor agonists, administered intraperitoneally, intravenously, subcutaneously, or orally, demonstrate analgesic efficacy (to greater or lesser degrees depending on the compound and model under investigation) across these models (Finn & Chapman, 2004; Pertwee, 2001) with a potency that is comparable with, or greater than, some opiates and cyclooxygenase inhibitors

(Bloom & Dewey, 1978; Smith, Cichewicz, Martin, & Welch, 1998; Sofia, Vassar, & Knobloch, 1975; Thorat & Bhargava, 1994). Many of the earlier studies used nonselective cannabinoid receptor agonists; however, the involvement of CB_1 and/or CB_2 receptors has been probed with selective antagonists, and more recent studies have assessed the efficacy of agonists with selectivity for CB_1 or CB_2 receptors. Interpretation of the results of studies employing systemic administration of cannabinoids can, however, sometimes be complicated by cannabinoid-mediated suppression of motor activity. To examine the specific sites and mechanisms through which cannabinoids reduce pain, studies have investigated the antinociceptive activity of cannabinoids and endocannabinoid system modulators administered supraspinally, spinally, and peripherally. These site-specific studies are the key focus of the present review.

2. ANATOMICAL LOCALIZATION OF THE ENDOCANNABINOID SYSTEM THROUGHOUT THE PAIN PATHWAY

Two major ascending pain pathways in mammals, the spinothalamic pathway and the spinoparabrachial pathway, encode the sensory-discriminatory and affective aspects of pain, respectively (see Fig. 1). In addition, the descending pain pathway originates in higher cortical regions and in the amygdala and hypothalamus, and projects (via the periaqueductal gray (PAG)) to the lower brain stem and spinal cord. Descending control of pain can be either inhibitory or facilitatory depending on the precise circuitry and receptors that are engaged (Millan, 2002; Ossipov, Morimura, & Porreca, 2014; Suzuki & Dickenson, 2005; Suzuki, Rygh, & Dickenson, 2004). The endocannabinoid system is expressed throughout the ascending and descending pain pathways at peripheral, spinal, and supraspinal sites (Fig. 1). CB_1 receptors are located on peripheral endings and central terminals of primary afferent neurons (Hohmann, Briley, & Herkenham, 1999; Hohmann & Herkenham, 1998, 1999a). CB_1 receptors are also found in the dorsal root ganglion (DRG) and in the superficial laminae of the spinal cord (Farquhar-Smith et al., 2000; Glass, Dragunow, & Faull, 1997; Herkenham et al., 1991; Hohmann & Herkenham, 1999b; Ross et al., 2001; Sanudo-Pena, Strangman, Mackie, Walker, & Tsou, 1999). Ahluwalia, Urban, Bevan, Capogna, and Nagy (2002) reported that 80% of CB_1R-expressing neurons either contained calcitonin gene-related peptide (CGRP), a marker for peptidergic neurons, or bound IB4, a marker

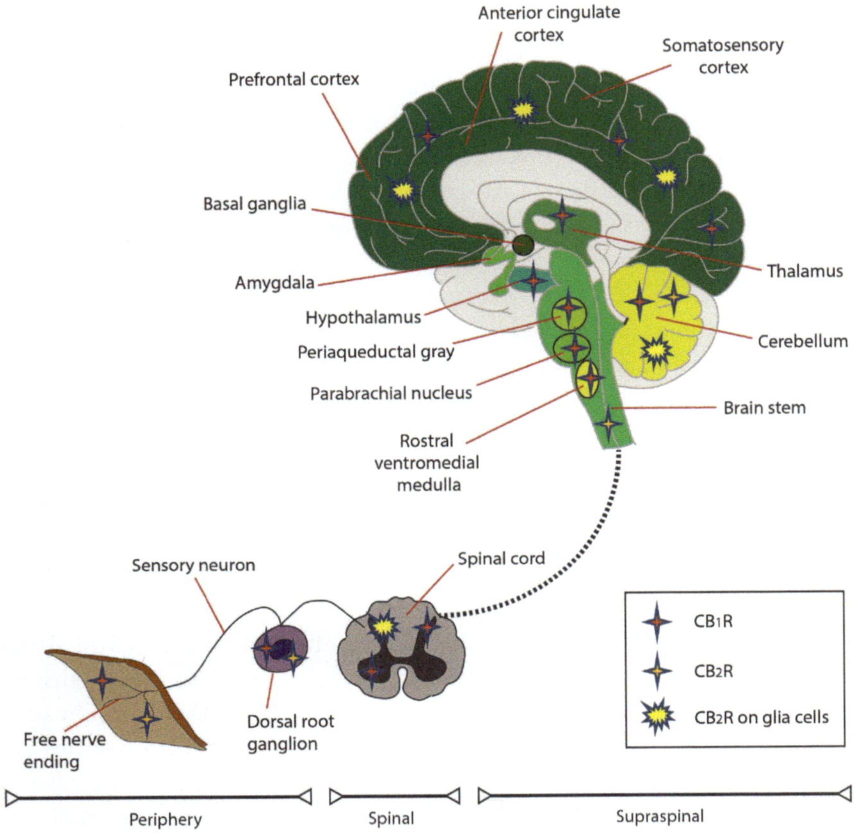

Fig. 1 Cannabinoid receptor distribution throughout the pain pathways. Cannabinoid receptors are present at all three levels of pain processing: (A) in the periphery: CB_1R is present in the peripheral sensory nerve endings, both CB_1R and CB_2R are expressed in the dorsal root ganglion (DRG); (B) in the spinal cord: CB_1R is found in the dorsolateral funiculus, in the surroundings of the central canal, and in the superficial dorsal horn. CB_2R is expressed on glial cells highly restricted to lumbar spinal cord; its expression coincides with the appearance of activated microglia, and (C) in the supraspinal sites: CB_1R is distributed in areas of the brain involved in pain processing, perception, and modulation, e.g., thalamus, amygdala, parabrachial nucleus, periaqueductal gray matter, and rostroventral medulla. They are also present in caudate nucleus and putamen (n. accumbens), basal ganglia, hypothalamus, and cerebellum. CB_2R is expressed in some neurons within the brain stem, and also on glial cells in the cerebellum and cortex. CB_1R and CB_2R distribution in regions involved in pain transduction, transmission, perception, and modulation provides the anatomical basis for the well-known ability of CB_1/CB_2R agonists to decrease pain.

for an unmyelinated neurons which express glycoproteins (Ahluwalia et al., 2002), suggesting a functional role for CB_1R on peripheral nerve terminals. However, there is also evidence that CB_1R mRNA is expressed predominantly in medium- and large-sized DRG neurons, with lower levels in DRG neurons expressing substance P or CGRP mRNA (Hohmann & Herkenham, 1999b). In addition to its peripheral and spinal localization, CB_1R is also located in all of the major brain regions involved in pain processing and modulation. Receptor autoradiography and immunohistochemistry studies have demonstrated the presence of CB_1R in the cortex, amygdala, hypothalamus, thalamus, PAG, parabrachial nucleus, and in brain stem regions including the rostral ventromedial medulla (RVM) (Glass et al., 1997; Herkenham et al., 1991, 1990; Mailleux, Parmentier, & Vanderhaeghen, 1992; Thomas, Wei, & Martin, 1992; Tsou, Brown, Sanudo-Pena, Mackie, & Walker, 1998). CB_1R localization is predominantly presynaptic, and its direct activation by synthetic agonists, or by endocannabinoids that signal retrogradely, inhibits the release of neurotransmitters including GABA and glutamate (Rea, Roche, & Finn, 2007).

The clinical utility of cannabinoids acting at CB_1R can be limited due to adverse central side effects and the development of tolerance (De Vry, Jentzsch, Kuhl, & Eckel, 2004; Gonzalez, Cebeira, & Fernandez-Ruiz, 2005). This has led to increased interest in the role of the CB_2R in pain. The CB_2R has been categorized classically as the peripheral cannabinoid receptor due to its presence on the cells and tissues of the immune, reproductive, cardiovascular, gastrointestinal, and respiratory systems and numerous reports which were unable to detect CB_2R transcripts in normal healthy brain (Derbenev, Stuart, & Smith, 2004; Facci et al., 1995; Griffin et al., 1999; Munro et al., 1993). However, more recent evidence suggests that CB_2R is present in the brain under normal and, in particular, under pathological/inflammatory conditions (Baek, Zheng, Darlington, & Smith, 2008; Concannon, Okine, Finn, & Dowd, 2015; Onaivi, Ishiguro, Gong, et al., 2006; Roche & Finn, 2010; Van Sickle et al., 2005; Zhang et al., 2014), although to a much lesser extent than the ubiquitously expressed CB_1R. CB_2R expression has been demonstrated within pain-related brain regions including the cerebral cortex, hippocampus, striatum, amygdala, thalamic nuclei, PAG, cerebellum, and several brain stem nuclei of the rodent brain (Ashton, Friberg, Darlington, & Smith, 2006; Brusco, Tagliaferro, Saez, & Onaivi, 2008; Gong et al., 2006; Onaivi et al., 2008; Onaivi, Ishiguro, Gong, et al., 2006; Onaivi, Ishiguro, Sejal, et al., 2006;

Suarez et al., 2008; Van Sickle et al., 2005). Although many studies have identified central CB_2R on glial and endothelial cells, there is also evidence to support the expression of CB_2R on subpopulations of neurons within the central nervous system (Ashton et al., 2006; Beltramo et al., 2006; Gong et al., 2006; Molina-Holgado et al., 2007; Onaivi, Ishiguro, Gong, et al., 2006; Palazuelos et al., 2006; Suarez et al., 2008; Van Sickle et al., 2005; Viscomi et al., 2009; Zhang et al., 2014). There is evidence for expression of CB_2R in DRG and in the dorsal horn of the spinal cord and upregulation during neuropathic or inflammatory pain (Anand et al., 2008; Hsieh et al., 2011; Romero-Sandoval & Eisenach, 2007; Romero-Sandoval, Nutile-McMenemy, & DeLeo, 2008; Ross et al., 2001; Svizenska, Brazda, Klusakova, & Dubovy, 2013; Wotherspoon et al., 2005; Zhang et al., 2003). The high expression of the CB_2R in tissues of the immune system including the spleen and thymus as well as on specific immune cells including B lymphocytes, natural killer cells, monocytes, neutrophils and T lymphocytes (Berdyshev, 2000; Howlett et al., 2002; Klein, Newton, & Friedman, 2001; Munro et al., 1993; Sugiura et al., 1995) has focused research on the viability of the CB_2R as a therapeutic target in inflammatory pain conditions in particular, but also neuropathic pain which can have a neuroinflammatory/neuroimmune component (Milligan et al., 2003; Watkins, Milligan, & Maier, 2003).

In addition to the cannabinoid receptors, other components of the endocannabinoid system are also present throughout the ascending and descending pain pathways. Thus, the endocannabinoids, *N*-acylethanolamines, and their metabolizing enzymes are localized in peripheral tissues innervated by primary afferent nociceptive neurons (Calignano, La Rana, Giuffrida, & Piomelli, 1998; Felder et al., 1996), spinal cord (Di Marzo et al., 2000; Egertova, Giang, Cravatt, & Elphick, 1998; Tsou, Nogueron, et al., 1998), and brain (Devane et al., 1992; Egertova et al., 1998; Hanus et al., 2001; Huang et al., 2002; Porter et al., 2002; Stella, Schweitzer, & Piomelli, 1997; Tsou, Nogueron, et al., 1998) tissues, including regions important in pain. Elegant in vivo microdialysis experiments demonstrated that intraplantar injection of the chemical irritant formalin evokes the release of AEA in the midbrain PAG (Walker, Huang, Strangman, Tsou, & Sanudo-Pena, 1999). The endocannabinoids and *N*-acylethanolamines also have affinity for, and activity at, a number of non-CB_1/non-CB_2 receptors, including TRPV1, GPR55 (putative CB_3 receptor), and the peroxisome proliferator-activated receptors (PPARs) (Alexander & Kendall, 2007; Wiley & Martin, 2002), all of which are also expressed throughout the pain pathways and likely play important roles in endocannabinoid-mediated regulation of pain. The remainder of this review will focus on functional in vivo studies of cannabinoids and the endocannabinoid system in models of acute, inflammatory, and neuropathic pain with a focus on supraspinal, spinal, and peripheral sites and mechanisms of action.

3. SUPRASPINAL SITES AND MECHANISMS OF ACTION

3.1 Evidence From Acute Pain Models

In the 1990s, it was demonstrated that the inhibitory effects of the cannabinoid receptor agonists CP-55,940, THC, and WIN55,212-2, administered systemically, on either tail-flick responding (Lichtman & Martin, 1991) or noxious-evoked responses of spinal neurons (Hohmann, Tsou, & Walker, 1999a) are abolished in rats following spinal transection, results that suggested an important role for descending inhibitory pathways in mediating cannabinoid-induced antinociception. The realization that CB_1R is present in moderate to high densities in brain regions which play an important role in nociceptive processing (see Section 2) also prompted investigation of supraspinal sites of action mediating cannabinoid-induced antinociception. Multiple studies have now shown that synthetic or plant-derived cannabinoid receptor agonists, or endogenous cannabinoid ligands, display antinociceptive activity in the mouse and rat tail-flick tests, following intracerebroventricular administration (Fang et al., 2012; Lichtman & Martin, 1997; Martin, Lai, Patrick, Tsou, & Walker, 1993; Pan et al., 2014; Raffa, Stone, & Hipp, 1999; Welch, 1994; Welch, Huffman, & Lowe, 1998; Welch, Thomas, & Patrick, 1995; Zheng et al., 2017).

Significant effort has also been directed at elucidating the specific brain regions that mediate the antinociceptive effects of cannabinoid receptor agonists (Corcoran, Roche, & Finn, 2015). In early work by Martin and colleagues, direct administration of WIN55,212-2 into a number of different brain regions including the amygdala, thalamus, superior colliculus, and A5 region was shown to be antinociceptive in the tail-flick test (Martin, Coffin, et al., 1999). Microinjection of the nonselective cannabinoid receptor agonists WIN55,212-2 and HU210 into the RVM also elevated tail-flick latencies in rats (Martin, Tsou, & Walker, 1998; Meng & Johansen, 2004). Moreover, the effects of HU210 were attenuated by co-administration with the CB_1R antagonist/inverse agonist rimonabant (Martin et al., 1998). Further evidence for the importance of the RVM in cannabinoid-induced attenuation of acute pain came from a study demonstrating that $GABA_A$

receptor agonist-mediated inactivation of the RVM prevented antinociceptive effects of systemically administered WIN55,212-2 in the rat tail-flick test (Meng, Manning, Martin, & Fields, 1998). In addition, it has been shown that the antinociceptive effects of intra-RVM administration of WIN55,212-2 in the tail-flick test are associated with inhibition of ON-cell activity and an increase in OFF-cell activity, effects blocked by rimonabant (Meng & Johansen, 2004). Within the RVM, the nucleus reticularis gigantocellularis pars alpha appears to be an important locus for cannabinoid-mediated antinociception (Monhemius, Azami, Green, & Roberts, 2001).

The PAG, another major component of the descending inhibitory pain pathway, is also an important locus for the antinociceptive effects of cannabinoids. Electrical stimulation of the dorsal or lateral columns of the PAG resulted in CB_1R-mediated antinociception in the rat tail-flick test which was accompanied by a marked increase in AEA release in the PAG (Walker et al. 1999). Intraplantar injection of formalin also resulted in increased AEA release, suggesting engagement of an endogenous cannabinergic pain modulatory system in this midbrain region. Direct administration of CP-55,940 into the ventrolateral (vl) PAG (Lichtman, Cook, & Martin, 1996) and of WIN55,212-2 into the dorsal (dl) PAG (Martin, Coffin, et al., 1999; Martin, Patrick, Coffin, Tsou, & Walker, 1995) had antinociceptive effects in the rat tail-flick test. In vitro studies of the mechanism of action of cannabinoids at the level of the PAG suggest that cannabinoids reduce neurotransmitter release from presynaptic terminals and inhibit GABAergic and glutamatergic transmission (Vaughan, Connor, Bagley, & Christie, 2000). Thus, the antinociceptive effects of cannabinoid agonists administered into the PAG may arise from the disinhibition of GABAergic interneurons and the activation of the descending inhibitory controls, with subsequent inhibition of excitatory transmission at the level of the spinal cord. There is also evidence for a CB_1–glutamatergic interaction in the dlPAG in mediating cannabinoid-induced antinociception in the plantar test in rats (Palazzo et al., 2001). The suppression of acute pain (tail-flick response) following exposure to acute stress (footshock) via the phenomenon of stress-induced analgesia has also been shown to be mediated by endocannabinoids acting at CB_1R in the dlPAG and RVM (Hohmann et al., 2005; Suplita, Farthing, Gutierrez, & Hohmann, 2005). There is also evidence that the cannabinoid receptor agonist HU210 can enhance the antinociceptive effects of morphine, and vice versa, with a site of action in the vlPAG (Wilson, Maher, & Morgan, 2008;

Wilson-Poe, Pocius, Herschbach, & Morgan, 2013). In addition to its activity at cannabinoid receptors, AEA also acts at TRPV1, a receptor that also plays an important role in supraspinal modulation of pain (Madasu, Roche, & Finn, 2015). The TRPV1 agonist capsaicin has been shown to induce initial hyperalgesia in the tail-flick test, followed by antinociception, when injected into the dlPAG (McGaraughty et al., 2003). Similarly, in the rat plantar test, biphasic effects of intra-dlPAG administration of capsaicin have been demonstrated (Palazzo et al., 2002) and intra-vlPAG administration of capsaicin results in glutamate release in the RVM, thereby activating OFF cells and producing antinociception (Starowicz et al., 2007). In further work using the rat plantar test, intra-vlPAG injection of a low dose of the FAAH inhibitor URB597 with the CB_1 receptor antagonist/inverse agonist AM251 converted the hyperalgesic effect of low dose URB597 to an antinociceptive effect, while coadministration of URB597 with both the TRPV1 antagonist capsazepine and AM251 abolished all effects (Maione et al., 2006). In comparison, the antinociceptive effect of high dose URB597 was converted to a hyperalgesic effect following TRPV1 antagonism. The URB597-induced antinociceptive effects (TRPV1 mediated) and pronociceptive effects (CB_1 receptor mediated) were associated with enhanced or reduced RVM OFF-cell activity, respectively, suggesting URB597-induced modulation of the activity of excitatory PAG output neurons (Maione et al., 2006). Intra-vlPAG injection of the dual FAAH inhibitor and TRPV1 antagonist AA-5-HT increased endocannabinoid levels and had an antinociceptive effect in the rat tail-flick test, with associated inhibition of RVM ON- and OFF-cell activity (de Novellis et al., 2008). These effects were blocked by the CB_1 receptor antagonist AM251 or the TRPV1 antagonist I-RTX and were mimicked by intra-vlPAG coadministration of the FAAH inhibitor URB597 with the TRPV1 antagonist I-RTX (de Novellis et al., 2008). Thus, activity of the descending pain pathway is regulated by the action of endocannabinoids at both CB_1R and TRPV1 in the vlPAG. For an excellent schematic of the possible mechanisms underlying endocannabinoid/endovanilloid-mediated control of nociception in the ventrolateral PAG and RVM, see scheme 1 within Maione et al. (2006). Recently, it has also been shown that intra-PAG administration of the GPR55 agonist lysophosphatidylinositol reduces the nociceptive threshold in the rat hot plate test, an effect blocked upon pretreatment with the GPR55 antagonist ML-193 (Deliu et al., 2015), thereby suggesting a role for this putative CB_3 receptor in the PAG in acute pain processing.

The amygdala is thought to play a role in the affective component of pain and is also a component of the descending pain pathway (Neugebauer, Galhardo, Maione, & Mackey, 2009; Neugebauer, Li, Bird, & Han, 2004). Direct administration of WIN55,212-2 into either the basolateral (BLA) or central (CeA) nucleus of the amygdala has been shown to increase tail-flick latency in rats (Hasanein, Parviz, Keshavarz, & Javanmardi, 2007; Martin, Coffin, et al., 1999). Intra-CeA, but not intra-BLA, administration of muscimol, significantly attenuated the antinociceptive effects of systemically administered WIN55,212-2 in rats (Manning, Martin, & Meng, 2003). Another study from the same group found that the amygdala also plays a role in cannabinoid-induced antinociception in nonhuman primates (Manning, Merin, Meng, & Amaral, 2001). Pharmacological blockade of CB_1R in the rat BLA attenuated the stress-induced suppression of nociceptive responding in the tail-flick test (Connell, Bolton, Olsen, Piomelli, & Hohmann, 2006). A role for CB_1R signaling in the rat prelimbic cortex in facilitation of stress-induced analgesia has also been demonstrated (Freitas, Salgado-Rohner, Hallak, Crippa, & Coimbra, 2013). Using fMRI, it has been shown that THC reduces the reported unpleasantness, but not the intensity of ongoing pain and hyperalgesia, induced by capsaicin in healthy human subjects, an effect positively correlated with amygdala activity. THC also reduced functional connectivity between the amygdala and primary sensorimotor areas during the ongoing-pain state (Lee et al., 2013).

3.2 Evidence From Inflammatory Pain Models

Some studies have investigated the effects of intracerebral administration of cannabinoids specifically in animal models of inflammatory pain. Direct microinjection of WIN55,212-2 into the nucleus reticularis gigantocellularis pars alpha, a major source of descending modulation, reduced formalin-evoked pain behavior, via the CB_1 receptor (Monhemius et al., 2001). Administration of the potent cannabinoid receptor agonist HU210 into the dlPAG inhibited formalin-evoked nociceptive behavior during the second phase and was antiaversive in rats (Finn et al., 2004, 2003). Intra-vlPAG administration of AA-5-HT to rats prevented the changes in ON- and OFF-cell firing activity induced by intraplantar injection of formalin and reversed the formalin-induced increase in locus coeruleus adrenergic cell activity (de Novellis et al., 2008). Injection of the CB_1 receptor antagonist AM251 into the PAG or RVM reverses metazinol-induced analgesia in the rat carrageenan model of inflammatory pain, suggesting a role for the endocannabinoid system in these brain regions in NSAID-induced analgesia (Escobar et al., 2012). These data provide additional evidence that the RVM and PAG are important brain regions mediating the antinociceptive effects of cannabinoids in animal models of inflammatory pain. Evidence that pharmacological blockade of CB_1R in the dlPAG attenuates conditioned fear-induced suppression of formalin-evoked nociceptive behavior (i.e., fear-conditioned analgesia) further substantiates the key role of the endocannabinoid system in the PAG in stress-induced analgesia (Olango, Roche, Ford, Harhen, & Finn, 2012). Conversely, anxiety and depression may exacerbate pain and are frequently found comorbid with chronic pain. Finn and coworkers have demonstrated that hyperalgesia to intraplantar formalin injection in Wistar–Kyoto rats that exhibit an anxiodepressive phenotype (vs Sprague–Dawley counterparts) is associated with impaired endocannabinoid–CB_1R signaling in the RVM (Rea et al., 2014). Recently, it has been shown that while CB_1R-mediated inhibition of GABAergic neurons in the RVM is reduced in the rat CFA model, CB_2R functionality in this region is increased in this model of persistent inflammatory pain (Li, Suchland, & Ingram, 2017), supporting the contention that CB_2R may represent a viable analgesic target.

Unilateral inactivation of the CeA reduced the suppression of formalin-evoked c-Fos expression by WIN55,212-2 in the superficial dorsal horn of the spinal cord (Manning et al., 2003). Furthermore, intra-BLA administration of WIN55,212-2 has also been shown to reduce formalin-evoked nociceptive behavior in rats, an effect attenuated by intra-BLA administration of the CB_1R antagonist AM251 (Hasanein et al., 2007). Interestingly, intra-BLA administration of rimonabant has also been reported to attenuate formalin-evoked nociceptive behavior and associated increases in c-Fos immunoreactivity in the hippocampus and RVM in rats (Roche, O'Connor, Diskin, & Finn, 2007; Roche et al., 2010), although intra-BLA administration of AM251 did not have this effect (Rea et al., 2013). In contrast, intra-BLA administration of AM251 (Rea et al., 2013), but not rimonabant (Roche et al., 2010, 2007), attenuated fear-conditioned analgesia in rats. The same doses of rimonabant and AM251 were microinjected into the BLA in these studies and under very similar methodological conditions. However, as discussed in Rea et al. (2013), discrepancies between the effects of the two CB_1R antagonists/inverse agonist may relate to dose–response differences between the two compounds when administered into this brain region or to differential activity of the two compounds at non-CB_1R targets expressed in the BLA (e.g., GPR55, TRPV1, or

PPARs). There is also evidence that fear-conditioned analgesia is mediated by endocannabinoid–CB_1R signaling in the ventral hippocampus (Ford, Kieran, Dolan, Harhen, & Finn, 2011).

In the rat kaolin/carrageenan intraarticular injection model of arthritis, coactivation of mGluR5 and CB_1R increased activity of prefrontal cortex neurons and inhibited pain-related neuronal activity in the CeA (Ji & Neugebauer, 2014). Further evidence for a role of the endocannabinoid system in the prefrontal cortex in arthritic conditions comes from work demonstrating that osteoarthritis pain is associated with increased 2-AG levels in the prefrontal cortex of mice in the monosodium iodoacetate model (La Porta et al., 2015). Recently, Finn and coworkers demonstrated that the antinociceptive effects of PEA injected into the anterior cingulate cortex in the rat formalin test are likely mediated by AEA-induced activation of CB_1R in this brain region arising from substrate competition between PEA and AEA at FAAH (Okine et al., 2016). A facilitatory role for PPARs and TRPV1 in the anterior cingulate cortex in formalin-evoked nociceptive behavior has also been suggested (Okine et al., 2016, 2014).

3.3 Evidence From Neuropathic Pain Models

Increased levels of AEA and 2-AG have been reported in the PAG and RVM of rats 7 days postchronic constriction injury (CCI) of the sciatic nerve, when hyperalgesia and mechanical allodynia were observed to be maximal (Petrosino et al., 2007). Partial sciatic nerve injury has been shown to reduce formalin-evoked pain behavior in rats (Monhemius et al., 2001). This effect was blocked by direct administration of rimonabant into the nucleus reticularis gigantocellularis pars, suggesting that increased endocannabinoid tone in neuropathic rats can modulate nociceptive behavior (Monhemius et al., 2001). In the thalamus, CB_1R mRNA is upregulated in a rat model of neuropathic pain (Siegling, Hofmann, Denzer, Mauler, & De Vry, 2001). Potentially, upregulation of thalamic CB_1R in neuropathic pain states may serve to enhance the analgesic effects of cannabinoids under these conditions. Interestingly, it has been shown that CB_2R plays a functional role in the modulation of responses of neurons in the ventral posterior nucleus of the thalamus in spinal nerve-ligated, but not sham-operated, rats (Jhaveri et al., 2008).

TRPV1 expression is increased in glutamatergic neurons of the medial prefrontal cortex following spared nerve injury (SNI) in rats (Giordano et al., 2012). Moreover, SNI-induced neuropathic pain is also associated with increased levels of endovanilloids and endocannabinoids in the medial prefrontal cortex and direct administration of AA-5-HT into the prelimbic and infralimbic cortices reduces nociceptive behavior in rats following SNI (de Novellis et al., 2011; Giordano et al., 2012).

4. SPINAL SITES AND MECHANISMS OF ACTION

4.1 Evidence From Acute Pain Models

Early evidence that the synthetic cannabinoid levonantradol produced a dose-dependent increase in the hot plate and tail-flick response latencies following intrathecal (i.t.) administration (Yaksh, 1981), followed by studies elucidating mechanisms of THC-induced analgesia (Smith & Martin, 1992), indicated a spinal component in the antinociceptive action of the cannabinoids. Behavioral (Smith & Martin, 1992; Yaksh, 1981), electrophysiological (Hohmann, Tsou, & Michael Walker, 1998; Johanek, Simone, & Lisa, 2005; Sokal, Elmes, Kendall, & Chapman, 2003), and neurochemical (Hohmann, Tsou, & Walker, 1999a, 1999b) studies have demonstrated that cannabinoids act at the spinal level to suppress nociceptive processing. In a model of tonic pain, immunocytochemistry for the protooncogene *c-fos* (a marker for the activation of nociceptive neurons in the spinal cord) was used to demonstrate that cannabinoids reduce behavioral responses to noxious stimuli by decreasing spinal processing of nociceptive inputs (Tsou, Martin, & Bereiter, 1996).

4.2 Evidence From Inflammatory Pain Models

The CB_1R has been suggested to be tonically active in the spinal cord under normal conditions, and its activity is increased in response to injections of CFA in the plantar surface of the rat hind paw (Martin, Loo, & Basbaum, 1999). The synthetic mixed CB_1R/CB_2R agonist WIN55,212-2 reverses inflammation-induced allodynia at doses that do not produce analgesia; additionally rimonabant differentially affects the pattern of Fos expression in the spinal cord, depending on the presence or absence of inflammation (Martin, Coffin, et al., 1999).

A functional inhibitory effect of i.t. administration of the CB_2R-selective agonists A-836339 and AM1241 has been demonstrated in CFA-induced chronic inflammatory pain (Hsieh et al., 2011). These data complement the findings that CB_2R mRNA is upregulated in the spinal cord only from rats under inflammatory conditions, suggesting that

CB_2R agonists may elicit analgesic effects by acting not only at peripheral DRG sites but also at central levels of the spinal cord, making CB_2 an attractive target for chronic pain treatment, avoiding the adverse psychotropic effects that can accompany CB_1R-based therapies. The antinociceptive effects of A-836339 were not sensitive to pretreatment with naloxone, and thus are not mediated by μ-opioid receptors. Interestingly, the blockade of AM1241 by naloxone was observed in the CFA model of inflammatory pain (Hsieh et al., 2011).

4.3 Evidence From Neuropathic Pain Models

Cannabinoids suppress C-fiber-evoked responses of dorsal horn neurons recorded in a rat model of neuropathic pain (Elmes, Jhaveri, Smart, Kendall, & Chapman, 2004). The synaptic processes that produce "windup," the phenomenon whereby repeated stimulation of cutaneous C-fibers at frequencies >0.3 Hz gives increasing responses of dorsal horn cells and withdrawal reflexes, are sufficient to produce central sensitization, which appears to be an important component of hyperalgesia and allodynia. The effect of cannabinoids, namely of the potent, synthetic cannabinoid receptor agonist WIN55,212-2 on windup of spinal dorsal horn neurons was investigated in 1999 (Strangman, Walker, & Strangman, 1999). Strangman and Walker provided the first direct evidence that cannabinoids inhibit the activity-dependent facilitation of spinal nociceptive responses. These authors suggested that cannabinoids may act as general inhibitors of central sensitization by inhibiting calcium entry (Strangman et al., 1999).

The effectiveness of cannabinoids is inconsistent in preclinical neuropathic pain models. WIN55,212-2 delivered i.t. is effective in mitigating mechanical allodynia in the CCI model (Lim, Sung, Ji, & Mao, 2003), while Costa et al. (2005) demonstrated that systemic administration of a CB_1R antagonist significantly reduces mechanical and thermal hyperalgesia in CCI rats and in mice. Others (Toniolo et al., 2014; Ueda et al., 2014) have also suggested that CB_1R expression and activation can be maladaptive. Very recent research indicates that CB_1R expression contributes to the development of persistent mechanical hypersensitivity, protects against the development of cold allodynia, but is not involved in motor impairment following SNI in mice (Sideris et al., 2016).

Although nerve injury increased CB_2R expression in spinal microglia (Zhang et al., 2003), CB_2R agonists suppressed microglial activation and reduced neuropathic pain symptoms (Wilkerson et al., 2012). I.t. delivery of the CB_2R agonist JWH-015 reverses hypersensitivity following nerve injury in a CB_2R- and not CB_1R-dependent manner (an effect blocked by AM630 but not AM281) (Romero-Sandoval & Eisenach, 2007). Interestingly, CB_2R knockout mice displayed increased microglial and astrocytic reactivity in the spinal cord and enhanced neuropathic pain symptoms, whereas transgenic mice overexpressing CB_2R showed attenuated glial reactivity and neuropathic pain (Racz et al., 2008). CB_2R is upregulated on both microglia and astrocytes following SNI in mice, and chronic systemic administration of the CB_2R agonist NESS400 reduces pain behavior, astrogliosis, microglial activation, and levels of proinflammatory cytokines, while promoting levels of antiinflammatory cytokines (Luongo et al., 2010).

Interestingly, the CB_2-selective agonists A-836339 and AM1241, which have previously been shown to counteract inflammatory pain, have also been proven to alleviate neuropathic pain in the rat spinal nerve ligation (SNL) model (Hsieh et al., 2011). As in the case of CFA-induced inflammation, A-836339 action was opioid insensitive, while the blockade of AM1241 by naloxone was not observed. The reason for the difference between two drugs is currently unknown. AM1241 may interact with additional targets that may contribute to the antinociceptive efficacy through the regulation of the opioid receptor pathway (Hsieh et al., 2011). However, there is some conflicting evidence in the literature, with a recent study reporting no effect of the CB_2 agonists GW-405,833 and JWH-133 on mechanical allodynia in CCI model of neuropathy (Brownjohn & Ashton, 2012). This study also reported no elevation of CB_2 at either the protein or mRNA level, probably due to the choice of neuropathic pain model (SNL or CCI).

The endocannabinoids AEA and 2-AG are also increased in the spinal cord following induction of a neuropathic pain state in a CCI model (Petrosino et al., 2007; Starowicz et al., 2012), suggesting that pharmacological manipulation of endocannabinoid accumulation or breakdown may suppress neuropathic nociception in rodents. Both FAAH and MAGL represent potential therapeutic targets for the development of pharmacological agents to treat chronic pain resulting from nerve injury. A significant reduction of neuropathic pain symptoms following inhibition of the AEA hydrolytic enzyme with URB597 in a rat CCI model was reported (Starowicz et al., 2013, 2012). Depending on the dose of URB597 used, and on the consequent lesser or higher elevation of endogenous AEA levels, analgesia was mediated via CB_1 or TRPV1 receptors, respectively. These data suggest that indirect modulation of TRPV1 function, as well as strengthening endogenous AEA signaling by inhibiting its enzymatic degradation, together hold promise for the development of novel multitarget pharmacological treatments. These studies highlight the importance of the endocannabinoid system as a potential therapeutic target for treatment of neuropathic pain.

5. PERIPHERAL SITES AND MECHANISMS OF ACTION

5.1 Evidence From Acute Pain Models

In behavioral experiments, administration of the endogenous CB_1R agonist, AEA, into the ipsilateral hind paw of the rat reduced formalin-induced nociception (Calignano et al., 1998), indicating that activation of peripheral CB_1R produces antinociception. PEA produced a similar effect by activating peripheral CB_2R. Furthermore, PEA was administered together with AEA, the two compounds acted synergistically. The peripheral actions of CB_1R agonists are attributed to an inhibition of both the sensitizing effects of NGF and CGRP release (Rice, Farquhar-Smith, & Nagy, 2002; Richardson, Kilo, & Hargreaves, 1998).

In 2001, it was demonstrated that selective activation of peripheral CB_2R results in antinociception (Malan et al., 2001). AM1241, the CB_2R-selective agonist, administered both locally and systematically (i.p.) produced thermal hypoalgesia, which was absent when the compound was coadministered with AM630, a CB_2R antagonist, but not AM251, the CB_1R antagonist. AM1241 administered locally to the contralateral paw did not elicit antinociception, which suggests a local site of action. Moreover, local administration of AM630 blocked the antinociceptive effect of AM1241 injected i.p., further implicating peripheral CB_2R as the main site of action. Ibrahim et al. (2005) reported that CB_2R activation produces antinociception by stimulating the release of β-endorphin from keratinocytes, which in turn acts at μ-opioid receptors on primary afferent neurons. Furthermore, it was also suggested that other mediators might be released from local cells after activation of CB_2R, contributing to its antinociceptive effects. Nonetheless, β-endorphin release was suggested to be critical for CB_2R-mediated antinociception because the effects of AM1241 were completely prevented by a β-endorphin-sequestering antiserum (Ibrahim et al., 2005).

Inhibition of endocannabinoid metabolism is considered a promising therapeutic target on its own. It has been demonstrated that blocking AEA degradation results in antinociceptive effects in the mouse hot plate test (Kathuria et al., 2003). The carbamate compound URB597 reduces pain-related behavior in the rat produced by prior i.p. injection of CFA in a manner blocked by a CB_1R but not a CB_2R antagonist (Wilson,

Clayton, Medhurst, Bountra, & Chessell, 2004). Also global deletion of FAAH results in lower inflammatory response to local administration of carrageenan (Lichtman et al., 2004). There is good evidence in the literature that CB_2R may regulate oedema and hyperalgesia in response to carrageenan (Holt, Comelli, Costa, & Fowler, 2005). Antioedemic effect of the CB_2R agonists, AM1241 and JTE-907, was demonstrated (Iwamura, Suzuki, Ueda, Kaya, & Inaba, 2001; Quartilho et al., 2003). Moreover, URB597 reduced oedema formation in a CB_2R-dependent manner (Holt et al., 2005).

5.2 Evidence From Inflammatory Pain Models

Studies have demonstrated that administration of the endogenous CB_1R agonist, AEA, into the ipsilateral hind paw of the rat reduces carrageenan-induced hyperalgesia (Richardson et al., 1998) and that administration of the PEA reduced oedema and inflammatory hyperalgesia (Mazzari, Canella, Petrelli, Marcolongo, & Leon, 1996). It was demonstrated that activation of CB_2R suppresses the development of inflammatory pain (Nackley, Makriyannis, & Hohmann, 2003). AM1241, when injected i.p., suppressed the development of carrageenan-evoked thermal and mechanical hyperalgesia as well as allodynia in a CB_2-dependent manner. Furthermore, intraplantar administration suppressed hyperalgesia and allodynia only on the inflamed paw and was inactive following administration in the contralateral (noninflamed) paw (Nackley et al., 2003).

As a result of systemic administration of the selective FAAH inhibitor, URB597, elevation in endogenous AEA levels reduced the mechanical allodynia and thermal hyperalgesia in an inflammatory pain model in both CB_1R- and CB_2R-dependent manner (Jayamanne et al., 2006). Moreover, two distinct inhibitors of MAGL (JZL184 and URB602) elicited local analgesia in the formalin-induced pain model that involved both CB_1R and CB_2R. URB602 produced regionally restricted increases in 2-AG levels in rat hind paw skin without altering AEA levels (Guindon, Guijarro, Piomelli, & Hohmann, 2011). The earlier findings indicate that increase in endocannabinoid tone blocks the development of inflammatory pain.

5.3 Evidence From Neuropathic Pain Models

Studies by Fox et al. (2001) and Elmes et al. (2004) showed that antinociceptive effects in the partial sciatic nerve ligation and SNL models were produced by the activation of peripheral CB_1R and CB_2R, respectively.

In particular, WIN55,212-2 reversed mechanical hyperalgesia following intraplantar administration into the ipsilateral hind paw (Fox et al., 2001). CB_1 mRNA is localized in DRG neurons, and CB_1R has been shown to undergo peripheral axonal flow in the sciatic nerve (Hohmann & Herkenham, 1999a, 1999b). Moreover, data form Hargreaves' group indicate that CB_1R activation inhibits sensory neuropeptide release from the skin of rat hind paws, demonstrating a functional inhibitory activity on peripheral sensory nerves (Richardson et al., 1998). JWH-133, a cannabinoid CB_2R agonist, also significantly reduced noxious mechanically evoked responses of wide dynamic range dorsal horn neurons following intraplantar injections (Elmes et al., 2004). Indeed CB_2 agonists offer promise in neuropathic pain management. CCI of the sciatic nerve-induced neuropathic pain behavior and bilateral elevation of both CB_2R protein and mRNA in lumbar L4–L5 as well as cervical C7–C8 DRG when compared with naive animals. CB_2R protein and mRNA were increased not only in DRG neurons but also in satellite glial cells. Such changes suggest propagation of neuroinflammation alongside the neuraxis and the neuroprotective effects of CB_2R (Svizenska et al., 2013). Work of Leichsenring et al. analyzed the effect of repeated i.p. administration of the CB_2R agonist GW-405,833 on mechanical allodynia, compared with the potent cannabinoid receptor agonist WIN55,212-2 (Leichsenring, Andriske, Bäcker, Stichel, & Lübbert, 2009). Both drugs, applied daily at a low nonpsychotropic dose, were equally effective in reducing mechanical allodynia induced by SNL. A reappearance of glial activation was also associated with return of neuropathic pain-related behavior in this study (Leichsenring et al., 2009). The involvement of peripheral CB_2R in neuropathic pain symptoms alleviation was also a subject of studies by Kinsey, Mahadevan, et al. (2011) and Kinsey, Naidu, et al. (2011). An ethyl sulfonamide THC analogue, O-3223, a selective CB_2 agonist, was reported to reduce thermal hyperalgesia in the CCI-induced neuropathic pain model. Its antihyperalgesic effects were blocked by pretreatment with the CB_2R-selective antagonist SR144528, but not by the CB_1R antagonist, rimonabant. In addition, O-3223 (unlike CP-55,940, CB_1R and CB_2R agonist) did not elicit hypothermia or motor disturbances, indicating it has significant antiinflammatory and antinociceptive effects in vivo, but does not cause CB_1R-mediated side effects.

The therapeutic utility of locally administered AEA for neuropathic pain was proven by Guindon and Beaulieu (2006). However, surprising data on the lack of antiallodynic and antihyperalgesic effects of URB597 in a neuropathic pain model were published by Jayamanne et al. (2006). In animals subjected to partial ligation of the sciatic nerve, i.p. administration of the selective FAAH inhibitor, URB597, produced no significant change in mechanical paw withdrawal latency. It has been suggested that repeated administration of URB597 may prove to be more efficacious in neuropathic pain models, as observed previously for exogenous cannabinoid receptor agonists (Costa et al., 2004). Moreover, acute administration of the irreversible FAAH inhibitor, URB597 and of the reversible FAAH inhibitor, OL-135, decreases allodynia in mouse CCI model of neuropathic pain (Kinsey et al., 2009). This attenuation was completely blocked by pre-treatment with either CB_1 or CB_2R antagonists. Given the neuro-inflammatory nature of the nerve injury in the CCI model, it is not surprising that both cannabinoid receptors play a role in modulating neuropathic pain.

Another FAAH inhibitor, PF-3845, characterized by an increased FAAH specificity and longer duration of in vivo activity (Kinsey, Long, Cravatt, & Lichtman, 2010) also showed an attenuation of CCI-induced mechanical and cold allodynia in wild-type mice (Kinsey et al., 2009). Subsequent work from the Lichtman group explored the contribution of CB_1R and/or CB_2R for the antiallodynic effects of the FAAH and the MAGL inhibitors in a mouse model of neuropathic pain (Kinsey et al., 2010) and further confirmed that both CB_1 and CB_2R are necessary for the anti-allodynic effects of FAAH inhibitors, while only CB_1R is necessary for the antiallodynic effects caused by MAGL inhibition. These data indicate that the endocannabinoids may affect different levels of the nociceptive and inflammatory pathways involved in neuropathic pain.

6. CONCLUSION

Cannabinoids exert a direct antinociceptive effect on pain of different origins. The CB_1R-mediated analgesic effects of cannabinoid ligands are well established, but limited by their side-effect profile. The observation that CB_2R activation produces desirable actions in a range of preclinical models (Han, Thatte, Buzard, & Jones, 2013; Leleu-Chavain et al., 2012) attracted considerable interest. However, despite very favorable efficacy in a range of preclinical models, CB_2 agonists have fared poorly in the clinic (Dhopeshwarkar & Mackie, 2014). The targeted manipulation of the endocannabinoid system might also be beneficial in the face of inflammation and chronic pain conditions. Interestingly investigations into the endocannabinoids and their effector sites, along with other noncannabinoid receptors, have exploded in recent years, and insights reveal this area of pharmacology to be highly complex and dynamic (Piscitelli & Di Marzo, 2012; Starowicz & Di Marzo, 2013). Data derived from complex and clinically relevant animal models highlight the question of effectiveness of dual-acting compounds (Aiello, Carullo, Badolato, & Brizzi, 2016; Ligresti et al., 2014; Malek & Starowicz, 2016) and support the case for multitarget pharmacological intervention for effective pain treatment.

CONFLICT OF INTEREST

The authors have no conflicts of interest to declare.

ACKNOWLEDGMENTS

This work was supported by grants from the National Science Center, Poland (SONATA BIS NCN/2012/07/E/NZ7/01269 and OPUS NCN/2014/13/B/NZ7/02311) to K.S. and a grant from Science Foundation Ireland (10/IN.1/B2976) to D.P.F. The authors wish to than Natalia Małek for her assistance in preparing the figure and table.

REFERENCES

Ahluwalia, J., Urban, L., Bevan, S., Capogna, M., & Nagy, I. (2002). Cannabinoid 1 receptors are expressed by nerve growth factor- and glial cell-derived neurotrophic factor-responsive primary sensory neurones. *Neuroscience*, *110*(4), 747–753.

Aiello, F., Carullo, G., Badolato, M., & Brizzi, A. (2016). TRPV1-FAAH-COX: The couples game in pain treatment. *ChemMedChem*, *11*(16), 1686–1694.

Alexander, S. P., & Kendall, D. A. (2007). The complications of promiscuity: Endocannabinoid action and metabolism. *British Journal of Pharmacology*, *152*(5), 602–623.

Anand, U., Otto, W. R., Sanchez-Herrera, D., Facer, P., Yiangou, Y., Korchev, Y., et al. (2008). Cannabinoid receptor CB2 localisation and agonist-mediated inhibition of capsaicin responses in human sensory neurons. *Pain*, *138*(3), 667–680.

Ashton, J. C., Friberg, D., Darlington, C. L., & Smith, P. F. (2006). Expression of the cannabinoid CB2 receptor in the rat cerebellum: An immunohistochemical study. *Neuroscience Letters*, *396*(2), 113–116.

Baek, J. H., Zheng, Y., Darlington, C. L., & Smith, P. F. (2008). Cannabinoid CB2 receptor expression in the rat brainstem cochlear and vestibular nuclei. *Acta Oto-Laryngologica*, *128*(9), 961–967.

Barnes, M. P. (2006). Sativex: Clinical efficacy and tolerability in the treatment of symptoms of multiple sclerosis and neuropathic pain. *Expert Opinion on Pharmacotherapy*, 7(5), 607–615.

Beltramo, M., Bernardini, N., Bertorelli, R., Campanella, M., Nicolussi, E., Fredduzzi, S., et al. (2006). CB2 receptor-mediated antihyperalgesia: Possible direct involvement of neural mechanisms. *The European Journal of Neuroscience*, *23*(6), 1530–1538.

Berdyshev, E. V. (2000). Cannabinoid receptors and the regulation of immune response. *Chemistry and Physics of Lipids*, *108*(1–2), 169–190.

Bicher, H. I., & Mechoulam, R. (1968). Pharmacological effects of two active constituents of marijuana. *Archives Internationales de Pharmacodynamie et de Thérapie*, *172*, 24–31.

Bjursell, M., Ryberg, E., Wu, T., Greasley, P. J., Bohlooly, Y. M., & Hjorth, S. (2016). Deletion of Gpr55 results in subtle effects on energy metabolism, motor activity and thermal pain sensation. *PLoS One*, *11*(12), e0167965.

Bloom, A. S., & Dewey, W. L. (1978). A comparison of some pharmacological actions of morphine and delta9-tetrahydrocannabinol in the mouse. *Psychopharmacology*, *57*(3), 243–248.

Boychuk, D. G., Goddard, G., Mauro, G., & Orellana, M. F. (2015). The effectiveness of cannabinoids in the management of chronic nonmalignant neuropathic pain: A systematic review. *Journal of Oral & Facial Pain and Headache*, *29*(1), 7–14.

Brownjohn, P. W., & Ashton, J. C. (2012). Spinal cannabinoid CB2 receptors as a target for neuropathic pain: An investigation using chronic constriction injury. *Neuroscience*, *203*, 180–193.

Brusco, A., Tagliaferro, P. A., Saez, T., & Onaivi, E. S. (2008). Ultrastructural localization of neuronal brain CB2 cannabinoid receptors. *Annals of the New York Academy of Sciences*, *1139*, 450–457.

Buckley, N. E. (2008). The peripheral cannabinoid receptor knockout mice: An update. *British Journal of Pharmacology*, *153*(2), 309–318.

Buckley, N. E., McCoy, K. L., Mezey, E., Bonner, T., Zimmer, A., Felder, C. C., et al. (2000). Immunomodulation by cannabinoids is absent in mice deficient for the cannabinoid CB(2) receptor. *European Journal of Pharmacology*, *396*(2–3), 141–149.

Calignano, A., La Rana, G., Giuffrida, A., & Piomelli, D. (1998). Control of pain initiation by endogenous cannabinoids. *Nature*, *394*(6690), 277–281.

Canadian Agency for Drugs and Technologies in Health. (2016). *Cannabinoid buccal spray for chronic non-cancer or neuropathic pain: A review of clinical effectiveness, safety, and guidelines*. Ottawa, ON.

Carey, L. M., Gutierrez, T., Deng, L., Lee, W. H., Mackie, K., & Hohmann, A. G. (2017). Inflammatory and neuropathic nociception is preserved in GPR55 knockout mice. *Scientific Reports*, 7(1), 944. http://dx.doi.org/10.1038/s41598-017-01062-2.

Carey, L. M., Slivicki, R. A., Leishman, E., Cornett, B., Mackie, K., Bradshaw, H., et al. (2016). A pro-nociceptive phenotype unmasked in mice lacking fatty-acid amide hydrolase. *Molecular Pain*, *12*, 1–23. http://dx.doi.org/10.1177/1744806916649192.

Castane, A., Celerier, E., Martin, M., Ledent, C., Parmentier, M., Maldonado, R., et al. (2006). Development and expression of neuropathic pain in CB1 knockout mice. *Neuropharmacology*, *50*(1), 111–122.

Concannon, R. M., Okine, B. N., Finn, D. P., & Dowd, E. (2015). Differential upregulation of the cannabinoid CB(2) receptor in neurotoxic and inflammation-driven rat models of Parkinson's disease. *Experimental Neurology*, *269*, 133–141.

Connell, K., Bolton, N., Olsen, D., Piomelli, D., & Hohmann, A. G. (2006). Role of the basolateral nucleus of the amygdala in endocannabinoid-mediated stress-induced analgesia. *Neuroscience Letters*, *397*(3), 180–184.

Corcoran, L., Roche, M., & Finn, D. P. (2015). The role of the brain's endocannabinoid system in pain and its modulation by stress. *International Review of Neurobiology*, *125*, 203–255.

Costa, B., Colleoni, M., Conti, S., Trovato, A. E., Bianchi, M., Sotgiu, M. L., et al. (2004). Repeated treatment with the synthetic cannabinoid WIN 55,212-2 reduces both hyperalgesia and production of pronociceptive mediators in a rat model of neuropathic pain. *British Journal of Pharmacology*, *141*(1), 4–8.

Costa, B., Trovato, A. E., Colleoni, M., Giagnoni, G., Zarini, E., & Croci, T. (2005). Effect of the cannabinoid CB1 receptor antagonist, SR141716, on nociceptive response and nerve demyelination in rodents with chronic constriction injury of the sciatic nerve. *Pain*, *116*(1–2), 52–61.

Cravatt, B. F., Demarest, K., Patricelli, M. P., Bracey, M. H., Giang, D. K., Martin, B. R., et al. (2001). Supersensitivity to anandamide and enhanced endogenous cannabinoid signaling in mice lacking fatty acid amide hydrolase. *Proceedings of the National Academy of Sciences of the United States of America*, *98*(16), 9371–9376.

de Novellis, V., Palazzo, E., Rossi, F., De Petrocellis, L., Petrosino, S., Guida, F., et al. (2008). The analgesic effect of N-arachidonoyl-serotonin, a FAAH inhibitor and TRPV1 receptor antagonist, associated with changes in rostral ventromedial medulla and locus coeruleus cell activity in rats. *Neuropharmacology*, *55*(7), 1105–1113.

de Novellis, V., Vita, D., Gatta, L., Luongo, L., Bellini, G., De Chiaro, M., et al. (2011). The blockade of the transient receptor potential vanilloid type 1 and fatty acid amide hydrolase decreases symptoms and central sequelae in the medial prefrontal cortex of neuropathic rats. *Molecular Pain*, 7, 7.

De Vry, J., Jentzsch, K. R., Kuhl, E., & Eckel, G. (2004). Behavioral effects of cannabinoids show differential sensitivity to cannabinoid receptor blockade and tolerance development. *Behavioural Pharmacology*, *15*(1), 1–12.

Deliu, E., Sperow, M., Console-Bram, L., Carter, R. L., Tilley, D. G., Kalamarides, D. J., et al. (2015). The lysophosphatidylinositol receptor GPR55 modulates pain perception in the periaqueductal gray. *Molecular Pharmacology*, *88*(2), 265–272.

Deng, L., Guindon, J., Cornett, B. L., Makriyannis, A., Mackie, K., & Hohmann, A. G. (2015). Chronic cannabinoid receptor 2 activation reverses paclitaxel neuropathy without tolerance or cannabinoid receptor 1-dependent withdrawal. *Biological Psychiatry*, 77(5), 475–487.

Derbenev, A. V., Stuart, T. C., & Smith, B. N. (2004). Cannabinoids suppress synaptic input to neurones of the rat dorsal motor nucleus of the vagus nerve. *The Journal of Physiology*, *559*(Pt. 3), 923–938.

Devane, W. A., Dysarz, F. A., 3rd, Johnson, M. R., Melvin, L. S., & Howlett, A. C. (1988). Determination and characterization of a cannabinoid receptor in rat brain. *Molecular Pharmacology*, *34*(5), 605–613.

Devane, W. A., Hanus, L., Breuer, A., Pertwee, R. G., Stevenson, L. A., Griffin, G., et al. (1992). Isolation and structure of a brain constituent that binds to the cannabinoid receptor. *Science*, *258*(5090), 1946–1949.

Dhopeshwarkar, A., & Mackie, K. (2014). CB2 cannabinoid receptors as a therapeutic target—What does the future hold? *Molecular Pharmacology*, *86*, 430–437.

Di Marzo, V., Breivogel, C. S., Tao, Q., Bridgen, D. T., Razdan, R. K., Zimmer, A. M., et al. (2000). Levels, metabolism, and pharmacological activity of anandamide in CB(1) cannabinoid receptor knockout mice: Evidence for non-CB(1), non-CB(2) receptor-mediated actions of anandamide in mouse brain. *Journal of Neurochemistry*, *75*(6), 2434–2444.

Egertova, M., Giang, D. K., Cravatt, B. F., & Elphick, M. R. (1998). A new perspective on cannabinoid signalling: Complementary localization of fatty acid amide hydrolase and the CB1 receptor in rat brain. *Proceedings. Biological Sciences*, *265*(1410), 2081–2085.

Elmes, S. J. R., Jhaveri, M. D., Smart, D., Kendall, D. A., & Chapman, V. (2004). Cannabinoid CB2 receptor activation inhibits mechanically evoked responses of wide dynamic range dorsal horn neurons in naïve rats and in rat models of inflammatory and neuropathic pain. *European Journal of Neuroscience*, *20*(9), 2311–2320.

Escobar, W., Ramirez, K., Avila, C., Limongi, R., Vanegas, H., & Vazquez, E. (2012). Metamizol, a non-opioid analgesic, acts via endocannabinoids in the PAG-RVM axis during inflammation in rats. *European Journal of Pain*, *16*(5), 676–689.

Facci, L., Dal Toso, R., Romanello, S., Buriani, A., Skaper, S. D., & Leon, A. (1995). Mast cells express a peripheral cannabinoid receptor with differential sensitivity to anandamide and palmitoylethanolamide. *Proceedings of the National Academy of Sciences of the United States of America*, *92*(8), 3376–3380.

Fang, Q., Han, Z. L., Li, N., Wang, Z. L., He, N., & Wang, R. (2012). Effects of neuropeptide FF system on CB(1) and CB(2) receptors mediated antinociception in mice. *Neuropharmacology*, *62*(2), 855–864.

Farquhar-Smith, W. P., Egertova, M., Bradbury, E. J., McMahon, S. B., Rice, A. S., & Elphick, M. R. (2000). Cannabinoid CB(1) receptor expression in rat spinal cord. *Molecular and Cellular Neurosciences, 15*(6), 510–521.

Felder, C. C., Nielsen, A., Briley, E. M., Palkovits, M., Priller, J., Axelrod, J., et al. (1996). Isolation and measurement of the endogenous cannabinoid receptor agonist, anandamide, in brain and peripheral tissues of human and rat. *FEBS Letters, 393*(2–3), 231–235.

Finn, D. P., & Chapman, V. (2004). Cannabinoids as analgesic agents: Evidence from in vivo studies. *Current Neuropharmacology, 2*(1), 75–89.

Finn, D. P., Jhaveri, M. D., Beckett, S. R., Kendall, D. A., Marsden, C. A., & Chapman, V. (2004). Cannabinoids modulate ultrasound-induced aversive responses in rats. *Psychopharmacology, 172*(1), 41–51.

Finn, D. P., Jhaveri, M. D., Beckett, S. R., Roe, C. H., Kendall, D. A., Marsden, C. A., et al. (2003). Effects of direct periaqueductal grey administration of a cannabinoid receptor agonist on nociceptive and aversive responses in rats. *Neuropharmacology, 45*(5), 594–604.

Ford, G. K., Kieran, S., Dolan, K., Harhen, B., & Finn, D. P. (2011). A role for the ventral hippocampal endocannabinoid system in fear-conditioned analgesia and fear responding in the presence of nociceptive tone in rats. *Pain, 152*(11), 2495–2504.

Fox, A., Kesingland, A., Gentry, C., McNair, K., Patel, S., Urban, L., et al. (2001). The role of central and peripheral cannabinoid 1 receptors in the antihyperalgesic activity of cannabinoids in a model of neuropathic pain. *Pain, 92*(1–2), 91–100.

Freitas, R. L., Salgado-Rohner, C. J., Hallak, J. E., Crippa, J. A., & Coimbra, N. C. (2013). Involvement of prelimbic medial prefrontal cortex in panic-like elaborated defensive behaviour and innate fear-induced antinociception elicited by GABAA receptor blockade in the dorsomedial and ventromedial hypothalamic nuclei: Role of the endocannabinoid CB1 receptor. *The International Journal of Neuropsychopharmacology, 16*(8), 1781–1798.

Giordano, C., Cristino, L., Luongo, L., Siniscalco, D., Petrosino, S., Piscitelli, F., et al. (2012). TRPV1-dependent and -independent alterations in the limbic cortex of neuropathic mice: Impact on glial caspases and pain perception. *Cerebral Cortex, 22*(11), 2495–2518.

Glass, M., Dragunow, M., & Faull, R. L. M. (1997). Cannabinoid receptors in the human brain: A detailed anatomical and quantitative autoradiographic study in the fetal, neonatal and adult human brain. *Neuroscience, 77*(2), 299–318.

Gong, J. P., Onaivi, E. S., Ishiguro, H., Liu, Q. R., Tagliaferro, P. A., Brusco, A., et al. (2006). Cannabinoid CB2 receptors: Immunohistochemical localization in rat brain. *Brain Research, 1071*(1), 10–23.

Gonzalez, S., Cebeira, M., & Fernandez-Ruiz, J. (2005). Cannabinoid tolerance and dependence: A review of studies in laboratory animals. *Pharmacology, Biochemistry, and Behavior, 81*(2), 300–318.

Griffin, G., Wray, E. J., Tao, Q., McAllister, S. D., Rorrer, W. K., Aung, M. M., et al. (1999). Evaluation of the cannabinoid CB2 receptor-selective antagonist, SR144528: Further evidence for cannabinoid CB2 receptor absence in the rat central nervous system. *European Journal of Pharmacology, 377*(1), 117–125.

Grinspoon, L., & Bakalar, J. B. (1993). *Marijuana, the forbidden medicine*. New Haven: Yale University Press.

Guindon, J., & Beaulieu, P. (2006). Antihyperalgesic effects of local injections of anandamide, ibuprofen, rofecoxib and their combinations in a model of neuropathic pain. *Neuropharmacology, 50*(7), 814–823.

Guindon, J., Guijarro, A., Piomelli, D., & Hohmann, A. G. (2011). Peripheral antinociceptive effects of inhibitors of monoacylglycerol lipase in a rat model of inflammatory pain. *British Journal of Pharmacology, 163*(7), 1464–1478.

Han, S., Thatte, J., Buzard, D. J., & Jones, R. M. (2013). Therapeutic utility of cannabinoid receptor type 2 (CB2) selective agonists. *Journal of Medicinal Chemistry*, *56*, 8224–8256.
Hanus, L., Abu-Lafi, S., Fride, E., Breuer, A., Vogel, Z., Shalev, D. E., et al. (2001). 2-Arachidonoyl glyceryl ether, an endogenous agonist of the cannabinoid CB1 receptor. *Proceedings of the National Academy of Sciences of the United States of America*, *98*(7), 3662–3665.
Hasanein, P., Parviz, M., Keshavarz, M., & Javanmardi, K. (2007). CB1 receptor activation in the basolateral amygdala produces antinociception in animal models of acute and tonic nociception. *Clinical and Experimental Pharmacology & Physiology*, *34*(5–6), 439–449.
Herkenham, M., Lynn, A. B., Johnson, M. R., Melvin, L. S., de Costa, B. R., & Rice, K. C. (1991). Characterization and localization of cannabinoid receptors in rat brain: A quantitative in vitro autoradiographic study. *The Journal of Neuroscience*, *11*(2), 563–583.
Herkenham, M., Lynn, A. B., Little, M. D., Johnson, M. R., Melvin, L. S., de Costa, B. R., et al. (1990). Cannabinoid receptor localization in brain. *Proceedings of the National Academy of Sciences of the United States of America*, *87*(5), 1932–1936.
Hohmann, A. G., Briley, E. M., & Herkenham, M. (1999a). Pre- and postsynaptic distribution of cannabinoid and mu opioid receptors in rat spinal cord. *Brain Research*, *822*(1–2), 17–25.
Hohmann, A. G., & Herkenham, M. (1998). Regulation of cannabinoid and mu opioid receptors in rat lumbar spinal cord following neonatal capsaicin treatment. *Neuroscience Letters*, *252*(1), 13–16.
Hohmann, A. G., & Herkenham, M. (1999a). Cannabinoid receptors undergo axonal flow in sensory nerves. *Neuroscience*, *92*(4), 1171–1175.
Hohmann, A. G., & Herkenham, M. (1999b). Localization of central cannabinoid CB1 receptor messenger RNA in neuronal subpopulations of rat dorsal root ganglia: A double-label in situ hybridization study. *Neuroscience*, *90*(3), 923–931.
Hohmann, A. G., Suplita, R. L., Bolton, N. M., Neely, M. H., Fegley, D., Mangieri, R., et al. (2005). An endocannabinoid mechanism for stress-induced analgesia. *Nature*, *435*(7045), 1108–1112.
Hohmann, A. G., Tsou, K., & Michael Walker, J. (1998). Cannabinoid modulation of wide dynamic range neurons in the lumbar dorsal horn of the rat by spinally administered WIN55,212-2. *Neuroscience Letters*, *257*(3), 119–122.
Hohmann, A. G., Tsou, K., & Walker, J. M. (1999a). Cannabinoid suppression of noxious heat-evoked activity in wide dynamic range neurons in the lumbar dorsal horn of the rat. *Journal of Neurophysiology*, *81*(2), 575–583.
Hohmann, A. G., Tsou, K., & Walker, J. M. (1999b). Intrathecal cannabinoid administration suppresses noxious stimulus-evoked Fos protein-like immunoreactivity in rat spinal cord: Comparison with morphine. *Zhongguo Yao Li Xue Bao*, *20*(12), 1132–1136.
Holt, S., Comelli, F., Costa, B., & Fowler, C. J. (2005). Inhibitors of fatty acid amide hydrolase reduce carrageenan-induced hind paw inflammation in pentobarbital-treated mice: Comparison with indomethacin and possible involvement of cannabinoid receptors. *British Journal of Pharmacology*, *146*(3), 467–476.
Howlett, A. C., Barth, F., Bonner, T. I., Cabral, G., Casellas, P., Devane, W. A., et al. (2002). International union of pharmacology. XXVII. Classification of cannabinoid receptors. *Pharmacological Reviews*, *54*(2), 161–202.
Hsieh, G. C., Pai, M., Chandran, P., Hooker, B. A., Zhu, C. Z., Salyers, A. K., et al. (2011). Central and peripheral sites of action for CB(2) receptor mediated analgesic activity in chronic inflammatory and neuropathic pain models in rats. *British Journal of Pharmacology*, *162*(2), 428–440.
Huang, S. M., Bisogno, T., Trevisani, M., Al-Hayani, A., De Petrocellis, L., Fezza, F., et al. (2002). An endogenous capsaicin-like substance with high potency at recombinant and

native vanilloid VR1 receptors. *Proceedings of the National Academy of Sciences of the United States of America*, *99*(12), 8400–8405.

Ibrahim, M. M., Porreca, F., Lai, J., Albrecht, P. J., Rice, F. L., Khodorova, A., et al. (2005). CB2 cannabinoid receptor activation produces antinociception by stimulating peripheral release of endogenous opioids. *Proceedings of the National Academy of Sciences of the United States of America*, *102*(8), 3093–3098.

Iskedjian, M., Bereza, B., Gordon, A., Piwko, C., & Einarson, T. R. (2007). Meta-analysis of cannabis based treatments for neuropathic and multiple sclerosis-related pain. *Current Medical Research and Opinion*, *23*(1), 17–24.

Iwamura, H., Suzuki, H., Ueda, Y., Kaya, T., & Inaba, T. (2001). In vitro and in vivo pharmacological characterization of JTE-907, a novel selective ligand for cannabinoid CB2 receptor. *The Journal of Pharmacology and Experimental Therapeutics*, *296*(2), 420–425.

Jayamanne, A., Greenwood, R., Mitchell, V. A., Aslan, S., Piomelli, D., & Vaughan, C. W. (2006). Actions of the FAAH inhibitor URB597 in neuropathic and inflammatory chronic pain models. *British Journal of Pharmacology*, *147*(3), 281–288.

Jhaveri, M. D., Elmes, S. J., Richardson, D., Barrett, D. A., Kendall, D. A., Mason, R., et al. (2008). Evidence for a novel functional role of cannabinoid CB(2) receptors in the thalamus of neuropathic rats. *The European Journal of Neuroscience*, *27*(7), 1722–1730. http://dx.doi.org/10.1111/j.1460-9568.2008.06162.x.

Ji, G., & Neugebauer, V. (2014). CB1 augments mGluR5 function in medial prefrontal cortical neurons to inhibit amygdala hyperactivity in an arthritis pain model. *The European Journal of Neuroscience*, *39*(3), 455–466.

Johanek, L. M., Simone, D. A., & Lisa, M. (2005). Cannabinoid agonist, CP 55, 940, prevents capsaicin-induced sensitization of spinal cord dorsal horn neurons. *Spinal Cord*, *93*, 989–997.

Kathuria, S., Gaetani, S., Fegley, D., Valiño, F., Duranti, A., Tontini, A., et al. (2003). Modulation of anxiety through blockade of anandamide hydrolysis. *Nature Medicine*, *9*(1), 76–81.

Kinsey, S. G., Long, J. Z., Cravatt, B. F., & Lichtman, A. H. (2010). Fatty acid amide hydrolase and monoacylglycerol lipase inhibitors produce anti-allodynic effects in mice through distinct cannabinoid receptor mechanisms. *Journal of Pain*, *11*(12), 1420–1428.

Kinsey, S. G., Long, J. Z., O'Neal, S. T., Abdullah, R. A., Poklis, J. L., Boger, D. L., et al. (2009). Blockade of endocannabinoid-degrading enzymes attenuates neuropathic pain. *The Journal of Pharmacology and Experimental Therapeutics*, *330*(3), 902–910.

Kinsey, S. G., Mahadevan, A., Zhao, B., Sun, H., Naidu, P. S., Razdan, R. K., et al. (2011a). The CB2 cannabinoid receptor-selective agonist O-3223 reduces pain and inflammation without apparent cannabinoid behavioral effects. *Neuropharmacology*, *60*(2–3), 244–251.

Kinsey, S. G., Naidu, P. S., Cravatt, B. F., Dudley, D. T., & Lichtman, A. H. (2011b). Fatty acid amide hydrolase blockade attenuates the development of collagen-induced arthritis and related thermal hyperalgesia in mice. *Pharmacology, Biochemistry, and Behavior*, *99*(4), 718–725.

Klein, T. W., Newton, C. A., & Friedman, H. (2001). Cannabinoids and the immune system. *Pain Research & Management*, *6*(2), 95–101.

La Porta, C., Bura, S. A., Aracil-Fernandez, A., Manzanares, J., & Maldonado, R. (2013). Role of CB1 and CB2 cannabinoid receptors in the development of joint pain induced by monosodium iodoacetate. *Pain*, *154*(1), 160–174.

La Porta, C., Bura, A. S., Llorente-Onaindia, J., Pastor, A., Navarrete, F., Garcia-Gutierrez, M. S., et al. (2015). Role of the endocannabinoid system in the emotional manifestations of osteoarthritis pain. *Pain*, *156*(1), 2001–2012.

Ledent, C., Valverde, O., Cossu, G., Petitet, F., Aubert, J. F., Beslot, F., et al. (1999). Unresponsiveness to cannabinoids and reduced addictive effects of opiates in CB1 receptor knockout mice. *Science*, *283*, 401–404.

Lee, M. C., Ploner, M., Wiech, K., Bingel, U., Wanigasekera, V., Brooks, J., et al. (2013). Amygdala activity contributes to the dissociative effect of cannabis on pain perception. *Pain*, *154*(1), 124–134.

Leichsenring, A., Andriske, M., Bäcker, I., Stichel, C. C., & Lübbert, H. (2009). Analgesic and antiinflammatory effects of cannabinoid receptor agonists in a rat model of neuropathic pain. *Naunyn-Schmiedeberg's Archives of Pharmacology*, *379*(6), 627–636.

Leleu-Chavain, N., Body-Malapel, M., Spencer, J., Chavatte, P., Desreumaux, P., & Millet, R. (2012). Recent advances in the development of selective CB2 agonists as promising anti-inflammatory agents. *Current Medicinal Chemistry*, *19*(21), 3457–3474.

Li, M. H., Suchland, K. L., & Ingram, S. L. (2017). Compensatory activation of cannabinoid CB2 receptor inhibition of GABA release in the rostral ventromedial medulla in inflammatory pain. *The Journal of Neuroscience*, *37*(3), 626–636.

Lichtman, A. H., Cook, S. A., & Martin, B. R. (1996). Investigation of brain sites mediating cannabinoid-induced antinociception in rats: Evidence supporting periaqueductal gray involvement. *The Journal of Pharmacology and Experimental Therapeutics*, *276*(2), 585–593.

Lichtman, A. H., & Martin, B. R. (1991). Spinal and supraspinal components of cannabinoid-induced antinociception. *The Journal of Pharmacology and Experimental Therapeutics*, *258*(2), 517–523.

Lichtman, A. H., & Martin, B. R. (1997). The selective cannabinoid antagonist SR 141716A blocks cannabinoid-induced antinociception in rats. *Pharmacology, Biochemistry, and Behavior*, *57*(1–2), 7–12.

Lichtman, A. H., Shelton, C. C., Advani, T., & Cravatt, B. F. (2004). Mice lacking fatty acid amide hydrolase exhibit a cannabinoid receptor-mediated phenotypic hypoalgesia. *Pain*, *109*(3), 319–327.

Ligresti, A., Martos, J., Wang, J., Guida, F., Allarà, M., Palmieri, V., et al. (2014). Prostamide F2α receptor antagonism combined with inhibition of FAAH may block the pro-inflammatory mediators formed following selective FAAH inhibition. *British Journal of Pharmacology*, *171*(6), 1408–1419.

Lim, G., Sung, B., Ji, R. R., & Mao, J. (2003). Upregulation of spinal cannabinoid-1-receptors following nerve injury enhances the effects of Win 55,212-2 on neuropathic pain behaviors in rats. *Pain*, *105*(1–2), 275–283.

Luongo, L., Palazzo, E., Tambaro, S., Giordano, C., Gatta, L., Scafuro, M. A., et al. (2010). 1-(2′,4′-Dichlorophenyl)-6-methyl-N-cyclohexylamine-1,4-dihy droindeno[1,2-c] pyrazole-3-carboxamide, a novel CB2 agonist, alleviates neuropathic pain through functional microglial changes in mice. *Neurobiology of Disease*, *37*(1), 177–185.

Lynch, M. E., & Ware, M. A. (2015). Cannabinoids for the treatment of chronic non-cancer pain: An updated systematic review of randomized controlled trials. *Journal of Neuroimmune Pharmacology*, *10*(2), 293–301.

Madasu, M. K., Roche, M., & Finn, D. P. (2015). Supraspinal TRPV1 in pain and psychiatric disorders. *Modern Trends in Pharmacopsychiatry*, *30*, 80–93.

Mailleux, P., Parmentier, M., & Vanderhaeghen, J. J. (1992). Distribution of cannabinoid receptor messenger RNA in the human brain: An in situ hybridization histochemistry with oligonucleotides. *Neuroscience Letters*, *143*(1–2), 200–204.

Maione, S., Bisogno, T., de Novellis, V., Palazzo, E., Cristino, L., Valenti, M., et al. (2006). Elevation of endocannabinoid levels in the ventrolateral periaqueductal grey through inhibition of fatty acid amide hydrolase affects descending nociceptive pathways via both cannabinoid receptor type 1 and transient receptor potential vanilloid type-1 receptors. *The Journal of Pharmacology and Experimental Therapeutics*, *316*(3), 969–982.

Malan, T. P., Jr., Ibrahim, M. M., Deng, H., Liu, Q., Mata, H. P., Vanderah, T., et al. (2001). CB2 cannabinoid receptor-mediated peripheral antinociception. *Pain*, *93*(3), 239–245.

Malek, N., & Starowicz, K. (2016). Dual-acting compounds targeting endocannabinoid and endovanilloid systems—A novel treatment option for chronic pain management. *Frontiers in Pharmacology*, 7, 257.

Manning, B. H., Martin, W. J., & Meng, I. D. (2003). The rodent amygdala contributes to the production of cannabinoid-induced antinociception. *Neuroscience*, *120*(4), 1157–1170.

Manning, B. H., Merin, N. M., Meng, I. D., & Amaral, D. G. (2001). Reduction in opioid- and cannabinoid-induced antinociception in rhesus monkeys after bilateral lesions of the amygdaloid complex. *Journal of Neuroscience*, *21*(20), 8238–8246.

Martin, W. J., Coffin, P. O., Attias, E., Balinsky, M., Tsou, K., & Walker, J. M. (1999a). Anatomical basis for cannabinoid-induced antinociception as revealed by intracerebral microinjections. *Brain Research*, *822*(1–2), 237–242.

Martin, W. J., Lai, N. K., Patrick, S. L., Tsou, K., & Walker, J. M. (1993). Antinociceptive actions of cannabinoids following intraventricular administration in rats. *Brain Research*, *629*(2), 300–304.

Martin, W. J., Loo, C. M., & Basbaum, A. I. (1999b). Spinal cannabinoids are anti-allodynic in rats with persistent inflammation. *Pain*, *82*(2), 199–205.

Martin, W. J., Patrick, S. L., Coffin, P. O., Tsou, K., & Walker, J. M. (1995). An examination of the central sites of action of cannabinoid-induced antinociception in the rat. *Life Sciences*, *56*(23–24), 2103–2109.

Martin, W. J., Tsou, K., & Walker, J. M. (1998). Cannabinoid receptor-mediated inhibition of the rat tail-flick reflex after microinjection into the rostral ventromedial medulla. *Neuroscience Letters*, *242*(1), 33–36.

Matsuda, L. A., Lolait, S. J., Brownstein, M. J., Young, A. C., & Bonner, T. I. (1990). Structure of a cannabinoid receptor and functional expression of the cloned cDNA. *Nature*, *346*(6284), 561–564.

Mazzari, S., Canella, R., Petrelli, L., Marcolongo, G., & Leon, A. (1996). N-(2-hydroxyethyl) hexadecanamide is orally active in reducing edema formation and inflammatory hyperalgesia by down-modulating mast cell activation. *European Journal of Pharmacology*, *300*(3), 227–236.

McCormick, M., et al. (2017). *The health effects of cannabis and cannabinoids: The current state of evidence and recommendations for research*. Washington, DC: The National Academies Press.

McGaraughty, S., Chu, K. L., Bitner, R. S., Martino, B., El Kouhen, R., Han, P., et al. (2003). Capsaicin infused into the PAG affects rat tail flick responses to noxious heat and alters neuronal firing in the RVM. *Journal of Neurophysiology*, *90*(4), 2702–2710.

Mechoulam, R., Ben-Shabat, S., Hanus, L., Ligumsky, M., Kaminski, N. E., Schatz, A. R., et al. (1995). Identification of an endogenous 2-monoglyceride, present in canine gut, that binds to cannabinoid receptors. *Biochemical Pharmacology*, *50*(1), 83–90.

Mechoulam, R., & Gaoni, Y. (1967). Isolation, structure and partial synthesis of an active constituent of hashish. *Journal of the American Chemical Society*, *86*, 1646–1647.

Meng, I. D., & Johansen, J. P. (2004). Antinociception and modulation of rostral ventromedial medulla neuronal activity by local microinfusion of a cannabinoid receptor agonist. *Neuroscience*, *124*(3), 685–693.

Meng, I. D., Manning, B. H., Martin, W. J., & Fields, H. L. (1998). An analgesia circuit activated by cannabinoids. *Nature*, *395*(6700), 381–383.

Millan, M. J. (2002). Descending control of pain. *Progress in Neurobiology*, *66*(6), 355–474.

Milligan, E. D., Twining, C., Chacur, M., Biedenkapp, J., O'Connor, K., Poole, S., et al. (2003). Spinal glia and proinflammatory cytokines mediate mirror-image neuropathic pain in rats. *The Journal of Neuroscience*, *23*(3), 1026–1040.

Molina-Holgado, F., Rubio-Araiz, A., Garcia-Ovejero, D., Williams, R. J., Moore, J. D., Arevalo-Martin, A., et al. (2007). CB2 cannabinoid receptors promote mouse neural stem cell proliferation. *The European Journal of Neuroscience*, *25*(3), 629–634.

Monhemius, R., Azami, J., Green, D. L., & Roberts, M. H. (2001). CB1 receptor mediated analgesia from the nucleus reticularis gigantocellularis pars alpha is activated in an animal model of neuropathic pain. *Brain Research*, *908*(1), 67–74.
Munro, S., Thomas, K. L., & Abu-Shaar, M. (1993). Molecular characterization of a peripheral receptor for cannabinoids. *Nature*, *365*(6441), 61–65.
Nackley, A. G., Makriyannis, A., & Hohmann, A. G. (2003). Selective activation of cannabinoid CB2 receptors suppresses spinal Fos protein expression and pain behavior in a rat model of inflammation. *Neuroscience*, *119*(3), 747–757.
Neugebauer, V., Galhardo, V., Maione, S., & Mackey, S. C. (2009). Forebrain pain mechanisms. *Brain Research Reviews*, *60*(1), 226–242.
Neugebauer, V., Li, W., Bird, G. C., & Han, J. S. (2004). The amygdala and persistent pain. *The Neuroscientist*, *10*(3), 221–234.
Nozaki, C., Markert, A., & Zimmer, A. (2015). Inhibition of FAAH reduces nitroglycerin-induced migraine-like pain and trigeminal neuronal hyperactivity in mice. *European Neuropsychopharmacology*, *25*(8), 1388–1396.
Okine, B. N., Madasu, M. K., McGowan, F., Prendergast, C., Gaspar, J. C., Harhen, B., et al. (2016). N-palmitoylethanolamide in the anterior cingulate cortex attenuates inflammatory pain behaviour indirectly via a CB1 receptor-mediated mechanism. *Pain*, *157*(12), 2687–2696.
Okine, B. N., Rea, K., Olango, W. M., Price, J., Herdman, S., Madasu, M. K., et al. (2014). A role for PPARalpha in the medial prefrontal cortex in formalin-evoked nociceptive responding in rats. *British Journal of Pharmacology*, *171*(6), 1462–1471.
Olango, W. M., Roche, M., Ford, G. K., Harhen, B., & Finn, D. P. (2012). The endocannabinoid system in the rat dorsolateral periaqueductal grey mediates fear-conditioned analgesia and controls fear expression in the presence of nociceptive tone. *British Journal of Pharmacology*, *165*(8), 2549–2560.
Onaivi, E. S., Ishiguro, H., Gong, J. P., Patel, S., Meozzi, P. A., Myers, L., et al. (2008). Brain neuronal CB2 cannabinoid receptors in drug abuse and depression: From mice to human subjects. *PLoS One*, *3*(2), e1640.
Onaivi, E. S., Ishiguro, H., Gong, J. P., Patel, S., Perchuk, A., Meozzi, P. A., et al. (2006a). Discovery of the presence and functional expression of cannabinoid CB2 receptors in brain. *Annals of the New York Academy of Sciences*, *1074*, 514–536.
Onaivi, E. S., Ishiguro, H., Sejal, P., Meozzi, P. A., Myers, L., Tagliaferro, P., et al. (2006b). Methods to study the behavioral effects and expression of CB2 cannabinoid receptor and its gene transcripts in the chronic mild stress model of depression. *Methods in Molecular Medicine*, *123*, 291–298.
Ossipov, M. H., Morimura, K., & Porreca, F. (2014). Descending pain modulation and chronification of pain. *Current Opinion in Supportive and Palliative Care*, *8*(2), 143–151.
Palazuelos, J., Aguado, T., Egia, A., Mechoulam, R., Guzman, M., & Galve-Roperh, I. (2006). Non-psychoactive CB2 cannabinoid agonists stimulate neural progenitor proliferation. *The FASEB Journal*, *20*(13), 2405–2407.
Palazzo, E., de Novellis, V., Marabese, I., Cuomo, D., Rossi, F., Berrino, L., et al. (2002). Interaction between vanilloid and glutamate receptors in the central modulation of nociception. *European Journal of Pharmacology*, *439*(1–3), 69–75.
Palazzo, E., Marabese, I., de Novellis, V., Oliva, P., Rossi, F., Berrino, L., et al. (2001). Metabotropic and NMDA glutamate receptors participate in the cannabinoid-induced antinociception. *Neuropharmacology*, *40*(3), 319–326.
Pan, J. X., Wang, Z. L., Li, N., Han, Z. L., Li, X. H., Tang, H. H., et al. (2014). Analgesic tolerance and cross-tolerance to the cannabinoid receptors ligands hemopressin, VD-hemopressin(alpha) and WIN55,212-2 at the supraspinal level in mice. *Neuroscience Letters*, *578*, 187–191.

Pertwee, R. G. (2001). Cannabinoid receptors and pain. *Progress in Neurobiology, 63*(5), 569–611.

Petrenko, A. B., Yamazaki, M., Sakimura, K., Kano, M., & Baba, H. (2014). Augmented tonic pain-related behavior in knockout mice lacking monoacylglycerol lipase, a major degrading enzyme for the endocannabinoid 2-arachidonoylglycerol. *Behavioural Brain Research, 271*, 51–58.

Petrosino, S., Palazzo, E., de Novellis, V., Bisogno, T., Rossi, F., Maione, S., et al. (2007). Changes in spinal and supraspinal endocannabinoid levels in neuropathic rats. *Neuropharmacology, 52*(2), 415–422.

Piscitelli, F., & Di Marzo, V. (2012). "Redundancy" of endocannabinoid inactivation: New challenges and opportunities for pain control. *ACS Chemical Neuroscience, 3*, 356–363.

Porter, A. C., Sauer, J. M., Knierman, M. D., Becker, G. W., Berna, M. J., Bao, J., et al. (2002). Characterization of a novel endocannabinoid, virodhamine, with antagonist activity at the CB1 receptor. *The Journal of Pharmacology and Experimental Therapeutics, 301*(3), 1020–1024.

Quartilho, A., Mata, H. P., Ibrahim, M. M., Vanderah, T. W., Porreca, F., Makriyannis, A., et al. (2003). Inhibition of inflammatory hyperalgesia by activation of peripheral CB2 cannabinoid receptors. *Anesthesiology, 99*(4), 955–960.

Racz, I., Nadal, X., Alferink, J., Baños, J. E., Rehnelt, J., Martín, M., et al. (2008). Interferon-gamma is a critical modulator of CB(2) cannabinoid receptor signaling during neuropathic pain. *The Journal of Neuroscience : The Official Journal of the Society for Neuroscience, 28*(46), 12136–12145.

Racz, I., Nent, E., Erxlebe, E., & Zimmer, A. (2015). CB1 receptors modulate affective behaviour induced by neuropathic pain. *Brain Research Bulletin, 114*, 42–48.

Raffa, R. B., Stone, D. J., Jr., & Hipp, S. J. (1999). Differential cholera-toxin sensitivity of supraspinal antinociception induced by the cannabinoid agonists delta9-THC, WIN 55,212-2 and anandamide in mice. *Neuroscience Letters, 263*(1), 29–32.

Rea, K., Olango, W. M., Harhen, B., Kerr, D. M., Galligan, R., Fitzgerald, S., et al. (2013). Evidence for a role of GABAergic and glutamatergic signalling in the basolateral amygdala in endocannabinoid-mediated fear-conditioned analgesia in rats. *Pain, 154*(4), 576–585.

Rea, K., Olango, W. M., Okine, B. N., Madasu, M. K., McGuire, I. C., Coyle, K., et al. (2014). Impaired endocannabinoid signalling in the rostral ventromedial medulla underpins genotype-dependent hyper-responsivity to noxious stimuli. *Pain, 155*(1), 69–79.

Rea, K., Roche, M., & Finn, D. P. (2007). Supraspinal modulation of pain by cannabinoids: The role of GABA and glutamate. *British Journal of Pharmacology, 152*(5), 633–648.

Rice, A. S., Farquhar-Smith, W. P., & Nagy, I. (2002). Endocannabinoids and pain: Spinal and peripheral analgesia in inflammation and neuropathy. *Prostaglandins, Leukotrienes, and Essential Fatty Acids, 66*(2–3), 243–256.

Richardson, J., Kilo, S., & Hargreaves, K. (1998). Cannabinoids reduce hyperalgesia and inflammation via interaction with peripheral CB1 receptors. *Pain, 75*(1), 111–119.

Roche, M., & Finn, D. P. (2010). Brain CB(2) receptors: Implications for neuropsychiatric disorders. *Pharmaceuticals (Basel), 3*(8), 2517–2553.

Roche, M., Johnston, P., Mhuircheartaigh, O. N., Olango, W. M., Mackie, K., & Finn, D. P. (2010). Effects of intra-basolateral amygdala administration of rimonabant on nociceptive behaviour and neuronal activity in the presence or absence of contextual fear. *European Journal of Pain, 14*(5), 487–495.

Roche, M., O'Connor, E., Diskin, C., & Finn, D. P. (2007). The effect of CB(1) receptor antagonism in the right basolateral amygdala on conditioned fear and associated analgesia in rats. *The European Journal of Neuroscience, 26*(9), 2643–2653.

Romero-Sandoval, A., & Eisenach, J. C. (2007). Spinal cannabinoid receptor type 2 activation reduces hypersensitivity and spinal cord glial activation after paw incision. *Anesthesiology, 106*(4), 787–794.
Romero-Sandoval, A., Nutile-McMenemy, N., & DeLeo, J. A. (2008). Spinal microglial and perivascular cell cannabinoid receptor type 2 activation reduces behavioral hypersensitivity without tolerance after peripheral nerve injury. *Anesthesiology, 108*(4), 722–734.
Ross, R. A., Coutts, A. A., McFarlane, S. M., Anavi-Goffer, S., Irving, A. J., Pertwee, R. G., et al. (2001). Actions of cannabinoid receptor ligands on rat cultured sensory neurones: Implications for antinociception. *Neuropharmacology, 40*(2), 221–232.
Russo, E. B. (2016). Current therapeutic cannabis controversies and clinical trial design issues. *Frontiers in Pharmacology, 7*, 309.
Sanudo-Pena, M. C., Strangman, N. M., Mackie, K., Walker, J. M., & Tsou, K. (1999). CB1 receptor localization in rat spinal cord and roots, dorsal root ganglion, and peripheral nerve. *Zhongguo Yao Li Xue Bao, 20*(12), 1115–1120.
Schlosburg, J. E., Blankman, J. L., Long, J. Z., Nomura, D. K., Pan, B., Kinsey, S. G., et al. (2010). Chronic monoacylglycerol lipase blockade causes functional antagonism of the endocannabinoid system. *Nature Neuroscience, 13*(9), 1113–1119.
Sideris, A., Piskoun, B., Russo, L., Norcini, M., Blanck, T., & Recio-Pinto, E. (2016). Cannabinoid 1 receptor knockout mice display cold allodynia, but enhanced recovery from spared-nerve injury-induced mechanical hypersensitivity. *Molecular Pain, 12*, 1–12. pii:1744806916649191.
Siegling, A., Hofmann, H. A., Denzer, D., Mauler, F., & De Vry, J. (2001). Cannabinoid CB1 receptor upregulation in a rat model of chronic neuropathic pain. *European Journal of Pharmacology, 415*(1), R5–R7.
Smith, F. L., Cichewicz, D., Martin, Z. L., & Welch, S. P. (1998). The enhancement of morphine antinociception in mice by delta9-tetrahydrocannabinol. *Pharmacology, Biochemistry, and Behavior, 60*(2), 559–566.
Smith, P. B., & Martin, B. R. (1992). Spinal mechanisms of Δ9-tetrahydrocannabinol-induced analgesia. *Brain Research, 578*(1–2), 8–12.
Sofia, R. D., Vassar, H. B., & Knobloch, L. C. (1975). Comparative analgesic activity of various naturally occurring cannabinoids in mice and rats. *Psychopharmacologia, 40*(4), 285–295.
Sokal, D. M., Elmes, S. J. R., Kendall, D. A., & Chapman, V. (2003). Intraplantar injection of anandamide inhibits mechanically-evoked responses of spinal neurones via activation of CB2 receptors in anaesthetised rats. *Neuropharmacology, 45*(3), 404–411.
Starowicz, K., & Di Marzo, V. (2013). Non-psychotropic analgesic drugs from the endocannabinoid system: "magic bullet" or "multiple-target" strategies? *European Journal of Pharmacology, 716*(1–3), 41–53.
Starowicz, K., Maione, S., Cristino, L., Palazzo, E., Marabese, I., Rossi, F., et al. (2007). Tonic endovanilloid facilitation of glutamate release in brainstem descending antinociceptive pathways. *The Journal of Neuroscience, 27*(50), 13739–13749.
Starowicz, K., Makuch, W., Korostynski, M., Malek, N., Slezak, M., Zychowska, M., et al. (2013). Full inhibition of spinal FAAH leads to TRPV1-mediated analgesic effects in neuropathic rats and possible lipoxygenase-mediated remodeling of anandamide metabolism. *PLoS One, 8*(4), e60040.
Starowicz, K., Makuch, W., Osikowicz, M., Piscitelli, F., Petrosino, S., Di Marzo, V., et al. (2012). Spinal anandamide produces analgesia in neuropathic rats: Possible CB 1- and TRPV1-mediated mechanisms. *Neuropharmacology, 62*(4), 1746–1755.
Staton, P. C., Hatcher, J. P., Walker, D. J., Morrison, A. D., Shapland, E. M., Hughes, J. P., et al. (2008). The putative cannabinoid receptor GPR55 plays a role in mechanical hyperalgesia associated with inflammatory and neuropathic pain. *Pain, 139*(1), 225–236.

Stella, N., Schweitzer, P., & Piomelli, D. (1997). A second endogenous cannabinoid that modulates long-term potentiation. *Nature, 388*(6644), 773–778.

Strangman, N. M., Walker, J. M., & Strangman, N. M. (1999). Cannabinoid WIN 55,212-2 inhibits the activity-dependent facilitation of spinal nociceptive responses. *Journal of Neurophysiology, 82*(1), 472–477.

Suarez, J., Bermudez-Silva, F. J., Mackie, K., Ledent, C., Zimmer, A., Cravatt, B. F., et al. (2008). Immunohistochemical description of the endogenous cannabinoid system in the rat cerebellum and functionally related nuclei. *The Journal of Comparative Neurology, 509*(4), 400–421.

Sugiura, T., Kondo, S., Sukagawa, A., Nakane, S., Shinoda, A., Itoh, K., et al. (1995). 2-Arachidonoylglycerol: A possible endogenous cannabinoid receptor ligand in brain. *Biochemical and Biophysical Research Communications, 215*(1), 89–97.

Suplita, R. L., 2nd, Farthing, J. N., Gutierrez, T., & Hohmann, A. G. (2005). Inhibition of fatty-acid amide hydrolase enhances cannabinoid stress-induced analgesia: Sites of action in the dorsolateral periaqueductal gray and rostral ventromedial medulla. *Neuropharmacology, 49*(8), 1201–1209.

Suzuki, R., & Dickenson, A. (2005). Spinal and supraspinal contributions to central sensitization in peripheral neuropathy. *Neurosignals, 14*(4), 175–181.

Suzuki, R., Rygh, L. J., & Dickenson, A. H. (2004). Bad news from the brain: Descending 5-HT pathways that control spinal pain processing. *Trends in Pharmacological Sciences, 25*(12), 613–617.

Svizenska, I. H., Brazda, V., Klusakova, I., & Dubovy, P. (2013). Bilateral changes of cannabinoid receptor type 2 protein and mRNA in the dorsal root ganglia of a rat neuropathic pain model. *The Journal of Histochemistry and Cytochemistry, 61*(7), 529–547.

Thomas, B. F., Wei, X., & Martin, B. R. (1992). Characterization and autoradiographic localization of the cannabinoid binding site in rat brain using [3H]11-OH-delta 9-THC-DMH. *The Journal of Pharmacology and Experimental Therapeutics, 263*(3), 1383–1390.

Thorat, S. N., & Bhargava, H. N. (1994). Evidence for a bidirectional cross-tolerance between morphine and delta 9-tetrahydrocannabinol in mice. *European Journal of Pharmacology, 260*(1), 5–13.

Toniolo, E. F., Maique, E. T., Ferreira, W. A., Heimann, A. S., Ferro, E. S., Ramos-Ortolaza, D. L., et al. (2014). Hemopressin, an inverse agonist of cannabinoid receptors, inhibits neuropathic pain in rats. *Peptides, 56*, 125–131.

Tsou, K., Brown, S., Sanudo-Pena, M. C., Mackie, K., & Walker, J. M. (1998a). Immunohistochemical distribution of cannabinoid CB1 receptors in the rat central nervous system. *Neuroscience, 83*(2), 393–411.

Tsou, K., Martin, W. J., & Bereiter, D. A. (1996). Suppression stimulus-evoked expression of Fos protein-like immunoreactivity in rat spinal cord by a selective agonist. *Neuroscience, 4522*(3), 791–798.

Tsou, K., Nogueron, M. I., Muthian, S., Sanudo-Pena, M. C., Hillard, C. J., Deutsch, D. G., et al. (1998b). Fatty acid amide hydrolase is located preferentially in large neurons in the rat central nervous system as revealed by immunohistochemistry. *Neuroscience Letters, 254*(3), 137–140.

Ueda, M., Iwasaki, H., Wang, S., Murata, E., Poon, K. Y. T., Mao, J., et al. (2014). Cannabinoid receptor type 1 antagonist, AM251, attenuates mechanical allodynia and thermal hyperalgesia after burn injury. *Anesthesiology, 121*(6), 1311–1319.

Valverde, O., Karsak, M., & Zimmer, A. (2005). Analysis of the endocannabinoid system by using CB1 cannabinoid receptor knockout mice. *Handbook of Experimental Pharmacology, 168*, 117–145.

Van Sickle, M. D., Duncan, M., Kingsley, P. J., Mouihate, A., Urbani, P., Mackie, K., et al. (2005). Identification and functional characterization of brainstem cannabinoid CB2 receptors. *Science*, *310*(5746), 329–332.

Vaughan, C. W., Connor, M., Bagley, E. E., & Christie, M. J. (2000). Actions of cannabinoids on membrane properties and synaptic transmission in rat periaqueductal gray neurons in vitro. *Molecular Pharmacology*, *57*(2), 288–295.

Vermersch, P. (2011). Sativex((R)) (tetrahydrocannabinol + cannabidiol), an endocannabinoid system modulator: Basic features and main clinical data. *Expert Review of Neurotherapeutics*, *11*(Suppl. 4), 15–19.

Viscomi, M. T., Oddi, S., Latini, L., Pasquariello, N., Florenzano, F., Bernardi, G., et al. (2009). Selective CB2 receptor agonism protects central neurons from remote axotomy-induced apoptosis through the PI3K/Akt pathway. *The Journal of Neuroscience*, *29*(14), 4564–4570.

Walker, J. M., Huang, S. M., Strangman, N. M., Tsou, K., & Sanudo-Pena, M. C. (1999). Pain modulation by release of the endogenous cannabinoid anandamide. *Proceedings of the National Academy of Sciences of the United States of America*, *96*(21), 12198–12203.

Watkins, L. R., Milligan, E. D., & Maier, S. F. (2003). Glial proinflammatory cytokines mediate exaggerated pain states: Implications for clinical pain. *Advances in Experimental Medicine and Biology*, *521*, 1–21.

Welch, S. P. (1994). Blockade of cannabinoid-induced antinociception by naloxone benzoylhydrazone (NalBZH). *Pharmacology, Biochemistry, and Behavior*, *49*(4), 929–934.

Welch, S. P., Huffman, J. W., & Lowe, J. (1998). Differential blockade of the antinociceptive effects of centrally administered cannabinoids by SR141716A. *The Journal of Pharmacology and Experimental Therapeutics*, *287*(3), 1301–1308.

Welch, S. P., Thomas, C., & Patrick, G. S. (1995). Modulation of cannabinoid-induced antinociception after intracerebroventricular versus intrathecal administration to mice: Possible mechanisms for interaction with morphine. *The Journal of Pharmacology and Experimental Therapeutics*, *272*(1), 310–321.

Whiting, P. F., Wolff, R. F., Deshpande, S., Di Nisio, M., Duffy, S., Hernandez, A. V., et al. (2015). Cannabinoids for medical use: A systematic review and meta-analysis. *JAMA*, *313*(24), 2456–2473.

Wiley, J. L., & Martin, B. R. (2002). Cannabinoid pharmacology: Implications for additional cannabinoid receptor subtypes. *Chemistry and Physics of Lipids*, *121*(1–2), 57–63.

Wilkerson, J. L., Gentry, K. R., Dengler, E. C., Wallace, J. A., Kerwin, A. A., Armijo, L. M., et al. (2012). Intrathecal cannabilactone CB 2R agonist, AM1710, controls pathological pain and restores basal cytokine levels. *Pain*, *153*(5), 1091–1106.

Wilson, A. W., Clayton, N. M., Medhurst, S. J., Bountra, C., & Chessell, I. P. (2004). The FAAH inhibitor URB597 reverses inflammatory pain through a CB1 receptor mediated mechanism. In *049P University of Newcastle Winter Meeting, December 2004, Copyright 2004.* The British Pharmacological Society.

Wilson, A. R., Maher, L., & Morgan, M. M. (2008). Repeated cannabinoid injections into the rat periaqueductal gray enhance subsequent morphine antinociception. *Neuropharmacology*, *55*(7), 1219–1225.

Wilson-Poe, A. R., Pocius, E., Herschbach, M., & Morgan, M. M. (2013). The periaqueductal gray contributes to bidirectional enhancement of antinociception between morphine and cannabinoids. *Pharmacology, Biochemistry, and Behavior*, *103*(3), 444–449.

Wotherspoon, G., Fox, A., McIntyre, P., Colley, S., Bevan, S., & Winter, J. (2005). Peripheral nerve injury induces cannabinoid receptor 2 protein expression in rat sensory neurons. *Neuroscience*, *135*(1), 235–245.

Yaksh, T. L. (1981). The antinociceptive effects of intrathecally administered levonantradol and desacetyllevonantradol in the rat. *The Journal of Clinical Pharmacology*, *21*(S1), 334S–340S.

Zhang, H. Y., Gao, M., Liu, Q. R., Bi, G. H., Li, X., Yang, H. J., et al. (2014). Cannabinoid CB2 receptors modulate midbrain dopamine neuronal activity and dopamine-related behavior in mice. *Proceedings of the National Academy of Sciences of the United States of America*, *111*(46), E5007–E5015.

Zhang, J., Hoffert, C., Vu, H. K., Groblewski, T., Ahmad, S., & O'Donnell, D. (2003). Induction of CB2 receptor expression in the rat spinal cord of neuropathic but not inflammatory chronic pain models. *The European Journal of Neuroscience*, *17*(12), 2750–2754.

Zheng, T., Zhang, T., Zhang, R., Wang, Z. L., Han, Z. L., Li, N., et al. (2017). Pharmacological characterization of rat VD-hemopressin(alpha), an alpha-hemoglobin-derived peptide exhibiting cannabinoid agonist-like effects in mice. *Neuropeptides*, *63*, 83–90.

Zimmer, A., Zimmer, A. M., Hohmann, A. G., Herkenham, M., & Bonner, T. I. (1999). Increased mortality, hypoactivity, and hypoalgesia in cannabinoid CB1 receptor knockout mice. *Proceedings of the National Academy of Sciences of the United States of America*, *96*(10), 5780–5785.

FURTHER READING

Di Marzo, V., Bifulco, M., & De Petrocellis, L. (2004). The endocannabinoid system and its therapeutic exploitation. *Nature Reviews Drug Discovery*, *3*(9), 771–784.

Richardson, J. (2001). Cannabinoids modulate pain by multiple mechanisms of action. *The Journal of Pain*, *1*, 2–14.

Salio, C., Doly, S., Fischer, J., Franzoni, M. F., & Conrath, M. (2002). Neuronal and astrocytic localization of the cannabinoid receptor-1 in the dorsal horn of the rat spinal cord. *Neuroscience Letters*, *329*(1), 13–16.